OSTEOARTHRITIS – DIAGNOSIS, TREATMENT AND SURGERY

Edited by **Qian Chen**

Osteoarthritis – Diagnosis, Treatment and Surgery
Edited by Qian Chen

Published by InTech
Janeza Trdine 9, 51000 Rijeka, Croatia

Publishing Process Manager Vana Persen

Technical Editor Teodora Smiljanic

Cover Designer InTech Design Team

Additional hard copies can be obtained from orders@intechopen.com

Osteoarthritis – Diagnosis, Treatment and Surgery, Edited by Qian Chen
p. cm.
978-953-51-0168-0

For EU product safety concerns:
IN TECH d.o.o., Prolaz Marije Krucifikse Kozulić 3, 51000 Rijeka, Croatia,
info@intechopen.com or visit our website at intechopen.com.

Meet the editor

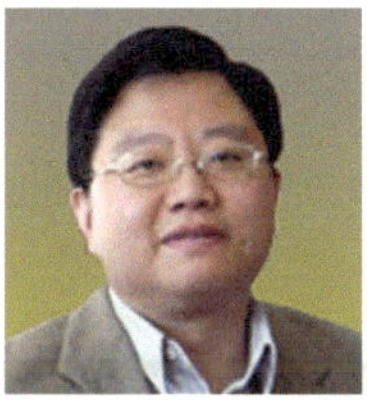

Dr Qian Chen is the Michael G. Ehrlich, MD Endowed Chair in Orthopaedic Research, Professor of Medical Science, and Vice Chair for Research in the Department of Orthopaedics at the Warren Alpert Medical School of Brown University. He is the director of Center of Biomedical Research Excellence in Skeletal Health and Repair in Rhode Island Hospital, a multi-disciplinary translational research center established by National Institute of Health. Dr Chen's research interest includes cartilage molecular biology, mechanotransduction, and osteoarthritis. Throughout Dr Chen's research career, he received the Independent Scientist Award from NIH, the Satterfield Arthritis Investigator Award from Arthritis Foundation, and the Kappa Delta Award from American Academy of Orthopaedic Surgeons. Dr Chen served on multiple NIH study sections and advisory panels. He served as an editor of the journal Current Opinions in Orthopaedics, and the topic Chair of Cartilage, Synovium, and Meniscus for the annual meeting of the Orthopaedic Research Society.

Contents

Preface

Osteoarthritis is one of the most debilitating diseases worldwide. Millions of people suffer from pain and disability associated with this disease. There are two major types of OA: primary and secondary. The primary OA is associated with aging. While people live longer and longer, the prevalence of OA becomes more prominent. It is expected that the percentage of the people who suffer from OA will continue to rise in the coming decades. The secondary OA is a consequence of injury to the joints. It is often associated with sports injury and/or other traumatic events. Thus, it often occurs in young people and adults who enjoy an active life style. Although the direct damage to the joint such as rapture of the ligaments is often repairable by surgery, the patients nevertheless would likely suffer from degeneration of the joint cartilage later in life.

My connection to OA is several fold. Because of the prevalence of OA, many of us know family members and/or friends who suffer from the disease. I am no exception. My mother suffered from both rheumatoid arthritis (RA) and OA. Although she also suffered from other diseases, she complained most about arthritis. Some of the other diseases might be more life-threatening; however, none of them brought as much pain and restrained her to bed on a daily basis as arthritis. She often said that life is not worth living if there is no quality. After her RA was brought under control by new drug therapy and both her knees were replaced by surgery, her pain became manageable and her mobility was regained. She was able to perform daily routine activities by herself that many of us take for granted, such as going to the bathroom, standing up after sitting, and walking the stairs. Her outlook on her life in the old age was brightened significantly because of the new treatment and surgery.

As a biomedical researcher, I was fascinated by the intricate process of cartilage development and aging since I was a young graduate student. The research was driven primarily by interest and curiosity. However, my mother's life experience and my interactions with other arthritis patients brought urgency as well as practicality into the basic research we were conducting. The basic knowledge gained from research must be translated into new methods of diagnosis, treatment, and surgery for patients. That is the most direct and effective way to improve the life quality of patients.

So far, there is no FDA approved disease modified drugs for OA. Joint replacement surgery remains the last, and perhaps the most effective way to restore the functions of the joint. Due to these circumstances, a multifaceted approach is needed to improve the current treatment as well as to develop new therapy for the future. We need to emphasize the improvement not only diagnosis and treatment of OA, but also the surgery to restore the function of the joint. We need to consider not only mechanistically driven research, but also alternative medicine that has been in practice in treating OA related symptoms in different parts of the world for long time.

Based on these guiding principles, we have included a variety of articles written by physicians and OA researchers from different parts of the world. The topics of the articles include general as well as alternative treatment of OA, diagnosis of OA in upper extremity (hand, wrist, shoulder, and elbow) as well as in lower extremity (hip, knee, and ankle), and common strategies for treatment as well as surgery of OA. We hope that this book serves as a comprehensive resource for professionals as well as patients who are interested in learning the state-of-the-art of OA diagnosis, treatment, and surgery. To borrow a Chinese proverb 抛砖引玉 (cast a brick to attract jade), we hope that this compilation of a variety of articles in this book, some of which are non-traditional or even provocative, may serve as a precursor to the breakthrough in developing new therapy and treatment of OA in the future.

Qian Chen, Ph.D.
Alpert Medical School of Brown University, Providence, RI,
USA

Part 1

General Treatment of OA

1

Long-Term Treatment of Osteoarthritis Pain: Achieving a Balance Between Efficacy and Tolerability for a Successful Chronic Therapy

Mila Etropolski
Johnson & Johnson Pharmaceutical Research & Development, L.L.C.
USA

1. Introduction

Throughout the world, in both developed and developing countries, arthritis is one of the most common causes of chronic pain (Catala et al., 2002; Elliott et al., 1999; Johannes et al., 2010; Tsang et al., 2008). The National Arthritis Data Workgroup estimates that 46.4 million adults in the United States have been diagnosed with some form of arthritis based on analyses of data from the third National Health and Nutrition Examination Survey (NHANES III; 1991-1994), the 2003 to 2005 National Health Interview Survey, and 2005 US Census Bureau population estimates (Helmick et al., 2008; Lawrence et al., 2008). Within this group, approximately 27 million adults have been diagnosed with osteoarthritis, making it the most common form of arthritis in the United States (Lawrence et al., 2008).

The prevalence of osteoarthritis increases with age (Kopec et al., 2007; Lawrence et al., 2008; Sakalauskiene & Jauniskiene, 2010; Shane & Loeser, 2010). Based on data from approximately 4 million patients seen over a 1-year period in British Columbia, Canada, the estimated prevalence of osteoarthritis increases from approximately 7% in patients between 40 and 44 years of age to 26% in patients between 60 and 64 years of age and to 49% in patients between 80 and 84 years of age (Kopec et al., 2007). The prevalence of knee osteoarthritis is particularly high in the elderly, and knee osteoarthritis is a major cause of disability in elderly patients (Shane & Loeser, 2010). Based on data from NHANES III and the Framingham Osteoarthritis Study, the prevalence of knee osteoarthritis in the United States is estimated to be 14% in adults 26 years of age or older, 19% in those 45 years of age or older, 37% in those 60 years of age or older, and 44% in those over 80 years of age (Dillon et al., 2006; Felson et al., 1987; Lawrence et al., 2008).

Osteoarthritis can have a negative impact on health-related quality of life and psychological well-being (Axford et al., 2008; Breedveld, 2004; de Bock et al., 1995; Jinks et al., 2007; Majani et al., 2005; Salaffi et al., 2005). Patients with osteoarthritis are often limited in their ability to participate in main daily activities (eg, household duties, employment, body care, ambulation, and sleep) and to maintain their independence (de Bock et al., 1995; Hunter et al., 2008; Jinks et al., 2007; Segal et al., 2004). Patients' mental health has been shown to decrease progressively over time, and patients with more severe osteoarthritis pain are most likely to experience depression and to have difficulty coping with their disease (Axford et al., 2008). In addition, patients with osteoarthritis have an increased risk of developing metabolic syndrome and cardiovascular disease (Breedveld, 2004; Puenpatom & Victor, 2009).

Osteoarthritis is also associated with a substantial economic cost (Kotlarz et al., 2009; Wagner, 2011; White et al., 2007). According to an analysis of a medical claims database of 32,043 privately insured patients from 1999 to 2004, the average annual direct cost of osteoarthritis was $11,543 per patient, including $8,602 in direct medical costs and $2,941 in drug costs (White et al., 2007). Based on results of the data from the Medical Expenditure Panel Survey, which was conducted over a 10-year period from 1996 to 2005, osteoarthritis was estimated to have increased aggregate annual healthcare expenditures by $185.5 billion per year (in 2007 dollars; Kotlarz et al., 2009).

Osteoarthritis can occur in any joint; however, it occurs most frequently in the knees, hips, and hands. Other commonly affected joints include those in the feet and the cervical or lumbar regions of the spine (Martel-Pelletier & Pelletier, 2010). Osteoarthritis is characterized by progressive degeneration of articular cartilage, bone remodeling and sclerosis, formation of osteophytes, synovial hypertrophy, and meniscal damage (Abramson & Attur, 2009; Felson, 2009; Hunter & Felson, 2006). The loss of articular cartilage, which is generally recognized as a defining characteristic of osteoarthritis, results from an imbalance in the dynamic equilibrium between the synthesis and degradation of the cartilaginous extracellular matrix (Abramson & Attur, 2009; Hinton et al., 2002; Michael et al., 2010). In normal articular cartilage, chondrocytes are responsible for the production and maintenance of the cartilaginous extracellular matrix; chondrocytes also act as mechano- and osmo-sensors, altering the rate of matrix synthesis or degradation in response to local physiochemical changes (Loeser, 2008; Martel-Pelletier & Pelletier, 2010; Shane & Loeser, 2010). However, in osteoarthritis, inflammatory and catabolic signals stimulate chondrocytes to synthesize proteolytic enzymes that actively degrade the articular cartilage matrix (Abramson & Attur, 2009; Shane & Loeser, 2010). In response to this increased degradation of cartilage matrix, chondrocytes trigger increased synthesis of the proteoglycan components of the matrix, but these newly synthesized proteoglycans are structurally altered and may have a reduced capacity to form new cartilage (Martel-Pelletier & Pelletier, 2010; Rizkalla et al., 1992). As osteoarthritis progresses, eventually chondrocytes are unable to synthesize enough proteoglycans to offset the degradation of the cartilage matrix. Irreversible matrix degradation and cartilage loss is followed by the development of synovitis, joint incongruence, and formation of subchondral cysts (Martel-Pelletier & Pelletier, 2010; Michael et al., 2010).

Although the loss of articular cartilage is considered to be the physiological hallmark of osteoarthritis, the destruction of cartilage is not directly responsible for the joint pain that is considered to be the clinical hallmark of the disease (Felson, 2009). The most likely sources of osteoarthritis pain are the bone, muscle, ligaments, periosteum, and synovium of the affected joints. Bone-related changes associated with osteoarthritis joint pain may include bone marrow lesions, sub-articular bone attrition, periostitis associated with osteophyte formation, subchondral microfractures, and bone angina. Osteoarthritis joint pain has also been linked to synovitis and joint effusions. In cases where osteoarthritis is secondary to joint injury with rupture of the ligaments, the nerves themselves may be a source of pain. Nerve fiber regrowth is typically abnormal and disorganized, comparable to that observed in animal models of nerve injury (Felson, 2009; Hunter et al., 2008).

Pain is usually the predominant symptom of osteoarthritis. Osteoarthritis pain is often described as deep and aching and is typically exacerbated by physical activity and relieved by rest. In advanced osteoarthritis, pain may become more constant and patients may experience pain while at rest, resulting in sleep disturbances that can further exacerbate pain (Hunter et al., 2008). Traditionally, osteoarthritis pain has been attributed to local tissue injury, which causes mechanical nociceptive pain (Gwilym et al., 2009; Hochman et al., 2010). However, results from several studies indicate that central sensitization (ie, increased response to stimulation mediated by amplification of signaling in the central nervous system) may also play a role in the pathophysiology of chronic osteoarthritis pain (Arendt-Nielsen et al., 2010; Courtney et al., 2010; Hochman et al., 2010; Kidd et al., 2007; Kosek & Ordeberg, 2000). In patients with chronic osteoarthritis, persistent joint damage, synovial inflammation, and subchondral bone changes are associated with chronic nociceptor stimulation. This stimulation can alter the mechanisms of nociceptive processing, resulting in modification of central pain-transmitting neurons and enhanced pain response (Arendt-Nielsen et al., 2010; Courtney et al., 2010; Hochman et al., 2010). Symptoms associated with central sensitization in patients with osteoarthritis include hypersensitivity to pain, skin sensitivity, and the spread of pain from the affected joint to large body areas (ie, referred pain; Arendt-Nielsen et al., 2010; Hochman et al., 2010; Hunter et al., 2008; Woolf, 2011).

2. Osteoarthritis management

There are currently no treatment options available for osteoarthritis that prevent or reverse disease progression or deterioration of the affected joints (Felson, 2006, 2009; Hinton et al., 2002; Michael et al., 2010). For that reason, osteoarthritis treatment strategies are generally targeted toward alleviating the painful symptoms of osteoarthritis, improving patient function and quality of life, and slowing disease progression (Felson, 2006, 2009; Hinton et al., 2002; Hunter & Felson, 2006; Michael et al., 2010). A combination of nonpharmacologic and pharmacologic measures is recommended for the management of osteoarthritis (Zhang et al., 2008). If these treatment options fail to provide adequate pain relief and functional improvement, then partial or total joint replacement surgery is considered (Michael et al., 2010; Zhang et al., 2008).

2.1 Nonpharmacologic measures

The most common nonpharmacologic measures used for the management of osteoarthritis pain are weight-loss and exercise programs (Jordan et al., 2003; Michael et al., 2010; Zhang et al., 2008). Some patients with osteoarthritis pain may also benefit from physical therapy, the use of mobility or orthopedic aids (eg, canes, crutches, wheeled walkers, knee braces, wedged shoe insoles), heat or cold therapy, transcutaneous electrical nerve stimulation, or acupuncture (American College of Rheumatology, 2000; Barron & Rubin, 2007; McHughes & Lipman, 2006; Zhang et al., 2008).

Obesity has been associated with an increased risk of development and progression of knee osteoarthritis and with an increased risk of falls; therefore, weight loss has been recommended to reduce pain and improve physical function and health status in patients with osteoarthritis (Felson et al., 2000; Klussmann et al., 2010; Messier, 2008). In a randomized controlled trial in overweight and obese patients with knee osteoarthritis who were 60 years of age or older (n = 252), modest weight loss due to changes in diet and exercise habits was associated with significant improvements in physical functioning and mobility (Messier et al., 2004). In a meta-analysis of changes in pain and physical function experienced by patients with osteoarthritis who lost weight (n = 454), Christensen and colleagues found that physical disability was significantly reduced in patients who lost more than 5.1% of their body weight at a rate of more than 0.24% per week (Christensen et al., 2007).

Current osteoarthritis treatment guidelines recommend that all patients participate in regular aerobic and muscle-strengthening exercise programs, which are intended to improve pain control, balance, strength, flexibility, and endurance (American College of Rheumatology, 2000; Coleman et al., 2010; Jordan et al., 2003; Zhang et al., 2008). The Physical Activity Guidelines Advisory Committee to the US Department of Health and Human Services found that there is strong evidence that moderate exercise, such as walking, can provide small to moderate improvements in pain relief and small improvements in function and disability in patients with osteoarthritis. These guidelines also state that patients with osteoarthritis can expect "significant improvements in pain, physical function, quality of life, and mental health" along with "delayed onset of disability" by engaging in low-impact physical activity 3 to 5 times per week for 30 to 60 minutes per session (Physical Activity Guidelines Advisory Committee, 2008). However, a recent systematic review of clinical trials of exercise therapy for managing hip osteoarthritis found little evidence that exercise therapy was effective for reducing osteoarthritis pain or improving joint function or quality of life (McNair et al., 2009). While the available evidence indicates that exercise can be beneficial for patients with knee osteoarthritis, the number of studies sufficiently powered to examine the effects of exercise on hip osteoarthritis is limited, and well-designed trials to determine joint-specific exercise recommendations are needed (McNair et al., 2009; Petrella, 2000).

2.2 Pharmacologic measures

Pharmacologic options for the management of osteoarthritis pain include acetaminophen, non-steroidal anti-inflammatory drugs (NSAIDs), intra-articular injections of hyaluronic acid or corticosteroids, the serotonin-norepinephrine reuptake inhibitor (SNRI) duloxetine, and opioids (Zhang et al., 2008). In addition, some nutritional supplements have shown efficacy in the reduction of osteoarthritis-related pain and may slow disease progression (Gregory et al., 2008; McAlindon et al., 2000). Topical capsaicin or lidocaine may also be used as adjunctive therapy for pain relief in combination with other therapies (Barron & Rubin, 2007; Jordan et al., 2003; Zhang et al., 2008).

2.2.1 Dietary supplements

A number of dietary supplements have been marketed for the management of osteoarthritis (Gregory et al., 2008). Supplements containing glucosamine sulfate, chondroitin sulfate, and/or *S*-adenosylmethionine may provide pain relief and functional improvement in patients with osteoarthritis, and these supplements may have structure-modifying effects that may slow disease progression. However, results from clinical studies of these supplements have been mixed (Gregory et al., 2008; McAlindon et al., 2000; Zhang et al., 2008; Zhang et al., 2010).

Glucosamine is a naturally occurring constituent of cartilage proteoglycans found in ligaments, synovial fluid, and other joint structures. In a pooled analysis of 20 randomized controlled trials in patients with knee osteoarthritis (n = 2,570), treatment with glucosamine was associated with a 28% improvement in pain and a 21% improvement in function using the Lequesne index. However, 5 of the 20 studies analyzed failed to show that glucosamine was superior to placebo (Towheed et al., 2005; Towheed & Anastassiades, 2007). The inconsistency of results from different trials of glucosamine may be due to the use of different products (ie, glucosamine sulfate vs glucosamine hydrochloride), different trial designs, and different analysis methods (Gregory et al., 2008; McAlindon et al., 2000). In 2 separate 3-year, randomized placebo-controlled trials of glucosamine sulfate (1,500 mg/day) in patients with knee osteoarthritis, patients who received glucosamine sulfate had no significant average change in joint-space width, while patients who received placebo had significant joint-space narrowing (Pavelka et al., 2002; Reginster et al., 2001). These results suggest that glucosamine sulfate may slow the progression of osteoarthritis in patients with mild to moderate disease (Zhang et al., 2008).

Chondroitin sulfate is a glycosaminoglycan involved in the formation of cartilage and other joint matrix structures. Evidence supporting the clinical benefits of chondroitin sulfate for the improvement of osteoarthritis symptoms is inconsistent (Reichenbach et al., 2007). In a recent meta-analysis of 10 large-scale placebo-controlled trials of chondroitin, glucosamine, or their combination (n = 3,803), Wandel and colleagues found that none of these therapies were associated with significant improvements in pain, as measured on a 10-cm visual analog scale, nor were they associated with any significant reduction in joint-space narrowing compared with placebo (Wandel et al., 2010).

S-Adenosylmethionine is a naturally occurring molecule involved in several different metabolic pathways. *S*-Adenosylmethionine may increase chondrocyte production and cartilage thickness and may decrease cytokine-induced chondrocyte damage, thus slowing the progression of osteoarthritis (Gregory et al., 2008). Results of clinical trials of *S*-adenosylmethionine have been consistently positive, showing that the efficacy of *S*-adenosylmethionine is superior to that of placebo and similar to that of NSAIDs; however, *S*-adenosylmethionine has a slower onset of action compared with NSAIDs (Hardy et al., 2003; Kim et al., 2009; Najm et al., 2004; Sander, 2003). *S*-Adenosylmethionine has a short shelf-life and may become unstable over time, and dose-escalation may be required to maintain efficacy (McHughes & Lipman, 2006). For these reasons and because no studies have been conducted comparing the risk/benefit ratio of *S*-adenosylmethionine with conventional therapies, current treatment guidelines do not recommend the use of *S*-adenosylmethionine for the management of osteoarthritis (Gregory et al., 2008; McHughes & Lipman, 2006).

2.2.2 Acetaminophen

Acetaminophen (up to 4 g/day) is recommended as the first-line oral analgesic therapy for the management of mild to moderate osteoarthritis pain (Altman, 2009; American College of Rheumatology, 2000; Jordan et al., 2003; Zhang et al., 2008). It can be used for the long-term management of osteoarthritis pain either alone or in combination with another analgesic (Jordan et al., 2003; Zhang et al., 2008).

The analgesic activity of acetaminophen is not fully understood, but is generally thought to result from the effects of acetaminophen on mediators of pain and inflammation in the central nervous system, possibly through interactions with nitric oxide, substance P receptors, or beta-endorphin. The anti-inflammatory properties of acetaminophen may block some of the inflammatory mechanisms involved in osteoarthritis pain (Flood, 2010).

In general, results from the published literature indicate that at standard recommended doses, pain relief achieved with acetaminophen is inferior to that achieved with most common NSAIDs (Boureau et al., 2004; Golden et al., 2004; Lee et al., 2004; Zhang et al., 2004); however, NSAIDs are associated with more severe side effects, especially when used at high doses for prolonged periods of time (Flood, 2010). A meta-analysis of data from 6 randomized placebo-controlled trials found that acetaminophen was safe and effective for the management of osteoarthritis pain; however, pain relief, clinical response rates, and health status were better with NSAIDs (including ibuprofen, diclofenac, rofecoxib, celecoxib, and naproxen) than with acetaminophen, and more patients preferred NSAIDs over acetaminophen. This meta-analysis also showed that the tolerability profile of acetaminophen was comparable to that of placebo, but NSAIDs were associated with more gastrointestinal side effects than acetaminophen or placebo (Zhang et al., 2004).

It should also be noted that although most studies of acetaminophen for the management of osteoarthritis pain have found that acetaminophen is associated with a low rate of adverse events (AEs; Flood, 2010), some studies have found associations between acetaminophen use and increased risks of upper gastrointestinal complications (Garcia Rodriguez & Hernandez-Diaz, 2001; Rahme et al., 2002) and renal toxicity (Fored et al., 2001). To date, these results are considered equivocal and have not resulted in changes to the recommendation that acetaminophen be used as first-line therapy for osteoarthritis pain management (Zhang et al., 2008).

2.2.3 NSAIDs

NSAIDs are recommended as a second-line treatment option in patients for whom acetaminophen treatment has failed to provide adequate pain relief (Jordan et al., 2003; Zhang et al., 2008). NSAIDs should be used at the lowest effective dose to avoid the risk of gastrointestinal and cardiovascular AEs, and long-term use should be avoided if possible (Zhang et al., 2008). In the United States, all marketed prescription NSAIDs carry a boxed warning about their potential to cause cardiovascular and gastrointestinal side effects (US Food and Drug Administration, 2005; Zhang et al., 2008).

NSAIDs are widely prescribed and are generally considered to be effective for the management of mild to moderate osteoarthritis pain. However, NSAIDs have a ceiling dose above which no additional analgesia can be achieved, which may limit their efficacy for the treatment of more severe pain (Fendrick & Greenberg, 2009). In a meta-analysis of the analgesic efficacy of NSAIDs for the short-term management of knee osteoarthritis pain (n = 10,845), Bjordal and colleagues observed that on average, NSAIDs reduced pain intensity by 10.1 mm (95% confidence interval [CI], 7.4-12.8) on a 10-cm visual analog scale, which was 15.6% better than placebo. Using a random-effects model, the authors determined that the effect size for pain reduction associated with NSAIDs was 0.32 (95% CI, 0.24-0.39; Bjordal et al., 2004).

Most common NSAIDs reduce inflammation through inhibition of the cyclo-oxygenase (COX) enzymes COX-1 and COX-2. COX-1 is expressed constitutively in many tissues and cells and may be involved in a number of physiologic functions, including protection of the gastrointestinal tract from its own acidity, platelet aggregation, and regulation of renal blood flow. In contrast, COX-2 is an inducible protein that is upregulated during inflammation and is primarily localized in inflamed tissue; COX-2 is not present in the stomach or small intestine (Crofford, 1997; Pham & Hirschberg, 2005). NSAIDs that inhibit both COX-1 and COX-2 are classified as nonselective NSAIDs (eg, ibuprofen, diclofenac, naproxen, nabumetone, indomethacin, aspirin, etc.), whereas NSAIDs that selectively inhibit COX-2 are classified as selective COX-2 inhibitors or coxibs (eg, celecoxib, etoricoxib; Altman, 2009).

The analgesic effects of NSAIDs are predominantly attributed to the inhibition of COX-2, while the gastrointestinal side effects are thought to be caused by inhibition of COX-1 (Fendrick & Greenberg, 2009). Thus, nonselective NSAIDs are associated with an increased risk of severe upper gastrointestinal complications, including gastrointestinal tract bleeding, peptic ulcer disease, obstruction, and perforation (Pham & Hirschberg, 2005). It is estimated that chronic use of nonselective NSAIDs increases a patient's risk of upper gastrointestinal complications by 3- to 5-fold compared with patients who do not take nonselective NSAIDs (Gabriel et al., 1991; Garcia Rodriguez & Hernandez-Diaz, 2001). For example, in a 5-year population-based cohort study of 958,397 persons in the United Kingdom, the relative risk of upper gastrointestinal bleeding and/or perforation was 2.4 (95% CI, 1.9-3.1) among patients who used low or medium doses of NSAIDs and 4.9 (95% CI, 4.1-5.8) among patients who used high doses of NSAIDs compared with non-users of NSAIDs. The use of gastroprotectants, such as proton pump inhibitors and misoprostol, reduces these risks (Garcia Rodriguez & Hernandez-Diaz, 2001), and many osteoarthritis treatment guidelines recommend the co-prescription of gastroprotectants when nonselective NSAIDs are used to manage pain, especially in patients who are at an increased risk of gastrointestinal complications (ie, elderly patients, patients with a history of gastrointestinal bleeding or ulcer disease, patients on a low-dose aspirin regimen, and patients with a history of alcohol consumption; Jordan et al., 2003; Pham & Hirschberg, 2005; Zhang et al., 2008). Because elderly patients have an increased risk of gastrointestinal complications associated with NSAIDs, the 2009 American Geriatrics Society Clinical Practice Guideline for the Pharmacological Management of Persistent Pain in Older Adults recommends that nonselective NSAIDs and COX-2 selective inhibitors be considered rarely, with caution, and only in highly selected individuals (American Geriatrics Society Panel on the Pharmacological Management of Persistent Pain in Older Persons, 2009).

Selective COX-2 inhibitors are associated with a substantially reduced risk of gastrointestinal complications relative to nonselective NSAIDs (Pham & Hirschberg, 2005). However, selective COX-2 inhibitors are associated with an increased risk of cardiovascular events (eg, myocardial infarction and stroke), and 2 widely used COX-2 inhibitors, rofecoxib and valdecoxib, were withdrawn from the market due to concerns about their cardiovascular safety (Altman, 2009; Andersohn et al., 2006; Caldwell et al., 2006). The cardiovascular risks associated with selective COX-2 inhibitors have been confirmed by the results of several studies (Bombardier et al., 2000; Bresalier et al., 2005; Graham et al., 2005; Nussmeier et al., 2005; Solomon et al., 2005), and in recent years these findings have been extended to nonselective NSAIDs, particularly diclofenac (Fosbol et al., 2009; Gislason et al., 2009; Hammad et al., 2008; McGettigan & Henry, 2006; Schjerning Olsen et al., 2011). In patients with a history of myocardial infarction, Schjerning Olsen and colleagues observed that NSAID treatment durations ranging from less than 7 days to more than 90 days were associated with significantly increased risks of death and recurrent myocardial infarction. All of the NSAIDs analyzed in this study (ie, rofecoxib, celecoxib, ibuprofen, diclofenac, naproxen, and other NSAIDs) were associated with a significantly increased risk of death. Diclofenac was associated with the earliest onset and highest relative risk of death/recurrent myocardial infarction, while the lowest risks were observed with naproxen (Schjerning Olsen et al., 2011).

NSAIDs are also available as topical preparations (Altman, 2010; Barthel & Oxford-Gatley, 2010). Topical formulations are believed to provide analgesia via the same mechanisms as oral NSAIDs, with similar efficacy but with reduced systemic exposure and, hence, fewer treatment-related side effects (Barthel & Oxford-Gatley, 2010). Osteoarthritis treatment guidelines issued by the UK National Institute for Health and Clinical Excellence recommend that topical NSAIDs, possibly in combination with acetaminophen, should be considered as second-line therapy after acetaminophen alone and before oral nonselective NSAIDs, selective COX-2 inhibitors, or opioids (The National Collaborating Centre for Chronic Conditions, 2008). In the United States, the only 2 topical NSAID formulations approved for the management of osteoarthritis pain are diclofenac sodium 1% gel and diclofenac sodium 1.5% in 45.5% dimethylsulfoxide (Altman & Smith, 2010; Barthel & Oxford-Gatley, 2010).

2.2.4 Intra-articular injections

Intra-articular injections of hyaluronic acid have demonstrated efficacy for the management of knee osteoarthritis pain; however, data on the use of intra-articular hyaluronic acid in hip and other types of osteoarthritis are limited (Goldberg & Buckwalter, 2005; Jordan et al., 2003; Neustadt, 2006). Hyaluronic acid is a high molecular weight glucosaminoglycan present in high concentrations in synovial fluid. It has lubricating and viscoelastic properties, which reduce articular cartilage friction. In osteoarthritis, the synthesis of hyaluronic acid is altered; ie, total concentration is decreased and molecular chain length is reduced. In patients with knee osteoarthritis, intra-articular injections of hyaluronic acid have been shown to reduce synovial fluid viscosity and to reduce pain by several different mechanisms. Hyaluronic acid may slow the progression of disease by improving synovite and chondrocyte function and by modifying the structure of damaged matrix proteins, collagen, and articular cartilage (Goldberg & Buckwalter, 2005). Injectable hyaluronic acid formulations are not associated with any major safety concerns; however, minor AEs, including transient injection-site pain, have been observed in clinical trials (Arrich et al., 2005; Bellamy et al., 2006b).

Intra-articular injections of corticosteroids have been used for more than 50 years for the treatment of osteoarthritis and other rheumatic diseases (Bannuru et al., 2011; Neustadt, 2006). Osteoarthritis treatment guidelines recommend that intra-articular corticosteroids should be considered in patients with moderate to severe pain who have not responded to oral analgesics (Jordan et al., 2003). Intra-articular corticosteroids often provide substantial and lasting osteoarthritis pain relief, and may reduce the inflammatory cell-mediated degradation of articular cartilage (Neustadt, 2006). The short-term benefits of intra-articular corticosteroids are well established; however, the long-term benefits remain unclear (Bellamy et al., 2006a). Intra-articular corticosteroids are generally well tolerated; the most common side effects associated with intra-articular corticosteroid use are post-injection flares of pain, crystal synovitis, haemarthrosis (Bellamy et al., 2006a), joint sepsis, and articular atrophy. These side effects are usually not serious (Bellamy et al., 2006a; Jordan et al., 2003). It is important that intra-articular corticosteroid injections are placed correctly to avoid the possible AEs of fat necrosis and para-articular tissue atrophy (Jones et al., 1993), and injections should not be repeated more than 4 times per year (Jordan et al., 2003).

In a meta-analysis comparing the analgesic efficacy of intra-articular hyaluronic acid versus intra-articular corticosteroids in patients with knee osteoarthritis, Bannuru and colleagues found that during the first 4 weeks of treatment, corticosteroids were more effective than hyaluronic acid (effect size at Week 2, −0.39 [95% CI, −0.65 to −0.12]), but by Week 4, the 2 treatments were not statistically different (effect size, −0.01 [95% CI, −0.23 to 0.21]). After more than 8 weeks of treatment, the efficacy of hyaluronic acid was superior to that of corticosteroids (effect size at Week 12, 0.35 [95% CI, 0.03-0.66]; at Week 26, 0.39 [95% CI, 0.18-0.59]; Bannuru et al., 2011).

2.2.5 SNRIs

Because osteoarthritis pain perception can have a central sensitization component (Arendt-Nielsen et al., 2010; Gwilym et al., 2009; Hochman et al., 2010; Woolf, 2011), recent studies have investigated the analgesic efficacy of the SNRI duloxetine for the management of chronic osteoarthritis pain (Chappell et al., 2009; Chappell et al., 2011; Sullivan et al., 2009). In 2 randomized, double-blind, placebo-controlled trials in patients with moderate to severe osteoarthritis knee pain (n = 231 and n = 256, respectively), 13 weeks of treatment with duloxetine (60-120 mg/day) was associated with significantly reduced weekly average 24-hour pain scores and significant improvements in Western Ontario and McMaster Universities (WOMAC) osteoarthritis index physical functioning scores (Chappell et al., 2009; Chappell et al., 2011). Duloxetine was associated with significantly higher incidences of nausea, constipation, and hyperhidrosis (all $P \leq 0.05$) and a significantly higher rate of discontinuation due to AEs ($P = 0.002$) compared with placebo (Chappell et al., 2011).

In August 2010, the Anesthetic and Life Support Drugs Advisory Committee (ALSDAC) of the US Food & Drug Administration (FDA) recommended approval of duloxetine hydrochloride (60 mg/day) for the management of chronic musculoskeletal pain by a vote of 8 to 6 (US Food and Drug Administration, 2010), and duloxetine is currently being marketed as a treatment for chronic osteoarthritis pain (CYMBALTA, 2011). However, at the same FDA meeting, the ALSDAC voted 9 to 4 (with 1 abstention) against the use of duloxetine for the management of chronic osteoarthritis pain. The committee expressed views that data from clinical trials in patients with chronic osteoarthritis pain did not provide adequate evidence supporting the analgesic efficacy of duloxetine in this population. The committee recommended that additional studies involving more patients should be conducted to confirm the efficacy of duloxetine for the management of chronic osteoarthritis pain (US Food and Drug Administration, 2010).

While the role of SNRIs in the management of osteoarthritis pain remains unclear, results from duloxetine trials published to date (Chappell et al., 2009; Chappell et al., 2011; Sullivan et al., 2009) suggest that central sensitization may play a significant role in pain perception in patients with chronic osteoarthritis pain.

2.2.6 Opioids

Weak opioid analgesics (eg, codeine, dihydrocodeine, tramadol) are recommended for the management of osteoarthritis pain in patients who have failed to respond to other pharmacologic or nonpharmacologic treatments, or when other analgesics are contraindicated (Zhang et al., 2008; Zhang et al., 2010). Strong opioids (eg, oxycodone, morphine, fentanyl, hydromorphone, oxymorphone, buprenorphine) are recommended for the management of severe osteoarthritis pain only when appropriate nonpharmacologic and pharmacologic treatments have been tried and referral for surgery has been considered (Zhang et al., 2008). Opioids can be used alone or in combination with acetaminophen or aspirin (Dominick et al., 2004; Jordan et al., 2003).

In recent years, the number of prescriptions for opioid analgesics for the management of chronic non-cancer pain has increased dramatically (Altman & Smith, 2010). According to the Trends and Risks of Opioid Use for Pain study, between 2000 and 2005, among patients with commercial health insurance who were diagnosed with chronic back pain, neck pain, joint/arthritis pain, headache pain, or pain associated with HIV/AIDS, the number of opioid prescriptions increased by 58%. During this time period, the number of eligible patients diagnosed with one of these painful conditions increased by 33%, from 18% (485,794/2,716,163) in 2000 to 24% (897,537/3,768,223) in 2005. Thus, the increase in opioid prescriptions is only partially explained by an increasing incidence of chronic pain conditions (Sullivan et al., 2008). Further, in a 1-year study of opioid prescriptions among patients in the Veterans Affairs healthcare system, of 3,061 patients who visited a physician for osteoarthritis, 41% had at least 1 opioid prescription (Dominick et al., 2004). These results suggest that opioids are increasingly gaining acceptance as a treatment option for chronic osteoarthritis pain (Altman & Smith, 2010; Dominick et al., 2004; Sullivan et al., 2008).

In clinical trials, opioids have demonstrated efficacy for the management of moderate to severe osteoarthritis pain (Altman & Smith, 2010; Avouac et al., 2007; Caldwell et al., 2002; Matsumoto et al., 2005; Nuesch et al., 2009; Roth et al., 2000). In a meta-analysis of 13 randomized placebo-controlled trials of orally or transdermally administered opioids (oxycodone, fentanyl, morphine sulfate, tramadol, tramadol/acetaminophen, or codeine) that included a total of 3,733 patients with osteoarthritis pain, the pooled effect size of opioids compared with placebo for pain intensity reduction was −0.79 (95% CI, −0.98 to −0.59) based on a random-effects model (Avouac et al., 2007).

Opioid treatment has also been associated with significant improvements in physical function and quality of life (Avouac et al., 2007; Caldwell et al., 2002; Hale et al., 2007; Matsumoto et al., 2005; Nuesch et al., 2009; Rosenthal et al., 2007; Roth et al., 2000). Improvements in WOMAC scores have been observed in studies of fentanyl, oxycodone, oxycodone/acetaminophen, morphine sulfate, oxymorphone, and hydromorphone for osteoarthritis pain (Caldwell et al., 2002; Hale et al., 2007; Katz et al., 2010; Langford et al., 2006; Matsumoto et al., 2005). In addition, improvements in sleep, mood, and enjoyment of life have been associated with opioid analgesic therapy for the management of chronic osteoarthritis pain (Rosenthal et al., 2007; Roth et al., 2000).

In spite of the improvements observed in pain intensity, physical function, and health-related quality of life associated with opioid analgesics, the long-term use of these agents may be limited by poor tolerability (Benyamin et al., 2008). In an open-label extension study lasting 6 to 18 months (following an initial 14-day placebo-controlled study) of oxycodone controlled release (CR; 10 or 20 mg bid) for the treatment of moderate to severe, chronic osteoarthritis pain, 57% (60/106) of patients discontinued treatment, and more than half of these discontinuations (32/60) were related to AEs (Roth et al., 2000). The most common AEs leading to discontinuation were constipation, nausea, pruritus, somnolence, and nervousness. These AEs were also among the most commonly reported treatment-emergent AEs (TEAEs). During this 6- to 18-month long-term extension trial, 52% (55/106) of patients taking oxycodone CR reported constipation, 30% (32/106) reported somnolence, 24% (25/106) reported nausea, 20% (21/106) reported pruritus, and 15% (16/106) reported nervousness (Roth et al., 2000).

In a Cochrane review of 10 trials (n = 2,268) that studied codeine, morphine, oxycodone, oxymorphone, or fentanyl for the management of osteoarthritis hip or knee pain, Nüesch and colleagues found that while opioids were more effective than controls (standardized mean difference, −0.36; 95% CI, −0.47 to −0.26), opioids were associated with a significantly increased risk of AEs (pooled risk ratio, 1.55; 95% CI, 1.41-1.70) and of dropout due to AEs (pooled risk ratio, 4.05; 95% CI, 3.06-5.38) compared with controls. The authors concluded that the small to moderate beneficial effects associated with opioids for the management of chronic osteoarthritis pain do not outweigh the significantly increased risk of AEs (Nuesch et al., 2009).

2.2.7 New treatment option: Tapentadol extended release, a μ-opioid receptor agonist and norepinephrine reuptake inhibitor

Tapentadol is a new, centrally acting analgesic that has μ-opioid receptor agonist and norepinephrine reuptake inhibitor activities (Tzschentke et al., 2006; Tzschentke et al., 2007). The opioid activity of tapentadol targets nociceptive pain at the joint level, while norepinephrine reuptake inhibition targets referred pain caused by central sensitization. In the United States, an extended-release formulation of tapentadol is in development for the management of moderate to severe chronic pain. In Europe, a prolonged-release formulation is indicated for the management of severe chronic pain in adults, which can be adequately managed only with opioid analgesics.

In preclinical studies, tapentadol has demonstrated efficacy in models of both neuropathic and nociceptive pain (Tzschentke et al., 2007). In addition, it has been observed that tapentadol's 2 mechanisms of action act synergistically to produce potent analgesia that is greater than the predicted additive effects of the 2 mechanisms. These synergistic effects are particularly notable in models of chronic pain, possibly because chronic pain is more likely than acute pain to have both noradrenergic and nociceptive components (Schroder et al., 2011). The 2 mechanisms of action of tapentadol affect both the ascending and descending pathways of central nervous system pain control, which may make it an appropriate treatment option for patients with chronic osteoarthritis who experience both nociceptive pain and pain caused by central sensitization.

The efficacy of tapentadol extended release (ER) has been demonstrated in patients with moderate to severe, chronic osteoarthritis pain (Afilalo et al., 2010). In a 15-week randomized, placebo- and active-controlled, phase 3 study in patients with moderate to severe, chronic osteoarthritis knee pain (n = 1,023), tapentadol ER (100-250 mg bid) provided significantly better pain relief compared with placebo (least-squares mean difference in average pain intensity from baseline to Week 12 measured on an 11-point numerical rating scale, −0.7; 95% CI, −1.04 to −0.33; Afilalo et al., 2010). Tapentadol ER was associated with significant improvements in overall heath, pain, and physical function compared with placebo based on the Short Form-36 (SF-36) and EuroQol-5 Dimension (EQ-5D) health status scores. Patients treated with tapentadol ER also scored significantly better on the global WOMAC and on pain and physical function WOMAC subscales compared with placebo, indicating that tapentadol ER treatment was associated with robust improvement in analgesia and overall physical function (Afilalo et al., 2010). In this study, the efficacy of tapentadol ER was particularly notable when it was administered to patients who had not received opioid analgesics within the 3 months prior to the study. Opioid-naive patients treated with tapentadol ER achieved statistically significant improvements from baseline in average pain intensity, while patients treated with oxycodone CR did not. In opioid-naive patients in the tapentadol ER and oxycodone CR groups, respectively, gastrointestinal TEAEs were reported by 47.7% and 67.5% of patients, and 19.6% and 48.3% of patients discontinued due to AEs (Etropolski et al., 2009).

In a 1-year, randomized, open-label, phase 3 long-term safety study in patients with moderate to severe, chronic osteoarthritis hip or knee pain or low back pain, tapentadol ER (100-250 mg bid) was shown to have comparable analgesic efficacy to oxycodone HCl CR (20-50 mg bid), but tapentadol ER was associated with better overall tolerability and lower incidences of side effects and TEAE-related discontinuations (Figure 1). Tapentadol ER was associated with particularly better gastrointestinal tolerability compared with oxycodone CR. Gastrointestinal TEAEs led to discontinuation in 8.6% (77/894) of patients in the tapentadol ER group compared with 21.5% (48/223) of patients in the oxycodone CR group (Wild et al., 2010).

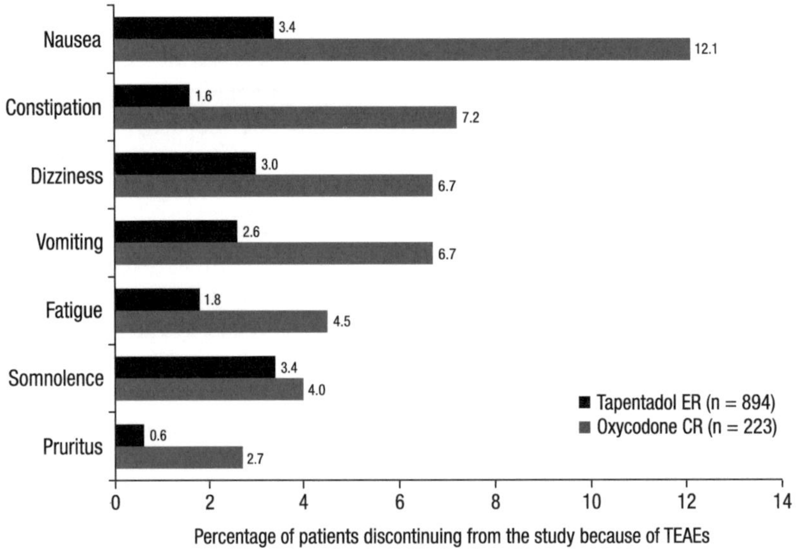

Fig. 1. TEAE-related discontinuations in a 1-year safety study of tapentadol ER (100-250 mg bid) compared with oxycodone HCl CR (20-50 mg bid). Reprinted from Pain Practice, Vol 10, Wild JE, et al, Long-term safety and tolerability of tapentadol extended release for the management of chronic low back pain or osteoarthritis pain, pp. 416-427 (2010), with permission from John Wiley and Sons. TEAE, treatment-emergent adverse event; ER, extended release; CR, controlled release.

In pooled analyses of data from 3 randomized, placebo- and active-controlled, phase 3 studies with 15 weeks of active treatment in patients with moderate to severe, chronic osteoarthritis knee pain (2 studies) or low back pain (1 study), the efficacy of tapentadol ER (100-250 mg bid) was non-inferior to that of oxycodone HCl CR (20-50 mg bid); however, tapentadol ER had a superior gastrointestinal tolerability profile relative to oxycodone CR (Lange et al., 2010). Tapentadol ER treatment was associated with fewer discontinuations from treatment compared with oxycodone CR and significant improvements in function and quality of life based on SF-36 and EQ-5D health status questionnaire results. Improvements observed in 7 of 8 SF-36 domains and the EQ-5D health status index score were significantly better with tapentadol ER (100-250 mg bid) compared with oxycodone HCl CR (20-50 mg bid, Lange et al., 2010).

The health status and WOMAC functional improvements observed in these studies are likely associated with the improved tolerability profile of tapentadol ER compared with oxycodone CR. The superior tolerability of tapentadol ER may have allowed patients to maintain their therapy and to sustain the achieved analgesic effect for a longer period of time compared with oxycodone CR. Oxycodone CR was associated with a higher rate of discontinuations and worse tolerability compared with tapentadol ER (Afilalo et al., 2010; Lange et al., 2010).

3. Conclusion

Nonpharmacologic approaches, including exercise and weight-loss programs, have been shown to reduce pain and psychological disability in patients with osteoarthritis, and should be an integral part of all osteoarthritis treatment plans (Felson et al., 2000; Klussmann et al., 2010; Messier, 2008; Physical Activity Guidelines Advisory Committee, 2008). Guidelines for the pharmacologic management of osteoarthritis pain recommend a stepwise approach to therapy, initiating with acetaminophen, then transitioning to NSAIDs and finally to opioids if prior therapy fails (Jordan et al., 2003; Zhang et al., 2008). However, the long-term utility of NSAIDs and opioid analgesics may be limited by safety and tolerability issues (Benyamin et al., 2008; Zhang et al., 2008).

Tapentadol ER provides effective pain control with good tolerability and improvements in quality of life (Afilalo et al., 2010; Lange et al., 2010; Wild et al., 2010). The favorable tolerability profile of tapentadol ER compared with oxycodone CR may allow patients to remain on treatment for longer periods of time, resulting in consistent, effective pain relief and long-term improvements in quality of life and health status. Because tapentadol acts as both a μ-opioid receptor agonist and as a norepinephrine reuptake inhibitor, tapentadol ER may relieve both nociceptive pain and neuropathic pain associated with central sensitization. Thus, tapentadol ER may be an effective treatment option that has better tolerability than pure μ-opioid analgesics in patients with moderate to severe, chronic osteoarthritis pain.

4. Acknowledgment

Editorial support for the writing of this chapter was provided by Megan Knagge, PhD, of MedErgy and was funded by Johnson & Johnson Pharmaceutical Research & Development, L.L.C. The author retained full editorial control over the content.

5. References

Abramson, S.B. & Attur, M. (2009). Developments in the Scientific Understanding of Osteoarthritis. *Arthritis Research & Therapy*, Vol.11, No.3, p. 227, ISSN 1478-6354

Afilalo, M., Etropolski, M.S., Kuperwasser, B., Kelly, K., Okamoto, A., Van, H., I, Steup, A., Lange, B., Rauschkolb, C. & Haeussler, J. (2010). Efficacy and Safety of Tapentadol Extended Release Compared With Oxycodone Controlled Release for the Management of Moderate to Severe Chronic Pain Related to Osteoarthritis of the

Knee: a Randomized, Double-Blind, Placebo- and Active-Controlled Phase III Study. *Clinical Drug Investigation*, Vol.30, No.8, pp. 489-505, ISSN 1173-2563

Altman, R.D. (2010). New Guidelines for Topical NSAIDs in the Osteoarthritis Treatment Paradigm. *Current Medical Research & Opinion*, Vol.26, No.12, pp. 2871-2876, ISSN 0300-7995

Altman, R.D. (2009). Practical Considerations for the Pharmacologic Management of Osteoarthritis. *American Journal of Managed Care*, Vol.15, No.8 Suppl, p. S236-S243, ISSN 1936-2692

Altman, R.D. & Smith, H.S. (2010). Opioid Therapy for Osteoarthritis and Chronic Low Back Pain. *Postgraduate Medicine*, Vol.122, No.6, pp. 87-97, ISSN 0032-5481

American College of Rheumatology. (2000). Recommendations for the Medical Management of Osteoarthritis of the Hip and Knee: 2000 Update. American College of Rheumatology Subcommittee on Osteoarthritis Guidelines. *Arthritis and Rheumatism*, Vol.43, No.9, pp. 1905-1915, ISSN 1529-0131

American Geriatrics Society Panel on the Pharmacological Management of Persistent Pain in Older Persons. (2009). Pharmacological Management of Persistent Pain in Older Persons. *Journal of the American Geriatrics Society*, Vol.57, No.8, pp. 1331-1346, ISSN 0002-8614

Andersohn, F., Suissa, S. & Garbe, E. (2006). Use of First- and Second-Generation Cyclooxygenase-2-Selective Nonsteroidal Antiinflammatory Drugs and Risk of Acute Myocardial Infarction. *Circulation*, Vol.113, No.16, pp. 1950-1957, ISSN 0009-7322

Arendt-Nielsen, L., Nie, H., Laursen, M.B., Laursen, B.S., Madeleine, P., Simonsen, O.H. & Graven-Nielsen, T. (2010). Sensitization in Patients With Painful Knee Osteoarthritis. *Pain*, Vol.149, No.3, pp. 573-581, ISSN 0304-3959

Arrich, J., Piribauer, F., Mad, P., Schmid, D., Klaushofer, K. & Mullner, M. (2005). Intra-Articular Hyaluronic Acid for the Treatment of Osteoarthritis of the Knee: Systematic Review and Meta-Analysis. *Canadian Medical Association Journal*, Vol.172, No.8, pp. 1039-1043, ISSN 0820-3946

Avouac, J., Gossec, L. & Dougados, M. (2007). Efficacy and Safety of Opioids for Osteoarthritis: a Meta-Analysis of Randomized Controlled Trials. *Osteoarthritis and Cartilage*, Vol.15, No.8, pp. 957-965, ISSN 1063-4584

Axford, J., Heron, C., Ross, F. & Victor, C.R. (2008). Management of Knee Osteoarthritis in Primary Care: Pain and Depression Are the Major Obstacles. *J Psychosom Res*, Vol.64, No.5, pp. 461-467, ISSN 0022-3999

Bannuru, R.R., Natov, N.S., Dasi, U.R., Schmid, C.H. & McAlindon, T.E. (2011). Therapeutic Trajectory Following Intra-Articular Hyaluronic Acid Injection in Knee Osteoarthritis - Meta-Analysis. *Osteoarthritis and Cartilage*, ISSN 1063-4584

Barron, M.C. & Rubin, B.R. (2007). Managing Osteoarthritic Knee Pain. *Journal of the American Osteopathic Association*, Vol.107, No.10 Suppl 6, p. ES21-ES27, ISSN 0098-6151

Barthel, H.R. & Oxford-Gatley, R.A. (2010). Topical Nonsteroidal Anti-Inflammatory Drugs for Osteoarthritis. *Postgraduate Medicine*, Vol.122, No.6, pp. 98-106, ISSN 0032-5481

Bellamy, N., Campbell, J., Robinson, V., Gee, T., Bourne, R. & Wells, G. (2006a). Intraarticular Corticosteroid for Treatment of Osteoarthritis of the Knee. *Cochrane Database of Systemic Reviews*, No.2, p. CD005328

Bellamy, N., Campbell, J., Robinson, V., Gee, T., Bourne, R. & Wells, G. (2006b). Viscosupplementation for the Treatment of Osteoarthritis of the Knee. *Cochrane Database of Systemic Reviews*, No.2, p. CD005321

Benyamin, R., Trescot, A.M., Datta, S., Buenaventura, R., Adlaka, R., Sehgal, N., Glaser, S.E. & Vallejo, R. (2008). Opioid Complications and Side Effects. *Pain Physician*, Vol.11, No.2 suppl, p. S105-S120, ISSN 1533-3159

Bjordal, J.M., Ljunggren, A.E., Klovning, A. & Slordal, L. (2004). Non-Steroidal Anti-Inflammatory Drugs, Including Cyclo-Oxygenase-2 Inhibitors, in Osteoarthritic Knee Pain: Meta-Analysis of Randomised Placebo Controlled Trials. *British Medical Journal*, Vol.329, No.7478, p. 1317, ISSN 0959-8138

Bombardier, C., Laine, L., Reicin, A., Shapiro, D., Burgos-Vargas, R., Davis, B., Day, R., Ferraz, M.B., Hawkey, C.J., Hochberg, M.C., Kvien, T.K., Schnitzer, T.J. & for the VIGOR Study Group. (2000). Comparison of Upper Gastrointestinal Toxicity of Rofecoxib and Naproxen in Patients With Rheumatoid Arthritis. *New England Journal of Medicine*, Vol.343, No.21, pp. 1520-1528, ISSN 0028-4793

Boureau, F., Schneid, H., Zeghari, N., Wall, R. & Bourgeois, P. (2004). The IPSO Study: Ibuprofen, Paracetamol Study in Osteoarthritis. A Randomised Comparative Clinical Study Comparing the Efficacy and Safety of Ibuprofen and Paracetamol Analgesic Treatment of Osteoarthritis of the Knee or Hip. *Annals of the Rheumatic Diseases*, Vol.63, No.9, pp. 1028-1034, ISSN 0003-4967

Breedveld, F.C. (2004). Osteoarthritis--the Impact of a Serious Disease. *Rheumatology (Oxford)*, Vol.43, No.suppl 1, p. i4-i8, ISSN 1462-0324

Bresalier, R.S., Sandler, R.S., Quan, H., Bolognese, J.A., Oxenius, B., Horgan, K., Lines, C., Riddell, R., Morton, D., Lanas, A., Konstam, M.A. & Baron, J.A. (2005). Cardiovascular Events Associated With Rofecoxib in a Colorectal Adenoma Chemoprevention Trial. *New England Journal of Medicine*, Vol.352, No.11, pp. 1092-1102, ISSN 0028-4793

Caldwell, B., Aldington, S., Weatherall, M., Shirtcliffe, P. & Beasley, R. (2006). Risk of Cardiovascular Events and Celecoxib: a Systematic Review and Meta-Analysis. *Journal of the Royal Society of Medicine*, Vol.99, No.3, pp. 132-140, ISSN 0141-0768

Caldwell, J.R., Rapoport, R.J., Davis, J.C., Offenberg, H.L., Marker, H.W., Roth, S.H., Yuan, W., Eliot, L., Babul, N. & Lynch, P.M. (2002). Efficacy and Safety of a Once-Daily Morphine Formulation in Chronic, Moderate-to-Severe Osteoarthritis Pain: Results From a Randomized, Placebo-Controlled, Double-Blind Trial and an Open-Label Extension Trial. *Journal of Pain and Symptom Management*, Vol.23, No.4, pp. 278-291, ISSN 0885-3924

Catala, E., Reig, E., Artes, M., Aliaga, L., Lopez, J.S. & Segu, J.L. (2002). Prevalence of Pain in the Spanish Population: Telephone Survey in 5000 Homes. *European Journal of Pain*, Vol.6, No.2, pp. 133-140, ISSN 1090-3801

Chappell, A.S., Desaiah, D., Liu-Seifert, H., Zhang, S., Skljarevski, V., Belenkov, Y. & Brown, J.P. (2011). A Double-Blind, Randomized, Placebo-Controlled Study of the Efficacy and Safety of Duloxetine for the Treatment of Chronic Pain Due to Osteoarthritis of the Knee. *Pain Practice*, Vol.11, No.1, pp. 33-41, ISSN 1530-7085

Chappell, A.S., Ossanna, M.J., Liu-Seifert, H., Iyengar, S., Skljarevski, V., Li, L.C., Bennett, R.M. & Collins, H. (2009). Duloxetine, a Centrally Acting Analgesic, in the

Treatment of Patients With Osteoarthritis Knee Pain: a 13-Week, Randomized, Placebo-Controlled Trial. *Pain*, Vol.146, No.3, pp. 253-260, ISSN 0304-3959

Christensen, R., Bartels, E.M., Astrup, A. & Bliddal, H. (2007). Effect of Weight Reduction in Obese Patients Diagnosed With Knee Osteoarthritis: a Systematic Review and Meta-Analysis. *Annals of the Rheumatic Diseases*, Vol.66, No.4, pp. 433-439, ISSN 0003-4967

Coleman, S., McQuade, J., Rose, J., Inderjeeth, C., Carroll, G. & Briffa, N.K. (2010). Self-Management for Osteoarthritis of the Knee: Does Mode of Delivery Influence Outcome? *BMC Musculoskeletal Disorders*, Vol.11, p. 56

Courtney, C.A., Kavchak, A.E., Lowry, C.D. & O'Hearn, M.A. (2010). Interpreting Joint Pain: Quantitative Sensory Testing in Musculoskeletal Management. *Journal of Orthopaedic and Sports Physical Therapy*, Vol.40, No.12, pp. 818-825, ISSN 0190-6011

Crofford, L.J. (1997). COX-1 and COX-2 Tissue Expression: Implications and Predictions. *Journal of Rheumatology Supplement*, Vol.49, pp. 15-19, ISSN 0380-0903

CYMBALTA® (Duloxetine Hydrochloride) Delayed-Release Capsules [Package Insert]. Indianapolis, In: Eli Lilly and Company; 2011

de Bock, G.H., Kaptein, A.A., Touw-Otten, F. & Mulder, J.D. (1995). Health-Related Quality of Life in Patients With Osteoarthritis in a Family Practice Setting. *Arthritis Care and Research*, Vol.8, No.2, pp. 88-93, ISSN 0893-7524

Dillon, C.F., Rasch, E.K., Gu, Q. & Hirsch, R. (2006). Prevalence of Knee Osteoarthritis in the United States: Arthritis Data From the Third National Health and Nutrition Examination Survey 1991-94. *Journal of Rheumatology*, Vol.33, No.11, pp. 2271-2279, ISSN 0315-162X

Dominick, K.L., Bosworth, H.B., Dudley, T.K., Waters, S.J., Campbell, L.C. & Keefe, F.J. (2004). Patterns of Opioid Analgesic Prescription Among Patients With Osteoarthritis. *Journal of Pain & Palliative Care Pharmacotherapy*, Vol.18, No.1, pp. 31-46, ISSN 1536-0288

Elliott, A.M., Smith, B.H., Penny, K.I., Smith, W.C. & Chambers, W.A. (1999). The Epidemiology of Chronic Pain in the Community. *Lancet*, Vol.354, No.9186, pp. 1248-1252, ISSN 0140-6736

Etropolski, M., Lange, B., Kuperwasser, B., Kelly, K., Okamoto, A., Steup, A., Van Hove, I., Weber, H. & Häussler, J. (2009). Efficacy and Safety of Tapentadol Extended Release Versus Oxycodone Controlled Release in Opioid-Naive and Opioid-Experienced Patients With Chronic Pain Associated With Osteoarthritis of the Knee. *Osteoarthritis and Cartilage*, Vol.17, No.suppl 1, p. S175

Felson, D.T. (2006). Clinical Practice. Osteoarthritis of the Knee. *New England Journal of Medicine*, Vol.354, No.8, pp. 841-848, ISSN 0028-4793

Felson, D.T. (2009). Developments in the Clinical Understanding of Osteoarthritis. *Arthritis Research & Therapy*, Vol.11, No.1, p. 203, ISSN 1478-6354

Felson, D.T., Lawrence, R.C., Dieppe, P.A., Hirsch, R., Helmick, C.G., Jordan, J.M., Kington, R.S., Lane, N.E., Nevitt, M.C., Zhang, Y., Sowers, M., McAlindon, T., Spector, T.D., Poole, A.R., Yanovski, S.Z., Ateshian, G., Sharma, L., Buckwalter, J.A., Brandt, K.D. & Fries, J.F. (2000). Osteoarthritis: New Insights. Part 1: the Disease and Its Risk Factors. *Annals of Internal Medicine*, Vol.133, No.8, pp. 635-646, ISSN 0003-4819

Felson, D.T., Naimark, A., Anderson, J., Kazis, L., Castelli, W. & Meenan, R.F. (1987). The Prevalence of Knee Osteoarthritis in the Elderly. The Framingham Osteoarthritis Study. *Arthritis and Rheumatism*, Vol.30, No.8, pp. 914-918, ISSN 0004-3591

Fendrick, A.M. & Greenberg, B.P. (2009). A Review of the Benefits and Risks of Nonsteroidal Anti-Inflammatory Drugs in the Management of Mild-to-Moderate Osteoarthritis. *Osteopathic Medicine and Primary Care*, Vol.3, p. 1

Flood, J. (2010). The Role of Acetaminophen in the Treatment of Osteoarthritis. *American Journal of Managed Care*, Vol.16 Suppl Management, p. S48-S54, ISSN 1088-0224

Fored, C.M., Ejerblad, E., Lindblad, P., Fryzek, J.P., Dickman, P.W., Signorello, L.B., Lipworth, L., Elinder, C.G., Blot, W.J., McLaughlin, J.K., Zack, M.M. & Nyren, O. (2001). Acetaminophen, Aspirin, and Chronic Renal Failure. *New England Journal of Medicine*, Vol.345, No.25, pp. 1801-1808, ISSN 0028-4793

Fosbol, E.L., Gislason, G.H., Jacobsen, S., Folke, F., Hansen, M.L., Schramm, T.K., Sorensen, R., Rasmussen, J.N., Andersen, S.S., Abildstrom, S.Z., Traerup, J., Poulsen, H.E., Rasmussen, S., Kober, L. & Torp-Pedersen, C. (2009). Risk of Myocardial Infarction and Death Associated With the Use of Nonsteroidal Anti-Inflammatory Drugs (NSAIDs) Among Healthy Individuals: a Nationwide Cohort Study. *Clinical Pharmacology and Therapeutics*, Vol.85, No.2, pp. 190-197, ISSN 0009-9236

Gabriel, S.E., Jaakkimainen, L. & Bombardier, C. (1991). Risk for Serious Gastrointestinal Complications Related to Use of Nonsteroidal Anti-Inflammatory Drugs. A Meta-Analysis. *Annals of Internal Medicine*, Vol.115, No.10, pp. 787-796, ISSN 0003-4819

Garcia Rodriguez, L.A. & Hernandez-Diaz, S. (2001). Relative Risk of Upper Gastrointestinal Complications Among Users of Acetaminophen and Nonsteroidal Anti-Inflammatory Drugs. *Epidemiology*, Vol.12, No.5, pp. 570-576, ISSN 1044-3983

Gislason, G.H., Rasmussen, J.N., Abildstrom, S.Z., Schramm, T.K., Hansen, M.L., Fosbol, E.L., Sorensen, R., Folke, F., Buch, P., Gadsboll, N., Rasmussen, S., Poulsen, H.E., Kober, L., Madsen, M. & Torp-Pedersen, C. (2009). Increased Mortality and Cardiovascular Morbidity Associated With Use of Nonsteroidal Anti-Inflammatory Drugs in Chronic Heart Failure. *Archives of Internal Medicine*, Vol.169, No.2, pp. 141-149, ISSN 0003-9926

Goldberg, V.M. & Buckwalter, J.A. (2005). Hyaluronans in the Treatment of Osteoarthritis of the Knee: Evidence for Disease-Modifying Activity. *Osteoarthritis and Cartilage*, Vol.13, No.3, pp. 216-224, ISSN 1063-4584

Golden, H.E., Moskowitz, R.W. & Minic, M. (2004). Analgesic Efficacy and Safety of Nonprescription Doses of Naproxen Sodium Compared With Acetaminophen in the Treatment of Osteoarthritis of the Knee. *American Journal of Therapeutics*, Vol.11, No.2, pp. 85-94, ISSN 1075-2765

Graham, D.J., Campen, D., Hui, R., Spence, M., Cheetham, C., Levy, G., Shoor, S. & Ray, W.A. (2005). Risk of Acute Myocardial Infarction and Sudden Cardiac Death in Patients Treated With Cyclo-Oxygenase 2 Selective and Non-Selective Non-Steroidal Anti-Inflammatory Drugs: Nested Case-Control Study. *Lancet*, Vol.365, No.9458, pp. 475-481, ISSN 0140-6736

Gregory, P.J., Sperry, M. & Wilson, A.F. (2008). Dietary Supplements for Osteoarthritis. *American Family Physician*, Vol.77, No.2, pp. 177-184, ISSN 0002-838X

Gwilym, S.E., Keltner, J.R., Warnaby, C.E., Carr, A.J., Chizh, B., Chessell, I. & Tracey, I. (2009). Psychophysical and Functional Imaging Evidence Supporting the Presence of Central Sensitization in a Cohort of Osteoarthritis Patients. *Arthritis and Rheumatism*, Vol.61, No.9, pp. 1226-1234, ISSN 0004-3591

Hale, M., Tudor, I.C., Khanna, S. & Thipphawong, J. (2007). Efficacy and Tolerability of Once-Daily OROS Hydromorphone and Twice-Daily Extended-Release Oxycodone in Patients With Chronic, Moderate to Severe Osteoarthritis Pain: Results of a 6-Week, Randomized, Open-Label, Noninferiority Analysis. *Clinical Therapeutics*, Vol.29, No.5, pp. 874-888, ISSN 0149-2918

Hammad, T.A., Graham, D.J., Staffa, J.A., Kornegay, C.J. & Dal Pan, G.J. (2008). Onset of Acute Myocardial Infarction After Use of Non-Steroidal Anti-Inflammatory Drugs. *Pharmacoepidemiology and Drug Safety*, Vol.17, No.4, pp. 315-321, ISSN 1053-8569

Hardy, M.L., Coulter, I., Morton, S.C., Favreau, J., Venuturupalli, S., Chiappelli, F., Rossi, F., Orshansky, G., Jungvig, L.K., Roth, E.A., Suttorp, M.J. & Shekelle, P. (2003). S-Adenosyl-L-Methionine for Treatment of Depression, Osteoarthritis, and Liver Disease. *Evidence Report - Technology Assessment (Summary)*, No.64, pp. 1-3, ISSN 1530-440X

Helmick, C.G., Felson, D.T., Lawrence, R.C., Gabriel, S., Hirsch, R., Kwoh, C.K., Liang, M.H., Kremers, H.M., Mayes, M.D., Merkel, P.A., Pillemer, S.R., Reveille, J.D. & Stone, J.H. (2008). Estimates of the Prevalence of Arthritis and Other Rheumatic Conditions in the United States. Part I. *Arthritis and Rheumatism*, Vol.58, No.1, pp. 15-25, ISSN 0004-3591

Hinton, R., Moody, R.L., Davis, A.W. & Thomas, S.F. (2002). Osteoarthritis: Diagnosis and Therapeutic Considerations. *American Family Physician*, Vol.65, No.5, pp. 841-848, ISSN 0002-838X

Hochman, J.R., French, M.R., Bermingham, S.L. & Hawker, G.A. (2010). The Nerve of Osteoarthritis Pain. *Arthritis Care & Research (Hoboken)*, Vol.62, No.7, pp. 1019-1023, ISSN 2151-464X

Hunter, D.J. & Felson, D.T. (2006). Osteoarthritis. *British Medical Journal*, Vol.332, No.7542, pp. 639-642, ISSN 0959-8146

Hunter, D.J., McDougall, J.J. & Keefe, F.J. (2008). The Symptoms of Osteoarthritis and the Genesis of Pain. *Rheumatic Diseases Clinics of North America*, Vol.34, No.3, pp. 623-643, ISSN 0889-857X

Jinks, C., Jordan, K. & Croft, P. (2007). Osteoarthritis As a Public Health Problem: the Impact of Developing Knee Pain on Physical Function in Adults Living in the Community: (KNEST 3). *Rheumatology (Oxford)*, Vol.46, No.5, pp. 877-881, ISSN 1462-0324

Johannes, C.B., Le, T.K., Zhou, X., Johnston, J.A. & Dworkin, R.H. (2010). The Prevalence of Chronic Pain in United States Adults: Results of an Internet-Based Survey. *Journal of Pain*, Vol.11, No.11, pp. 1230-1239, ISSN 1526-5900

Jones, A., Regan, M., Ledingham, J., Pattrick, M., Manhire, A. & Doherty, M. (1993). Importance of Placement of Intra-Articular Steroid Injections. *British Medical Journal*, Vol.307, No.6915, pp. 1329-1330, ISSN 0959-8138

Jordan, K.M., Arden, N.K., Doherty, M., Bannwarth, B., Bijlsma, J.W., Dieppe, P., Gunther, K., Hauselmann, H., Herrero-Beaumont, G., Kaklamanis, P., Lohmander, S., Leeb, B., Lequesne, M., Mazieres, B., Martin-Mola, E., Pavelka, K., Pendleton, A., Punzi, L., Serni, U., Swoboda, B., Verbruggen, G., Zimmerman-Gorska, I. & Dougados, M. (2003). EULAR Recommendations 2003: an Evidence Based Approach to the Management of Knee Osteoarthritis: Report of a Task Force of the Standing

Committee for International Clinical Studies Including Therapeutic Trials (ESCISIT). *Annals of the Rheumatic Diseases*, Vol.62, No.12, pp. 1145-1155, ISSN 0003-4967

Katz, N., Hale, M., Morris, D. & Stauffer, J. (2010). Morphine Sulfate and Naltrexone Hydrochloride Extended Release Capsules in Patients With Chronic Osteoarthritis Pain. *Postgraduate Medicine*, Vol.122, No.4, pp. 112-128, ISSN 0032-5481

Kidd, B.L., Langford, R.M. & Wodehouse, T. (2007). Arthritis and Pain. Current Approaches in the Treatment of Arthritic Pain. *Arthritis Research & Therapy*, Vol.9, No.3, p. 214, ISSN 1478-6354

Kim, J., Lee, E.Y., Koh, E.M., Cha, H.S., Yoo, B., Lee, C.K., Lee, Y.J., Ryu, H., Lee, K.H. & Song, Y.W. (2009). Comparative Clinical Trial of S-Adenosylmethionine Versus Nabumetone for the Treatment of Knee Osteoarthritis: an 8-Week, Multicenter, Randomized, Double-Blind, Double-Dummy, Phase IV Study in Korean Patients. *Clinical Therapeutics*, Vol.31, No.12, pp. 2860-2872, ISSN 0149-2918

Klussmann, A., Gebhardt, H., Nubling, M., Liebers, F., Quiros, P.E., Cordier, W., von Engelhardt, L.V., Schubert, M., David, A., Bouillon, B. & Rieger, M.A. (2010). Individual and Occupational Risk Factors for Knee Osteoarthritis: Results of a Case-Control Study in Germany. *Arthritis Research & Therapy*, Vol.12, No.3, p. R88, ISSN 1478-6354

Kopec, J.A., Rahman, M.M., Berthelot, J.M., Le, P.C., Aghajanian, J., Sayre, E.C., Cibere, J., Anis, A.H. & Badley, E.M. (2007). Descriptive Epidemiology of Osteoarthritis in British Columbia, Canada. *Journal of Rheumatology*, Vol.34, No.2, pp. 386-393, ISSN 0315-162X

Kosek, E. & Ordeberg, G. (2000). Abnormalities of Somatosensory Perception in Patients With Painful Osteoarthritis Normalize Following Successful Treatment. *European Journal of Pain*, Vol.4, No.3, pp. 229-238, ISSN 1090-3801

Kotlarz, H., Gunnarsson, C.L., Fang, H. & Rizzo, J.A. (2009). Insurer and Out-of-Pocket Costs of Osteoarthritis in the US: Evidence From National Survey Data. *Arthritis and Rheumatism*, Vol.60, No.12, pp. 3546-3553, ISSN 0004-3591

Lange, B., Kuperwasser, B., Okamoto, A., Steup, A., Haufel, T., Ashworth, J. & Etropolski, M. (2010). Efficacy and Safety of Tapentadol Prolonged Release for Chronic Osteoarthritis Pain and Low Back Pain. *Advances in Therapy*, Vol.27, No.6, pp. 381-399, ISSN 0741-238X

Langford, R., McKenna, F., Ratcliffe, S., Vojtassak, J. & Richarz, U. (2006). Transdermal Fentanyl for Improvement of Pain and Functioning in Osteoarthritis: a Randomized, Placebo-Controlled Trial. *Arthritis and Rheumatism*, Vol.54, No.6, pp. 1829-1837, ISSN 0004-3591

Lawrence, R.C., Felson, D.T., Helmick, C.G., Arnold, L.M., Choi, H., Deyo, R.A., Gabriel, S., Hirsch, R., Hochberg, M.C., Hunder, G.G., Jordan, J.M., Katz, J.N., Kremers, H.M. & Wolfe, F. (2008). Estimates of the Prevalence of Arthritis and Other Rheumatic Conditions in the United States. Part II. *Arthritis and Rheumatism*, Vol.58, No.1, pp. 26-35, ISSN 0004-3591

Lee, C., Straus, W.L., Balshaw, R., Barlas, S., Vogel, S. & Schnitzer, T.J. (2004). A Comparison of the Efficacy and Safety of Nonsteroidal Antiinflammatory Agents Versus Acetaminophen in the Treatment of Osteoarthritis: a Meta-Analysis. *Arthritis and Rheumatism*, Vol.51, No.5, pp. 746-754, ISSN 0004-3591

Loeser, R.F. (2008). Molecular Mechanisms of Cartilage Destruction in Osteoarthritis. *Journal of Musculoskeletal and Neuronal Interactions*, Vol.8, No.4, pp. 303-306, ISSN 1108-7161

Majani, G., Giardini, A. & Scotti, A. (2005). Subjective Impact of Osteoarthritis Flare-Ups on Patients' Quality of Life. *Health and Quality of Life Outcomes*, Vol.3, p. 14

Martel-Pelletier, J. & Pelletier, J.P. (2010). Is Osteoarthritis a Disease Involving Only Cartilage or Other Articular Tissues? *Eklem Hastalik Cerrahisi*, Vol.21, No.1, pp. 2-14, ISSN 1305-8282

Matsumoto, A.K., Babul, N. & Ahdieh, H. (2005). Oxymorphone Extended-Release Tablets Relieve Moderate to Severe Pain and Improve Physical Function in Osteoarthritis: Results of a Randomized, Double-Blind, Placebo- and Active-Controlled Phase III Trial. *Pain Medicine*, Vol.6, No.5, pp. 357-366, ISSN 1526-2375

McAlindon, T.E., LaValley, M.P., Gulin, J.P. & Felson, D.T. (2000). Glucosamine and Chondroitin for Treatment of Osteoarthritis: a Systematic Quality Assessment and Meta-Analysis. *JAMA: The Journal of the American Medical Association*, Vol.283, No.11, pp. 1469-1475, ISSN 0098-7484

McGettigan, P. & Henry, D. (2006). Cardiovascular Risk and Inhibition of Cyclooxygenase: a Systematic Review of the Observational Studies of Selective and Nonselective Inhibitors of Cyclooxygenase 2. *JAMA: The Journal of the American Medical Association*, Vol.296, No.13, pp. 1633-1644, ISSN 0098-7484

McHughes, M. & Lipman, A.G. (2006). Managing Osteoarthritis Pain When Your Patient Fails Simple Analgesics and NSAIDs and Is Not a Candidate for Surgery. *Current Rheumatology Reports*, Vol.8, No.1, pp. 22-29, ISSN 1523-3774

McNair, P.J., Simmonds, M.A., Boocock, M.G. & Larmer, P.J. (2009). Exercise Therapy for the Management of Osteoarthritis of the Hip Joint: a Systematic Review. *Arthritis Research & Therapy*, Vol.11, No.3, p. R98, ISSN 1478-6354

Messier, S.P. (2008). Obesity and Osteoarthritis: Disease Genesis and Nonpharmacologic Weight Management. *Rheumatic Diseases Clinics of North America*, Vol.34, No.3, pp. 713-729, ISSN 0889-857X

Messier, S.P., Loeser, R.F., Miller, G.D., Morgan, T.M., Rejeski, W.J., Sevick, M.A., Ettinger, W.H., Jr., Pahor, M. & Williamson, J.D. (2004). Exercise and Dietary Weight Loss in Overweight and Obese Older Adults With Knee Osteoarthritis: the Arthritis, Diet, and Activity Promotion Trial. *Arthritis and Rheumatism*, Vol.50, No.5, pp. 1501-1510, ISSN 0004-3591

Michael, J.W., Schluter-Brust, K.U. & Eysel, P. (2010). The Epidemiology, Etiology, Diagnosis, and Treatment of Osteoarthritis of the Knee. *Deutsches Arzteblatt International*, Vol.107, No.9, pp. 152-162

Najm, W.I., Reinsch, S., Hoehler, F., Tobis, J.S. & Harvey, P.W. (2004). S-Adenosyl Methionine (SAMe) Versus Celecoxib for the Treatment of Osteoarthritis Symptoms: a Double-Blind Cross-Over Trial. [ISRCTN36233495]. *BMC Musculoskeletal Disorders*, Vol.5, p. 6

Neustadt, D.H. (2006). Intra-Articular Injections for Osteoarthritis of the Knee. *Cleveland Clinic Journal of Medicine*, Vol.73, No.10, pp. 897-4, 906, ISSN 0891-1150

Nuesch, E., Rutjes, A.W., Husni, E., Welch, V. & Juni, P. (2009). Oral or Transdermal Opioids for Osteoarthritis of the Knee or Hip. *Cochrane Database of Systemic Reviews*, No.4, p. CD003115

Nussmeier, N.A., Whelton, A.A., Brown, M.T., Langford, R.M., Hoeft, A., Parlow, J.L., Boyce, S.W. & Verburg, K.M. (2005). Complications of the COX-2 Inhibitors Parecoxib and Valdecoxib After Cardiac Surgery. *New England Journal of Medicine*, Vol.352, No.11, pp. 1081-1091, ISSN 0028-4793

Pavelka, K., Gatterova, J., Olejarova, M., Machacek, S., Giacovelli, G. & Rovati, L.C. (2002). Glucosamine Sulfate Use and Delay of Progression of Knee Osteoarthritis: a 3-Year, Randomized, Placebo-Controlled, Double-Blind Study. *Archives of Internal Medicine*, Vol.162, No.18, pp. 2113-2123, ISSN 0003-9926

Petrella, R.J. (2000). Is Exercise Effective Treatment for Osteoarthritis of the Knee? *British Journal of Sports Medicine*, Vol.34, No.5, pp. 326-331, ISSN 0306-3674

Pham, K. & Hirschberg, R. (2005). Global Safety of Coxibs and NSAIDs. *Current Topics in Medicinal Chemistry*, Vol.5, No.5, pp. 465-473, ISSN 1568-0266

Physical Activity Guidelines Advisory Committee. (2008). Physical Activity Guidelines Advisor Committe Report, 2008, 16.05.2011, Available from: http://www.health.gov/PAguidelines/Report/pdf/CommitteeReport.pdf

Puenpatom, R.A. & Victor, T.W. (2009). Increased Prevalence of Metabolic Syndrome in Individuals With Osteoarthritis: an Analysis of NHANES III Data. *Postgraduate Medicine*, Vol.121, No.6, pp. 9-20, ISSN 0032-5481

Rahme, E., Pettitt, D. & LeLorier, J. (2002). Determinants and Sequelae Associated With Utilization of Acetaminophen Versus Traditional Nonsteroidal Antiinflammatory Drugs in an Elderly Population. *Arthritis and Rheumatism*, Vol.46, No.11, pp. 3046-3054, ISSN 0004-3591

Reginster, J.Y., Deroisy, R., Rovati, L.C., Lee, R.L., Lejeune, E., Bruyere, O., Giacovelli, G., Henrotin, Y., Dacre, J.E. & Gossett, C. (2001). Long-Term Effects of Glucosamine Sulphate on Osteoarthritis Progression: a Randomised, Placebo-Controlled Clinical Trial. *Lancet*, Vol.357, No.9252, pp. 251-256, ISSN 0140-6736

Reichenbach, S., Sterchi, R., Scherer, M., Trelle, S., Burgi, E., Burgi, U., Dieppe, P.A. & Juni, P. (2007). Meta-Analysis: Chondroitin for Osteoarthritis of the Knee or Hip. *Annals of Internal Medicine*, Vol.146, No.8, pp. 580-590, ISSN 0003-4819

Rizkalla, G., Reiner, A., Bogoch, E. & Poole, A.R. (1992). Studies of the Articular Cartilage Proteoglycan Aggrecan in Health and Osteoarthritis. Evidence for Molecular Heterogeneity and Extensive Molecular Changes in Disease. *Journal of Clinical Investigation*, Vol.90, No.6, pp. 2268-2277, ISSN 0021-9738

Rosenthal, M., Moore, P., Groves, E., Iwan, T., Schlosser, L.G., Dziewanowska, Z. & Negro-Vilar, A. (2007). Sleep Improves When Patients With Chronic OA Pain Are Managed With Morning Dosing of Once a Day Extended-Release Morphine Sulfate (AVINZA): Findings From a Pilot Study. *Journal of Opioid Management*, Vol.3, No.3, pp. 145-154, ISSN 1551-7489

Roth, S.H., Fleischmann, R.M., Burch, F.X., Dietz, F., Bockow, B., Rapoport, R.J., Rutstein, J. & Lacouture, P.G. (2000). Around-the-Clock, Controlled-Release Oxycodone Therapy for Osteoarthritis-Related Pain: Placebo-Controlled Trial and Long-Term Evaluation. *Archives of Internal Medicine*, Vol.160, No.6, pp. 853-860, ISSN 0003-9926

Sakalauskiene, G. & Jauniskiene, D. (2010). Osteoarthritis: Etiology, Epidemiology, Impact on the Individual and Society and the Main Principles of Management. *Medicina (Kaunas)*, Vol.46, No.11, pp. 790-797, ISSN 1010-660X

Salaffi, F., Carotti, M., Stancati, A. & Grassi, W. (2005). Health-Related Quality of Life in Older Adults With Symptomatic Hip and Knee Osteoarthritis: a Comparison With Matched Healthy Controls. *Aging Clinical and Experimental Research*, Vol.17, No.4, pp. 255-263, ISSN 1594-0667

Sander, O. (2003). Review: S-Adenosylmethionine Treats Osteoarthritis As Effectively As Nonsteroidal Anti-Inflammatory Drugs With Fewer Adverse Effects. *American College of Physicians Journal Club*, Vol.138, No.1, p. 21, ISSN 1056-8751

Schjerning Olsen, A.M., Fosbol, E.L., Lindhardsen, J., Folke, F., Charlot, M., Selmer, C., Lamberts, M., Bjerring, O.J., Kober, L., Hansen, P.R., Torp-Pedersen, C. & Gislason, G.H. (2011). Duration of Treatment With Nonsteroidal Anti-Inflammatory Drugs and Impact on Risk of Death and Recurrent Myocardial Infarction in Patients With Prior Myocardial Infarction: a Nationwide Cohort Study. *Circulation*, Vol.123, No.20, pp. 2226-2235, ISSN 0009-7322

Schroder, W., Tzschentke, T.M., Terlinden, R., De, V.J., Jahnel, U., Christoph, T. & Tallarida, R.J. (2011). Synergistic Interaction Between the Two Mechanisms of Action of Tapentadol in Analgesia. *Journal of Pharmacology and Experimental Therapeutics*, Vol.337, No.1, pp. 312-320, ISSN 0022-3565

Segal, L., Day, S.E., Chapman, A.B. & Osborne, R.H. (2004). Can We Reduce Disease Burden From Osteoarthritis? *Medical Journal of Australia*, Vol.180, No.5 Suppl, p. S11-S17, ISSN 0025-729X

Shane, A.A. & Loeser, R.F. (2010). Why Is Osteoarthritis an Age-Related Disease? *Best Pract Res Clin Rheumatol*, Vol.24, No.1, pp. 15-26, ISSN 1521-6942

Solomon, S.D., McMurray, J.J., Pfeffer, M.A., Wittes, J., Fowler, R., Finn, P., Anderson, W.F., Zauber, A., Hawk, E. & Bertagnolli, M. (2005). Cardiovascular Risk Associated With Celecoxib in a Clinical Trial for Colorectal Adenoma Prevention. *New England Journal of Medicine*, Vol.352, No.11, pp. 1071-1080, ISSN 0028-4793

Sullivan, M.D., Bentley, S., Fan, M.Y. & Gardner, G. (2009). A Single-Blind, Placebo Run-in Study of Duloxetine for Activity-Limiting Osteoarthritis Pain. *Journal of Pain*, Vol.10, No.2, pp. 208-213, ISSN 1526-5900

Sullivan, M.D., Edlund, M.J., Fan, M.Y., Devries, A., Brennan, B.J. & Martin, B.C. (2008). Trends in Use of Opioids for Non-Cancer Pain Conditions 2000-2005 in Commercial and Medicaid Insurance Plans: the TROUP Study. *Pain*, Vol.138, No.2, pp. 440-449, ISSN 0304-3959

The National Collaborating Centre for Chronic Conditions. (2008). *Osteoarthritis: National Clinical Guideline for Care and Management in Adults*, Royal College of Physicians, London

Towheed, T.E. & Anastassiades, T. (2007). Glucosamine Therapy for Osteoarthritis: an Update. *Journal of Rheumatology*, Vol.34, No.9, pp. 1787-1790, ISSN 0315-162X

Towheed, T.E., Maxwell, L., Anastassiades, T.P., Shea, B., Houpt, J., Robinson, V., Hochberg, M.C. & Wells, G. (2005). Glucosamine Therapy for Treating Osteoarthritis. *Cochrane Database of Systemic Reviews*, No.2, p. CD002946

Tsang, A., Von, K.M., Lee, S., Alonso, J., Karam, E., Angermeyer, M.C., Borges, G.L., Bromet, E.J., de, G.G., de, G.R., Gureje, O., Lepine, J.P., Haro, J.M., Levinson, D., Oakley Browne, M.A., Posada-Villa, J., Seedat, S. & Watanabe, M. (2008). Common Chronic Pain Conditions in Developed and Developing Countries: Gender and Age

Differences and Comorbidity With Depression-Anxiety Disorders. *Journal of Pain*, Vol.9, No.10, pp. 883-891, ISSN 1526-5900

Tzschentke, T.M., Christoph, T., Kögel, B., Schiene, K., Hennies, H.-H., Englberger, W., Haurand, M., Jahnel, U., Cremers, T.I., Friderichs, E. & De Vry, J. (2007). (-)-(1*R*,2*R*)-3-(3-Dimethylamino-1-Ethyl-2-Methyl-Propyl)-Phenol Hydrochloride (Tapentadol HCl): a Novel M-Opioid Receptor Agonist/Norepinephrine Reuptake Inhibitor With Broad-Spectrum Analgesic Properties. *Journal of Pharmacology and Experimental Therapeutics*, Vol.323, No.1, pp. 265-276, ISSN 0022-3565

Tzschentke, T.M., De Vry, J., Terlinden, R., Hennies, H.H., Lange, C., Strassburger, W., Haurand, M., Kolb, J., Schneider, J., Buschmann, H., Finkam, M., Jahnel, U. & Friderichs, E. (2006). Tapentadol HCl. *Drugs of the Future*, Vol.31, No.12, pp. 1053-1061, ISSN 0377-8282

US Food and Drug Administration. (2005). COX-2 Selective (Includes Bextra, Celebrex, and Vioxx) and Non-Selective Non-Steroidal Anti-Inflammatory Drugs (NSAIDs). April 7, 2005., 18.05.11 A.D., Available from:
http://www.fda.gov/drugs/drugsafety/postmarketdrugsafetyinformationforpatientsandproviders/ucm103420.htm

US Food and Drug Administration. (2010). Meeting of the Anesthetic and Life Support Drugs Advisory Committee (ALSDAC): Summary Minutes From the August 19, 2010 Meeting, 23.05.2011, Available from:
http://www.fda.gov/downloads/AdvisoryCommittees/CommitteesMeetingMaterials/Drugs/AnestheticAndLifeSupportDrugsAdvisoryCommittee/UCM236241.pdf

Wagner, E. (2011). [Direct Costs of Osteoarthritis]. *Wiener Medizinische Wochenschrift*, Vol.161, No.1-2, pp. 44-52, ISSN 0043-5341

Wandel, S., Juni, P., Tendal, B., Nuesch, E., Villiger, P.M., Welton, N.J., Reichenbach, S. & Trelle, S. (2010). Effects of Glucosamine, Chondroitin, or Placebo in Patients With Osteoarthritis of Hip or Knee: Network Meta-Analysis. *British Medical Journal*, Vol.341, p. c4675, ISSN 0959-8138

White, A.G., Birnbaum, H.G., Buteau, S., Janagap, C. & Schein, J.R. (2007). Cost of Pain Therapy for Osteoarthritis in a Privately Insured Population in the United States. *Value in Health*, Vol.10, No.3, p. A117

Wild, J.E., Grond, S., Kuperwasser, B., Gilbert, J., McCann, B., Lange, B., Steup, A., Häufel, T., Etropolski, M.S., Rauschkolb, C. & Lange, R. (2010). Long-Term Safety and Tolerability of Tapentadol Extended Release for the Management of Chronic Low Back Pain or Osteoarthritis Pain. *Pain Practice*, Vol.10, No.5, pp. 416-427, ISSN 1530-7085

Woolf, C.J. (2011). Central Sensitization: Implications for the Diagnosis and Treatment of Pain. *Pain*, Vol.152, No.3 Suppl, pp. S2-15, ISSN 0304-3959

Zhang, W., Doherty, M., Peat, G., Bierma-Zeinstra, M.A., Arden, N.K., Bresnihan, B., Herrero-Beaumont, G., Kirschner, S., Leeb, B.F., Lohmander, L.S., Mazieres, B., Pavelka, K., Punzi, L., So, A.K., Tuncer, T., Watt, I. & Bijlsma, J.W. (2010). EULAR Evidence-Based Recommendations for the Diagnosis of Knee Osteoarthritis. *Annals of the Rheumatic Diseases*, Vol.69, No.3, pp. 483-489, ISSN 0003-4967

Zhang, W., Jones, A. & Doherty, M. (2004). Does Paracetamol (Acetaminophen) Reduce the Pain of Osteoarthritis? A Meta-Analysis of Randomised Controlled Trials. *Annals of the Rheumatic Diseases*, Vol.63, No.8, pp. 901-907, ISSN 0003-4967

Zhang, W., Moskowitz, R.W., Nuki, G., Abramson, S., Altman, R.D., Arden, N., Bierma-Zeinstra, S., Brandt, K.D., Croft, P., Doherty, M., Dougados, M., Hochberg, M., Hunter, D.J., Kwoh, K., Lohmander, L.S. & Tugwell, P. (2008). OARSI Recommendations for the Management of Hip and Knee Osteoarthritis, Part II: OARSI Evidence-Based, Expert Consensus Guidelines. *Osteoarthritis and Cartilage*, Vol.16, No.2, pp. 137-162, ISSN 1063-4584

2

Characterization of Live and Experimentally Degenerated Hyaline Cartilage with Thermal Analysis

Gellért Sohár[1], Piroska Szabó-Révész[2], Kálmán Tóth[1] and Zoltán Aigner[2]
[1]*Department of Orthopaedics, University of Szeged, Faculty of Medicine, Szeged,*
[2]*Department of Pharmaceutical Technology, University of Szeged, Faculty of Pharmacy, Szeged, Hungary*

1. Introduction

Osteoarthritis (OA), the most prevalent joint disease, is characterized by the progressive loss of articular cartilage that leads to chronic pain and functional restrictions in affected joints [Goldring & Goldring, 2007]. The prior notion of OA as a bland disease related to aging and "wear and tear" of the joint has given way to views of a dynamic system with multiple pathogenic contributors, as local factors, as well as crystals and inflammation [Brandt et al., 2006]. OA represents a major therapeutic challenge to medical and health-care providers. In part, this is because OA is a chronic condition in which symptoms evolve over long periods of time and in which symptomatic episodes are frequently separated by lengthy asymptomatic periods. It is likely, however, that alterations in joint structure and function continue during these relative periods of clinical quiescence. In addition, limited tools are available for the assessment of the progression of structural changes in joint tissues in association with the development of osteoarthritis. Importantly, the correlation between structural alterations and symptoms is contradictory. There is a significant difference in the expression levels of cartilage relevant molecules between specimens showing histological alterations and control samples [Lorenz et al., 2006]. A total breakdown in synthesis of matrix molecules leads to the end stage OA with further progression of cartilage loss.

A number of OA models, e.g. aging animals, genetically modified mice, as well as animals with surgically, enzymatically, or chemically induced OA [van den Berg, 2001] have been developed to investigate the pathogenesis of OA and evaluate the potentials of new disease/structure-modifying drugs [Oegema et al., 2002]. Among these, monosodium iodoacetate (MIA, iodoacetic acid) model has been widely used to analyze the histological and biochemical changes observed during the progression of OA [Ameye, & Young, 2006]. Injection of the metabolic inhibitor, MIA, into joints inhibits glyceraldehye-3-phosphate dehydrogenase activity in chondrocytes, resulting in disruption of glycolysis and eventual cell death [Kalbhen, 1987]. The progressive loss of chondrocytes results in histologic and morphologic changes to the articular cartilage, closely resembling those seen in human OA [Janusz et al., 2001]. In addition, the model has been utilized by a number of investigators to test pharmacologic agents for their ability to preserve cartilage structure [Janusz et al., 2001].

Glucosamine, a naturally-occurring amino monosaccharide, is present in the polysaccharides of the connective and cartilage tissues, and contributes to maintaining the strength, flexibility, and elasticity of these tissues. Thus, glucosamine has been widely used for more than two decades in humans to treat osteoarthritis [Crolle, 1980]. Several short- and long-term clinical trials in osteoarthritis have shown the significant symptom-modifying effect of glucosamine [Reginster, et al., 2001]. Moreover, the updated Osteoarthritis Research Society International (OARSI) recommendations for management of hip and knee OA have recently suggested that glucosamine has symptom-relieving and structure modifying effects in knee OA [Zhang et al. 2008]. Importantly, it has been previously revealed in vitro that glucosamine can inhibit the degradation and stimulate the synthesis of glycosaminoglycans (proteoglycans), thereby possibly exhibiting chondroprotective action [Fenton et al., 2000]. Moreover, glucosamine has been shown to reduce radiographic progression of joint space narrowing in knee OA [Reginster, et al., 2001]. On the other hand, Glucosamine/chondroitin Arthritis Intervention Trial reported that glucosamine did not reduce pain effectively in patients with OA [Clegg et al., 2006], and the nonsufficient number of trials cannot confirm statistically that glucosamine sulphite has no effect [Vlad et al., 2007]. Thus, the effect of glucosamine on OA is still controversial [McAlindon, 2003].

Thermal analysis comprises a group of techniques in which a physical property of a substance is measured as a function of temperature, while the substance is subjected to a controlled temperature programme. Differential scanning calorimetry (DSC) has been widely used for determining physicochemical transformations that occur during thermal degradation [Collett & Brown, 1998]. Calorimetry can be used to determine most thermodynamic properties; e.g. enthalpy changes for reactions (ΔH) and for phase changes [Aigner et al., 2009; Than & Lőrinczy, 2003]. The usefulness of calorimetric examination in the characterization of biological samples has been demonstrated by previous studies [Than et al., 2000; Wiegand et al., 2009]. Prior studies have demonstrated the usefulness of calorimetric examination in the characterization of cartilage degeneration [Wiegand et al., 2010]. We have extended the use of thermal analysis by introducing thermogravimetric investigations. Thereby new information on the physicochemical properties of normal and OA tissues has been acquired.

An increasing number of papers have been published with the use of calorimetric techniques in the examination of degenerative [Mécs et al., 2009], rheumatoid arthritis [Tóth et al., 2009], and healthy human hyaline cartilage [Aigner et al., 2009]. P. Than et al. investigated first animal hyaline cartilage using differential scanning calorimetric method [Than et al., 2000]. They have concluded that structural manifestation of OA causes a remarkable change of thermal stability of hyaline cartilage. The healthy cartilage samples used in these studies were of cadaver origin as waste material, pathological cartilage was derived as intraoperative tissue fragments. The samples were washed in sterile phosphate-buffered saline and stored in complex solution containing fetal bovine serum, antibiotic, antimycotic solution, and amino acids. The measurements were conducted in 48 hours of sample deriving. The reported data on the calorimetric enthalpy changes proved to be inconsistent. In severely affected osteoarthritis, the ΔH has increased almost twofold, while in an earlier study, enthalpy changes in the intact hyaline cartilage altered from higher to lower levels in some cases [Than et al., 2000; Than et al., 2004].

The aim of these studies was to further characterize the altered metabolisms in OA that promotes disease progression. Based on previous studies, we hypothesized that thermodynamic findings may clearly differentiate normal and degenerated human hyaline `cartilage. Physicochemical transformations may provide information on the role of water content in OA, and enthalpy change of the process, initiated by the temperature change, might represent potential marker of the disease activity. Under experimental circumstances, calorimetric examinations were used to differentiate normal and degenerated rat hyaline cartilage and the effect of oral glucosamine-sulphate pre-treatment in OA was also studied. The purpose of this study was to elucidate complex deviations that are developed from the normal matrix composition during OA and OA with glucosamine-sulphate treatment in contributing to disease progression.

2. Conceptual background

2.1 Pathology

Articular cartilage has been the focus of research into OA for decades and the literature is extensive. The role of the chondrocytes has been reviewed [Hunziker, 2002], and some key features are also briefly summarized. The mechanical properties of cartilage, including viscoelasticity and high resistance against load and shear stress, are controlled through the metabolic balance within the matrix collagen-proteoglycan network. Water is the main composite (60–80%) of the extracellular matrix [Armstrong & Mow, 1982; Mankin & Thrasher, 1975; Sandell & Hering, 2001]. Proteoglycans induce a high osmotic pressure and have a high water binding capacity. Between 5 and 10% of the cartilage mass are proteoglycans, mostly aggrecan [Eyre, 2002]. Collagen (90% collagen type II) is responsible for the high resistance against tensional forces. Collagen type II contributes to up to 60% of the dry weight [Mayne, 1989]. During inflammation or slow degeneration, the homeostasis within the collagen-proteoglycan network in the chondral matrix is disordered [Sandell & Hering, 2001].

Theoretical and computational analyses of the contact response of cartilage under various loading conditions have predicted that more than 90% of the load transmitted across articular layers is supported by the pressurized interstitial fluid, with the remnant contributed by the collagen-proteoglycan solid matrix. Since the pressure of this fluid is a hydrostatic stress, and since cartilage has been shown to be nearly incompressible at physiological levels of pressures, it has become evident that the interstitial fluid shields the solid matrix from excessive deformations [Park et al., 2003; Soltz & Ateshian, 1998].

2.2 Thermal analysis

Thermal analysis comprises a group of techniques in which a physical property of a substance measured as a function of temperature, while the substance is subjected to a controlled temperature programme. Differential scanning calorimetry (DSC) and thermogravimetric (TG) analysis have been widely used for determining physicochemical transformations that occur during thermal degradation [Bihari-Varga 1982; Collett & Brown, 1998]. These techniques measure net changes in enthalpy and weight as a result of many reactions taking place simultaneously and are particularly useful for indicating the temperature range and the rate of thermal processes as well as giving considerable information on physical and chemical changes [O'Neill, 1964; Richardson, 1997]. Not many papers have been published on the thermal properties of human hyaline cartilage.

Understanding the response of drugs and their formulations to thermal stresses is an integral part of the development of stable medicinal products. Thermal analytical methods have thus become important tools for the development of modern medicines. These are precise and accurate techniques with low sample requirements, and can provide detailed information about new chemical entities even at the very earliest stages of drug discovery and development [Clas et al., 1999].

2.2.1 Thermogravimetry

Thermogravimetric analysis (TGA) is an analytical technique used to determine a material's thermal stability and its fraction of volatile components by monitoring the weight change that occurs as a specimen is heated [Gill, 1992]. The measurement is normally carried out in air or in an inert atmosphere, such as Argon, and the mass is recorded as a function of increasing temperature. Sometimes, the measurement is performed in a lean oxygen atmosphere (1 to 5% O_2 in N_2 or He) to slow down oxidation. In addition to mass changes, some instruments also record the temperature difference between the specimen and one or more reference pans (differential thermal analysis, or DTA) or the heat flow into the specimen pan compared to that of the reference pan (differential scanning calorimetry, or DSC). The latter can be used to monitor the energy released or absorbed via chemical reactions during the heating process.

In most cases, TG analysis is performed in an oxidative atmosphere (air or oxygen and inert gas mixtures) with a linear temperature ramp. The maximum temperature is selected so that the specimen mass is stable at the end of the experiment, implying that all chemical reactions are completed (i.e., all of the carbon is burnt off leaving behind metal oxides). This approach provides two important numerical informations: ash content (residual mass, M_{res}) and oxidation temperature (T_o). While the definition of ash content is unambiguous, oxidation temperature can be defined in many ways, including the temperature of the maximum in the weight loss rate (dm/dT_{max}) and the weight loss onset temperature (T_{onset}). The former refers to the temperature of the maximum rate of oxidation, while the latter refers to the temperature when oxidation just begins. The ability of TG to generate fundamental quantitative data from almost any class of materials, has led to its widespread use in every field of science and technology [Riesen, 1998; Rouquerol, 1989].

2.2.2 Calorimetry

Differential scanning calorimetry (DSC) is a thermoanalytical technique for measuring the energy necessary to establish a nearly zero temperature difference between a substance and an inert reference material, as the two specimens are subjected to identical temperature regimes in an environment heated or cooled at a controlled rate. In heat-flux DSC, the sample and reference are connected by a low-resistance heat-flow path (a metal disc). The assembly is enclosed in a single furnace (Fig. 1).

Enthalpy or heat capacity changes in the sample cause a difference in its temperature relative to the reference; the resulting heat flow is small as compared to that of in differential thermal analysis (DTA) because the sample and reference are in good thermal contact. The temperature difference is recorded and related to enthalpy change in the sample using calibration experiments [O'Neill, 1964].

DSC is a frequently preferred thermal analytical technique because of its ability to provide detailed information about both the physical and energetic properties of a substance. This information cannot be obtained accurately, easily, or quickly using any other technique. With the development of sophisticated, modulated temperature programs, it is likely that DSC will retain its place at the forefront of the pharmaceutical thermal analytical sciences for some time to come [Clas et al., 1999].

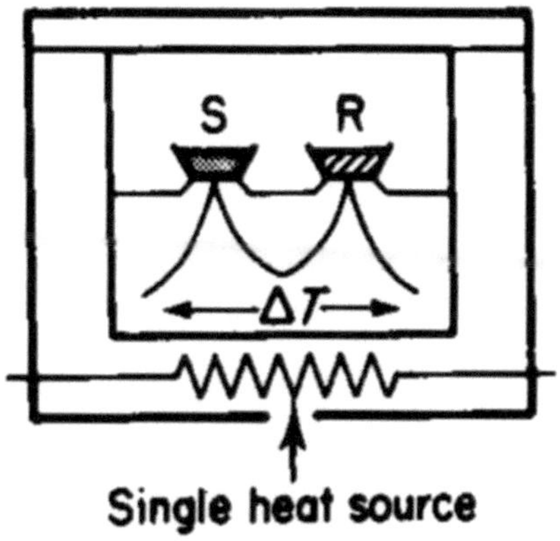

Fig. 1. Heat flux DSC (S: substance, R: reference material)

Calorimetry can be used to determine most thermodynamic properties; e.g. enthalpy changes for reactions (ΔH) or phase changes. Calorimetry can also be used for qualitative and quantitative analyses. ΔH can often be determined for an unknown reaction in a complex system, and the value of ΔH can then be used to assist in identifying the reaction [Jones, 1997]. Since calorimetry directly measures the instantaneous rate of the process, calorimetry is a particularly advantageous method for determination of the kinetics of slow processes. Calorimetric parameters provide a description of the system as a function of the experimental variables. Calorimetric data can also be used to gain fundamental insight into a process or property of a material [Hansen & Russell, 2006].

2.3 Thermal analysis of biological systems

Biological samples are often expensive and scarce due to the difficulty of their isolation and purification [Collett & Brown, 1998; Privalovand & Plotnikov, 1989]. The biological system represents an aqueous environment and the water present in the specimen limits the amount of sample that can be investigated, when studying the bulk properties of a sample. Analysis of the conformational and structural changes of molecules requires the solutions to be sufficiently dilute so that the inter-molecular contributions can be ignored. Advantages of thermal analysis in biological studies: the thermal behavior of tissues, as opposed to tissue components, can be readily studied by thermal analysis. No preparation procedures are required and so the basic molecular structures can be preserved for the analysis [Burroughs et al., 1980]. Initially, thermal transitions were only used to gain insight into the structures of compounds, but subsequently, applications have also been extended to give physiological data [Collett & Brown, 1998; Melchior & Steim, 1976]. These interactions are probably best studied by thermodynamic methods. Of all the thermal analysis techniques applied to biological samples, DSC and TGA are the most commonly used. These applications of thermal analysis to the study of biological systems have obvious medical advantages [Melchior & Steim, 1976].

2.4 Thermal analysis of connective tissue

Connective tissue may be classified as a semifluid gel in order to explain its properties and functions. Thermal analysis of the material requires no preparation procedures. The material could thus be studied without complicated purification procedures which means that the basic molecular structure can be preserved [Bihari-Varga, 1982]. Bihari-Varga concluded that connective tissue, like other tissue, shows considerable changes as the body passes to older age, and that, it is affected by pathological conditions. The study revealed that both the amount of structurally bound water and the concentration of glycosaminoglycan's (GAG) decrease significantly with age in various types of connective tissues.

More than 35 years ago in Bihari-Varga's experiments [Bihari-Varga et al., 1975] complex thermoanalytical methods [Paulik et al., 1958] were applied to study various collagen-proteoglycan-glycoprotein complexes prepared from different connective tissues. Thermal analysis was successfully used in their investigations for the quantitative determination of polysaccharides, for the characterization of protein structure, and for the estimation of age-related [Simon et al., 1969] and pathological [Biró & Bihari-Varga, 1972] changes in proteoglycan- and collagen-containing biological tissues. The study was extended to investigate the effect of drugs on the osteoarthritic tissue [Farkas et al., 1974].

More recently, thermal stability and structure of cancellous bone mineral from the femoral head of patients with OA or osteoporosis (OP) was investigated by Mkukuma et al. [Mkukuma et al. 2005]. Thermogravimetric analysis was linked to mass spectrometry (MS) to investigate the thermal decomposition of the matrix and hence its mineral content. Thermal stability of the bone matrix or the mineral phase alone, was little altered by disease, though OA bone contained less mineral than OP or control normal bone [Mkukuma et al. 2005].

2.5 Cartilage water content

Simple collagen-water systems have been examined with nuclear magnetic resonance (NMR) spectroscopy. It was shown that water molecules exist either as bulk water or as interior hydration water molecules [Chae et al., 2009]. Water within collagen fibrils consists of molecules involved in both inter- and intrahelical hydrogen bond formation. Based on a single endothermic DSC peak in cartilage, Bagratashvili et al. [Bagratashvili et al. 1997] found that the proportion of bound water in cartilage is around 4% using differential microcalorimetry and FTIR spectroscopy. Water diffusion through the tissue and from bound to free water transformation controlled water molecule liberation and adsorption. Alternating breakage and reformation of weak bonds between water molecules and proteoglycans directs movement of water in cartilage tissue. Both the extrafibrillar and most of the intrafibrillar water is freely exchangeable and behaves towards small solutes as available water has been independently shown by Katz and Li [Katz & Li, 1973] for other collagenous tissues. Furthermore Maroudas and Schneiderman have shown that the very major fraction of cartilage water is free, therefore the water in cartilage is completely exchangeable under a variety of experimental conditions [Maroudas & Schneiderman, 1987].

3. Experimental

3.1 Materials

3.1.1.1 Patients

In order to conduct the thermoanalytical study, 23 samples were collected from live surgeries of OA patients between October 2005 and April 2006. During hip arthroplasty procedures performed at the Orthopedic Department, University of Szeged, 16 OA human hyaline cartilage samples and normal cartilage from 7 knee were obtained. There was no clinical meaningful difference in age between OA patients (64 ± 5.2) and controls (61 ± 4.2). There were no considerable sex differences between OA patients (75% females) and controls (70% females); Chi-square P = 0.54.

Usually, total knee arthroplasty is performed in OA of both medial and lateral knee compartments. When only one compartment is affected and ligamental stability is intact, unicondylar prosthesis is implanted. We were able to obtain normal cartilage samples from those patients where one compartment of the same knee was degenerated, and the other one was normal. Therefore, the unaffected femoral condyle had to be sacrificed for the procedure because ligamental instability was the indication for total knee arthroplasty.

3.1.1.2 Patients grading

Preoperatively, the diagnosis of the patients were established on the basis of the patient history, clinical signs, laboratory tests, and radiological findings. The state of the hyaline cartilage was determined intraoperatively. All patients in the osteoarthritic group were considered to be 5-6 articular surface degeneration by Osteoarthritis Research Society International (OARSI) grade. OARSI Grade 5-6 OA is characterized by deformation and change in the contour of the articular surface [Pritzker et al., 2006]. This results not only from articular plate fractures, but also from increased metabolic activity of the articular bone plate, as well as from activation of connective tissue at the lateral and, sometimes, central cartilage/bone interfaces. Samples were considered to be normal when hyaline articular cartilage was uninvolved with OA (OARSI Grade 0). In these results, the cartilage surface is smooth, no enlargement, distortion, and no proliferative changes are observed.

3.1.1.3 Human sample preparation for thermal analysis

After the operation, a disc (5mm in diameter) was removed from the unhealthy and healthy cartilage surfaces. The samples were taken under sterile conditions, excess bone was removed, and only the remaining full thickness cartilage was used. The disc was first washed in sterile saline, then stored in 20 ml saline for transportation at room temperature. Mean storage time was 6 hours (min: 1 hour, max: 26 hour), 29 samples out of 35 were studied within four hours of preparation. Six samples were stored overnight at 5 °C. Preemptive control examinations did not show any change in the calorimetric and thermogravimetric properties after storage for 26 hours at 5 °C.

3.1.1.4 Animal model

Animal experiments were performed at the Physiology Department, Faculty of Medicine, University of Szeged. Adult male Wistar rats (Charles River strain; Bioplan, Budapest, Hungary), weighing 470±6 g were housed individually in ventilated cages on a 12-hour day/night cycle at a temperature of 22±1 °C. Water and food were provided ad libitum. The experiments were performed in accordance with the US National Institutes of Health Guidelines for the Care and Use of Laboratory Animals, and with the approval of the Animal Welfare Committee of the University of Szeged. Four groups of animals were defined as follows:

GA, non-osteoarthritic negative control rats injected with saline but pre-treated with oral glucosamine-sulphate;

Sham, non-osteoarthritic negative control rats injected with saline and not pre-treated with oral glucosamine-sulphate;
MIA, rats injected with monosodium iodioacetate and not pretreated with oral glucosamine-sulphate;
MIA+GA, rats injected with monosodium iodoacetate but pretreated with oral glucosamine-sulphate.

3.1.1.5 Compounds

Monosodium iodoacetate was obtained from Sigma-Aldrich Kft. Budapest and dissolved in 0.9% NaCl (Baxter) solution to get the required concentrations.
Glucosamine sulphate was supplied by Rottapharm S.p.A., Italy.

3.1.1.6 Induction of osteoarthritis

Animals were briefly anesthetized with an isoflurane/O2 gas mixture and the left knee was shaved and disinfected with 70% ethanol followed by povidone-iodide. Osteoarthritis was induced by the intraarticular injection of 50 µl of 40 mg/ml monosodium iodoacetate solution using a 300 µl syringe fitted with a 29 G needle, as described earlier [Guingamp et al., 1997]. The animals of the GA and Sham groups underwent the same procedure, but were injected with 50 µl of 0.9% NaCl solution.

3.1.1.7 Glucosamine-sulphate pre-treatment

Glucosamine sulphate solution dissolved in distilled water was administered to the rat through a cannula daily for 8 weeks through a gastric tube (500 mg/kg dose per day in 2 ml volume). The control group received the same volume of distilled water. The first administration was applied two weeks after the MIA injection.

3.1.1.8 Animal sample preparation

For sample preparation, the rats were anesthetized and a disc (2 mm in diameter) was removed from the unhealthy and healthy cartilage surfaces. The samples were taken under sterile conditions, excess bone and adipose tissue was removed, and only the remaining full thickness cartilage was used for the experiments. The disc was first washed in sterile saline, then stored in 20 ml saline for transportation at room temperature for immediate examination. Before the measurements, all water from the surface was removed. Mean storage time was 4 hours (min: 1 hour, max: 12 hours), all samples were examined the same day of preparation. Preemptive control examinations did not show any changes in the calorimetric properties after storage for 24 hours at 5 °C.

3.2 Thermal measurements

The success of the thermal experiments depends on the careful preparation of samples and the judicious selection of the appropriate experimental conditions (such as scanning rate and sample size). In general, DSC samples are analyzed in small metal pans, designed for optimal thermal conductivity and minimum reaction with the samples (for example, aluminum alloy, platinum, stainless steel, or silver) [Clas et al., 1999]. For accurate quantitative work, the thermal mass of the sample and reference pans were matched.
The calorimetric properties of samples were determined by DSC method (Mettler-Toledo DSC 821e apparatus, Mettler-Toledo GmbH, Switzerland). Samples were heated from 0 to 80 °C. The heating rate was 0.3 °C/min. Conventional Hastelloy batch vessels were used with

40 µl sample volume. All the DSC measurements were preceded in Ar atmosphere, and the flow rate was 100 ml/min. From the DSC curves, the decomposition temperature (onset temperature), the transition temperature range (endset temperature), and the total calorimetric enthalpy change were calculated. Well-defined standards and calibration procedures are particularly important, therefore high care was taken in calibrating the instrument as close to the transition temperatures of interest as possible.

The thermogravimetric analysis was performed with the use of a MOM Derivatograph (MOM, Budapest, Hungary), and the TG, DTG, and DTA curves were determined. The temperature (T) curve shows the linear increase of temperature during the process. DTG curve represents the first derivative of the mass change [Riesen, 1998; Rouquerol, 1989]. Heating was linear from 25 to 150 °C and the rate of heating was 5 °C/min. Al_2O_3 was used as reference material. In the first step, the total water loss and kinetic parameters were calculated. The kinetic parameters calculated by the derivatograph are the following: the reaction order (n), the activation energy (E_a), and the pre-exponential factor (A) [Arnold et al., 1987].

3.3 Statistics

SPSS for Windows statistical program was used to compare enthalpy changes in the different groups. Data are presented as mean, ±SD, ±SEM. Statistical significance was assessed by the unpaired two t-test and the level of confidence interval. The results were considered significant, if $p < 0.05$.

3.4 Ethics

All tissues were yielded in accordance to legal regulation, international ethical concerns, and patients' consent. The Human Investigation Review Board of the University of Szeged has decided (2006.09.18.) that the experiments comply with the ethics of research and the declaration of the Medical World Federation.

4. Results

4.1. Human hyaline cartilage study

4.1.1 Thermogravimetry

TG, DTG and DTA curves of the normal samples are presented on Fig. 2. Many information can be obtained from the T, TG, DTG and DTA curves. The temperature (T) curve shows the linear increase of temperature during the process.

It was found, that the average total water content of intact (normal) cartilage is 81%, which was probably the interstitial water. To remove the cartilage extracellular water content, 52 kJ/M energy was needed.

Total water content of the OA samples was 87%, and 73 kJ/M energy was used for the removal of the fluid content (Table 1 and Fig. 3).

Loss of water content in both groups are presented with a sharp step on the TG curve, starting on average temperature of 37 °C and ending at 116 °C. Linear part of the TG curve begun at around 57 °C and ended at around 104 °C (Table 1). Placing a line on this portion of the curve, the slope of the curve can be calculated which represents the speed of the water content loss (Table 2). The slope of the linear region correlated in both groups.

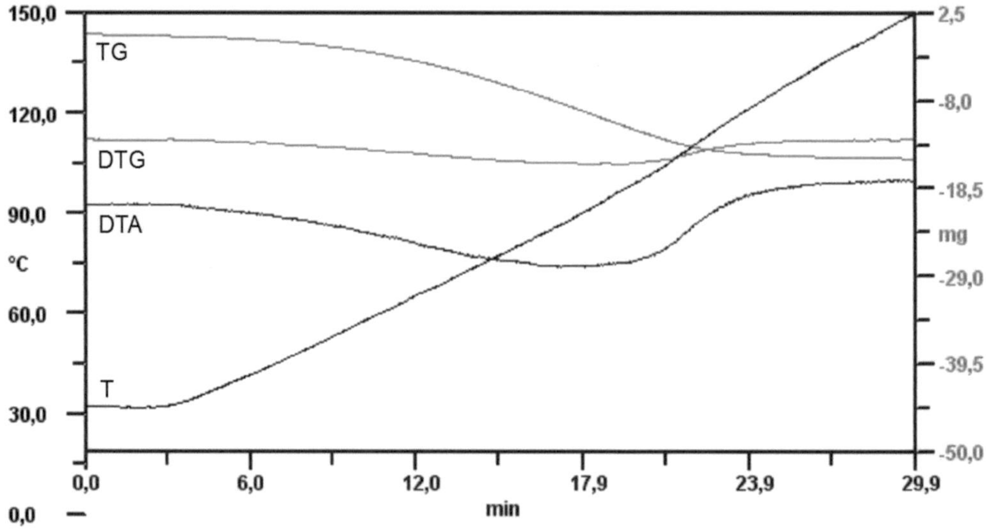

Fig. 2. Thermogravimetric curves of a normal sample

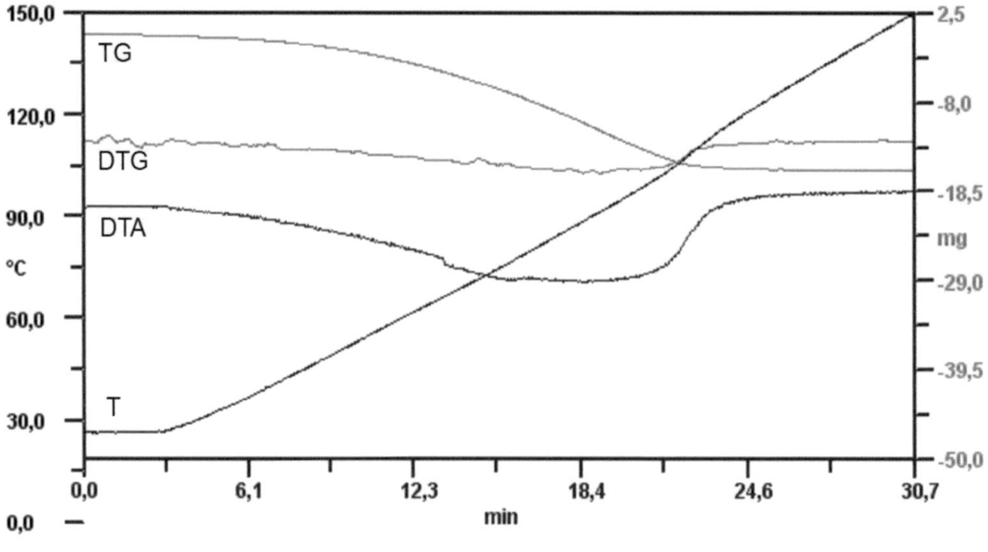

Fig. 3. Thermogravimetric curves of an osteoarthritic sample

Sample group	Sample number	TG step (°C)	Total mass loss (%) (p=0.05)	E_{act} (kJ M-1)
Normal	7	39.1-113.8	80.79 SD: 7.09	52.33 SD: 6.68
OA	16	36.4-121.9	86.71 SD: 7.84	72.72 SD: 23.46

Table 1. Average mass loss and activation energy of normal and degenerated samples.

In case of the normal hyaline cartilage, 0.196 mg of fluid content release was observed (average mass of the normal samples was 15.48 mg) with increase of temperature by 1 °C, therefore 1.3% $°C^{-1}$ loss was detected. In the osteoarthritic samples (average mass: 17.02 mg), 0.242 mg decrease was measured which represents 1.4% $°C^{-1}$ mass reduction. The resulting amount of mass lost in the linear region was recounted from these results (Table 2).

Sample Group	Sample number	TG step linear region (°C)	Mass loss (%)	Reaction order (n)	Slope of linear region
Normal	7	62.67-102.25	-51.45	1 SD: 0.203	-0.039
OA	16	58.0-104.6	-65.24	1.03 SD: 0.27	-0.048

Table 2. Reaction kinetic parameters of normal and degenerated samples.

4.1.2 Calorimetry

With the rise of temperature, an endothermic reaction was observed in all of the cases (Fig. 4). The enthalpy change of the process initiated by the temperature change showed noticeable difference between the normal and pathological groups. (Table 3)

Sample group	Sample number	ΔH (J/g) (-)	DSC peak (°C)	Beginning (°C)	Ending (°C)
Normal	7	788.346 SD: 83.181	50.18 SD: 3.31	≈32.5 SD: 3.45	57.09 SD: 5.35
OA	16	543.838 SD: 88.572	50.34 SD: 2.937	≈33.8 SD: 4.3	≈33.8 SD: 4.3

Table 3. Thermal parameters of denaturation (mean ±SD) of normal and degenerated samples.

Greater change in the enthalpy was observed in normal cartilage: 788.346 J/g (SD = 83.18). In case of osteoarthritis 543.838 J/g (SD = 88.57) was measured (Table 3). Therefore, denaturation caused by heating was larger in the normal human hyaline cartilage. Consequently these samples required the largest amount of energy for decomposition. Statistical tests proved these calculations to be significant (Fisher LSD method, $p<0.05$). Denaturation peak in normal cartilage was at 50.18 °C (SD = 3.31), and it was similar in osteoarthritis 50.34 °C (SD = 2.93). to that of the control results (Fig. 4).

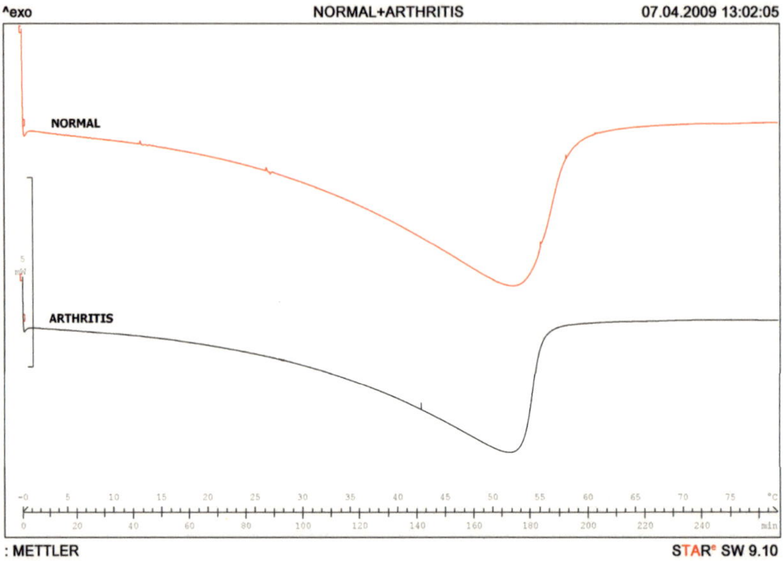

Fig. 4. DSC curve of normal and osteoarthritic human hyaline cartilage samples, the average change in the enthalpy in normal cartilage: 788.346 J/g (SD = 83.18) and OA 543.838 J/g (SD = 88.57) respectively. (The downwards deflection means endothermic effect)

4.2 Animal model

With the rise of temperature an endothermic reaction was observed in all of the cases (Figure 5).

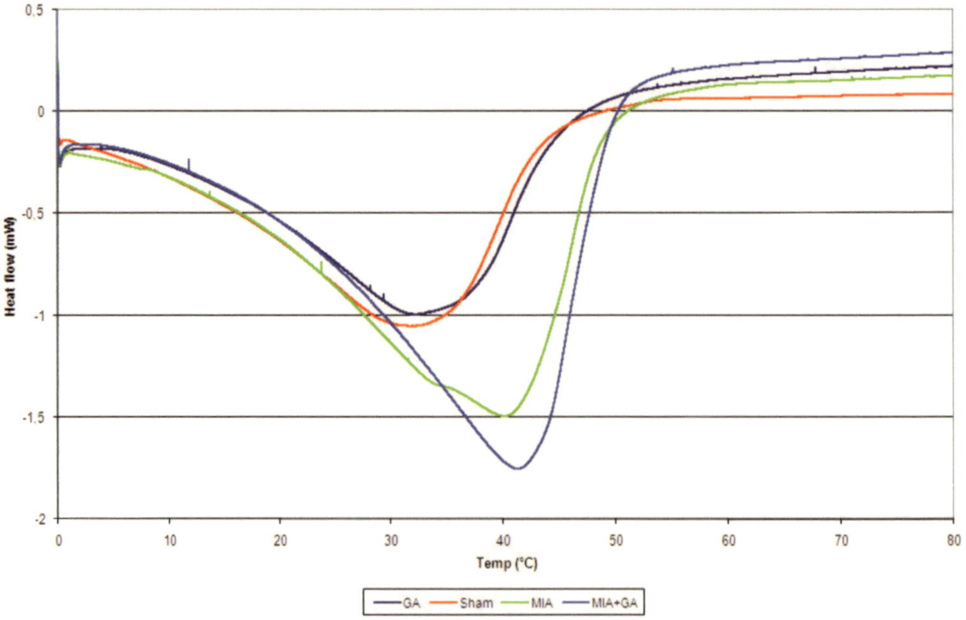

Fig. 5. DSC curve of cartilage samples. (the downwards deflection means endothermic effect)

The enthalpy change of the process initiated by the temperature change did show marked difference between the normal and pathological groups (Table 4).

Sample group	Sample Number	ΔH (kJ/kg)
Sham	7	-783.65 SD: 63.44 SEM: 23.98
GA	8	-848.86 SD: 177.53 SEM: 62.77
MIA	8	-1150.19 SD: 137.63 SEM: 48.66
MIA+GA	7	-1402.92 SD: 90.74 SEM: 34.29

Table 4. Thermal parameters (mean, ±SD, ±SEM) of all samples

Change in enthalpy was observed in normal cartilage at -783.65 kJ/kg (SD = 63.44), and in case of pre-treatment with Glucosamine-sulphate, a slight increase was seen at -848.86 kJ/kg (SD = 177.53). In the non-treated OA samples (MIA), the change of enthalpy was -1150.19 kJ/kg (SD = 137.63). Further increase of the thermal parameters was measured in the OA group that was pre-treated with Glucosamine-sulphate (MIA+GA) -1402.92 kJ/kg (SD = 90.74). Therefore, enthalpy change caused by the loss of water content by heating was lower in the normal samples than in the OA sample groups.

The ΔH mean value of the normal samples statistically did not differ significantly from the treated normal group ($p=0.3752$). On the other hand, statistically extremely significant difference ($p<0.0001$) was observed when the calorimetric properties of the normal non-treated hyaline samples were evaluated against either the MIA or the MIA+GA groups. (Table 5) Furthermore, even the low end of the confidence interval represents a difference large enough to be considered biologically important.

Compared groups	95% confidence interval (from-to)	two-tailed P value
Sham/MIA	-489.3105 to -243.7645	< 0.0001
Sham/MIA+GA	-710.4533 to -528.0925	<0.0001
MIA/MIA+GA	-385.0286 to -120.4421	0.0012

Table 5. Statistical parameters

Further analysis showed additional statistically significant ($p<0.0012$) increase in the mean value of the enthalpy change of the non-treated OA group to the treated OA groups. But the size of the confidence interval range difference is inconclusive (Table 5).

5. Conclusion

OA development takes place in consecutive steps of breakdown and attempted regeneration. Though the comprehension about OA has grown enormously over the last years, there is still need to extend our knowledge about the basic context of OA genesis and development. Several biochemical and biomechanical factors are considered for the pathogenesis [Abramson & Attur, 2009]. The data up to date show, however, that OA is a very complex disease procedure, and it can be speculated, that the context leading to the progressive process is not finally resolved. There might still be molecules involved which have not yet been studied or even identified [Kumar et al., 2001].

OA is widely believed to result from local mechanical factors acting within the context of systemic susceptibility [Goldring & Goldring, 2007]. Molecular pathology of osteoarthritis is under intense investigation since biomechanical factors result in chemical alteration within the joint. Rearrangements of intra- and intermolecular bonds in collagen molecule and disaggregation of proteoglycans and their elimination from OA cartilage found to be responsible for water accumulation [Loeuille et al., 2002]. It was also shown that the most part of water is free water and its quantity is increased in the osteoarthritis of the hyaline cartilage [Nikolaeva et al., 2000].

We observed increase in water content of the cartilage matrix in all cases of the investigated degenerative cartilages [Sohár et al., 2007]. Based on our results, it can be stated that water content is higher in impaired samples, meanwhile water interstitial bonding was stronger in these cases. Rise in water adherence was well distinguishable since higher energy was needed for removal. Activation energy correlated considerably with water content in the samples. Denaturation caused by heating was larger in the normal cartilage than in the diseased ones, therefore normal samples required larger amount of energy for decomposition [Tóth et al., 2007].

The purpose of our study was also to clarify the previously reported studies in the literature [Than & Kereskai, 2005]. By acquiring normal cartilage from live surgery and by performing the investigation in a relatively short period of time compared to the earlier reports [Sohár et al., 2007; Than et al., 2004; Than & Kereskai, 2005], similar sample environment was provided as with the degenerarative samples. This way, we minimized the extracorpal degeneration. All samples we used showed a clear denaturation peak on the calorimetric curve, therefore volume of the curve was easily calculated giving the enthalpy change of the sample. These changes correlated with the water content of the samples. Due to the increased number of samples acquired for our studies, the results were much better reproducible than results in the literature, and the difference between the normal and diseased samples was significant [Sohár et al., 2007; Tóth et al., 2007].

The newly established thermogravimetric protocol that we used was sufficient for compositional thermoanalytical study of normal and degenerative human hyaline cartilage. Water content elevation contributing to disease progression was observed in OA. Previously, this method has not been used for this type of investigations. The main goal of the thermogravimetric measurements was to identify the nature and quantity of water molecules in the investigated samples. Water molecules' binding mode may have an important consequence in pharmacokinetics. The reaction order turned out to be approximately 1 in all the cases (normal and OA), and the standard deviation was low (Table 2). The TG curve's slope of the linear region showed, that the rate of water loss depends on the water amount remaining in the tissue. Comparing the data in the presented tables (Tables 1, 2) (Total mass loss: normal: 80.79% and OA: 86.71%), it can be concluded that the higher water content in the degenerative samples bound stronger to the matrix. However, the reaction order and the slope of the linear region correlated in both groups. This first order kinetic means that the rate of water loss depends on the water amount remaining in the tissue, namely if the amount of water decreases in the tissue, the rate of loss also decreases.

DSC as part of thermal analysis was a reliable method for differentiating normal hyaline cartilage from degenerated samples. The available calorimeter proved to be adequate for these measurements. DSC techniques are still developing and many new variants and applications are reported each year. Combined techniques [Elder, 1994] with microscopic or spectroscopic instruments are of obvious value to the pharmaceutical scientist, although commercially available units are not widely used and have limited pharmaceutical applications. With the rapid development of atomic and molecular scale microscopy, hyphenated micro-thermal analysis techniques, such as atomic force microscopy-DSC, are also becoming commercially available. There may be many future applications of micro-DSC measurements to pharmaceutical problems, although these are likely to be limited to basic research applications in the next few years until the full potential of the technique has been demonstrated.

Our study has had several limitations, as many other studies on OA. First, the sample size was not large enough to arrive at definitive conclusions. Additional measurements are needed to affirm the results of our study. Secondly, we investigated those patients for normal cartilage samples of the knee, who underwent surgery for the other compartment OA. This was the only ethical and technical way of acquiring normal tissues from living persons for our experiments. Previous thermoanalytical studies used cadaver samples for the investigation as normal human hyaline cartilage. All samples that were extracted for our studies were obtained during live surgeries and were macroscopically intact [Sohár et al., 2007; Tóth et al., 2007]. There is no previous report in the literature of examining normal cartilage from live surgery. Only full thickness cartilage was used for the normal analysis. A new protocol had to be established before the detailed investigation of human tissues could be performed. Most of the known changes in the extracellular matrix in OA come from animal models in the literature since human samples for investigation are not widely available for experiments.

The promise of biomarkers has yet to be fulfilled in OA. Although numerous clinical studies have suggested that specific biomarkers or their combinations can have predictive value in terms of the presence and severity of the disease [Poole, 2003]. The wide variability in these values limits their use for individual patients. Whereas, the use of thermal analysis could be a simple and effective method for controlling the relationship between these markers and disease progression. The revised protocol for sample taking during live surgeries eliminates the presence of disturbing substances during the examination.

Characterization of the altered metabolism in cartilage that promotes disease progression should lead to future treatment options that can prevent structural damage. Since damaged articular cartilage has a very limited potential for healing, prevention is fundamental in treatment. However, prevention is not possible without the knowledge of the basic pathomorphological mechanism leading to cartilage degeneration. With better understanding of the exact amount of water in matrix and its binding characteristics, preventive measures can be developed. These therapeutic steps can be adequately tested and monitored with thermal measurements. The use of these methods can also determine the effectiveness of currently used medications (Glucosamin, Chondroitin) for resolving cartilage matrix degeneration.

The results of the experimental OA calorimetric examinations showed that physicochemical properties of normal samples are clearly statistically different from the MIA induced OA groups (treated and non-treated alike). This inequality even at the low end of the 95% confidence interval represents a difference large enough to be considered biologically important. Therefore, it can be concluded that there is a difference between treatment means and that the variation is large enough to be scientifically relevant. Interestingly the rats injected with monosodium iodoacetate and pretreated with oral glucosamine-sulphate showed significantly higher increase in the value of the enthalpy change than the non-treated, but OA induced cartilage samples. However, at 95% confidence interval range (from -385.0286 to -120.4421) a strong conclusion can not be drawn. Therefore more data needs to be obtained to draw a clear conclusion.

Further understanding of the initiating events in cartilage destruction, the relationship between the different pathologic influences, and the role of the chondrocyte in maintaining extracellular matrix homeostasis is necessary to reveal potential targets of therapy. Clinical trials are currently underway for a number of potential disease modifying agents that may significantly change the treatment approach for OA. With the use of disease-modifying OA drugs (DMOADs), the necessity for instruments that are sensitive to changes has become very apparent in clinical trials [Qvista, 2008].

6. Acknowledgment

Study was supported by „TÁMOP-4.2.1/B-09/1/KONV-2010-0005 - Creating the Center of Excellence at the University of Szeged" is supported by the European Union and co-financed by the European Regional Development Fund.

We would like to thank the orthopedic surgeon colleagues of the Orthopedic Department, University of Szeged for their gracious support in providing samples for our study from their arthroplasty procedures. We acknowledge laboratory assistants of the Department of Pharmaceutical Technology and the Department of Physiology, University of Szeged for technical assistance.

7. References

Abramson, S.B. & Attur, M. (2009). Developments in the scientific understanding of osteoarthritis. *Arthritis Research & Therapy*, 11(3): 227.

Aigner, Z.; Mécs, L.; Sohár, G.; Wellinger, K.; Szabó-Révész, P. & Tóth, K. (2009). Novel calorimetric investigation of different degenerative disorders of the human hyaline cartilage. *J. Thermal Anal. and Calorim.*, 95(3), 801-804.

Ameye, L.G. & Young, M.F. (2006). Animal models of osteoarthritis: lessons learned while seeking the "Holy Grail". *Current Opinion in Rheumatology*, 18 (5), pp. 537–547.

Armstrong, C.G. & Mow, V.C. (1982). Variations in the intrinsic mechanical properties of human articular cartilage with age, degeneration, and water content. *J. Bone Joint. Surg. Am.*, 64: 88-94.

Arnold, M.; Somogyvári, P.; Paulik, J. & Paulik, F. (1987). Derivatograph-C-a microcomputer-controlled simultaneous TG, DTG, DTA, TD and EGA apparatus. *J. Therm. Anal.*, 32: 679-683.

Bagratashvili, V.; Sobol, E.; Sviridov, A.; Popov, V.; Omel'chenko A. & Howdle, S. (1997). Thermal and diffusion processes in laser-induced stress relaxation and reshaping cartilage. *J. Biomech.*, 30:813-817.

Bihari-Varga, M. Sepulchre, C. & Moczár, E. (1975). Thermoanalytical studies on protein-polysaccharide complexes of connective tissues. *Journal of Thermal Analysis*, 7:675-683.

Bihari-Varga, M. (1982). The application of thermoanalytical methods in the investigation of biological substances. *J. Therm. Anal.*, 23:7-13.

Biró, T. & Bihari-Varga, M. (1972). Thermoanalytical Studies of Tendon Healing. *Connective Tissue Res.*, 1:305-309.

Brandt, K.D.; Radin, E.L.; Dieppe, P.A. & van de Putte, L. (2006). Yet more evidence that osteoarthritis is not a cartilage disease. *Ann. Rheum. Dis.*, 65, 1261-1264.

Burroughs, P.; Paterson, E. & Pope, M.I. (1980). Purity determination by differential scanning calorimetry. *Anal. Proc.*, 17: 231-234.

Chae, Y.; Protsenko, D.; Lavernia, E.J. & Wong, B.J.F. (2009). Effect of water content on enthalpic relaxations in porcine septal cartilage. *J. Thermal Anal. and Calorim.*, 95(3): 937-943.

Clas, S.D.; Dalton, C.R. & Hancock, B.C. (1999). Differential scanning calorimetry: applications in drug development. *Pharm. Sci. Techn. Today*, 2: 311-320.

Clegg, D.O.; Reda, D.J.; Harris, C.L.; Klein, M.A.; O'Dell, J.R.; Hooper, M.M.; Bradley, J.D.; Bingham, C.O. 3rd; Weisman, M.H.; Jackson, C.G.; Lane, N.E.; Cush, J.J.; Moreland, L.W.; Schumacher, H.R. Jr.; Oddis, C.V.; Wolfe, F.; Molitor, J.A.; Yocum, D.E.; Schnitzer, T.J.; Furst, D.E.; Sawitzke, A.D.; Shi, H.; Brandt, K.D.; Moskowitz, R.W. & Williams, H.J. (2006). Glucosamine, chondroitin sulfate, and the two in combination for painful knee osteoarthritis. *N Engl J Med.*, 23;354(8), 795-808.

Collett, L.A.; Brown, M.E. (1998). Biochemical and biological applications of thermal analysis. *J. Therm. Anal.*, 51, 693-726.

Crolle, G. (1980). Glucosamine sulphate for the management of arthrosis: a controlled clinical investigation. *D'Este E Curr Med Res Opin.*, 7(2), 104-9.

Elder, J.P. (1994). Thermophysical characterization studies of pharmaceutical hydrates. *Thermochim. Acta*,234: 153-164.

Eyre, D. (2002). Collagen of articular cartilage. *Arthritis Res.*, 4: 30-35.

Farkas, T. & Bihari-Varga, M. & Biró, T. (1974). Thermoanalytical and histological study of intra-articular papain-induced degradation and repair of rabbit cartilage. I. Immature animals. *Ann Rheum Dis.*, 33:385-390.

Fenton, J.I.; Chlebek-Brown, K.A.; Peters, T.L.; Caron, J.P. & Orth, M.W. (2000). Glucosamine HCl reduces equine articular cartilage degradation in explant culture. *Osteoarthritis Cartilage*, 8(4), 258-65.

Gill, P.S., Sauerbrunn, S.R. & Crowe, B.S. (1992). High resolution thermogravimetry. *J. Therm. Anal.*, 38: 255-266.

Goldring, M.B. & Goldring, S.R. (2007). Osteoarthritis. *J. Cell. Physiol.*, 213, 626-634.

Guingamp, C.; Gegout-Pottie, P.; Philippe, L.; Terlain, B.; Netter, P. & Gillet, P. (1997). Mono-iodoacetate-induced experimental osteoarthritis: a dose-response study of loss of mobility, morphology, and biochemistry. Arthritis Rheum., 40(9): 1670-9.

Hansen, L.D. & Russell, D.J. (2006). Which calorimeter is best? A guide for choosing the best calorimeter for a given task. *Thermochim. Acta,* 450: 71-72.

Hunziker, E. B. (2002). Articular cartilage repair: basic science and clinical progress. A review of the current status and prospects. *Osteoarthritis and Cartilage,* 10(6), 432-63.

Janusz, M.J.; Hookfin, E.B.; Heitmeyer, S.A.; Woessner, J.F.; Freemont, A.J. & Hoyland, J.A. (2001). Moderation of iodoacetate-induced experimental osteoarthritis in rats by matrix metalloproteinase inhibitors. *Osteoarthritis and Cartililage,* 9, 751–60.

Jones, K.J. (1997). The origin and interpretation of the signals of MTDSC. *Thermochim. Acta,* 304/305: 187-199.

Kalbhen, D.A. (1987). Chemical model of osteoarthritis—a pharmacological evaluation. *Rheumatology,* 14, 130–1.

Katz, E.P. & Li, S.T. (1973). The intermolecular space of reconstituted collagen fibrils. *J. Mol. Biol.,* 73:351-369.

Kumar, S.; Connor, J.R.; Dodds, R.A.; Halsey, W.; Van Horn, M.; Mao, J.; Sathe, G.; Mui, P.; Agarwal, P.; Badger, A.M.; Lee, J.C.; Gowen, M. & Lark, M.W. (2001). Identification and initial characterization of 5000 expressed sequenced tags (ESTs) each from adult human normal and osteoarthritic cartilage cDNA libraries. *Osteoarthritis and Cartilage,* 9: 641-653.

Loeuille, D.; Olivier, P.; Watrin, A.; Grossin, L.; Gonord, P.; Guillot, G.; Etienne, S.; Blum, A.; Netter, P. & Gillet, P. (2002). Some biochemical characteristics and water exchange in human articular cartilage in osteoarthrosis. *Bull. Exp. Biol. Med.,* 133, 484-487.

Lorenz, H.; Wenz, W.; Ivancic, M.; Steck, E. & Richter, W. (2005). Early and stable upregulation of collagen type II, collagen type I and YKL40 expression levels in cartilage during early experimental osteoarthritis occurs independent of joint location and histological grading. *Arthritis Res. Ther.,* 7(1), R156-165.

Mankin, H.J. & Thrasher, A.Z. (1975) Water content and binding in normal and osteoarthritic human cartilage. *J. Bone Joint. Surg. Am.,* 57: 76-80.

Maroudas, A. & Schneiderman, R. (1987). "Free" and "Exchangeable" or "Trapped" and "Non-exchangeable" Water in Cartilage. *J. of Orthop. Res.,* 5:133-138.

Mayne, R. (1989). Cartilage collagens. What is their function, and are they involved in articular disease? *Arthritis Rheum.,* 32: 241-246.

McAlindon, T. (2003). Why are clinical trials of glucosamine no longer uniformly positive? *Rheum Dis Clin N Am,* 29 789–801.

Mécs, L.; Aigner, Z.; Sohár, G.; Szabó-Révész, P. & Tóth, K. (2009). Characterization of human cartilage in degenerated spine disease with differntial scanning calorimetry. *J. Thermal Anal. and Calorim.,* 95(3), 809–811.

Melchior, D.L. & Steim, J.M. (1976). Thermotropic Transitions in Biomembranes *Ann. Rev. Biophys. Bioeng.,* 5:205-238.

Mkukuma, L.D.; Imrie, C.T.; Skakle, J.M.S.; Hukins, D.W.L. & Aspden, R.M. (2005). Thermal stability and structure of cancellous bone mineral from the femoral head of patients with Osteoarthritis or osteoporosis. *Ann Rheum Dis.,* 64:222-225.

Nikolaeva, S.S.; Chkhol, K.Z.; Bykov, V.A.; Roshchina, A.A.; Iakovleva, L.V.; Koroleva, O.A.; Omel'ianenko, N.P. & Rebrov, L.B. (2000). Water-exchange processes in hyaline cartilage and its basic components in a normal state and in osteoarthritis. *Vopr. Med. Khim.*, 6, 81-90.

Oegema, Jr.; Deloria, L.B.; Sandy, J.D. & Hart, D.A. (2002). Effect of oral glucosamine on cartilage and meniscus in normal and chymopapain-injected knees of young rabbits. *Arthritis & Rheumatism*, 46 (9), pp. 2495–2503.

O'Neill, M.J. (1964). The analysis of a temperature-controlled scanning calorimeter. *Anal. Chem.*, 36: 1238-1245.

Park, S.; Krishnan, R.; Nicoll, S.B. & Ateshian, G.A. (2003). Cartilage interstitial fluid load support in unconfined compression. *J. Biomechanics*,36: 1785–1796.

Paulik, F.; Paulik, J. & Erdey, L. (1958). Der Derivatograph - I. Mitteilung Ein automatisch registrierender Apparat zur gleichzeitigen Ausführung der Differentialthermoanalyse, der thermogravimetrischen und der derivativ-thermogravimetrischen Untersuchungen. *Fresenius' Zeitschrift für Analytische Chemie.*, 160:241-252.

Poole, A. (2003). Biochemical/immunochemical biomarkers of osteoarthritis: utility for prediction of incident or progressive osteoarthritis. *Rheumatic Disease Clinics of North America*, 29: 803-818.

Pritzker, K.P.H.; Gay, S.; Jimenez, S.A.; Ostergaard, K.; Pelletier, J.P.; Revell, P.A.; Salter, D. & van den Berg, W.B. (2006). Osteoarthritis cartilage histopathology: grading and staging. *Osteoarthritis and Cartilage*, 14: 13-29.

Privalovand, P.L.& Plotnikov, V.V. (1989). Three generations of scanning microcalorimeters for liquids. *Thermochim. Acta.*, 139:257-277.

Qvista, P.; Bay-Jensena, A.C.; Christiansena, C.; Erik, B.D.; Pastoureaub, P. & Morten, A.K. (2008). The disease modifying osteoarthritis drug (DMOAD): Is it in the horizon? *Pharm. Res.*, 58, 1-7.

Reginster, J.Y. (2001). Long-term effects of glucosamine sulphate on osteoarthritis progression: a randomised, placebo-controlled clinical trial. *The Lancet*, 357, 251-256.

Richardson, M.J. (1997). Quantitative aspects of differential scanning calorimetry. *Thermochim. Acta*, 300: 15-28.

Riesen, R. (1998). Adjustment of heating rate for maximum resolution in TG and TMA (MaxRes). *J. Therm. Anal.* 53: 365-374.

Rouquerol, J. (1989). Controlled transformation rate thermal analysis: The hidden face of thermal analysis. *Thermochim. Acta*, 144: 209-224.

Sandell, L.J. & Hering, T.M. (2001) Biochemistry and molecular and cell biology of articular cartilage in osteoarthritis. In: *Osteoarthritis. Diagnosis and medical/surgical management*, Moskowitz, R.W.; Howell, D.S.; Altman, R.D. Buckwalter, J.A. Goldberg, V.M. pp. 115-143, WB Sauders Company, Philadelphia.

Simon, J.; Bihari-Varga, M.; Erdey, L. & Gerő, S. (1969). Thermal investigations on structural glycosaminoglycans and proteins. 1. The influence of age on the thermal decomposition of aortic intima. *Acta Biochim. Biophys. Acad. Sci. Hung.*, 3:273-278.

Sohár, G.; Pallagi, E.; Szabó-Révész, P. & Tóth, K. (2007). New thermogravimetric protocol for the investigation of normal and damaged human hyaline cartilage. *J. Therm. Anal. Cal.*, 89: 853-856.

Soltz, M.A. & Ateshian, G.A. (1998). Experimental verification and theoretical prediction of cartilage interstitial fluid pressurization at an impermeable contact interface in confined compression. *J. Biomechanics*, 31: 927-934.

Than, P.; Domán, I. & Lőrinczy, D. (2004). Differential scanning calorimetry in the research of degenerative musculoskeletal disorders. *Thermochim. Acta*, 415: 83-87.

Than, P. & Kereskai, L. (2005). Thermal analysis of the osteoarthritic human hyaline cartilage. *J. Therm. Anal. Cal.*, 82: 213-216.

Than, P.; Vermes, C.; Schäffer, B. & Lőrinczy, D. (2000). Differential scanning calorimetric examination of the human hyaline cartilage. A preliminary study. *Thermochim. Acta*, 346: 147-151.

Than, P. & Lőrinczy, D. (2003). Differential scanning calorimetric examination of the osteoarthritic hyaline cartilage in rabbits. *Thermochim. Acta*, 404, 149-153.

Tóth, K., Sohár, G., Pallagi, E. & Szabó-Révész, P. (2007). Further characterization of degenerated human cartilage with differential scanning calorimetry. *Thermochim. Acta*, 464: 75-77.

Tóth, K.; Sohár, G.; Aigner, Z.; Greksa, F. & Szabó-Révész, P. (2009). Novel Calorimetric properties of human cartilage samples in rheumatoid arthritis. *J. Thermal Anal. and Calorim.*, 95(3), 813-815.

van den Berg, W.B. (2001). Lessons from animal models of osteoarthritis. *Current Opinion in Rheumatology*, 13 (5), pp. 452–456.

Vlad, S.C.; LaValley, M.P.; McAlindon, T.E. & Felson, D.T. (2007) Glucosamine for pain in osteoarthritis: why do trial results differ? *Arthritis Rheum.*, 56(7), 2267-77. Review.

Wiegand, N.; Vámhidy, L.; Kereskai, L. & Lőrinczy, D. (2010). Differential scanning calorimetric examination of the ruptured Achilles tendon in human. *Thermochimica Acta*, 498. 7-10.

Wiegand, N.; Vámhidy, L.; Patczai, B.; Dömse, E.; Kereskai, L. & Lőrinczy, D. (2009). Differential scanning calorimetric examination of the human skeletal muscle in a compartment syndrome of the lower extremities. *J. Thermal Anal. Calorim.*, 98, 177-182.

Zhang, W.; Moskowitz, R.W.; Nuki, G.; Abramson, S.; Altman, R.D.; Arden, N.; Bierma-Zeinstra, S.; Brandt, K.D.; Croft, P.; Doherty, M.; Dougados, M.; Hochberg, M.; Hunter, D.J.; Kwoh, K.; Lohmander, L.S. & Tugwell, P. (2008). OARSI recommendations for the management of hip and knee osteoarthritis, Part II: OARSI evidence-based, expert consensus guidelines. *Osteoarthritis Cartilage*, 16(2), 137-62.

3

Topical and Regional Treatment for Osteoarthritis

Leena Patel[1] and Charles Mackworth-Young[2]
[1]*Department of Rheumatology, Whipps Cross University Hospital, London*
[2]*Department of Rheumatology, Charing Cross Hospital, London, UK*

1. Introduction

Osteoarthritis (OA) is the most common joint-related disorder. The prevalence rises steeply with age and is a major cause of pain and disability. In the over 65-year-old population, 12% suffer from symptomatic knee OA (1) while 13– 26 % suffer from symptomatic OA in at least one hand joint (2). Hip OA is much less common. The prevalence of radiographic change is much higher; in the elderly population 75% have evidence of hand OA and 30% of knee OA on plain radiographs (3).

The term "osteoarthritis" is used to refer to a number of related conditions that can be broadly classified into two groups. Primary OA, which can be localised or generalised and more commonly affects peri-menopausal woman (especially involving the hand inter-phalangeal joints); or secondary OA which has an underlying cause such as an inflammatory arthritis (e.g. rheumatoid arthritis or crystal arthritis), mechanical damage (e.g. articular fractures), a congenital or developmental disorder or a metabolic or endocrine condition (4). An osteoarthritic joint may show varying degrees of inflammatory change, detectable clinically and histologically. It is uncertain to what degree these (and other) subdivisions of OA are useful in terms of therapy.

This chapter addresses therapies for all forms of OA of limb joints. Much of the evidence that will be considered here does not distinguish between the various types, although where possible, efficacy in knee, hip and hand OA is described separately due to the differing natural history and prognosis of OA at these sites.

Treatments for OA are limited. They consist of a combination of non- pharmacological and pharmacological approaches, which should be tailored to the individual according to their needs and stage of disease. They aim to relieve pain and stiffness and thereby improve function. It is recognised that pain arises from both intra-articular structures (bone or synovial tissue) and from peri-articular structures such as entheses, bursae or tendons. Sensitisation of peripheral nerves and central nervous system changes can also contribute to the persistence of pain over time.

All patients should be offered education, advice and access to information in combination with physical approaches (e.g. strengthening exercises and physiotherapy, including aerobic fitness training) and lifestyle changes (e.g. weight reduction and dietary manipulation) as appropriate. Additional therapies include systemic drugs (e.g. analgesics, anti-inflammatory agents, supplements, and, recently, disease modifying treatment such as hydroxychloroquine) and surgery.

This chapter focuses on treatments that are administered to the joint itself, or in the region of the joint. Pain management techniques such as nerve block and transcutaneous electrical stimulation are beyond the scope of the article.

2. Specific therapies

2.1 Splinting/support

Orthoses (or braces) are external devices mainly prescribed to modulate mechanical stress on a symptomatic joint compartment. They are used in knee and hand OA but not in hip OA. For knee OA, they include rest orthoses, knee sleeves and unloading braces. For hand OA they include thumb and wrist splints. Insoles are used in hip and knee OA: they include cushioned or neutral insoles, which act as shock absorbers; and wedged insoles, which also modulate mechanical stress.

For lower limb OA, the main purpose of orthoses and insoles is to support an unstable joint and to help correct alignment (5). In doing so, they reduce pain, reduce load bearing and improve physical function. They can also improve proprioception (6) and possibly slow disease progression (7). They are particularly recommended in mild or moderate unicompartmental knee OA (8,9,10) where varying degrees of frontal or sagittal instability and varus or valgus mal-alignment occur, and ideally should be used in combination with other therapeutic approaches. The different interventions are described individually below.

1. **Rest orthoses** are made from a stiff composite and are intended for joint immobilization. They are rarely used in practice however, and there are no clinical trial data to suggest effectiveness. Whether they would be helpful in transiently immobilising a swollen knee remains uninvestigated (11).
2. **Knee sleeves** are functional elastic non-adhesive orthoses that can be used alone or in association with various devices and are aimed at patellar alignment or frontal femoro-tibial stabilisation. Simple neoprene knee sleeves used in medial compartment OA have been shown to reduce pain on activity and stiffness but not physical disability in the short term (6 months) when compared with no sleeve (12). This does not appear related to a local thermic effect. They have also been shown to increase static and dynamic balance, which might help prevent falls (13). Heat retaining sleeves (worn for 12 hours per day for 4 weeks) do not offer additional therapeutic benefit over standard devices (14). Medial patellar strapping has also been shown to reduce pain significantly in patello-femoral OA associated with patellar mal-alignment (15).
3. **Unloading knee braces** are functional devices indicated in patients with mal-alignment secondary to medial or lateral unicompartmental OA. They are composed of external stems, hinges and straps and are designed to decrease the compressive load transmitted to the diseased compartment by applying an external valgus or varus force respectively. Analgesic effect is achieved by improved stability, increased joint opening and possibly by reduction in local muscle contractions during gait (7).

   A single randomized controlled trial (RCT) of 110 patients showed that a valgus brace significantly improved pain, functional status and disease-specific quality of life at six months compared with no intervention in patients with medial compartment knee OA, and was more effective than a neoprene sleeve (12). However, a further RCT did not confirm its efficacy in pain reduction (16). A subset of patients in this trial found the varus brace effective for lateral compartment OA; this is the only trial result supporting efficacy of varus bracing. Unloading braces have been shown to improve isokinetic

quadriceps strength and gait symmetry (11) and while they significantly improve joint proprioception, this does not appear to improve postural control (6).
The main drawbacks with unloading braces are a variable response rate (39 to 93% of patients notice improvement) (11), and discomfort due to heaviness, heat and mobility of the device. The latter can also lead to persistent joint instability. In a three-year follow up study of 22 patients, the most common complaint was skin irritation affecting 41% of patients (17). Long-term compliance is therefore a problem: 20% of patients discontinue their brace at 6 months and many discontinue treatment within 1 to 2 years (18). Long term efficacy is therefore unknown. The most serious reported side effect is venous thromboembolism.

4. **Insoles.** There are limited data for the effectiveness of insoles (either laterally wedged or neutral) in reducing the symptoms of OA. In one study there was significant decrease in non-steroidal anti-inflammatory drug (NSAID) consumption and significantly better compliance in the laterally wedged insole group at 6 and 24 months compared to the neutral wedge group but there was no significant difference in pain, stiffness and function (19). Another study has shown that elastic subtalar strapping significantly reduces pain and femoro-tibial angulation at 6 and 24 months compared with traditional laterally wedged insoles (20). Adverse effects include low back, popliteal and foot sole pain (21). However, given their low cost and relatively better compliance, attention to footwear with shock-absorbing properties is worth considering (22).
5. **Thumb Splints.** In patients with hand OA, pain and its anticipation is a major factor in loss of hand function. Pain reduction should therefore be the primary goal of treatment. It appears that 1st carpo-metacarpal (CMC) joint OA contributes more to pain and disability than inter-phalangeal joint OA (23). As heavy stresses are placed on the 1st CMC joint during pinching and grasping, thumb splints are useful especially if the patient has difficulty in performing daily tasks.

Their efficacy was shown in a systematic review in 2010, which found high to moderate evidence for thumb CMC joint immobilization in improving pain and function and moderate evidence in improving grip strength (24). A multi-centre trial also showed strong evidence for efficacy at twelve months (but not at one month) in terms of improved pain and disability (25). There are several different designs of thumb CMC splints (from a short opponens splint which supports the 1st CMC and metacarpo-phalangeal (MCP) joint, to a much larger long opponens splint which includes both the MCP and wrist joint) (26). As yet it is unclear which are considered most comfortable for patients and thus will be worn long term, and what degree of support is required at what stage of OA in order to improve pain and function effectively (22).

2.2 Topical non-steroidal anti-inflammatory drugs

Direct application of topical non-steroidal anti-inflammatory drugs (NSAIDs) in the region of a painful joint is a common and recommended treatment in mild to moderate OA (8,9,10,22). This treatment is particularly useful in the management of a single painful osteoarthritic joint (especially the knee), or when a few hand joints are involved. It can provide a safe and effective alternative to systemic anti-inflammatory therapy.
Topical NSAIDs act primarily through inhibition of cyclo-oxygenases responsible for prostaglandin biosynthesis at the site of pain and inflammation, but might also work through peripheral and central desensitisation (27). Unlike other topical treatments, the act

of local rubbing appears less important in achieving a therapeutic effect. Topical NSAIDs can be applied over the affected joint up to 2 to 4 times a day depending on the drug, but currently are not recommended for continuous use beyond one month.

There are several different preparations of topical NSAID available, which differ in the active drug (diclofenac, ibuprofen, ketoprofen, piroxicam and felbinac), formulation (gel, solution, cream, plaster and patch) and the presence of a penetration enhancer to improve drug delivery (45.5% dimethylsulfoxide [DMSO] or menthol). The most commonly studied preparations are diclofenac sodium 1% gel (DSG) and diclofenac sodium 1.5% in 45.5% DMSO solution (Pennsaid).

To be effective, a topical NSAID needs to penetrate the skin and enter the circulation or additionally be absorbed into the underlying tissue. The formulation with respect to its lipid and aqueous solubility (requirements for passing through the stratum corneum and epidermal layer respectively) determines the degree of dermal penetration (28). Formulations of gels and sprays are more effective than creams.

Studies show that penetration of the topical NSAID into the intra- and peri-articular structures via the local bloodstream gives rise to therapeutic concentrations within these tissues without significant systemic absorption (28,29). This accounts for their superior safety profile over oral therapy with respect to systemic renal, cardiovascular and gastrointestinal toxicity.

Peak concentrations in the skin are achieved 2 hours after application, with a second peak 10 hours after application, which is attributed to the systemic circulation. The skin appears to act as a 'reservoir' from which the drug is distributed to deeper tissues (30). Only 3-7% of the applied dose is systemically absorbed (29) and mean plasma concentrations are typically 5% or less of the level reached following oral administration (31,32). Low systemic absorption is evidenced further by the lack of symptom relief in other joints distant to the site of application (33).

With respect to knee osteoarthritis, up until recently there was no research evidence to support the long-term use (greater than a month) of topical NSAIDs; a systematic review in 1998 (34) and two meta-analyses in 2004 (35,36) confirmed that topical NSAIDs were superior to placebo for up to two weeks in the treatment of chronically painful conditions but not longer. Later trials have however shown more long term efficacy, benefit beyond 4 weeks was confirmed in a meta-analysis of trials assessing efficacy between 4 and 12 weeks (37), and two further recent large high quality RCTs have demonstrated a sustained response maintained up to 12 weeks with diclofenac ("DSG" (33) and "Pennsaid" (38)) when compared with placebo. A recent RCT has also found topical ibuprofen to be as effective as oral ibuprofen and other NSAIDs for 12 months (39).

Currently there is insufficient evidence to compare efficacy of topical to oral administration of the same NSAID. The meta-analysis of RCTs in 2004 found that overall topical NSAIDs were less effective than oral NSAIDs (36). Two recent studies comparing topical diclofenac (in DMSO) with oral diclofenac in patients with knee OA have however demonstrated equivalent efficacy (40,41).

Placebo controlled trials and head to head studies with oral NSAIDs also show efficacy of topical NSAIDs in finger joint OA: hence they are preferred to systemic therapy, especially for mild to moderate OA and when few joints are involved (42).

The main side effect of topical anti-inflammatory treatment is local application site reactions such as dry skin, rash, pruritis and burning (36,37). They are short-lived and minor however, and usually resolve when application is discontinued. Studies show that local adverse events are reported with equal frequency for topical NSAIDs and placebo preparations; hence they appear not to be related to the NSAID itself (35). Safety between different topical agents has not been studied. However, three 12-week trials showed a greater incidence (5 to 8 fold higher) of local application site reactions with diclofenac in DMSO solution (26-42%) compared with DSG (5.1%) (33).

Compared to oral NSAIDs, topical therapy is associated with fewer systemic adverse events and gastro-intestinal side effects (33,35,40,41). However, data regarding gastro-intestinal safety and tolerability of topical NSAIDs in older patients (over the age of 50 years) are conflicting. Some studies report minor side effects to be infrequent, including the two-year RCT comparing topical to oral ibuprofen (39,43); but a recent systemic review has demonstrated gastro-intestinal adverse events in 15% and local skin reactions in 39.3% of patients receiving topical NSAIDs including skin sensitivity, contact dermatitis and photodermatitis (44).

While topical NSAIDs should be considered with paracetamol as first line treatment ahead of oral NSAIDs, COX-2 inhibitors or opioids in view of their efficacy and relative safety, further studies are needed to confirm their long-term efficacy and use in bilateral knee OA. Their use in older patients also might still require a degree of caution until further data demonstrating their safety profile in this age group become available.

2.3 Topical counter-irritants

Topical counter-irritants or rubefacients are agents that are frequently applied locally to relieve musculoskeletal pain in the extremities. The most commonly used rubefacient is salicylate, but this class of agent also includes nicotinate esters. Topical capsaicin is commonly considered to be a rubefacient; however its mechanism of action is sufficiently different for this treatment to be described separately.

The principal action of rubefacients is to act as a skin irritant. This results in reddening from vasodilatation and increased blood flow, but also leads to a soothing sensation of warmth i.e. counter-irritation. It is still unclear whether topical salicylates additionally relieve pain via cyclo-oxygenase inhibition, but there is little evidence that there is significant systemic absorption (45). This is consistent with the fact that no benefit is found using a rubefacient applied distal to the site of pain (46). Pain may also be offset or altered in the underlying muscle, joint and tendon by irritation of the sensory nerve endings (47). More recently there is evidence to suggest that salicylates and other rubefacients may act via the transient receptor potential (TRP) ion channels involved in thermal and pain sensation (48,49).

Although topical rubefacients containing salicyclate are widely used in England (almost 1.8 million prescriptions issued in 2006) (50), there is currently no evidence to support their prescription for chronic musculoskeletal pain. A Cochrane analysis in 2009 of six studies of rubefacients in chronic conditions such as osteoarthritis has shown that they produced significant benefit compared with placebo at 14 days, with 1 in 6 individuals achieving 50% pain relief (51). This compares poorly with topical NSAIDs however, where the number needed to treat (NNT) is 3.1 compared to placebo. Additionally their efficacy may be over-estimated as adequate blinding is not possible with any trial involving a rubefacient, the mechanism of action is through local irritation and any sham preparation, which attempts to mimic this, would be a rubefacient itself. However, placebo gels in trials were rubbed on to the skin in the same way as the active treatment overcoming any additional therapeutic effect of rubbing (52).

Based on limited data, rubefacients appear well tolerated and local adverse effects are uncommon in the short term (2% of patients) (51,52). Currently they are usually used as adjuvants to other therapies, such as oral analgesics, support bandages, rest, ice, and compression, and may be useful for patients who cannot tolerate oral analgesics (52). RCTs are needed to support their clinical use with respect to long-term efficacy and safety especially in osteoarthritis, which is a chronically painful condition. Most trials have lasted 14 days only and the longest trial spanned 28 days (52). Consequently rubefacients are not recommended in the UK in osteoarthritis although this recommendation has been based on a small number of limited studies (22).

2.4 Topical capsaicin

Topical capsaicin (0.025%) cream can be used to treat pain from osteoarthritis and rheumatoid arthritis. A higher dose (0.075%) is used in the treatment of neuropathic pain. The preparations contain capsaicin, a lipophilic alkaloid extracted from chilli peppers that has an extremely potent irritant effect. They work by initially selectively activating and sensitising c-nociceptors in the skin by binding the transient receptor vanilloid type 1 (TRPV 1) cation channel (53). Substance P is released which causes local irritation; however with repeated applications, levels are depleted leading to reversible desensitization of pain fibres and eventual degeneration of epidermal nerve fibres resulting in hypoalgesia (54). Although topical capsaicin is better than placebo for treatment of chronic pain, a meta-analysis of topical capsaicin (0.025%) or plaster for chronic musculoskeletal pain calculated the NNT at 4 weeks to be 8.1 for a 50% reduction in pain suggesting that capsaicin is only marginally effective (55).

In general therefore topical capsaicin is best employed as an adjunct to other modes of therapy. It should be used for 3 to 4 weeks (applied 4 times daily) to achieve maximal benefit. A transient local burning sensation (which can be intense), stinging or erythema at the application site are common (40%) (10), and lead to 1 in 10 patients discontinuing the treatment (55) however. Systemic events are rare.

2.5 Thermotherapy

The local application of heat or cold (cryotherapy) to a painful joint has been used for many years in the rehabilitation of patients with OA to relieve pain, stiffness and oedema. Cryotherapy is usually administered by application of cold packs or massage with ice over painful areas or acupoints (56). Cold application helps to reduce pain and swelling by causing temporary vasoconstriction and a reduction in local blood flow. This may in turn help improve range of motion and function (57). Heat therapy is used to reduce pain and stiffness by possibly improving circulation and relaxing muscles. However there are concerns that increased blood flow may worsen inflammation and oedema. Common methods of superficial heat administration are electrical heating pads, application of hot packs, towels or wax, or immersion in warm water or wax baths.

Supporting evidence for the efficacy of this mode of treatment remains very limited. For knee osteoarthritis, ice massage may be a useful adjunct for pain relief and cold packs may be used to lessen knee oedema (Cochrane review of three RCTs in 2003, involving 179 patients) (58). Ice massage for 20 minutes, 5 times a week for 3 weeks had a clinically significant effect on knee strength (29% improvement) with a statistically significant improvement in range of movement (8% relative difference) and function (11% relative difference) after two weeks of treatment (59) but not at three weeks given three times a week (60). Ice packs did not affect pain significantly compared to controls; however ice massage did have a significant effect. Cold packs also lead to a significant reduction in knee swelling but this has not been seen with hot packs (61). Some studies have shown that heat therapy for knee OA used for 20 minutes every other day for four weeks can significantly improve pain and disability but not stiffness (62). There have been no controlled trials of cryotherapy in hip OA.

There are no experimental studies to examine the role of cryotherapy in hand osteoarthritis. However, a systematic review in 2010 found three studies that had examined the role of heat therapy in 174 patients (63). There is weak evidence for the role of paraffin wax in pain reduction, improved range of movement and function, and moderate level evidence to support the use of low level continuous heat wrap and steam treatments for pain reduction and improved grip strength (64). Local application of heat prior to exercise may be helpful in knee OA; however direct research evidence for the benefit of local application of heat as a pretreatment or in combination with other physical therapies for hand OA is lacking (42).

Although further studies are required to determine their efficacy, heat and cold therapies are easy, non-invasive treatments with very few adverse events, and therefore can be considered as an adjunct to core treatment in hand and knee OA.

2.6 Joint aspiration

Aspiration of synovial fluid from a swollen joint (e.g. aspiration of knee) can provide temporary relief in pain and stiffness, although effusions usually re-accumulate unless steroid is injected. Aspiration of cystic fluid in cystic OA of joints similarly often provides symptomatic relief, but again fluid tends to re-accumulate.

2.7 Intra-articular corticosteroid

Intra-articular (IA) corticosteroid injections have been widely used to treat symptomatic peripheral joint OA for many years. The corticosteroid exerts its anti-inflammatory effect by interrupting the immune and inflammatory cascade at several levels. Local delivery of high doses of corticosteroid minimises systemic toxicity and can result in rapid improvement in symptoms during acute or severe symptom flares, especially in knee and hand OA.

Corticosteroid preparations differ in solubility and potency: more soluble preparations have a shorter duration of action, e.g. hydrocortisone acetate, compared to longer acting emulsion based preparations, which are only slightly soluble, e.g. methlyprednisolone acetate (MPA) or relatively insoluble, e.g.triamcinolone acetonide (TCA). Longer acting preparations are more effective for intra-articular injections as they remain in the joint longer, but there are few randomised, controlled trials comparing different IA corticosteroids. In a double blind RCT of 57 patients with symptomatic knee OA comparing TCA 20mg with MPA 40mg, there was a greater reduction in pain compared with baseline at 3 weeks with TCA compared to MPA, but this was only maintained at 8 weeks in the MPA group despite TCA being less soluble (65). In practice the choice of agent is usually based on local availability and cost. The dose-response relationship has not been systematically studied.

Most manufacturers advise against corticosteroid dilution with local anaesthetic (e.g. lignocaine) because of the risk of clumping and precipitation of steroid crystals. However this remains common practice and provides additional benefits: there is early temporary relief of symptoms; it verifies delivery of steroid to site of pain (66); and it dilutes the suspension, enabling even distribution within the joint, (especially in shoulder joint injections), and hence avoids placement of highly concentrated fluid into a single area.

Several randomised controlled trials (67-70) and one Cochrane systematic review (71) have shown significant short-term efficacy (between 1 to 4 weeks) in terms of pain reduction for a single IA corticosteroid (TCA, MPA and cortivazol) over placebo in knee OA although effects on function appear less marked. There was no significant benefit at 4 to 24 weeks post injection. Hence IA corticosteroids work rapidly, but the effects are mostly short-lived. The lack of a sustained response over placebo in these studies might relate to lower than recommended steroid doses used, and a strong beneficial effect seen in patients receiving IA placebo injection. In clinical practice, IA steroid injections provide rapid short-term pain relief to settle flares of pain and permit patients to begin other interventions such as quadriceps strengthening exercises.

The benefit of IA corticosteroid injections to the hip remains inconclusive. One small RCT of 35 patients examining the role of TCA in patients awaiting hip replacement showed good pain relief at one month, but this was not maintained, and in 8.5% symptoms deteriorated (72). Another RCT showed significant improvement by IA MPA 40mg at 2 weeks compared with placebo 0.9% saline injection, but efficacy was lost at 3 months (73).

The efficacy of IA 1st CMC joint injection was evaluated in a trial of 40 patients with primary moderate to severe OA, randomized to either 0.25mls TCA (5mg) or an equivalent volume of 0.9% saline. No clinical benefit was gained compared to placebo injection (74). A further prospective study of 30 patients with radiographically staged hand OA has shown long-term benefit (18 months) with a single IA 1st CMC joint injection and subsequent splinting for 3 weeks, in 80% of patients with early radiographic disease i.e preserved joint space and minimal other changes. In patients with more radiographically advanced OA with osteophytes and joint space narrowing, sustained pain relief was less reliably achieved (75).

While IA corticosteroids have marked anti-inflammatory effects and reduce the volume of synovitis in OA (73), disease factors which might relate to the presence of inflammation have not been found to determine clinical response including local heat and synovial thickening (70), and synovial fluid (SF) volume and leucocyte count (69). Furthermore the presence of a knee effusion does not appear to predict response either (67,70). In one study prior synovial fluid aspiration did lead to a greater reduction in pain (69); however this may have been related to less steroid dilution by synovial fluid and more accurate placement of the IA injection confirmed by prior synovial fluid aspiration (76). Hence the presence of a knee effusion is not necessarily an indication for corticosteroid injection unless it causes significant restriction in movement. (22)

Additionally a steroid response is not confined to joints with clinical evidence of inflammation (70). This appears not to be related to inaccuracy in detecting inflammation on clinical examination; a recent ultrasound scanning study showed that patients with non-inflammatory features on ultrasound derived more prolonged benefit compared to patients with inflammatory features (77).

The risks in IA steroid injection are generally small but the following potential side effects can occur:

1. Post-injection crystal-induced synovitis can occur in 2 to 6% of patients. It is usually observed within 24 hours of injection, and spontaneously resolves in 1 to 3 days (78). It is usually managed by analgesic therapy or ice packs. Flares have also been reported following saline injection suggesting that other factors such as injection technique may be responsible (67,69).
2. Iatrogenic infection is rare, with a reported incidence between 1 in 3000 to 1 in 50 000 (79). Symptoms usually occur within 3 to 4 days of injection. Aseptic technique and withholding injection in at risk patients should minimise this potential serious complication.
3. Lipoatrophy secondary to subcutaneous deposition of steroid is more common with less soluble preparations and was found to occur in 0.6% of patients in a prospective study of intra- and peri-articular injections of methylprednisolone acetate (80). Hence longer acting preparations are generally avoided in small joint injections where accurate placement is technically difficult.
4. Local effects including tendon weakening/ rupture, muscle wasting, skin pigmentation changes, nerve and blood vessel damage can be minimised by more accurately directed injections.
5. Systemic effects vary. Facial flushing is relatively frequent (40% in one study) (81) and may occur after a few hours. Diabetic control may be temporarily disturbed but not significantly (82). Corticosteroid-induced osteoporosis does not appear to be a major concern due to lack of net impact on bone resorption. Anaphylaxis is extremely rare (81).

Concern regarding long-term effects of repeated injection, such as risk of progressive articular cartilage damage, has limited the number of injections given to any particular joint: the general consensus is for no more than 3 to 4 per year. While animal studies have shown steroid induced chondrocyte degeneration (83), data to support this recommendation in clinical practice are lacking. In a randomised prospective trial of patients receiving TCA injections every 3 months for up to 2 years for knee osteoarthritis, no evidence of increased loss of joint space was observed (84). Similarly there are very few reports of osteonecrosis, with no convincing causal relationship identified. Unpublished experience does however suggest that there may be an increased risk of osteonecrosis of the femoral head following such injections into the hip joint.

Repeated intra-articular corticosteroid injections do not provide long-term benefit (76), and it is generally accepted that other treatment modalities should be sought if patients require frequent or numerous injections.

2.8 Intra-articular hyaluronic acid/ hyaluronan

Endogenous hyaluronan, previously known as hyaluronic acid (HA), is a large linear glycosamino-glycan. It is a major non-structural component of both the synovial and cartilage extracellular matrix and of synovial fluid. Key functions in the joint are to confer viscoelasticity and lubrication, and to help maintain tissue hydration and protein homeostasis by preventing large fluid movements (22). OA is associated with a decrease of HA content in the synovial fluid (85). The therapeutic goal of intra-articular viscosupplementation with HA is therefore to restore the natural protective function of hyaluronan in the joint.

The mechanism by which HA exerts its therapeutic effect, if any, is not certain. Intra-articular residency is short (hours), but the reported benefit is long (months). The short-term mode of action might be based on the pain relieving effect of the viscoelastic fluid in the affected joint. In the long term a sequence of events might be triggered which restores the trans-synovial flow and subsequently the metabolic and rheological homeostasis of the joint (86). However there is minimal evidence for a role in long term disease modification (8).

Commercial preparations of HA have the same structure as endogenous HA, although cross-linked HA molecules (known as hylans) were later engineered in order to obtain greater elasto-viscosity and intra-articular dwell-time. There are several formulations available (Artz, BioHy, Durolane, Hyalgan, Synvisc, Suvenyl, Orthovisc, Replasyn and Suplasyn) which vary in their molecular weight (2 to over 7 million KDA). This difference is thought to be of importance with respect to the volume and number of injections needed, and the length of time the preparation remains in the joint. Higher molecular weight preparations, such as Hylan G-F 20 (Synvisc), seem to be more effective than lower-molecular-weight preparations in this respect (87).

Although there are a large number of studies in the literature, evidence for the efficacy of HAs is difficult to interpret because studies have used different molecular weights of HA and different injection schedules, and because of poor trial design. In addition, the benefit from placebo saline injections was high in some of the studies. Overall, hyaluronans and hylan derivatives seem to be superior to placebo in terms of efficacy (including pain relief, function and patient global assessment) and quality of life outcomes in patients with knee OA at different post-injection periods, but especially at 5 to 13 weeks after the last of a series of 3 to 5 injections (86). Clinical trials do not suggest that sub-groups of osteoarthritis patients may have greater benefit; however this would be of research interest given the high cost of this particular treatment (22). Data from the Cochrane meta-analysis suggest that IA therapy with hyaluronans may have a more prolonged effect than IA corticosteroids (86). Adverse effects are rare but include a transient increase in pain and very rarely a frank arthritis flare with knee effusion. There do not appear to be any systemic side effects.

In hip OA, no significant differences between hyaluronans and placebo were reported at any time point by a RCT evaluating efficacy and function outcomes, but the effect was better in patients without an effusion (88). There was no significant difference between hyaluronan and corticosteroid injection either (88). Similarly, hyaluronan and corticosteroid injections perform similarly with respect to efficacy and function in hand OA (89).

Overall the evidence for HA efficacy is mostly in knee OA, with a slower onset of action but a more durable response than IA corticosteroid injection. It is a safe treatment. However its widespread use is limited by cost. It is usually offered to patients who are not fit for or would like to delay surgical intervention, and in patients who require repeated IA corticosteroid injections.

2.9 Acupuncture

Accupuncture is a recommended modality of therapy for symptomatic treatment of patients with knee and hip OA. It involves treatment with fine filiform stainless steel needles of 0.25-0.35mm diameter. Typically six needles are placed near the painful area and possibly elsewhere and are either manipulated to produce a 'needle sensation' or stimulated electrically (electroacupuncture) for up to 20 minutes. A course of treatment usually consists of six or more sessions. The response can be variable, the reasons for which are not well understood. Potential underlying neurophysiological mechanisms are complex. The 'gate control theory' and release of endogenous opioids are possible explanations for the apparent analgesic effect (10).

Although an earlier systematic review of acupuncture in patients with OA at various peripheral sites did not show it to be any better than sham controls (90), several randomized trials report benefit in knee OA over sham acupuncture (91-93) and standard treatment (94). A systematic review in 2001 of 7 RCTs including 393 patients (95) found that acupuncture significantly improved pain compared with sham acupuncture, but not function (92,93). However, it was not found to be more effective than physical therapy or than being on a waiting list to receive acupuncture (94,96). The benefit appears short to medium term (6-12 weeks); the few studies with long-term follow up did not show benefit at 26 weeks (91,94). Combining acupuncture with a course of advice and exercise has not been shown to provide any additional benefit (97). Acupuncture of peripheral joints appears safe (98). Mild adverse effects occur in 7% of patients (99,100), but serious side effects are rare (101).

2.10 Trigger point injection

In many forms of arthritis, localised areas of thickening and tenderness in cutaneous and other soft tissues can be found. These have been referred to by a number of different names, including interstitial fibrositis, myofasciitis and myofascial trigger points (102-104). They are also well described by acupuncturists (105). Some are found clinically in cutaneous and subcutaneous tissue at sites near to or distant from inflamed or painful joints, typically in areas of a limb proximal to an affected joint, such as in the upper part of the rectus femoris in patients with knee pain, and in paraspinal regions in the cervical and lumbar areas (106).

The term trigger point injection (TPI) refers to direct injection of a substance into the trigger point itself, or into the skin or soft tissue over the trigger point (indirect needling); or to dry needling of either of these areas. The main objective is to inactivate the trigger point thereby reducing pain and restoring function. However, the aetiology and pathogenesis of trigger points have yet to be elucidated, and the precise mechanism by which TPI inactivates the trigger point is still unknown (107).

Optimal technique and treatment regimen for TPI varies between practitioners, and is largely based on clinical experience. Treatment begins with identifying the trigger point; the area of maximal tenderness and immobilising the muscle between the thumb and forefinger. Generally a sterile small gauge needle is then introduced into the trigger point. Correct identification is supported by a twitch in the affected muscle, exacerbation of pain and the presence of referred pain (108).

Clinicians have used local anaesthetic, anti-inflammatory agents (long-acting corticosteroid, acetylsalicylate and ketorolac), saline and water (104,108-113). Injecting a trigger point is painful and the addition of a local anaesthetic to the injected fluid can help reduce pain and irritation (114,115).

A systematic review of the efficacy of TPI to treat chronic non-malignant musculoskeletal pain (such as whiplash syndrome or chronic head, neck, shoulder, and back pain) of more than three months' duration found that TPI relieved symptoms when used as a sole treatment for patients, regardless of the injectant used, but was not more effective than other less invasive treatments such as laser and ultrasound (107).

The efficacy of TPI as a treatment for osteoarthritis is not well described; and as most studies have looked at its role as a sole treatment rather than in the adjunct capacity in which it is routinely used in clinical practice, its effectiveness might be underestimated. One study showed that intra-articular injection combined with lidocaine TPI of any of the 15 leg muscle trigger points was more effective than intra-articular injection alone in relieving pain and improving knee function in a highly selected group of older patients with knee osteoarthritis (116). Except for the rare occurrence of muscle atrophy at the injection site, very few adverse events are reported with TPI and it is currently recommended as an adjunct therapy in osteoarthritis.

2.11 Subcutaneous sodium salicylate injection

Trigger point injection using sodium salicyclate has also been studied. In a large uncontrolled study Fox reported a good response from injecting 0.5% sodium salicylate into superficial areas of tender soft tissue thickening: using multiple injections, he recorded an improvement in symptoms in 79% of patients at 12 weeks (117). Most of these subjects had osteoarthritis.

Following similar preliminary observations in our group, we performed a pilot study, in which 16 patients with OA of the first (thumb) CMC joint were treated with injections of 0.5% sodium salicylate or saline into similar areas of superficial soft tissue thickening (118). There was a significant improvement in pain score in both groups. The improvement was better maintained in the patients that received salicylate. A subsequent double-blind study of 40 patients with the same condition showed superiority of sodium salicylate injections over sham injections (119). Pain and tenderness during follow up were both significantly lower in the active treatment group compared with the sham group.

The chief limitation in studies of this kind is the imperfect nature of the control treatment. However, in the sham-controlled study, the improvement in the active treatment group was sustained for as long as 13 weeks, suggesting that an effect greater than placebo was being observed. Furthermore, there was no significant correlation in the active group between the pain of the injections and response in terms of pain in the joint.

The mechanism of action of this treatment is uncertain. The injected patches are distant from the affected joint. It is possible that the salicylate causes a change in the control of pain, perhaps through a modification of central sensitisation. This would be consistent with reports by patients of improvement in symptoms within minutes. The treatment could modify the neurogenic control of inflammation, which may be disturbed in musculoskeletal disease (120,121). One way in which this might occur could be through changes in the expression or transport of neurogenic peptides (122), brought about by an irritant effect of the salicylate, similar to that of topical capsaicin (55,123). A systemic anti-inflammatory effect is unlikely, since similar injections of salicylate at other sites fail to produce any effect on the symptoms of osteoarthritis (Mackworth-Young C.G., personal observation).

It could be that sodium salicylate injection therapy acts in a manner similar to acupuncture, but achieves a more prolonged effect because a substance is injected into the tissues that results in a sustained stimulus. Many of the injected patches occur at standard acupuncture sites.

Sodium salicylate therapy is inexpensive, and can be administered by general practitioners and trained nurses. The studies on this treatment also suggest areas for further scientific enquiry in the regulation of pain and inflammation in osteoarthritis.

3. Conclusions

There are many local therapies available for the treatment of patients with limb joint OA. Some are well established, such as intra-articular corticosteroid. Some are relatively new, and show promise for further development.

Most of them are primarily symptomatic treatments, which need to be tailored to the individual's preference and tolerance. Many of them function well as adjuncts to other treatments, such as systemic analgesics or anti-inflammatory agents. Given the chronicity of OA however, they are likely to be required over long periods of time, either continuously or as episodic treatment during symptom flares. Long-term efficacy data are largely missing, although the therapies appear to be generally safe. Furthermore studies for costly interventions with proven efficacy such as hyaluronan injections are needed to identify subsets of patients who would benefit most from the treatment to allow more targeted use.

It is uncertain if some treatments may modify medium or long-term outcome. For example in inflammatory OA of small finger joints, it is not clear whether intra-articular steroid injection hastens the settling down of the inflammation (which tends to happen anyway), and thus reduces the amount of joint damage. Similarly, effects of topical NSAIDs, acupuncture and subcutaneous sodium salicyclate injections on disease modulation are unknown. Longitudinal studies on these treatments may answer these questions.

4. References

[1] Felson DT, Zhang Y. An update on the epidemiology of knee and hip osteoarthritis with a view to prevention. Arthritis Rheum 1998; 41(8): 1343-55.

[2] Zhang Y, Niu J, Kelly-Hayes M, Chaisson CE, Aliabadi P, Felson DT. Prevalence of symptomatic hand osteoarthritis and its impact on functional status among the elderly: The Framingham Study. Am J Epidemiol. 2002; 156(11): 1021-7.

[3] Arden N, Nevitt M. Oeseoarthritis: Epidemiology. Best Pract Res Clin Rheumatol. 2006; 20(1): 3-25.

[4] Haq I, Murphy E, Dacre J. Osteoarthritis. Postgrad Med J. 2003; 79(933): 377-83.

[5] Rannou F, Poiraudeau S, Beaudreuil J. Role of bracing in the management of knee osteoarthritis. Curr Opin Rheumatol. 2010; 22(2): 218-22.

[6] Birmingham TB, Kramer JF, Kirkley A, Inglis JT, Spaulding SJ, Vandervoort AA. Knee bracing for medial compartment osteoarthritis: effects on proprioception and postural control. Rheumatology (Oxford). 2001; 40(3): 285–9.

[7] Ramsey DK, Briem K, Axe MJ, Snyder-Mackler L. A mechanical theory for the effectiveness of bracing for medial compartment osteoarthritis of the knee. J Bone Joint Surg Am. 2007; 89(11): 2398–407.

[8] Jordan KM, Arden NK, Doherty M, *et al.* EULAR Recommendations 2003: an evidence-based approach to the management of knee osteoarthritis: Report of a Task Force of the Standing Committee for International Clinical Studies Including Therapeutic Trials (ESCISIT). Ann Rheum Dis. 2003; 62(12): 1145–1155.

[9] Recommendations for the medical management of osteoarthritis of the hip and knee: 2000 update. American College of Rheumatology Subcommittee on Osteoarthritis Guidelines. Arthritis Rheum. 2000; 43(9): 1905–15.

[10] Zhang W, Moskowitz RW, Nuki G, et al. OARSI recommendations for the management of hip and knee osteoarthritis, Part II: OARSI evidence-based, expert consensus guidelines. Osteoarthritis Cartilage. 2008; 16(2): 137–162.

[11] Beaudreuil J, Bendaya S, Faucher M, Coudeyre E, Ribinik P, Revel M, Rannou F. Clinical practice guidelines for rest orthosis, knee sleeves, and unloading knee braces in knee osteoarthritis. Joint Bone Spine. 2009; 76(6): 629-36.

[12] Kirkley A, Webster-Bogaert S, Litchfield R, Amendola A, MacDonald S, McCalden R, Fowler P. The effect of bracing on varus gonarthrosis. J Bone Joint Surg. 1999; 81(4): 539–48.

[13] Chuang SH, Huang MH, Chen TW, Weng MC, Liu CW, Chen CH. Effect of knee sleeve on static and dynamic balance in patients with knee osteoarthritis. Kaohsiung J Med Sci. 2007; 23(8): 405–11.

[14] Mazzuca SA, Page MC, Meldrum RD, Brandt KD, Petty-Saphon S. Pilot study of the effects of a heat- retaining knee sleeve on joint pain, stiffness, and function in patients with knee osteoarthritis. Arthritis Rheum. 2004; 51(5): 716–21.

[15] Warden SJ, Hinman RS, Watson MA Jr, Avin KG, Bialocerkowski AE, Crossley KM. Patellar taping and bracing for the treatment of chronic knee pain: a systematic review and meta-analysis. Arthritis Rheum. 2008; 59(1): 73–83.

[16] Brouwer RW, van Raaij TM, Verhaar JA,Coene LN, Bierma-Zeinstra SM. Brace treatment for osteoarthritis of the knee: a prospective randomized multicentre trial. Osteoarthritis Cartilage. 2006; 14(8): 777–83.

[17] Pollo FE, Otis JC, Backus SI, Warren RF, Wickiewicz TL. Reduction of medial compartment loads with valgus bracing of the osteoarthritic knee. Am J Sports Med. 2002; 30 (3): 414–21.

[18] Giori NJ. Load-shifting brace treatment for osteoarthritis of the knee: a minimum 2 1/2-year follow-up study. J Rehabil Res Dev. 2004; 41(2) : 187–94.

[19] Maillefert JF, Hudry C, Baron G, Kieffert P, Bourgeois P, Lechevalier D, et al. Laterally elevated wedged insoles in the treatment of medial compartment osteoarthritis: a prospective randomized controlled trial. Osteoarthritis Cartilage. 2001; 9(8): 738–45.

[20] Toda Y, Tsukimura N. A 2-year follow up of a study to compare the efficiency of lateral wedged insoles with subtalar strapping and in- shoe lateral wedged insoles in patients with varus deformity osteoarthritis of the knee. Osteoarthritis and Cartilage. 2006; 14(3): 231–7.

[21] Brouwer RW, Jakma TS, Verhagen AP, Verhaar JA, Bierma- Zeinstra SM. Braces and orthoses for treating osteoarthritis of the knee. Cochrane Database Syst Rev. 2005; Jan 25; (1): CD004020.

[22] National Institute for Health and Clinical Excellence. Osteoarthritis: national clinical guideline for care and management in adults London: NICE, 2008. www.nice.org.uk/CG059.

[23] Bijsterbosch J, Visser W, Kroon HM, Stamm T, Meulenbelt I, Huizinga TW, Kloppenburg M. Thumb base involvement in symptomatic hand osteoarthritis is associated with more pain and functional disability. Ann Rheum Dis. 2010; 69(3): 585–7.

[24] Kristin Valdes and Tambra Marik. A Systematic Review of Conservative Interventions for Osteoarthritis of the Hand. J Hand Ther. 2010; 23(4): 334–50.

[25] Rannou F, Dimet J, Boutron I, et al. Splint for base-of-thumb osteoarthritis: a randomized trial. Ann Intern Med. 2009; 150(10): 661-9.

[26] Batra S, Kanvinde R. Osteoarthritis of the thumb trapeziometacarpal joint. Current Orthopaedics. 2007; 21, 135–44.

[27] Doherty M, Jones A. Topical NSAIDs. In: Brandt K, Doherty M, Lohmander S, Osteoarthritis. 2nd ed. Oxford: Oxford University Press, 2003:291-5.

[28] Haroutiunian S, Drennan DA, Lipman AG. Topical NSAID therapy for musculoskeletal pain. Pain Med. 2010 Apr; 11(4): 535-49.

[29] Anon. Topical analgesics: A review of reviews and a bit of perspective. www.jr2.ox.ac.uk/Bandolier/Extraforbando/ Topextra3.pdf 2005.

[30] Sioufi A, Pommier F, Boschet F, Godbillon J, Lavoignat D, Salliere D. Percutaneous absorption of diclofenac in healthy volunteers after single and repeated topical application of diclofenac Emulgel. Biopharm Drug Dispos. 1994; 15(6): 441- 9.

[31] Massey T, Derry S, Moore RA, McQuay HJ. Topical NSAIDs for acute pain in adults. Cochrane Database Syst Rev. 2010 Jun 16;(6): CD007402

[32] Brunner M, Dehghanyar P, Seigfried B, Martin W, Menke G, Müller M. Favourable dermal penetration of diclofenac after administration to the skin using a novel spray gel formulation. Br J Clin Pharmacol. 2005; 60(5): 573–7.

[33] Barthel HR, Haselwood D, Longley S 3rd, Gold MS, Altman RD. Randomized controlled trial of diclofenac sodium gel in knee osteoarthritis. Semin Arthritis Rheum. 2009; 39(3): 203-12.

[34] Moore RA, Tramer MR, Carroll D, Wiffen PJ, McQuay HJ. Quantitative systematic review of topical applied non-steroidal anti-inflammatory drugs. BMJ. 1998; 316(7168): 333-8.

[35] Mason L, Moore RA, Edwards JE, Derry S, McQuay HJ. Topical NSAIDs for chronic musculoskeletal pain: systematic review and metaanalysis. BMC Musculoskeletal Disord. 2004; Aug 19;5: 28.

[36] Lin J, Zhang W, Jones A, Doherty M. Efficacy of topical non-steroidal anti-inflammatory drugs in the treatment of osteoarthritis: meta-analysis of randomised controlled trials. BMJ. 2004; 329(7461): 324.

[37] Biswal S, Medhi B, Pandhi P. Longterm efficacy of topical nonsteroidal antiinflammatory drugs in knee osteoarthritis: Metaanalysis of randomized placebo controlled clinical trials. J Rheumatol. 2006; 33(9): 1841–4.

[38] Roth SH, Shainhouse JZ. Efficacy and safety of a topical diclofenac solution (Pennsaid) in the treatment of primary osteoarthritis of the knee: a randomized, double-blind, vehicle-controlled clinical trial. Arch Intern Med. 2004; 164(18): 2017-23.

[39] Underwood M, Ashby D, Cross P, Hennessy E, Letley L, Martin J, Mt-Isa S, Parsons S, Vickers M, Whyte K. Advice to use topical or oral ibuprofen for chronic knee pain in older people: randomised controlled trial and patient preference study. BMJ. 2008; 336(7636): 138-42.

[40] Tugwell PS, Wells GA, Shainhouse JZ. Equivalence study of a topical diclofenac solution (pennsaid) compared with oral diclofenac in symptomatic treatment of osteoarthritis of the knee: A randomized controlled trial. J Rheumatol. 2004; 31(10): 2002–12.

[41] Simon LS, Grierson LM, Naseer Z, Bookman AA, Zev Shainhouse J. Efficacy and safety of topical diclofenac containing dimethyl sulfoxide (DMSO) compared with those of topical placebo. DMSO vehicle and oral diclofenac for knee osteoarthritis. Pain. 2009; 143(3): 238-45.

[42] Zhang W, Doherty M, Leeb BF et al. EULAR evidence based recommendations for the management of hand osteoarthritis: report of a Task Force of the EULAR Standing Committee for International Clinical Studies Including Therapeutics (ESCISIT). Ann Rheum Dis. 2007; 66(3): 377-88.

[43] Baraf HS, Gloth FM, Barthel HR, Gold MS, Altman RD. Safety and efficacy of topical diclofenac sodium gel for knee osteoarthritis in elderly and younger patients: pooled data from three randomized, double-blind, parallel-group, placebo-controlled, multicentre trials. Drugs Aging. 2011; 28 (1): 27-40.
[44] Makris UE, Kohler MJ, Fraenkel L. Adverse effects of topical non-steroidal anti-inflammatory drugs in older adults with osteoarthritis: a systematic literature review.J Rheumatol. 2010; 3(6): 1236-43.
[45] Martin D, Valdez J, Boren J, Mayersohn M. Dermal absorption of camphor, menthol, and methyl salicylate in humans. J of Clin Pharmacol. 2004; 44(10): 1151–7.
[46] Shackel NA, Day RO, Kellett B, Brooks PM. Copper-salicylate gel for pain relief in osteoarthritis: a randomised controlled trial. Med J of Aust. 1997; 167(3): 134–6.
[47] Morton I, Hall J. The Royal Society of Medicine: Medicines. 6th Edition. London: Bloomsbury, 2002.
[48] Nilius B, Owsianik G, Voets T, Peters JA. Transient receptor potential cation channels in disease. Physiol Rev. 2007; 87(1): 165–217.
[49] Stanos SP. Topical agents for the management of musculoskeletal pain. J of Pain and Symptom Manage. 2007; 33(3): 342–55.
[50] Prescription Cost Analysis, England. 2006ISBN: 1-84636-035-6 2006.
[51] Matthews P, Derry S, Moore RA, McQuay HJ. Topical rubefacients for acute and chronic pain in adults. Cochrane Database Syst Rev. 2009 Jul 8; (3): CD007403.
[52] Mason L, Moore RA, Edwards JE, McQuay HJ, Derry S, Wiffen PJ. Systematic review of efficacy of topical rubefacients containing salicylates for the treatment of acute and chronic pain. BMJ. 2004 Apr 24; 328(7446): 995.
[53] Baron R. Capsaicin and nociception: from basic mechanisms to novel drugs. Lancet. 2000; 356(9232): 785-7.
[54] Nolano M, Simone DA, Wendelschafer-Crabb G, Johnson T, Hazen E, Kennedy WR. Topical capsaicin in humans: parallel loss of epidermal nerve fibres and pain sensation. Pain 1999; 81(1-2): 135-45.
[55] Mason L, Moore RA, Derry S, Edwards JE, McQuay HJ. Systematic review of topical capsaicin for the treatment of chronic pain. BMJ. 2004; 328(7446): 991-94.
[56] Cameron MH. Physical agents in rehabilitation. From research to practice. Philadelphia: WB Saunders Company, 1999.
[57] Arthritis Foundation. Conditions and treatments. Disease Centre. http://www.arthriitis.org/conditions/DiseaseCenter? Oa.asp., 2003
[58] Brosseau L, Yonge KA, Robinson V, Marchand S, Judd M, Wells G, Tugwell P. Thermotherapy for treatment of osteoarthritis. Cochrane Database Syst Rev 2003; (4): CD004522.
[59] Yurtkuran M, Kocagil T. TENS, Electroacupuncture and Ice Massage: Comparison of Treatment for Osteoarthritis of the Knee. Am J of Acupunct. 1999; 27(3-4): 133–40.
[60] Clarke GR, Willis LA, Stenner L, Nichols PJR. Evaluation of Physiotherapy in the Treatment of Osteoarthrosis of the Knee. Rheumatol Rehabil. 1974; 13(4): 190–7.
[61] Hecht PJ, Backmann S, Booth RE, Rothman RH. Effects of Thermal Therapy on Rehabilitation after Total Knee Arthroplasty : A Prospective Randomized Study. Clinical Orthopadics and Related Research 1983; 178: 198–201.

[62] Yildirim N, Filiz Ulusoy M, Bodur H. The effect of heat application on pain, stiffness, physical function and quality of life in patients with knee osteoarthritis. J Clin Nurs. 2010; 19(7-8): 1113-20.
[63] Valdes K, Marik T. A systematic review of conservative interventions for osteoarthritis of the hand. J Hand Ther. 2010; 23(4): 334-50.
[64] Boustedt C, Nordenskiold U, Nilsson AL. Effects of a hand joint protection programme with an addition of splinting and exercise. Clin Rheumatol. 2009; 28: 793–9.
[65] Pyne D, Ioannou Y, Mootoo R, Bhanji A. Intra-articular steroids in knee osteoarthritis: a comparative study of triamcinolone hexacetonide and methylprednisolone acetate. Clin Rheumatol. 2004; 23(2): 116-20.
[66] Schumacher HR. Aspiration and injection therapies for joints. Arthritis Rheum. 2003; 49(3): 413-20.
[67] Friedman DM & Moore ME. The efficacy of intra-articular steroids in osteoarthritis: a double blind study. J Rheumatol. 1980; 7(6): 850-6.
[68] Dieppe PA, Sathapatayavongs B, Jones HE, Bacon PA, Ring EF. Intra-articular steroids in osteoarthritis. Rheumatol Rehab. 1980; 19(4): 212-17.
[69] Gaffney K, Ledingham J, Perry JD. Intra-articular triamcinolone hexacetonide in knee osteoarthritis: factors influencing the clinical response. Ann Rheum Dis. 1995; 54(5): 379-81.
[70] Jones A & Doherty M. Intra-articular corticosteroids are effective in osteoarthritis but there are no clinical predictors of response. Ann Rheum Dis. 1996; 55(11): 829-32.
[71] Bellamy N, Campbell J, Robinson V, Gee T, Bourne R, Wells G. Intra-articular corticosteroids for osteoarthritis of the knee. Cochrane Database Syst Rev. 2006 Apr 19; (2): CD005328.
[72] Flanagan J, Casale FF, Thomas TL, Desai KB. Intra-articular injection for pain relief in patients awaiting hip replacement. Ann R Coll Surg Engl. 1988; 70(3): 156-7.
[73] Qvistgaard E, Christensen R, Torp-Pedersen S, Bliddal H. Intra-articular treatment of hip osteoarthritis: a randomized trial of hyaluronic acid, corticosteroid, and isotonic saline. Osteoarthritis Cartilage. 2006; 14(2): 163-70.
[74] Meenagh GK, Patton J, Kynes C, Wright GD. A randomised controlled trial of intra-articular corticosteroid injection of the carpometacarpal joint of the thumb in osteoarthritis. Ann Rheum Dis. 2004; 63(10): 1260–3.
[75] Day CS, Gelberman R, Patel AA, Vogt MT, Ditsios K, Boyer MI. Basal joint osteoarthritis of the thumb: a prospective trial of steroid injection and splinting. J Hand Surg. 2004; 29(2): 247–51.
[76] Ayral X. Injections in the treatment of osteoarthritis. Best Pract Res Clin Rheumatol. 2001; 15(4), 609-26.
[77] Chao J, Wu C, Sun B, Hose MK, Quan A, Hughes TH, Boyle D, Kalunian KC. Inflammatory characteristics on ultrasound predict poorer longterm response to intraarticular corticosteroid injections in knee osteoarthritis. J Rheumatol. 2010; 37(3): 650-5.
[78] Schumacher HR, Chen LX. Injectable corticosteroids in treatment of arthritis of the knee. Am J Med 2005; 118(11): 1208-14.
[79] Creamer P. Intra-articular corticosteroid treatment in osteoarthritis. Curr Opin Rheumatol. 1999; 11(5): 417-21.

[80] Kumar N, Newman RJ. Complications of intra- and peri-articular steroid injections. Br J Gen Pract. 1999; 49(443): 465-6.
[81] Pattrick M, Doherty M. Facial flushing after intra-articular injection of bupivacaine and methylprednisolone. BMJ. 1987; 295(6610): 1380.
[82] Slotkoff A, Clauw D, Nashel D. Effect of soft tissue corticosteroid injection on glucose control in diabetics. Arthritis Rheum. 1994; 37(suppl 9): S347.
[83] Papacrhistou G, Anagnostou S, Katsorhis T. The effect of intraarticular hydrocortisone injection on the articular cartilage of rabbits. Acta Orthop Scand. Suppl. 1997; 275: 132-4.
[84] Raynauld JP, Buckland-Wright C, et al. Safety and efficacy of long-term intraarticular steroid injections in osteoarthritis of the knee: a randomized, double-blind, placebo-controlled trial. Arthritis Rheum. 2003; 48(2): 370-7.
[85] Fife R. Osteoarthritis: A. Epidemiology, pathology and pathogenesis. In: Klippel JH, editor. Primer on the rheumatic diseases. 11th edition. Atlanta: The Arthritis Foundation; 1997. p. 216-7.
[86] Bellamy N, Campbell J, Robinson V, Gee T, Bourne R, Wells G. Viscosupplementation for the treatment of osteoarthritis of the knee. Cochrane Database Syst Rev. 2006 Apr 19; (2): CD005321.
[87] Wobig M, Bach G, Beks P, et al. The role of elastoviscosity in the efficacy of viscosupplementaion for osteoarthritis of the knee: A comparison of hylan G-F 20 and a lower molecular weight hyaluronan. Clin Ther. 1999; 21(9): 1549–62.
[88] Qvistgaard E, Christensen R, Torp-Pedersen S, Bliddal H. Intra-articular treatment of hip osteoarthritis: a randomized trial of hyaluronic acid, corticosteroid, and isotonic saline. Osteoarthritis Cartilage. 2006; 14(2): 163-70.
[89] Fuchs S, Mönikes R, Wohlmeiner A, Heyse T. Intra-articular hyaluronic acid compared with corticoid injections for the treatment of rhizarthrosis. Osteoarthritis Cartilage. 2006; 14(1): 82-8.
[90] Ernst E. Acupuncture as a symptomatic treatment of osteoarthritis. A systematic review. Scand J Rheumatol. 1997; 26(6): 444–7.
[91] C Witt, B Brinkhaus, S Jena, et al. Acupuncture in patients with osteoarthritis of the knee: a randomised trial. Lancet. 2005; 366(9480): 136–43.
[92] Molsberger A, Böwing G, Jensen KU, Lorek M.[Accupuncture treatment for the relief of gonarthrosis pain-a controlled clinical trial]. Der Schmerz 1994; 8(1): 37–42. German.
[93] Petrou P, Winkler V, Genti G, Balint G. Double blind trial to evaluate the effect of acupuncture treatment on knee osteoarthritis. Scand J Acupunct. 1988; 3: 112–15.
[94] Berman BM, Singh BB, Lao L, et al. A randomized trial of acupuncture as an adjunctive therapy in osteoarthritis of the knee. Rheumatology (Oxford). 1999; 38(4): 346–54.
[95] Ezzo J, Hadhazy V, Birch S, Kaplan G, Hochberg M, Berman B. Acupuncture for osteoarthritis of the knee: a systematic review. Arthritis Rheum. 2001; 44(4): 819–25.
[96] Christensen BV, Luhl IU, Vilbek H, Bulow HH, Dreijer NC, Rasmussen HF. Acupuncture treatment of severe knee osteoarthrosis: a long-term study. Acta Anaesthesiol Scand. 1992; 36(6): 519–25.
[97] Foster NE, Thomas E, Barlas P, Hill JC, Young J, Mason E, et al. Acupuncture as an adjunct to exercise based physiotherapy for osteoarthritis of the knee: randomised controlled trial. BMJ 2007; 335(7617): 436.

[98] Yamashita H, Tsukayama H, Hori N, Kimura T, Tanno Y. Incidence of adverse reactions associated with acupuncture. J Altern Complement Med. 2000; 6(4): 345–50.
[99] Melchart D, Weidenhammer W, Streng A Reitmayr S, Hoppe A, Ernst E, Linde K. Prospective investigation of adverse effects of acupuncture in 97733 patients. Arch Intern Med. 2004; 164(1): 104–5.
[100] Berman BM, Lao L, Langenberg P, Lee WL, Gilpin AM, Hochberg MC. Effectiveness of Acupuncture as Adjunctive Therapy in Osteoarthritis of the Knee. Ann Intern Med. 2004; 141(12): 901-10.
[101] Ernst E, White A. Acupuncture: safety first. BMJ. 1997; 314(7091): 1362.
[102] Steindler A and Luck JV. Differential diagnoses of pain in the low back. J. Amer. Med. Assoc. 1938; 110:106-113.
[103] Travell JG, Simons DG (eds.) Myofascial Pain and Dysfunction: the Trigger Point Manual. Williams & Wilkins, Baltimore, MD, USA, 1983: 2-18.
[104] Cailliet R. Chronic pain concept. In: Soft Tissue Pain and Disability. FA Davis, Philadelphia, PA, USA, 1977: 25-40.
[105] Mann F: Acupuncture: the Ancient Chinese Art of Healing. Heinemann, London, 1971: 28-30.
[106] Fox WW and Freed DLJ. Understanding arthritis. Macmillan, London, 1990.
[107] Scott NA, Guo B, Barton PM, Gerwin RD. Trigger point injections for chronic non-malignant musculoskeletal pain: a systematic review. Pain Med. 2009; 10(1): 54-69.
[108] Kim PS. Role of injection therapy: review of indications for trigger point injections, regional blocks, facet joint injections, and intra-articular injections. Curr Opin Rheumatol. 2002; 14(1): 52-7.
[109] Sidel N and Abrams MI. Treatment of chronic arthritis; results of vaccine therapy with saline injections used as controls. J. Am. Med. Assoc. 1940; 11:1740-1742.
[110] Traut EF, Passarelli EW. Study in the controlled therapy of degenerative arthritis. Arch. Intern. Med. 1956; 98(2): 181-186.
[111] Frost FA, Jessen B, Siggaard-Andersen J. A controlled, double-blind comparison of mepivacaine versus saline injection for myofascial pain. Lancet. 1980; 1(8167): 499-500.
[112] Frost FA. Diclofenac versus lidocaine as injection therapy in myofascial pain. Scand J Rheumatol. 1986; 15: 153-156.
[113] Byrn C, Olsson I, Falkheden L et al. Subcutaneous sterile water injections for chronic neck and shoulder pain following whiplash injuries. Lancet. 1993; 341(8843): 449-52.
[114] Fricton JR. Management of masticatory myofascial pain. Semin Orthod 1995; 1: 229–43.
[115] Fischer AA. Algometry in the daily practice of pain management. J Back Musculoskelet Rehabil 1997; 8: 151–63.
[116] Yentür EA, Okcu G, Yegul I. The role of trigger point therapy in knee osteoarthritis. Pain Clinic 2003; 15: 385–90.
[117] Fox WW: Arthritis therapy. In Machtey I (ed.) Progress in Rheumatology Golda Medical Centre, Peta-Tigva, 1987; 3: 242-5.
[118] Mackworth-Young CG. Treatment of osteoarthritis by cutaneous injection of salicylate or saline: a pilot study. J Orthop Med. 2000; 22: 75-80.

[119] Smith AS, Doré CJ, Dennis L, Julius A, Mackworth-Young CG. A randomised controlled trial of subcutaneous sodium salicylate therapy for osteoarthritis of the thumb. Postgrad Med J. 2010; 86(1016): 341-5.

[120] Kidd BL, Urban LA. Mechanisms of inflammatory pain. Br J of Anaesth. 2001; 87(1): 3-11.

[121] Schaible HG, Ebersberger A, Von Banchet GS. Mechanisms of pain in arthritis. Ann N Y Acad Sci. 2002; 966: 343-54.

[122] Holzer P. Local effector functions of capsaicin-sensitive sensory nerve endings: involvement of tachykinins, calcitonin gene-related peptide and other neuropeptides. Neuroscience 1988; 24(3): 739-68.

[123] McCarthy GM, McCarty DJ Effect of topical capsaicin in the therapy of painful osteoarthritis of the hands. J. Rheumatol. 1992; 19: 604-607

4

Intra-Articular Injections for the Treatment of Osteoarthritis: Focus on the Clinical Use of Several Regimens

Dong Rak Kwon and Gi Young Park
Departments of Rehabilitation Medicine, Catholic University of Daegu School of Medicine, Daegu, South Korea

1. Introduction

Osteoarthritis is the most common joint disease, and is characterized by progressive loss of articular cartilage, subchondral bone sclerosis, osteophyte formation, synovial membrane changes, and an increase in synovial fluid with decreased viscosity and lubrication properties. Mechanical, biochemical, and genetic factors are all involved in pathogenesis of osteoarthritis (Chevalier, 2002; Wearing et al., 2006).

Given the chronic and non-life-threatening nature of osteoarthritis, a good safety profile is essential. Characteristics of osteoarthritis vary across patients, and several definite clinical patterns have been identified. The choice of a suitable treatment strategy for a patient depends on clinical history, contraindications to specific therapies, and overall tolerability and acceptability of the considered treatment. This is especially true in the elderly, the major targeted people for osteoarthritis therapy, for whom one must consider the risk of upper gastrointestinal or adverse renal effects and the diverse array of concomitantly used medications. Intra-articular injection into osteoarthritic joints may play an important role in the therapeutic plan. Osteoarthritis of weight-bearing joints, such as knee osteoarthritis, is more a local mechanical driven disease than a generalized one. In order to reach a non-vascularized tissue, such as cartilage, local intra-articular administration of drugs should be considered.

Intra-articular injections are one of the clinician's many tools for treatment of osteoarthritis. Injection should be contemplated as an adjunct to the overall treatment plan-never as the sole component of therapy. Injections may be used diagnostically as well as therapeutically and are generally "safe" when used judiciously by a skilled practitioner.

At this time, no targeted treatments for osteoarthritis have been developed. Therefore, preclinical and clinical research studies using other pharmacologic agents that might provide additional benefit are currently underway. A review of these investigational approaches — hyaluronic acid, recombinant human growth hormone, and platelet rich plasma — will be presented here.

1.1 Rationale for intraarticular injection of osteoarthritis

While some patients present with generalized osteoarthritis, which is thought to be strongly influenced by genetic factors, much of osteoarthritis of weight bearing joints can be regarded as a local disease driven by abnormal mechanical stress.

Osteoarthritis, distinct from many other diseases, is amenable to local intraarticular treatment as well as systemic treatment. Though most efforts so far have concentrated on development of systemic treatments, the agents used bear considerable risk of systemic side effects, such as the cardiovascular events and gastrointestinal adverse effects observed in association with most non-steroidal anti-inflammatory drugs and cyclooxygenase-2 inhibitors for treatment of joint pain (Petit-Zeman, 2004; Topol, 2004). The chronic nature of the disease requires development of drugs suitable for chronic systemic treatment with minimal side effects, which is a challenging goal. Local drug application, i.e., injection of drugs directly into the affected joint, is an option for treatment of osteoarthritis which is already frequently used and has the potential to deliver the desired profile.

In summary, progression of knee osteoarthritis results from local factors, which include synovial membrane inflammation, chondrocyte activation, and bone remodeling. Therefore, it appears logical to favor an intra-articular route for treatment of knee (as well as hip) osteoarthritis.

1.2 Advantages and disadvantages of intraarticular administration compared to systemic administration

The main advantage of intraarticular administration is that the drug reaches the cartilage, which includes no blood vessels, and, therefore, is not exposed to circulating drugs (Gerwin et al., 2006). Drugs given by systemic administration may also penetrate the joint fluid from blood via diffusion through the synovium, particularly in cases of active synovitis, as in rheumatoid arthritis. Because the superficial cartilage is altered in osteoarthritis, drugs present in high concentrations in the joint fluid may be able to penetrate within the cartilage by passive diffusion. However, short residence time due to rapid uptake by circulation imposes a major challenge in intra-articular delivery of solutions and correlates with the severity of synovitis (which accelerates drug clearance) (Gerwin et al., 2006). For instance, most hyaluronic acid preparations remain in the joint for only a few hours (half-life, 17 h) (Brandt et al., 2000). This emphasizes the need for development of sustained-release formulas that support continuous release of the drug from a depot in the joint space over a period of several weeks to months.

In the effort to achieve an increase in drug residence time in the synovial cavity, drug delivery systems may be used. Among them, thermally responsive elastin-like polypeptide gels capable of spontaneous aggregation after intraarticular injection represent a simple and innovative way to prolong the intraarticular half-life of a drug. These aggregating elastin-like polypeptides form a drug-depot, resulting in a 25-fold longer half-life than drugs administered with a non-aggregating protein (Betre et al., 2006). Besides the thermo-gelling approach, which is used to increase the retention time of a drug formulation in the joint, pH-sensitive gels are interesting tools. For instance, an intra-articularly injected sustained-release vehicle, such as gelatin hydrogel microspheres, for platelet rich plasma appeared to stimulate cartilage matrix metabolism, suggesting its potential for use in osteoarthritis treatment (Saito et al., 2009).

Aspiration and injection into the knee or other joints is a common technique for both diagnostic and therapeutic purposes, in spite of practical difficulties, such as the lack of accessibility of the joint, and, thus, obstructed needle placement (Jackson et al., 2002). Although rare, complications of intraarticular injections, such as infection, post-injection flare, crystal-induced synovitis, cutaneous atrophy, and steroid arthropathy (Neustadt,

2001), could result in dramatic side effects. The incidence of septic joints related to local steroid injection is about 1 in 10 000 injections, while for post-injection flare, a frequency of around 2% has been reported. Inappropriate injection technique, inexact needle placement, and blockage of synovial outflow by viscous injections have all been suggested as causative factors for development of acute pseudoseptic arthritis (Chen et al., 2002) Therefore, proper needle placement within the intraarticular joint deserves careful attention.

1.3 Technical consideration of intraarticular administration

Although an intra-articular injection of the knee is not a complex procedure, assessment of whether the tip of the needle lies free in the joint or is embedded in synovium or soft tissue before administration of the preparation of medication could be difficult. Some recent studies have called into question the ability of physicians to accurately localize such injections, finding that almost a third of knee injections are inaccurate (Jones & Doherty, 2003). This finding emphasizes the importance of proper needle placement. Needle placement is easily confirmed when an effusion is present. The return of synovial fluid documents intra-articular placement of the needle. In the absence of an effusion, needle placement requires the use of anatomic landmarks and tactile feed-back to help the operator in positioning of the needle. Prior to performance of an injection, all landmarks for entry into the joints were outlined with a marking pen (Fig. 1.).

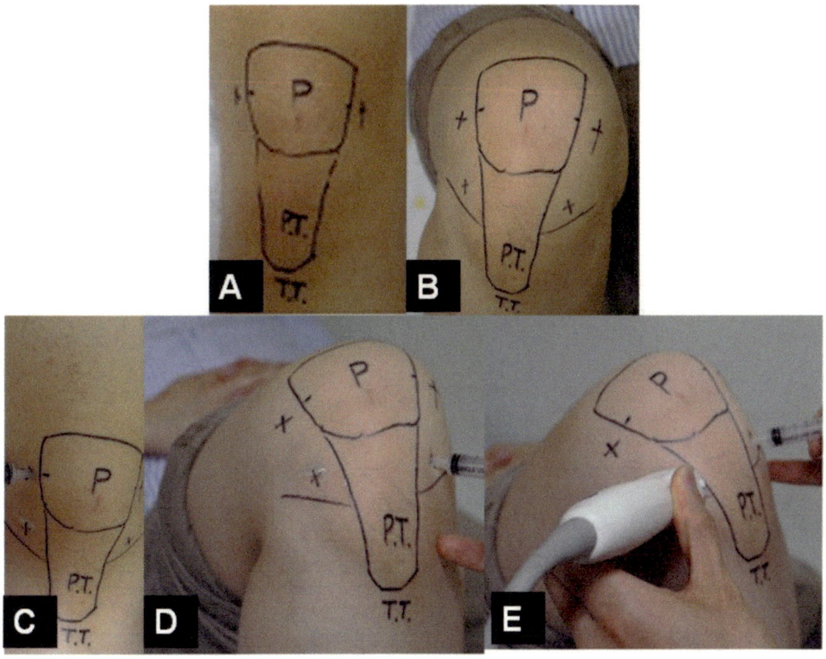

Fig. 1. All landmarks were outlined with a marking pen. A. Landmarks for lateral and medial mid-patellar injections sites. B. Landmarks for anteriomedial and anteriolateral injections sites. C. Lateral mid-patellar injection were performed with the lower limb extended on the examination table. D. Anteriolateral injection were performed with the knee in flexed position. E. Anteriolateral injection via ultrasound guidance were performed with the knee in flexed position.

The operator then stands level with the other knee. With one hand, the patella is pushed up and toward the operator, which causes the lateral/medial edge to become more prominent. Lateral mid-patella and medial mid-patella injections were administered with the lower extremity extended on the examination table. The needle was advanced transversely between the articular surfaces of the patellofemoral joint at the midpoint of the patella. Jackson et al. evaluated the accuracy of needle placement in 80 obese patients undergoing treatment for symptomatic degenerative joint disease (Jackson et al., 2002). They reported difficulty in establishing anatomical landmarks about the knee due to obesity. A large quantity of subcutaneous fat also increases the distance between the skin and the joint space. They used anteromedial, anterolateral, and lateral mid-patella portals. Results of their study demonstrated that injection through the lateral mid-patella approach had an accuracy of 93%. They explained that, when this route is used, the needle passes through a minimal amount of soft tissue in order to reach the intra-articular space; therefore, they recommended use of the lateral mid-patella portal with the knee extended. The extended leg lateral midpatellar approach has been shown to be highly accurate (93%) (Fig. 1.) (Jackson et al., 2002). In patients with severe osteoarthritis, the midpatellar approach may be impractical due to hindrance of the injection pathway by patellofemoral osteophytes (Jackson et al., 2002). To overcome this problem, anteriolateral and anteriomedial injections were performed with the patient's leg hanging over the side of the examination table with the knee flexed to approximately 90 degrees (Fig. 1). On the basis of careful palpation of anatomical landmarks, the injection site was selected inferior to the patella, one finger breadth proximal to the joint surface, and either medial or lateral to the patellar tendon. The needle was directed obliquely toward the intercondylar notch. While accessing the anteriolateral and anteriomedial approach with the patient in the sitting position with the knee bent, these approaches provide only 71-75% accuracy (Neustadt, 2006). Improvement of accuracy has been attempted through use of ultrasound techniques; the operator placed the long axis of the ultrasound transducer over the anteriomedial portion of the knee (Fig. 1.). The modified anteriolateral bent knee approach has been reported to be an effective, accurate, and equivalent alternative to the standard lateral midpatellar approach for intraarticular injection of the knee (Chavez-Chiang et al., 2011). Therefore, any of these approaches might be preferred, depending on the experience of the physician. On the other hand, 100% accuracy could not be obtained through any approach, which should be kept in mind when treating knee problems with intra-articular injections. Injections were administered using a 5 ml syringe, with a 4 cm long needle. Injection and aspiration of the knee is commonly used for both diagnostic and therapeutic purposes. Determination of whether the needle tip lies freely within the joint or is embedded in the synovium or other intra-articular tissues may be difficult. In addition, clinical experience has shown that intra-articular injection is more painful when the tip of the needle is placed in Hoffa's fat pad.

2. Special focus on three intraarticular administration regimens

2.1 Current most available intraarticular injection fromulation for treatment of osteoarthritis: Hyaluronic acid

2.1.1 Basic concept of hyaluronic acid

Hyaluronic acid is a very long polysaccharide chain, consisting of repeating disaccharide units of N-acetyl-glucosamine and glucuronic acid. The average molecular weight of synovial fluid hyaluronic acid is 5 to 7 × 10^6 d, or 12,500 disaccharide units (Balazs &

Denlinger, 1993). Endogenous hyaluronic acid is synthesized by type B synoviocytes and fibroblasts in the synovium and released into the joint space. Hyaluronic acid is a major component of synovial fluid and articular cartilage, and is an important contributor to joint homeostasis (Balazs & Denlinger, 1993). The viscoelasticity and rheology of synovial fluid is due entirely to its hyaluronic acid content.

Hyaluronic acid contributes to the viscous and elastic properties, affording the synovial fluid the peculiar capacity to function differently under distinct loading conditions (Simon, 1999). Viscosity is defined as the ability to dissipate mechanical energy as heat during low shear stress; elasticity is the ability of a molecule to absorb mechanical energy under increased loads. In the presence of low shear forces with slow joint movements, the hyraluronic acid solution exhibits high viscosity with reduced elasticity and acts as a joint lubricant. With increased rates of joint motion (high shear), this is reversed as the synovial fluid becomes more elastic and acts as a shock absorber (Balazs & Denlinger, 1993). The normal adult knee contains approximately 2 mL of synovial fluid, with a hyaluronic acid concentration of 2.5 to 4.0 mg/mL (Watterson & Esdaile, 2000). In patients with osteoarthritis, the concentration and molecular weight of hyaluronic acid in synovial fluid is reduced by a factor of 2 or 3, owing to both degradation and dilution. Furthermore, the molecular weight of the hyaluronate that is present is reduced to as low as 2×10^5 d (Balazs & Denlinger, 1993). These consequences lead to dramatic changes in the viscoelastic properties of the synovial fluid, and, thus, altered joint mechanics. Decreased lubrication leads to increased stress upon the already diseased cartilage, further disrupting the collagen network and the integrity of the chondral surface (Marshall, 2000). Cartilage nutrition and waste removal are also adversely affected. Beyond these mechanical properties, hyaluronic acid has been reported to serve other significant functions within the joint (See Table 1-hyruan injection review). Higher molecular weight hyaluronic acid has been shown to influence a variety of leukocyte functions, including migration, chemotaxis, phagocytosis, adherence, and proliferation. In vitro studies have further demonstrated effects on levels of prostaglandins and cyclic AMP in synovial fluid. In addition to these anti-inflammatory properties, analgesic activity of hyaluronic acid has been demonstrated in both in vitro and animal studies (Ghosh, 1994). This may be mediated both directly via inhibition of nociceptors and indirectly through decrease of synthesis of or binding to bradykinin, substance P, and other hyperalgesic compounds.

Hyaluronic acid may have a chondroprotective effect, inhibiting degradation of cartilage, as well as encouraging its healing and repair. Ghosh (Ghosh, 1994) conducted de novo HA biosynthesis by fibroblasts upon in vitro exposure to exogenous hyaluronic acid. The efficacy of intra-articular injection can be influenced by the concentration and molecular weight of exogenous hyaluronic acid, with molecular weights greater than 5×10^6 being the most effective. Lower molecular weight hyaluronic acid compounds did not elicit a significant biosynthetic response. The author also reported that high molecular weight cross-linked derivatives of hyaluronic acid (hylans) provided a protective effect on chondrocytes exposed to cytokines (IL-1), oxygen-derived free radicals, or leukocyte proteinases. This effect was reversible and viscosity dependant; higher molecular weight hyaluronic acid may yield more superior protection than those with lower molecular weights.

2.1.2 History and development of HA

In the late 1960s, Balazs and coworkers (Balazs & Denlinger, 1993) conducted extensive research into joint fluid rheology and hyaluronic acid, which resulted in definition of the concept of "viscosupplementation". Nearly 2 decades would pass before clinical application was achieved. Original source material for study was derived from both human umbilical cord tissue and rooster combs. Subsequently, the noninflammatory fraction of sodium hyaluronan (NIF-NaHA) was developed for therapeutic use in both joint viscosupplementation and ophthalmic viscosurgery. This product (marketed as Healon or Hyartil-Vet) was subsequently used, with some reported success, for treatment of traumatic joint injury in race horses beginning in 1975 (Marshall, 2000). In the late 1980s, 2 NIF-NaHA products, Artz (Seikagaku, Japan) and Hyalgan (Fidia,Italy), were placed on the market overseas for use in human arthritic joints. Because both formulations were lower in molecular weight, clinical recommendations were for 5 weekly injections. Hylans has been reported to improve viscoelastic properties and increase residual time within the joint, as a function of cross-linking. Two forms, a fluid (hylan A) and a gel (hylan B), were produced. Exogenous hylan A has been demonstrated to remain in the knee joint for approximately 1 week after injection; hylan B may be present for as long as 30 days after injection. Hylan G-F 20 (Synvisc) was the first (and remains the only) commercially available cross-linked hyaluronic acid in the United States. Hylan G-F 20 consists of a combination of the fluid and gel forms at a 4:1 ratio (or 20% gel). Its molecular weight is 6×10^6 d, similar to that of hyaluronic acid in a healthy joint. By comparison, the molecular weight of Hyalgan is significantly less (between 5.0 and 7.3×10^5 d). Viscosupplementation with intra-articular hyaluronic acid was first approved by the Food and Drug Administration in 1997. Several different formulations of hyaluronic acid from diverse sources, and with varying composition and molecular weight, are available in the United States for intra-articular injection. By obtaining approval under the category of a "biologic device," these agents are indicated for treatment of pain in patients with osteoarthritis who have failed to respond to conservative treatment, such as non-pharmacological therapy and simple analgesics. Each of these agents (Table 2) has distinct properties, dosing instructions, cost, and, possibly, clinical outcomes. Viscosupplementation is currently indicated only for treatment of patients with osteoarthritis of the knee. It has been accepted as part of the American College of Rheumatology guidelines for treatment of osteoarthritis and the American Academy of Orthopedic Surgeons guidelines for treatment of osteoarthritis of the knee.

Hyraluronic acid formulations can be obtained by prescription or directly from the clinician's office, and are dispensed in 2 mL vials or 2 mL prefilled syringes. Currently, the recommended injection schedules are 1 injection weekly for 3 weeks for the cross linked higher molecular weight injection, such as hylan G-F 20. All of these products, except for Euflexxa, are contraindicated in patients with a hypersensitivity to poultry. Any knee effusion should be aspirated before injection in order to prevent dilution of the viscosupplement (Vad et al., 2003). Excessive weight-bearing and activity are limited for 48 to 72 hours after each injection. Repeat courses of viscosupplementation are Food and Drug Administration approved, and have generally led to a 6-month interval period between injections (Raynauld et al., 2005)

2.1.3 Safety profile of hyraluronic acid

The safety profile of intra-articular hyaluronans is very favorable, and, because they are used as a local therapy, there are no known drug interactions-an advantage for patients receiving treatment for comorbid conditions. The total incidence of side effects has been reported to be approximately 1% to 4% per injection (Hammesfahr et al., 2003). The most frequent adverse effect is local reaction in the injected knee, including mild pain, swelling, warmth, and/or redness at the site of injection. Such reactions are usually temporary, lasting 1 or 2 days, and generally respond well to physiotherapy and non-steroidal anti-inflammatory drugs. In one large, retrospective review of viscosupplementation with hylan G-F 20 (Synvisc), local adverse reactions developed in 28 of 336 patients, with an overall rate of 2.7% per injection. Incidence of adverse events was found to be significantly affected by the injection technique, with a side effects response rate of 5.2% with a medial approach in a flexed knee, versus 1.7% when injected laterally in extension (Hammesfahr et al., 2003). Adverse reactions may be related more to the accuracy of intra-articular injection than the substance itself. As previously mentioned, injection technique is very important. There is growing evidence that hylan G-F 20 in particular may be associated with an adverse event, which has been termed pseudosepsis, or a severe acute inflammatory reaction (Goldberg & Coutts., 2004). This phenomenon has been associated with cross-linked hyaluroic acid. This clinical entity appears to be distinct from previously described minor local inflammatory reactions uncommonly seen with all hyaluronic acid preparations. Pseudosepsis presents as a severe inflammatory process of the joint, with a large effusion, and significant pain occurring within 1 to 3 days of injection. Differential diagnosis is requested from true sepsis or inflammatory arthritis, requiring synovial aspiration and examination. Aspirates of patients with pseudosepsis typically show a moderate cell count with high numbers of mononuclear cells (eosinophils, neutrophils, and macrophages), and the absence of organisms or calcium pyrophosphate crystals.

Pseudosepsis characteristically occurs after previous injection, such as upon receiving the second or third injection in the first course. One report documented a 10-fold increase in the rate of reactions in patients

undergoing a repeat course of hylan G-F 20 viscosupplementation (Leopold et al., 2002). As a result, some authors have supposed an immunologic etiology for this process (Leopold et al., 2002). However, in a recent prospective study comparing aspirates from 16 patients who presented with a severe acute inflammatory reaction after Synvisc treatment with 20 aspirates from control patients with osteoarthritis, analysis was notably more consistent with a type 4 (cell-mediated) hypersensitivity reaction than with an antibody-mediated reaction (Marino et al., 2006). The frequent presence of eosinophils further supports these findings. To date, sodium hyaluronates (Hyalgan, etc) have not been reported to trigger this process, suggesting a link between pseudosepsis and chemical cross-linking modification of the hyaluronic acid molecule in hylan synthesis (Synvisc). Pseudosepsis requires symptomatic treatment, including use of modalities, activity modification, analgesics, and non-steroidal anti-inflammatory drugs. Arthrocentesis is recommended in order to rule out sepsis, and can be helpful in palliation. Once infection has been excluded, intra-articular steroids may be of value (Goldberg & Coutts., 2004).

2.1.4 Preclinical studies

Chondroprotective effects of hyaluronic acid were observed in vitro, e.g., that it stimulates production of tissue inhibitors of matrix metalloproteinases by chondrocytes, inhibits neutrophil-mediated cartilage degradation, and attenuates interleukin-1 induced matrix degeneration and chondrocyte cytotoxicity (Brockmeier & Shaffer, 2006). In several studies hyaluronic acid was found to enhance prostaglandin synthesis and to decrease prostaglandin breakdown and release from cartilage matrix (Moreland, 2003). In addition, it was shown to normalize endogenous hyaluronic acid synthesis by synoviocytes (Vuorio et al., 1982).

There has been considerable controversy with regard to whether hyaluronic acid has structure-modifying effects. A number of animal models have been conducted for experimental induction of changes associated with osteoarthritis, such as degradation of collagen and proteoglycans of articular cartilage, and increased inflammation. The most commonly studied models have been total or partial meniscectomy and anterior cruciate ligament transection; it should be noted that these models are quite aggressive in that degenerative changes can occur within a few months after induction. Using these approaches, potential structure-modifying activities of exogenously added hyaluronic acid have been demonstrated in several species. Wiig et al. (Wiig et al., 1990) reported that administration of a single injection of Healon_(sodium hyaluronate, MW 1900 - 3900 kDa) (Pharmacia & Upjohn, Uppsala, Sweden) immediately after anterior cruciate ligament transection in rabbits resulted in significantly decreased inflammation, increased collagen synthesis, increased angiogenesis, and enhanced tissue repair, compared with a single injection of saline.

The structure-modifying effects of hyaluronic acid have been investigated using a meniscectomy model in rabbits and sheep. Injection of Artz (Supartz, sodium hyaluronate, MW 620 - 1170 kDa) after partial meniscectomy in rabbits or sheep resulted in significantly inhibited cartilage degeneration (Kikuchi et al., 1996; Armstrong et al., 1994). Five weekly intraarticular injections of sodium hyaluronate, initiated immediately after partial or total meniscectomy, resulted in significantly enhanced collagen remodeling, compared with saline injections (Sonoda et al., 1997, 2000). A course of 5 weekly injections of Artz (Supartz, sodium hyaluronate, MW 620 - 1170 kDa) was found to protect chondrocytes from apoptotic cell death following anterior cruciate ligament transection in a rabbit model (Takahashi et al, 2000).

Following administration to either rabbits or dogs after anterior cruciate ligament transaction, Artz (Supartz, sodium hyaluronate, MW 620 - 1170 kDa) was also found to decrease the degree of damage to femoral cartilage and aided in preservation of articular cartilage and integrity of synovial tissue (Yoshioka et al., 1997; Shimizu et al., 1998).

In a study for evaluation of the effects of Synvisc (hylan G-F 20, MW >6000 kDa) (Biomatrix, Montreal, Canada) in a dog anterior cruciate ligament transection model, gross morphological and histological damage within joints that received injections was significantly milder than that seen in control joints (Marshall et al., 2000). Similar results were obtained in rabbits and dogs using Hyalgan (sodium hyaluronate, MW 500 - 730 kDa). A course of 5 weekly Hyalgan injections, starting at 4 or 13 weeks after anterior cruciate ligament transection, resulted in a significantly reduced degree of articular degeneration at evaluations performed 26 weeks after surgery. In this study, rabbits who received 10 injections showed less disease progression than did rabbits treated with five injections, suggesting that a sequential course of Hyalgan therapy may provide long-term benefits for altering the disease course (Amiel et al., 2003). In dogs, initiation of weekly IA injections of sodium hyaluronate starting at 3, 6, or 12 weeks after anterior cruciate ligament transection (the Pond-Nuki model of osteoarthritis) resulted in significantly inhibited formation of a fibroblast-like cell layer on the articular cartilage and increased mean chondrocyte density and area in the middle and deep layer of the articular cartilage (Schiavinato et al., 1989). When given starting at 3, 6, or 12 weeks after anterior cruciate ligament transection in dogs, Hyalartz (sodium hyaluronate, MW 500 - 750 kDa) was found to induce a significant reduction in cartilaginous lesions (Pond-Nuki model of osteoarthritis) (Wenz et al., 2000).

On the other hand, injection of hyaluronic acid into sheep joints subjected to meniscectomy resulted in significantly more extensive osteophytosis and cartilage fibrillation and reduction in proteoglycan synthesis. A striking reduction in proteoglycan concentration in cartilage was also observed in dogs with anterior cruciate ligament transection who received prophylactic treatment with a series of hyaluronic acid injections. These findings raised concerns that hyaluronic acid treatment could aggravate joint damage in osteoarthritis. Safety and efficacy of intraarticular hyaluronic acid for treatment of pain of osteoarthritis of the knee have been demonstrated; preliminary work supports use of hyarluronic acid for osteoarthritis pain relief in other joints as well. Based on preclinical data, there is evidence to support the notion that all hyaluronic acids approved in the US may have some structure-modifying characteristics. Work in these areas is ongoing.

2.1.5 Clinical studies

The first human clinical trial of intra-articular hyaluronic acid for treatment of arthritis was published by Peyron and Balazs in 1974.

A large number of clinical trials have been conducted with different hyaluronic acid preparations, several of which involve large, multicenter, blinded, randomized, placebo-controlled studies. Early clinical trials attempted to establish the clinical safety of intra-articular hyaluronic acid and its clinical superiority in comparison with placebo (Table 2). Some of these studies have provided evidence that hyaluronic acid preparations are more effective than placebo in reducing pain associated with osteoarthritis (Dixon et al., 1988; Dougados et al., 1993) In contrast, others were unable to demonstrate any significant difference when compared with placebo groups (Henderson et al., 1993; Dahlberg et al., 1994).

Recent attention has focused on comparison of intra-articular viscosupplementation with other osteoarthritis treatment methods (such as oral anti-inflammatories and intra-articular steroid injections). In a multicenter trial in Canada, Adams et al compared the 3 treatment arms: oral non-steroidal anti-inflammatory drugs alone, hylan G-F 20 treatment (3 weekly injections), and combined oral non-steroidal anti-inflammatory drugs and hylan G-F 20 treatment. Patients took their "usual" non-steroidal anti-inflammatory drugs in the appropriate arms. At 12 weeks, all 3 of the groups showed improvement, but no statistical difference was observed between groups. However, at the 26-week time point, both the hylan G-F 20 only and combined non-steroidal anti-inflammatory drugs and hylan G-F 20 groups were statistically superior to the non-steroidal anti-inflammatory drugs only group (Adams et al., 1995). In another large, prospective study, Altman et al compared 5 weekly injections of sodium hyaluronate with a placebo group and with a group of patients treated with oral Naproxen. On the basis of visual analog scores and the Western Ontario and McMaster University Osteoarthritis Index, the hyaluronate group was found to be superior to the placebo group at 26 weeks. The hyaluronic acid group also tended to show improved outcomes, compared with the non-steroidal anti-inflammatory drugs group; however, this finding did not show statistical significance (Altman et al., 1998). Three recent prospective studies have been conducted for comparison of intra-articular hyaluronic acid to intra-articular corticosteroids. In 1 randomized, blinded comparative trial, 63 patients were stratified to receive 5 weekly injections of sodium hyaluronate or 1 injection of triamcinolone followed by 4 placebo injections. Patients were followed for 6 months with VAS assessments of pain with trends suggesting some benefit of viscosupplementation over intra-articular steroids. However, due to a high drop-out rate, the findings were not statistically significant (Jones et al,, 1995). Leopold et al conducted a prospective comparison of 2 cohorts of patients with knee osteoarthritis. Patients in the first group received 3 weekly injections with hylan G-F 20, whereas those in the second group received 1 injection of intra-articular betamethasone, and were able to request 1 additional corticosteroid injection if needed, over the course of the study. Although both groups showed improvement, at 6 months, no significant difference was noted between the 2 cohorts with respect to WOMAC scores, VAS, or the Knee Society Scoring System (Leopold et al., 2003). In a more recent report from the Synvisc 901 study group, Caborn et al used the Western Ontario and McMaster University Osteoarthritis Index and Visual analogue scores pain scores to compare the 2 groups of patients who received either 3 weekly injections of hylan G-F 20 or 1 isolated injection of triamcinolone. This study was not blinded. In their study, maximal benefit was noted at week 2 for the steroid group and at week 12 for the hylan G-F 20 group. From week 12 through week 26, significantly superior outcomes were observed in patients treated with hylan G-F 20 when compared with those treated with intra-articular steroids (Caborn et al., 2004).

In the most recent meta-analysis from the Cochrane database, one research study obtained 76 randomized placebo-controlled trials that fulfilled strict study design and methodology criteria. On the basis of their analysis of the literature, the authors concluded that viscosupplementation is an effective treatment for osteoarthritis of the knee, with favorable effects on pain, function, and patient global assessment, particularly during weeks 5 to 13 after the injection period (Bellamy et al., 2006).

Conservative treatments for osteoarthritis may be characterized as symptom-modifying or disease-modifying drugs. As defined by the Osteoarthritis Research Society, disease-modifying drugs are those that are intended to prevent, retard, stabilize, or reverse development of morphological changes of osteoarthritis (Altman et al., 1996). At present, no pharmacological treatments for osteoarthritis have been approved for the indication of modifying the rate of osteoarthritis disease progression. Intra-articular hyaluronic acid is currently indicated only as a symptom-modifying treatment for osteoarthritis of the knee.

However, evaluation of novel agents and agents with established symptom-modifying activity for disease-modifying effects has become a major focus of research on osteoarthritis. In an effort to obtain evidence for disease-modifying efficacy of hyaluronic acid injections, a large number of clinical trials have been conducted with different hyaluronic acid preparations over the past 25 years. However, there is substantial evidence to suggest that hyaluronic acid in certain patient populations can also have disease modifying activity. This possibility was initially suggested by the finding that the pain-relieving benefit of intraarticular hyaluronic acid generally persists for considerably longer than its half-life within the injected joint, which has been estimated in animal studies to be as short as 18 to 24 h (Sakamoto et al., 1984). For example, clinical efficacy in randomized, controlled trials has been demonstrated to last for at least 26 weeks for Hyalgan®(sodium hyaluronate, average molecular weight 500 -730 kDa) (Altman et al., 1998) and may last as long as a year or more in some patients (Kotz & Kolarz, 1999). Similarly, Synvisc_ (hylan G-F 20, average MW >6000 kDa) (Wobig et al., 1998) (Genzyme Biosurgery, Cambridge, MA), and Supartz® (sodium hyaluronate, average MW 630 - 1120 kDa) (Puhl et al., 1993) (Seikagaku Corporation, Tokyo, Japan) have also demonstrated months of pain relief. Although many of these studies were well designed, the results are difficult to interpret due to a number of

factors. A number of these studies used highly subjective, non-validated rating scales. Different formulations and treatment regimens were often used, limiting study comparisons. Patient treatment groups were often heterogenous, leading to stratified outcomes based on characteristics such as age and disease severity.
The ideal candidate for intra-articular hyaluronic acid has yet to be clearly defined. Despite clinical evaluations, age, symptoms, and disease severity have not proven helpful in identifying patients who may best benefit. One early placebo-controlled trial indicated increased benefit among older patients with more significant osteoarthritis. (Lohmander et al., 1996)
In another study, Dahlberg et al evaluated a group of patients with normal radiographs and early arthritic changes observed at arthroscopy. They reported no significant benefit from 5 weekly injections of sodium hyaluronate (compared with placebo) (Dahlberg et al., 1994). Despite failure to identify the optimal cohort, there is reason to believe that the greatest potential benefit of hyaluronic acid would likely be among younger patients, as some clinical data have suggested that younger patients are more likely to respond. In a meta-analysis by Wang et al, 35 patients older than 65 years of age and those with the most advanced stages of arthritic change (ie, complete loss of joint space) were found to be less likely to show improvement with hyaluronic acid therapy. Jubb et al., in a large, randomized study for evaluation of the disease-modifying effects of sodium hyaluronate in knee osteoarthritis, demonstrated that viscosupplementation, compared with placebo, significantly reduced the radiographic progression of joint space loss in the subset of patients with a higher joint space area at study entry. Currently, intra-articular hyaluronic acid therapy should be considered in patients who have failed standard non-pharmacologic and pharmacologic treatment options, those who have a contraindication to non-steroidal anti-inflammatory drugs, and those who are trying to delay or are poor candidates for surgical treatment. (Jubb et al., 2003)

2.2 Candidate drugs for disease-modifying intraarticular injection regimens

Metabolism of mature articular cartilage is regulated by a number of growth factors that are delivered from cellular production within the cartilage, as well as from the synovial fluid and surrounding tissues. As the mechanisms of action for these growth factors are obtained through well-defined in vitro studies, it is becoming clear that growth factors may eventually serve to augment current cartilage repair techniques.
Chemotactic growth factors may be used to encourage cell migration to an injury site. Cell numbers can be increased and matrix production up-regulated by release of appropriate local growth factors via scaffolds or other methods of intra-articular administration.
Growth factors are a group of biologically active polypeptides produced by the body, which can stimulate cellulardivision, growth, and differentiation. In articular cartilage, numerous growth factors work in concert to regulate development and homeostasis of articular cartilage throughout life (Goldring et al., 2009). Therefore, growth factors offer promising treatments for enhanced regeneration of cartilage in situations of widespread cartilage loss, such as those that occur in osteoarthritis. When considering an osteoarthritic joint, the effects of any treatment, such as growth factors, on cartilage, synovial lining, ligaments, tendons, meniscus, any exposed subchondral bone, as well as on mesenchymal stem cells that gain access to the articular environment should be collectively considered. Numerous anabolic growth factors stimulate chondrocyte synthesis of proteoglycans, aggrecan, and

type II collagen, induce synoviocyte and mesenchymal stem cell proliferation, drive chondrogenic differentiation of mesenchymal stem cells, and decrease the catabolic effects of cytokines, such as interleukin-1 and matrix metalloproteinases. In addition to being proanabolic and anticatabolic to restoration of cartilage in naturally occurring disease, an ideal growth factor for general cartilage tissue engineering or regeneration in osteoarthritis would be effective regardless of the patient's age or the presence of osteoarthritis and would have no detrimental effects on either cartilage or the synovial lining.

Historically, most growth factors have been evaluated on an independent basis, rather than in combination, in order to assess their effects on cartilage homeostasis in vitro or in vivo. Given the array and interactions of growth factors necessary for proper cartilage development and homeostasis, it is unlikely that any single growth factor will lead to complete cartilage repair or affect the arthritic milieu, but rather a combination approach will be required.

In the following review, some key players are portrayed comprehensively. Obviously, the collected insights indicate a major potential for regulation of cartilage and chondrocytes in disease and regeneration within the organism and in tissue engineering if the structural properties and dynamics of natural hormone activity are carefully considered. Individual characteristics of growth factors are described.

Transforming Growth Factor-b1 stimulates chondrocyte synthetic activity and decreases the catabolic activity of interleukin-1 (Blaney et al., 2007). In vitro, Transforming Growth Factor-b1 stimulates chondrogenesis of synovial lining and bone marrow-derived mesenchymal stem cells (Fan et al., 2010; Kurth et al., 2007). In addition, promising studies in rabbits have demonstrated Transforming Growth Factor-b1-enhanced repair of cartilage defects (Diao et al., 2009). However, in mouse and rabbit animal studies, numerous deleterious side effects of Transforming Growth Factor-b1 supplementation have been announced, including stimulation of synovial proliferation and fibrosis, attraction of inflammatory leukocytes to the synovial lining, and induction of osteophyte formation (Bakker et al., 2001; Blaney et al., 2007). Given these serious safety concerns, which are not components of other growth factor-based strategies, Transforming Growth Factor-b1 therapy is not presently a suitable option for use in the articular environment.

Insulin like growth factor is a circulating cytokine that reaches articular cartilage through the synovial fluid. Insulin like growth factor is a single polypeptide with protein sequencing similar to that of insulin. Insulin like growth factor -1 is the main anabolic growth factor for articular cartilage.

It plays a key role in cartilage homeostasis, balancing proteoglycan synthesis and breakdown by chondrocytes. In vitro studies have demonstrated that Insulin like growth factor -1 stimulates proteoglycan production in a dose-dependent manner, as evidenced by increased [35S]-sulfate incorporation (Coutts et al., 1997). Similarly, Insulin like growth factor -1 has been shown to slow proteoglycan catabolism in a dose-dependent fashion (Hickey et al., 2003).

The role of Insulin like growth factor -I in articular cartilage metabolism in both health and disease has been extensively evaluated (Denko et al., 1994; MaQuillan et al., 1986; Middleton et al., 1996; Posever et al., 1995; Wang et al., 1995). When added exogenously to monolayer or explant cultures of normal articular cartilage from a variety of species, Insulin like growth factor-I induces a plethora of anabolic effects and decreases catabolic responses (Sah et al., 2008; Schalkwijk et al., 1989; Tyler 1989). Chondrogenic differentiation of mesnechymal stem cells is induced by Insulin like growth factor-I, but is enhanced when Insulin like growth factor -I and Transforming Growth Factor-b1 are used in combination (Longobardi et al., 2006; Worster et al., 2001). The premise that Insulin like growth factor-I is required for maintenance of articular cartilage integrity is supported by an in vivo study in rats in which chronic Insulin like growth factor-I deficiency led to development of articular cartilage lesions (Ekenstedt et al., 2006). In animal models, Insulin like growth factor-I has led to enhanced repair of extensive cartilage defects and protection of the synovial membrane from chronic inflammation (Fortier & Miller, 2006; Goodrich et al., 2007). However, studies of human articular cartilage indicate that serum Insulin like growth factor-1 levels and chondrocyte responsiveness to Insulin like growth factor-1 diminish progressively with age (Ashton & Matheson, 1979; Boehm et al., 2007; Fortier & Miller, 2006; Loeser et al., 2002; Loeser et al., 2000; Martin et al., 1997; Trippel, 1995) This finding suggests that a simultaneous decrease in the amount of Insulin like growth factor-1 available and a reduced ability of cells to respond to the remaining Insulin like growth factor may produce cartilage that is less capable of maintaining its structural and functional integrity. Insulin like growth factor non-responsiveness has been further observed to exist in chondrocytes from arthritic cartilage or in the presence of inflammation (Verschure et al., 1996). The cellular response to Insulin like growth factor-1 is receptor mediated and Insulin like growth factor binding proteins in synovial fluid appear to regulate the amount of free Insulin like growth factor-1 available for receptor binding (Trippel, 1995).

Age-related decline in the responsiveness of chondrocytes to Insulin like growth factor-1 appears to be due at least in part to overexpression of Insulin like growth factor binding proteins. Chondrocytes from patients with osteoarthritis have been observed to generate excessive levels of Insulin like growth factor-1 binding proteins (Martin et al., 1997; van den Berg et al., 1999). It has also been suggested that a defect in Insulin like growth factor receptor binding or postreceptor signaling may contribute to Insulin like growth factor non-responsiveness in aged and arthritic cartilage (Verschure et al., 1996; coutts et al., 2003; Hickey et al., 2003).

Evidence suggests an uncoupling of Insulin like growth factor-I responsiveness in osteoarthritis with Insulin like growth factor-I having the ability for robust simulation of matrix synthesis with an inability to decrease matrix catabolism (Morales, 2008). Despite the diminished ability of Insulin like growth factor-I to decrease catabolism in aged and osteoarthritis cartilage, studies have suggested that a combination of Insulin like growth factor-I and bone morphogenetic protein-7 results in greater potential for repair than either growth factor alone (Chubinskaya et al., 2007; Loeser et al., 2003). These studies demonstrated that, in general, bone morphogenetic protein-7 was more potent than Insulin like growth factor-I in stimulating matrix synthesis in aged and osteoarthritis cells; however, the greatest increase in matrix synthesis was observed after combination treatment with bone morphogenetic protein-7 and Insulin like growth factor-I.

Platelet-derived growth factor is a locally produced and locally acting growth factor. It is synthesized by smooth muscle cells, fibroblasts, endothelial cells, and macrophages and is stored primarily in platelets (Lee, 2000).

Platelet-derived growth factor plays a fundamental role in the wound healing cascade. It is present in high concentrations in platelets and in fluids generated during the early stage of wound healing (Spindler et al., 1995). Platelet-derived growth factor is a potent mitogenic and chemotactic factor for cells of mesenchymal origin, including fibroblasts, osteoblasts, and chondrocytes, and is thus believed to be capable of enhancing tissue regeneration and repair. Platelet-derived growth factor receptors have been identified on a number of cell types, including chondrocytes, and the number of receptors is up-regulated by the presence of inflammatory cytokines, such as interleukin-1 (Smith et al., 1991).

Indirect evidence for the role of Platelet-derived growth factor and other growth factors active in the wound healing process can be seen from the healing response in cartilage defects treated with microfracture. This procedure involves creation of microperforations in subchondral bone with an arthroscopic awl in and around a chondral lesion (Steadman et al., 2001). The mechanical integrity of the bone is maintained through careful placement of holes. The awl is driven to a depth of 2-4 mm to ensure that the marrow space is accessed and bleeding is observed. A clot forms in the defect, which is anchored to the bone by the increased surface roughness produced by the microperforations. Growth factors such as Platelet-derived growth factor are released into the defect site, exerting chemotactic and mitogenic effects on cells in the surrounding cartilage and infiltrating mesenchymal stem cells. This provides an enriched environment for new tissue formation, which may be augmented by placement of a scaffold seeded with autologous cells (Breinan et al., 2000; Dorotka et al., 2005).

Platelet-derived growth factor exists as a homodimer (Platelet-derived growth factor-AA or Platelet-derived growth factor-BB) or a heterodimer (Platelet-derived growth factor-AB). Evidence to support the use of Platelet-derived growth factor in cartilage repair has been extrapolated from the role of Platelet-derived growth factor in wound healing or stimulation of matrix synthesis in growth plate chondrocytes (Schmidt et al., 2006). In vivo, when injected into the knee of skeletally immature rats, no adverse effects were noted in the cartilage or synovial membrane (Hulth et al., 1996). Presently, the most commonly used form of Platelet-derived growth factor is within the milieu of platelet-rich plasma, as discussed subsequently.

2.2.1 Growth hormone

Growth and homeostasis of cartilage tissue, particularly chondrocytes, during embryogenesis, postnatal development, and adulthood is governed by a significant number of humoral factors. Those factors may also be used during intrinsic or artificial repair and induced regeneration. Unfortunately, many of them also appear to accompany degenerative disease processes, such as osteoarthritis, and the question remains as to what extent they are involved in disease processes or whether they are actually a signature of ongoing endogenous repair pathways (Gaissmaier et al., 2008).

Paracrine components can be delivered through typical nutrient supply mechanisms, ie, fluid flow under compressive loading, which also delivers blood based hormones, such as insulin and cytokines. Alternatively, certain elements are retained in the extracellular matrix, including Insulin-like growth factor Insulin like growth factor-1 and Insulin like growth factor-binding proteins, or ions, like potassium, which is the major counter ion for sulfate residues on glycosaminoglycans, and calcium (which is stored in mineralized cartilage) bound in part to matrix vesicles and chondrocalcin (collagen type II C-propeptide) (Gaissmaier et al., 2008). The insulin-like growth factor signaling axis is involved in maintenance of matrix metabolism in articular cartilage (McQuillan et al., 1986) A demise in metabolic control of cartilage matrix content is the hallmark of degenerative osteoarthritis (Mankin et al., 2000).

Growth hormone is an important regulator of skeletal growth and bone mineral density. It also stimulates cartilage growth, probably through local and systemic Insulin like growth factor-1 production, and possibly by direct stimulation of cartilage cell proliferation. Circulating Growth hormone or one of its mediators may accelerate healing of osteochondral defects through stimulation of osseous and chondral tissue formation (Adam et al., 1995).

Until recently, the effect of exogenous Growth hormone administration in the process of skeletal repair has remained controversial. Bak *et al.* studied 36 rats with closed diaphyseal tibial fractures with intramedullary nailing. In this study, all rats received subcutaneous injections of recombinant human Growth hormone (1 mg) twice per day. Significant improvement in maximal stiffness and ultimate load-bearing were observed during evaluation performed after 40 days of healing (Bak et al., 1990). Kolbeck *et al.* studied 23 dogs with experimentally-induced 3 cm ulnar bone defects and intramedullary fixation. Dogs were injected with recombinant bovine Growth hormone (1 mg), and several of these Growth hormone -treated dogs showed closure of these bone defects, while the remainder demonstrated healing. They reported that administration of homologous Growth hormone stimulates callus formation and ossification in the early phase of bone healing, which consequently results in increased mechanical strength and stiffness (Kolbeck et al., 2003). On the contrary, Growth hormone administration showed no measurable effects on fracture healing in a standardized tibia osteotomy rabbit model (Carpenter et al., 1992).

Morphoangiogenesis was initially identified in the knees of adult rabbits undergoing intra-articular Growth hormone injections for articulophyseal cartilage regeneration (Dunn, 2002). In this experiment, the regeneration cascade resulted in transformation of central arteries in subchondral osteones into tortuous, thin-walled fenestrated capillary structures containing erythrocytes, histiocytes, stem cells, and chondrocytes. This morphoangiogenesis might promote generative and constructive action in joints. The exact mechanisms of intra-articular growth hormone are unclear; however, synovial fluid growth hormone could enhance proliferation, matrix synthesis, and differentiation of bone and cartilage cells *in vitro* (Goldspink & Goldberg, 1975).

Kim et al. conducted a study of 30 rabbits with collagenase-induced osteoarthritis. After intra-articular collagenase injection, mature New Zealand white rabbits (n=30) were divided into 3 groups. Group 1 (control rabbits) received once-weekly intra-articular saline injections for 4 weeks. Group 2 rabbits received 6 mg hyaluronic acid injections, and group 3 rabbits were injected with 6 mg hyaluronic acid and 3 mg recombinant human growth hormone. These injections were initiated 4 weeks after collagenase injections. Lameness was observed for 9 weeks after collagenase injections. Macroscopic and histopathological knee joint findings were also evaluated at the end of 9 weeks after collagenase injections. Although all animals had lameness after collagenase injections, the duration and severity of lameness were significantly shorter and less severe in group 3 than in groups 1 and 2 ($P<0.01$) (Fig. 2.) Macroscopic scores showed that femoral condyles of group 3 rabbits received significantly less cartilage damage than those of rabbits in groups 1 and 2 ($P<0.01$) (Fig. 2.) Histopathological score was also the lowest in group 3 ($P<0.01$) (Fig. 2.)

They reported that co-injection of intra-articular HA and recombinant human growth hormone may be more effective than hyaluronic acid injections alone in an osteoarthritis model. Novel combined therapy of hyaluronic acid with chondrocyte protective functions and recombinant human growth hormone with generative and constructive actions in osteoarthritis-affected joints may be a promising treatment option for osteoarthritis (Kim et al., 2011). The recombinant human growth hormone used in this study is a sustained-release formula, which induced continuous serum Insulin like growth factor-1 elevation for 6 days after a single injection. This product also exhibited greater than 95% bioavailability. Sustained release growth hormone was used in this study. Previously-marketed daily injections have provided distinct peaks and troughs of growth hormone concentrations over a period of 24 hours. The pharmacokinetic profile of recombinant Growth hormone differs from that of normal physiologic growth hormone, with distinct bursts (Laursen et al., 1995). Using poly lactic glycolic acid microparticles for the first time, Genentech and Alkermes developed the Nutropin Depot® as a sustained-release human growth hormone formulation. Nutropin Depot® appeared to achieve stable therapeutic Insulin like growth factor-1 target levels for at least 14 days with higher efficacy and without supraphysiological growth hormone concentrations at all times. Nutropin Depot® required the fewest number of injections for achievement of growth hormone levels within the target range, and appealed to patients in its convenience and compliance. However, the poly lactic glycolic acid particle size of microspheres was too large for efficient suspension in an injection medium. Therefore, injections through a 21 to 23 gauge are inevitable. Complexities with a long-acting protein delivery system using poly lactic glycolic acid include inflammation and protein denaturation by hydrophobic interactions and harsh acidic microenvironments. These complexities decrease the bioavailability of Nutropin Depot® (Fu et al., 2000). However, recombinant human growth hormone in medium chain triglycerides can be easily injected through a 26 to 27 gauge needle due to the small particle size and localized lecithin on the microparticle surfaces.

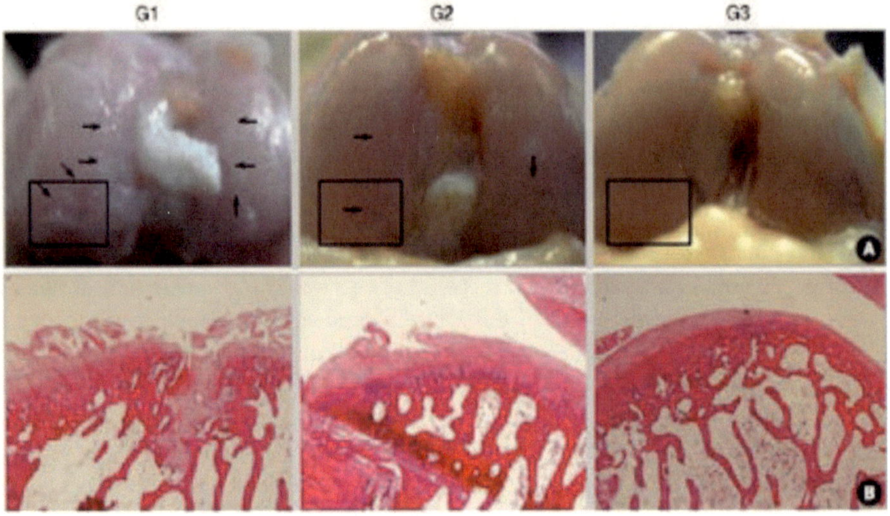

Fig. 2. (A) Gross findings of the femoral condyles in Group 1 (G1), Group 2 (2), and Group 3 (3) rabbits. (B) histologic findings of axial sections obtained at the rectangular areas shown in column A photographs (H&E staining, × 40). The loss of cartilage is seen on the femoral condyle (black arrows). (From Kim SB, Kwon DR, Kwak H, Shin YB, Han HJ, Lee JH, Choi SH. Additive effects of intra-articular injection of growth hormone and hyaluronic acid in rabbit model of collagenase-induced osteoarthritis. J Korean Med Sci. 2010 May;25(5):776-780; with permission.)

Lis evaluated diagnostic usefulness of Insulin like growth factor-1 and human growth hormone serum level in osteoarthritis. Twenty five patients with coxarthrosis and 16 healthy persons were enrolled for measurement of Insulin like growth factor-1 and human growth hormone concentration in serum. Insulin like growth factor-1 and human growth hormone serum level were assayed by enzyme-linked immunosorbent assay. No significant correlation was observed between human growth hormone and Insulin like growth factor-1 in serum. Insulin like growth factor-1 concentration in patient serum was found to be significantly lower than that in the control group. They reported that serum concentration of Insulin like growth factor-1 appears to be a useful laboratory marker of osteoarthritis (Lis, 2008).

As previously mentioned, studies of human articular cartilage indicate that serum Insulin like growth factor-1 levels and chondrocyte responsiveness to Insulin like growth factor-1 diminish progressively with age (Ashton & Matheson, 1979; Boehm et al., 2007; Fortier & Miller, 2006; Loeser et al., 2002; Loeser et al., 2000; Martin et al., 1997; Trippel, 1995) This suggests that a simultaneous decrease in the amount of Insulin like growth factor-1 available and a reduced ability for cells to respond to the remaining Insulin like growth factor may cause cartilage to be less capable of maintaining its structural and functional integrity. Insulin like growth factor non-responsiveness has been further observed to exist in chondrocytes from arthritic cartilage or in the presence of inflammation (Verschure et al., 1996). Growth hormone stimulates cartilage growth, probably through production of local and systemic Insulin like growth factor-1.

Recombinant human growth hormone is produced in laboratories. Several well known pharmaceutical companies manufacture recombinant human growth hormone. Recombinant human growth hormone is pure and free of all viruses. Recombinant human growth hormone has been manufactured for several years and is approved by the Food and Drug Administration for several uses, such as inducing growth of short children to a normal size. However, it has not yet been approved by the Food and Drug Administration for injection in joints, which is an "off-label" use. There is interest in the use of growth hormone as a potential osteoarthritis disease-modifying treatment; however, few studies of its effects in humans have been conducted.

2.3 Platelet Rich Plasma (PRP)

2.3.1 Basic science of PRP

Platelets were thought to act solely in the clotting cascade. In addition to local hemostasis at sites of vascular injury, platelets contain an abundance of growth factors and cytokines that are crucial in soft tissue healing and bone mineralization (Anitua et al., 2006). Besides, we know that platelets also discharge many bioactive proteins responsible for attracting macrophages, mesenchymal stem cells, and osteoblasts, which not only promote scavenging of necrotic tissue but also facilitate tissue regeneration and healing (Sampson, 2008). The concept that application of PRP would result in improvement of cartilage repair is based on the physiological role of platelets in wound healing (Nurden et al., 2008). Platelet rich plasma is composed of 3-8 times the concentration of platelets contained in whole blood; therefore, it contains a hyperphysiological content of autologous growth factors. Of note, a universally accepted definition of platelet rich plasma in terms of concentration does not exist. Giusti et al., postulated that the most efficacious concentration of platelets for stimulation of angiogenesis in vitro was 1.5×10^6 platelets/L. In an adult, the normal platelet count is approximately 150,000-450,000 platelets/L. (Giusti et al., 2009) There are classification schemes that categorize platelet concentrates based on relative concentrations of platelets, leucocytes, and fibrin, and, although it is important to recognize and understand that there are obvious differences between types of platelet concentrates that are being used, the general term/abbreviation, PRP, is used herein (Dohan Ehrenfest et al., 2009). Several centrifuge devices (harvest SmartPReP APC+TM, Huons®sPRP etc) are commercially available for use in physicians' offices. These devices achieve varying concentrations, with whole blood-to-platelet ratios ranging from 1:2 to 1:8. The ratio of white blood cell content also varies with the device. Obviously, the ratio of plasma to platelets in autologous blood is 1:1. Due to a lack of high-quality studies, the ideal ratio of plasma to platelets and the ideal amount of white blood cell concentrate is not well established at this time.

In response to tissue injury, clots rich in platelets and fibrin form a scaffold for subsequent healing. There are over 1500 proteins within platelets, and, among them, are growth factors stored in platelets as granules, which are known to play important roles in the normal healing response, including Platelet-derived growth factor, vascular endothelial growth factor, transforming growth factor-b, fibroblast growth factor, and epidermal growth factor (Qureshi et al., 2009). Through modulation of the inflammatory response, promotion of local angiogenesis, attraction of fibroblasts and local stem cells to the site of injury, and induction of autocrine growth factor production by uninjured adjacent cells, platelets and their products are instrumental in repair and regeneration of normal tissue.

In addition to the growth factors mentioned, there are several others that have been evaluated for their role in chondrogenesis, and it could be concluded that these factors will therefore be important during cartilage regeneration or repair. Clearly, numerous growth factors are needed for proper sequencing of chondrogenesis, and it is likely that more than a single growth factor will be needed for achievement of hyaline cartilage tissue in a reparative procedure. It is becoming increasingly clear that growth factors can work synergistically to enhance cartilage matrix synthesis, as in the case of bone morphogenetic protein-7 and Insulin like growth factor-I (Loeser et al., 2003), and Insulin like growth factor-I, fibroblast growth factor-2, and transforming growth factor-b differentially regulate their own and each other's gene expression and protein production in vitro (Shi et al., 2009). Based on the concept that a combination of bioactive growth factors is likely necessary for cartilage repair, and the increasing application of autogenous biologics for tissue engineering, recent attention has been given to the use of platelet rich plasma in cartilage repair techniques. Another advantage of platelet rich plasma is that on clotting; platelets form three-dimensional scaffolds to fill the cartilage defect and act as a guide for neochondrogenesis in situ. Although these issues are not insurmountable, the agents most likely to succeed in this regard are likely to include the polygrowth factor environment provided by platelet rich plasma products.

2.3.2 History and development of PRP

In the 1930s, Schultz demonstrated an injection technique that successfully induced tightening of loose temporomandibular joints; the solution injected was derived from psyllium seed. In the 1950s, Hackett named this technique prolotherapy to imply proliferation of fibrous tissue. In the early 1990s, his work was updated with articles on proposed mechanisms of action and use of prolotherapy (using other injectants, such as dextrose and morrhuate sodium) in essentially all joints of the body. More recently, prolotherapy has been defined as the injection of growth factors or growth factor production stimulants to facilitate growth and repair of normal cells and tissue. A proliferant is any solution injected with the intent of growth or repair. Growth factors produced or provided with proliferant injection are those that are increased during the repair phase in soft tissue of various types; thus, connective tissue is the target for treatment. Linetsky et al proposed the term regenerative injection therapy to describe treatments with this goal.

Autologous platelet rich plasma was first used in 1987 by Ferrari et al., following open heart surgery in order to avoid excessive transfusion of homologous blood products. Rationale: reversal of the blood ratio through decrease of red blood cell to 5% and increase of platelets to 94% for stimulation of recovery; defined as a volume of the plasma fraction of autologous blood having a platelet concentration above baseline; clinical efficacy with above 1 million platelets/ul.

In the late 1990s, surgeons began adding platelet rich plasma to fibrin glue, forming a gel for placement in surgical sites. The goal was to improve healing, anchoring of implantable materials, and speed of recovery. In the early part of this century, physicians began injection of platelet rich plasma as a proliferant. The first published, nonsurgical report was a case series published in the podiatry field. Since 2005, the Hackett-Hemwall Foundation and the University of Wisconsin have sponsored an annual research forum focused on regenerative injection treatments. The mode of action of these therapies has been a major focus of discussion. Banks (Banks, 1991) has proposed that the common end point of regenerative therapy is formation of new collagen fibers. Growth factor stimulation by lipids released from cell membrane rupture and microbleeding with release of platelets have been proposed as potential mechanisms for such an effect (Reeves et al., 2008). Rabago et al discussed these proposed mechanisms of action in their review of 4 injection therapies, including dextrose/sodium morrhuate, polidocanol, autologous whole blood, and platelet rich plasma injections. They reported that the common goal of these injections is to stimulate a normal tissue repair cascade resulting in organized collagen fibers, not scars. Regenerative biomedicine is receiving progressive attention in medicine. Advancements in the study of these innovative bioactive therapies, such as the use of platelet rich plasma, mesenchymal stem cells, extracorporeal shock wave therapy, sclerosing agents, nitric oxide, and matrix metalloproteinase etc, have taken place during the past 2 decades.

2.3.3 Preparation and safety of PRP

Platelet rich plasma is prepared by centrifuging autologous, anticoagulated whole blood. The range of ideal concentrations is based primarily on opinion, and most publications differ on the platelet rich plasma concentrations cited. Citrate can be used for inhibition of the clotting cascade by binding ionized calcium. Centrifugation separates the following: (1) plasma (top layer) from (2) platelets and white blood cells (buffy coat, middle layer) and (3) red blood cells (bottom layer) (Fig. 3.) as a result of differences in specific gravity.

In order to further concentrate the preparation, a second centrifugation separates the platelet rich plasma from platelet-poor plasma. Of note, the use of 2 spins versus 1 spin is controversial. Although a second spin will certainly concentrate the platelets further, the question of whether this step is necessary remains a subject of discussion. The platelet rich plasma (middle layer) is then drawn off, and addition of calcium chloride or thrombin activates the platelet rich plasma and results in prompt release of 70% of the growth factors from the granules within 10 minutes (and nearly all of the contents within an hour). The issue of pre-activation is also controversial, and not all clinicians include this step. Presently, a number of different manufacturers have introduced systems for platelet rich plasma preparation, allowing for both intraoperative and outpatient use of platelet rich plasma for a variety of orthopaedic pathologies (Hall et al., 2009). The volume of platelet rich plasma and concentration of platelets yielded from a volume of whole blood can differ based on the preparation system used (Foster et al., 2009; Mishra et al., 2009; Hall et al., 2009). For example, in our clinic, we use the Huons® sPRP system (Huons®, Gyeonggido, Korea) (Fig. 3.). The procedure utilizes a 50 ml venous blood sample, which is drawn using aseptic technique from the anticubital vein. Use of an 18-19 gauge butterfly needle is advised, in an effort to avoid irritation and trauma to platelets. Blood is then placed in a Korean Food and Drug Administration approved device (Huons®, Gyeonggido, Korea), centrifuged for 3 min at 3,200 rpm, and separated into platelet poor plasma, PRP, and RBC. Platelet poor plasma is extracted through a special port and discarded from the device. Afterward, the platelet rich plasma is withdrawn. Approximately 5.5 or 6.0 cc of platelet rich plasma is available.

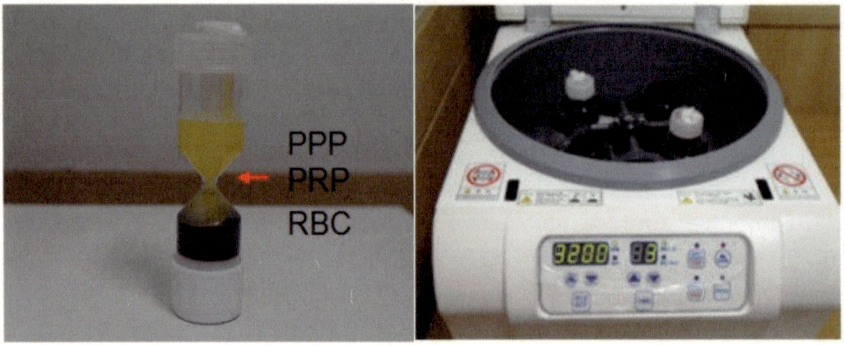

Fig. 3. Platelet rich plasma preparation. (1) Platelet poor plasma (top layer) (2) platelets and white blood cells (buffy coat, middle layer) and (3) red blood cells (bottom layer). PPP; platelet poor plasma, PRP; platelet rich plasma, RBC; red blood cell. Photo courtesy of Huons® Technoloogies, sPRP kit.

Platelet rich plasma is prepared from autologous blood; therefore, any concerns regarding immunogenic reactions or disease transfer are eliminated. Growth factors act on cell membranes, rather than on the cell nucleus, and activate normal gene expression. Growth factors are not mutagenic and act naturally through gene regulation and normal wound healing feed-back control mechanisms.

2.3.4 Preclinical studies

In a rabbit model, osteochondral defects were treated with either autogenous platelet rich plasma in a poly-lacticglycolic acid carrier, poly-lacticglycolic acid alone, or left untreated (Sun et al., 2010). The platelet rich plasma group demonstrated a higher extent of cartilage regeneration as well as increased production of glycosaminoglycans in the extracelluar matrix.

Osteoarthritis models have also been used in study of the effects of platelet rich plasma on synovial cell biology. Cells from 10 patients were cultured and exposed to either a platelet-poor or platelet-rich solution. Investigators found that the platelet rich solution in growth

factors enhanced hyaluronic acid secretion; therefore, they concluded that intra-articular injections of platelet-released growth factor may be useful in maintenance of joint homeostasis by contributing to hyaluronic acid restoration (Anitua et al., 2007).
In the animal literature, results of several studies have demonstrated evidence of osteogenesis and formation of cartilaginous tissue with platelet rich plasma combined with chondrocytes or a collagen matrix (Qi et al., 2009). Sustained-release platelet rich plasma intra-articular injections also resulted in increased cartilage matrix metabolism (Saito et al., 2009). Although chondrocytes and platelet rich plasma appeared to stimulate chondrogenesis subcutaneously, demineralized bone matrix and platelet rich plasma did not stimulate osteogenesis intramuscularly (Ranly et al., 2007) which prompts further questions about the substrates with which platelet rich plasma may have synergistic effects and the environment in which the composite is placed. Intra-articularly injected sustained-release vehicles for platelet rich plasma appeared to stimulate cartilage matrix metabolism, which suggests potential uses in osteoarthritis management (Saito et al., 2009). In a canine model, a composite was created when platelet rich plasma was combined with bone marrow stromal cells and demineralized bone matrix, and then subsequently wrapped in a muscle flap containing blood vessels. This combination appeared to enhance osteogenesis and vascularization (Li et al., 2009).
In a study of porcine mandibular bone defects, platelet rich plasma combined with bone marrow was found to stimulate osteogenesis (Lopez-Lopez et al., 2009). In another study, platelet rich plasma was combined with bone graft and stimulated osteogenesis in rabbit calvarium defects (Nagata et al., 2009). Chondrogenesis was demonstrated in rabbit knee cartilage defects when platelet rich plasma was used with a scaffold (Sun et al., 2010). platelet rich plasma alone also has been found to enhance the healing of diabetic fractures in rats (Gandhi et al., 2006).

2.3.5 Clinical studies

Blood-derived growth factors have already been studied for their potential to aid in cartilage repair and have been documented in the literature in both preclinical and clinical studies (Saito et al., 2009; Wu et al., 2007). In particular, Baltzer et al. (Tamoto et al., 1994) conducted an analysis of the effect of autologous conditioned serum in treatment of patients with knee osteoarthritis. In their prospective, randomized patient- and observer-blinded, placebo-controlled trial, they demonstrated that autologous conditioned serum injections induced considerable improvement of the clinical signs and symptoms of osteoarthritis with results that are even superior to those of hyaluronic acid. Recently, there has been increasing interest in the use of another autologous blood product, platelet rich plasma, which might provide cellular and humoral mediators to promote tissue healing in a variety of applications. The rationale is based on the activity of blood growth factors carried in platelets, many of which have been shown to take part in regulation of articular cartilage (Kobayashi et al., 1994). Platelets contain storage pools of growth factors in their a-granules (Larsen et al., 1977), including Platelet-derived growth factor, Transforming Growth Factor-b, Insulin like growth factor-1, fibroblast growth factor, and many others, as well as cytokines and chemokines (Sanzhez et al., 2009). Platelet rich plasma is derived from centrifugation of autologous whole blood and contains a platelet concentration that is 4 to 5 times higher than that of normal blood, thus offering a high concentration of growth factors in physiological proportions. Some research findings have suggested a possible role for platelet rich plasma in treatment of cartilage lesions (Saito et al., 2009). In an observational retrospective cohort study using hyaluronan injections as a control, Sanchez et al. (Sanchez et al., 2008) showed interesting preliminary results using intra-articular injections of an autologous preparation rich in growth factors for treatment of knee osteoarthritis. These studies suggest that these potent biological regulators of chondrocytes have an important role in cartilage repair. However, for the time being, evidence for clinical use of platelet rich plasma is still in its infancy, particularly regarding treatment of degenerative knee conditions via multiple platelet rich plasma injections. A study was performed to explore this novel approach for treatment of articular cartilage degenerative lesions. The preliminary results indicated that this procedure was safe and had the potential to relieve pain and improve knee function and quality of life in younger patients with a low degree of articular cartilage degeneration.

A number of studies investigating the use of platelet rich plasma and autologous blood have received attention in the popular press. However, there is still a lack of high-quality, prospective research providing definitive assistance to physicians in the appropriate use of these agents (Nguyen et al., 2011). That being said, early use of these agents for conditions that are often resistant to other treatments has been encouraging (Kazemi et. Al., 2010). In addition, platelet rich plasma and autologous blood have shown less potential for serious side effects, such as tendon rupture and fat necrosis, than corticosteroids. Autologous blood treatment protocols involve injection of a local anesthetic in the affected region and then performance of venipuncture and re-injection of the patient's blood into the abnormal tissue. To date, no randomized controlled trials have been conducted in this area. We found an observational, retrospective clinical study that used hyaluronan as a control. The investigators used serial intra-articular platelet rich plasma injections, with modest outcomes. Another clinical study was prospective and showed more positive results, but did not include a control group. Investigators found promising results in patients of younger ages, patients with a lower body mass index, males, and cases of milder severity (Filardo et al., 2010). Application of platelet rich plasma in cartilage repair is relatively new; therefore, there have been limited publications investigating its use. Chondrocytes and mesenchymal stem cells exposed to platelet rich plasma have shown both increased cell proliferation and cartilage extracellular matrix synthesis of proteoglycans and collagen type II, compared with controls (Akeda et al., 2006). Synoviocytes from patients with osteoarthritis cultured in platelet rich plasma demonstrated increased hyaluronic acid production and secretion, suggesting that platelet rich plasma could potentially serve as an endogenous source of chondroprotection and joint lubrication after intra-articular application (Anitua et al., 2007). In a cohort of 30 patients for comparison of injections of platelet rich plasma with hyaluronic acid in management of osteoarthritis, the success rate for the pain subscale reached 33.4% for the platelet rich plasma group, compared with 10% for the hyaluronic acid group ($p = 0.004$) (Sanchez et al., 2008). In addition, percent reductions in the physical function subscale and overall Westren Ontario and McMaster Universities (Bellamy et al., 1988) at 5 weeks were also associated solely with treatment modality in favor of platelet rich plasma, with $p = 0.043$ and $p = 0.010$, respectively. Kon et al. reported results of a large, prospective case series using intraarticular platelet rich plasma injection in patients with degenerative chondral lesions of the knee, as seen on magnetic resonance image (Kellgren o, n = 58 knees) or clear osteoarthrosis on radiograph (Kellgren I-III, n = 33; Kellgre IV, n = 24. Injection of 5 mL PRP (via a lateral approach without guidance) was administered every 21 days for a total of 3 treatments. Calcium chloride was added for activation of platelets. A substantial improvement in International Knee Documentation Committee (Irrgang et al., 2001) and EuroQol-visual analogue scale scores (EuroQol, 2007) was noted at the end of therapy and at both the 6- and 12-month time points. International Knee Documentation Committee subjective scores as well as the EuroQol-visual analogue scale score also demonstrated major improvements at the end of therapy. The authors concluded that treatment with platelet rich plasma is safe and effective for improvement of pain, function, and quality of life in patients with degenerative articular pathology. No follow-up imaging was reported.

The initial hypothesis was that the use of platelet rich plasma might stimulate chondral anabolism and produce a reduction in catabolic processes, thus leading to chondroprotective and chondroregenerative actions, and, therefore, symptomatic improvement. However, the clinical nature of this study makes it difficult to assess the disease-modifying properties of this approach. Moreover, despite the initial considerable improvement in clinical signs and symptoms of knee cartilage degeneration, the marked worsening observed at the 24-month follow-up indicates that improvement due to platelet rich plasma injections is mostly symptomatic, at least with this procedure. Platelet rich plasma probably influences overall joint homoeostasis, also through reduction of synovial membrane hyperplasia and modulation of the cytokine level, thus leading to the observed improvement in the clinical outcome, albeit only temporarily, and maybe without affecting cartilage tissue structure or progression of joint degeneration (Saito et al., 2009). Further studies will determine whether or not other application modalities, with different platelet/growth factor concentrations and injection times, may allow for achievement of better and more durable results.

Treatment is most effective in younger male patients, with lower body mass index and lower degrees of chondral degeneration. The interesting results obtained regarding the safety, feasibility, and short-term efficacy of this treatment suggest that it may represent a minimally invasive and safe procedure that may be cyclically repeated in order to improve knee function and quality of life.

Despite early optimism and the positive safety profile of platelet rich plasma and autologous blood, most insurance companies are reluctant to cover the use of these agents due to a lack of high-quality randomized, double-blinded studies.

3. Conclusion

When treating a patient with osteoarthritis, it is best to start with non-interventional approaches, such as physiotherapy, ice, and analgesics. If conservative treatment fails, injectable agents may help. Corticosteroid injections are effective in reducing pain associated with osteoarthritis and in treatment of conditions in which inflammation is present. When corticosteroid treatment is not effective for osteoarthritis, intra-articular injections with hyaluronic acid are another option. Hyaluronic acid injections provide longer-lasting pain relief than corticosteroids for patients with osteoarthritis; however, they are much more expensive. Growth hormone has not yet received Food and Drug Administration approval for injection in joints, which is an "off-label" use. There is interest in the use of growth hormone as a potential osteoarthritis disease-modifying treatment; however, studies of its effects in humans are lacking. Platelet-rich plasma and/or autologous blood injections are safer and may be more effective than corticosteroids for treatment of osteoarthritis.

However, physicians need to understand that high-quality prospective evidence as to the appropriate use of some of these treatments for certain conditions is lacking. Considering the limited data, no clear definition of a standardized platelet rich plasma treatment protocol has been established to date. Further research is needed.

4. Acknowledgment

This book chapter is dedicated to my family; my wife, Mi Sung Kim, my daughter, Hyun Jo Kwon, and my son, Eun Sang Kwon for their love, support and patience through this special effort.

5. References

Wearing SC, Henning EM, Byrne NM, Steele JR, & Hills AP. (2006). Musculoskeletal disorders associated with obesity: a biomechanical perspective. *Obes Rev.*, 7(3), 239-250, 1467-7881

Chevalier X. Physiopathogenesis of osteoarthritis. (1998). The arthritis cartilage. *Presse Med.*, 27(2), 81-87, 0755-4982

Topol EJ. (2004). Failing the public health-rofecoxib, Merck, and the FDA. *N. Engl. J. Med.*, 351(17), 1707-1709, 0028-4793

Petit-Zeman S. (2004). Characteristics of COX2 inhibitors questioned. *Nat Rev Drug Discov.*, 3(9), 726-727, 1474-1776

Gerwin N, Hops C, Lucke A. (2006). Intraarticular drug delivery in osteoarthritis. *Adv Drug Deliv Rev.*, 58(2), 226-242, 0169-409X

Brandt KD, Smith GN Jr, Simon LS. (2000). Intra-articular injection of hyaluronan as treatment for knee osteoarthritis: what is the evidence? *Arthritis Rheum.*, 43(6), 1192-1203, 0004-3591

Betre H, Liu W, Zalutsky MR, Chilkoti A, Kraus VB, Setton LA. (2006). A thermally responsive biopolymer for intra-articular drug delivery. *J Control Release.*, 115(2), 175-182, 0168-3659

Saito M, Takahashi KA, Arai Y, Inoue A, Sakao K, Tonomura H, Honjo K, Nakagawa S, Inoue H, Tabata Y, Kubo T. (2009). Intraarticular administration of platelet-rich plasma with biodegradable gelatin hydrogel microspheres prevents osteoarthritis progression in the rabbit knee. *Clin Exp Rheumatol.*, 27(2), 201-207, 0392-856X

Chen AL, Desai P, Adler EM, Di Cesare PE. (2002). Granulomatous inflammation after Hylan G-F 20 viscosupplementation of the knee : a report of six cases. *J Bone Joint Surg Am.*, 84(7), 1142-1147, 0021-9355

Jackson DW, Evans NA, Thomas BM. (2002). Accuracy of needle placement into the intra-articular space of the knee. *J Bone Joint Surg Am.*, 84(9), 1522-1527, 0021-9355

Neustadt DH. (2006). Intra-articular injections for osteoarthritis of the knee. *Cleve Clin J Med.*, 73(10), 897-898, 901-904, 906-911, 0891-1150

Chavez-Chiang CE, Sibbitt WL Jr, Band PA, Chavez-Chiang NR, Delea SL, Bankhurst AD. (2011). The highly accurate anteriolateral portal for injecting the knee. *Sports Med Arthrosc Rehabil Ther Technol.*, 3(1), 6, 1758-2555

Jones A, Doherty M. (2003). *Osteoarthritis (2nd edition)*, Oxford University Press, 0198509677, New York

Ayral X. (2001). Injections in the treatment of osteoarthritis. *Best Pract Res Clin Rheumatol.*, 15(4), 609-626, 1521-6942

Neustadt DH. (2001). *Osteoarthritis: Diagnosis and Medical/Surgical Management (3rd edition)*, W.B. Saunders Company, 0721684394, Philadelphia

Balazs EA, Denlinger JL. (1993). Viscosupplementation: a new concept in the treatment of osteoarthritis. *J Rhematol Suppl.*, 39: 3-9, 0380-0903

Simon LS. (1999). Viscosupplementation therapy with intra-articular hyaluronic acid. Fact or fantasy?. *Rhem Dis Clin North Am.*,25(2), 345-358, 0889-857X

Marshall KW. (2000). Intra-articular hyaluronan therapy. *Curr Opin Rheumatol.*, 12(5), 468-474, 1040-8711

Ghosh P. (1994). The role of hyaluronic acid in health and disease: interactions with cells, cartilage, and components of synovial fluid. *Clin Exper Rheum.*, 12(1), 75-82, 0392-856X

Vad VB, Bhat AL, Sculco TP, Wickiewicz TL. (2003). Management of knee osteoarthritis: knee lavage combined with hylan versus hylan alone. *Arch Phys Med Rehabil.*, 84(5), 634-637, 0003-9993

Raynauld JP, Goldsmith CH, Bellamy N, Torrance GW, Polisson R, Belovich D, Pericak D, Tugwell P. (2005). Effectiveness and safety of repeat courses of hylan G-F 20 in patients with knee osteoarthritis. *Osteoarthritis Cartilage*,13(2), 111-119, 1063-4584

Hammesfahr JF, Knopf AB, Stitik T. (2003). Safety of intra-articular hyaluronates for pain associated with osteoarthritis of the knee. *Am J orthop.*, 32(6), 277-283, 1078-4519

Leopold SS, Warme WJ, Pettis PD, Shott S. (2002). Increased frequency of acute local reaction to intra-articular hylan GF-20 (synvisc) in patients receiving more than one course of treatment. *J Bone Joint Surg Am.*, 84(9), 1619-1623, 0021-9355

Marino AA, Waddell DD, Kolomytkin OV, Pruett S, Sadasivan KK, Albright JA. (2006). Assessment of immunologic mechanisms for flare reactions to Synvisc. *Clin Orthop Relat Res.*, 442, 187-194, 0009-921X

Brockmeier SF, Shaffer BS. (2006). Viscosupplementation therapy for osteoarthritis. Sports Med Arthrosc., 14(3),155-162, 1062-8592

Moreland LW. (2003). Intra-articular hyaluronan (hyaluronic acid) and hylans for the treatment of osteoarthritis: mechanisms of action. *Arthritis Res. Ther.*, 5(2), 54-67, 1478-6354

Vuorio E, Einola S, Hakkarainen S, Penttinen R. (1982). Synthesis of underpolymerized hyaluronic acid by fibroblasts cultured from rheumatoid and non-rheumatoid synovitis. *Rheumatol Int.*, 2(3), 97-102, 0172-8172

Kikuchi T, Yamada H, Shimmei M. (1996). Effect of high molecular weight hyaluronan on cartilage degradation in a rabbit model of osteoarthritis. *Osteoarthritis Cartilage*, 4(2), 99-110, 1063-4584

Armstrong S, Read R, Ghosh P. (1994). The effects of intraarticular hyaluronan on cartilage and subchondral bone changes in an ovine model of early osteoarthritis. *J Rheumatol.*, 21(4), 680-688, 0315-162X

Sonoda M, Harwood FL, Wada Y, Moriya H, Amiel D. (1997). The effects of hyaluronan on the meniscus and on the articular cartilage after partial meniscectomy. *Am J Sports Med.*, 25(6), 755-762, 0363-5465

Sonoda M, Harwood FL, Amiel ME, Moriya H, Temple M, Chang DG, et al. (2000). The effects of hyaluronan on tissue healing after meniscus injury and repair in a rabbit model. *Am J Sports Med.*, 28(1), 90-97, 0363-5465

Wiig ME, Amiel D, VandeBerg J, Kitabayashi L, Harwood FL, Arfors KE. (1990). The early effect of high molecular weight hyaluronan (hyaluronic acid) on anterior cruciate ligament healing: an experimental study in rabbits. *J Orthop Res.*, 8(3), 425-434, 0736-0266

Takahashi K, Hashimoto S, Kubo T, Hirasawa Y, Lotz M, Amiel D. (2000). Effect of hyaluronan on chondrocyte apoptosis and nitric oxide production in experimentally induced osteoarthritis. *J Rheumatol.*, 27(7), 1713-1720, 0315-162X

Schiavinato A, Lini E, Guidolin D, Pezzoli G, Botti P, Martelli M, et al. (1989). Intraarticular sodium hyaluronate injections the Pond-Nuki experimental model of osteoarthritis in dogs. II. Morphological findings. *Clin*

Orthop., 241, 286-299, 0009-921X

Wenz W, Breusch SJ, Graf J, Stratmann U. (2000). Ultrastructural findings after intraarticular application of hyaluronan in a canine model of arthropathy. *J Orthop Res.*, 18(4), 604-612, 0736-0266

Yoshioka M, Shimizu C, Harwood FL, Coutts RD, Amiel D. (1997). The effects of hyaluronan during the development of osteoarthritis. *Osteoarthritis Cartilage,* 5(4), 251-260, 1063-4584

Shimizu C, Yoshioka M, Coutts RD, Harwood FL, Kubo T, Hirasawa Y, et al. (1998). Long-term effects of hyaluronan on experimental osteoarthritis in the rabbit knee. *Osteoarthritis Cartilage,* 6(1), 1-9, 1063-4584

Marshall KW, Manolopoulos V, Mancer K, Staples J, Damyanovich A. (2000). Amelioration of disease severity by intraarticular hylan therapy in bilateral canine osteoarthritis. *J Orthop Res.*, 18(3), 416-425, 0736-0266

Amiel D, Toyoguchi T, Kobayashi K, Bowden K, Amiel ME, Healey RM. (2003). Long-term effect of sodium hyaluronate (Hyalgan) on osteoarthritis progression in a rabbit model. *Osteoarthritis Cartilage,*11(9), 636-643, 1063-4584

Dixon AS, Jacoby RK, Berry H, Hamilton EB. (1988). Clinical trial of intra-articular injection of sodium hyaluronate in patients with osteoarthritis of the knee. *Curr Med Res Opin.*, 11(4), 205-213, 0300-7995

Dougados M, Nguyen M, Listrat V, Amor B. (1993). High molecular weight sodium hyaluronate (hyalectin) in osteoarthritis of the knee: a 1 year placebo-controlled trial. *Osteoarthritis Cartilage,* 1(2), 97-103, 1063-4584

Henderson EB, Smith EC, Pegley F, Blake DR. (1994). Intra-articular injections of 750 kD hyaluronan in the treatment of osteoarthritis: a randomized single centre double-blind placebo-controlled trial of 91 patients demonstrating lack of efficacy. *Ann Rhem Dis.*, 53(8), 529-534, 0003-4967

Dahlberg L, Lohmander S, Ryd L. (1994). Intraarticular injections of hyaluronan in patients with cartilage abnormalities and knee pain: a one-year double-blind, placebo-controlled study. *Arthritis Rhem.*, 37(4), 521-528, 0004-3591

Bellamy N, Campbell J, Robinson V, Gee T, Bourne R, Wells G. (2006). Viscosupplementation for the treatment of osteoarthritis of the knee. *Cochranc Database syst Rev.*, 19(2), CD005321, 1469-493X

Adams ME, Atkinson MH, Lussier AJ, Schulz JI, Siminovitch KA, Wade JP, Zummer M. (1995). The role of viscosupplementation with hylan G-F 20 in the treatment of osteoarthritis of the knee: a Canadian multicenter trial comparing hylan G-F 20 alone, hylan G-F 20 with non-steroidal anti-inflammatory drugs (NSAIDs) and NSAIDs alone. *Osteoarthritis Cartilage,* 3(4), 213-225, 1063-4584

Altman RD, Moskowitz R. (1998). Intraarticular sodium hyaluronate in the treatment of patients wth osteoarthritis of the knee: a randomized clinical trial. *J Rheum.,* 25(11), 2203-2212, 0315-162X

Jones AC, Pattrick M, Doherty S, Doherty M. (1995). Intra-articular hyaluronic acid compared to intra-articular triamcinolone hexacetonide in inflammatory knee osteoarthritis. *Osteoarthritis Cartilage,* 3(4), 269-273, 1063-4584

Leopold SS, Redd BB, Warme WJ, Wehrle PA, Pettis PD, Shott S. (2003). Corticosteroid compared with hyaluronic acid injections for the treatment of osteoarthritis of the knee: a prospective, randomized trial. *J Bone Joint Surg Am.,* 85(7), 1197-1203, 0021-9355

Caborn D, Rush J, Lanzer W, Parenti D, Murray C. (2004). A randomized, single-blind comparison of the efficacy and tolerability of hylan G-F 20 and triamcinolone hexacetonide in patients with osteoarthritis of the knee. *J Rheum.,* 31(2), 333-343, 0315-162X

Altman R, Brandt K, Hochberg M, Moskowitz R. (1996). Design and conduct of clinical trials in patients with osteoarthritis: recommendations from a task force of the Osteoarthritis Research Society. *Osteoarthritis Cartilage,* 4(4), 217-243, 1063-4584

Goldring MB, Tsuchimochi K, Ijiri K. (2006). The control of chondrogenesis. *J Cell Biochem.,* 97(1), 33–44, 0730-2312

Blaney Davidson EN, van der Kraan PM, van den Berg WB. (2007). TGF-beta and osteoarthritis. *Osteoarthritis Cartilage,* 15(6), 597–604, 1063-4584

Fan J, Gong Y, Ren L, Varshney RR, Cai D, Wang DA. (2010). In vitro engineered cartilage using synovium-derived mesenchymal stem cells with injectable gellan hydrogels. *Acta Biomater.,* 6(3), 1178–1185, 1742-7061

Kurth T, Hedbom E, Shintani N, Sugimoto M, Chen FH, Haspl M, Martinovic S, Hunziker EB. (2007). Chondrogenic potential of human synovial mesenchymal stem cells in alginate. *Osteoarthritis Cartilage,* 15(10), 1178–1189, 1063-4584

Bakker AC, van de Loo FA, van Beuningen HM, Sime P, van Lent PL, van der Kraan PM, Richards CD, van den Berg WB. (2001). Overexpression of active TGF-beta-1 in the murine knee joint: evidence for synovial-layer-dependent chondro-osteophyte formation. *Osteoarthritis Cartilage,* 9(2), 128–136, 1063-4584

Diao H, Wang J, Shen C, Xia S, Guo T, Dong L, Zhang C, Chen J, Zhao J, Zhang J. (2009). Improved cartilage regeneration utilizing mesenchymal stem cells in TGF-beta1 gene-activated scaffolds. *Tissue Eng Part A.,* 15(9), 2687–2698, 1937-3341

Coutts RD, Sah RL, Amiel D. (1997). Effects of growth factors on cartilage repair. Instr Course Lect., 46, 487-494, 0065-6895

Hickey DG, Frenkel SR, Di Cesare PE. (2003). Clinical applications of growth factors for articular cartilage repair. *AmJ Orthop.*, 32(2), 70-76, 1078-4519

Ashton IK, Matheson JA. (1979). Change in response with age of human articular cartilage to plasma somatomedin activity. *Calcif Tiss Int.*, 29(2), 89–94, 0171-967X

Boehm AK, Seth M, Mayr KG, Fortier LA. (2007). Hsp90 mediates insulin-like growth factor 1 and interleukin-1beta signaling in an age-dependent manner in equine articular chondrocytes. *Arthritis Rheum.*, 56(7), 2335–2343, 0004-3591

Denko CW, Boja B, Moskowitz RW. (1994). Growth promoting peptides in osteoarthritis and diffuse idiopathic skeletal hyperostosis—insulin, insulin-like growth factor-I, growth hormone. *J Rheumatol.*, 21(9), 1725–1730, 0315-162X

Dore S, Pelletier J, DiBattista JA, Tardif G, Brazeau P, Martel-Pelletier J. (1994). Human osteoarthritic chondrocytes possess an increased number of insulin-like growth factor 1 binding sites but are unresponsive to its stimulation: possible role of IGF-1 binding proteins. *Arthritis Rheum.*, 37(2), 253–263, 0004-3591

Ekenstedt KJ, Sonntag WE, Loeser RF, Lindgren BR, Carlson CS. (2006). Effects of chronic growth hormone and insulin-like growth factor 1 deficiency on osteoarthritis severity in rat knee joints. *Arthritis Rheum.*, 54(12), 3850–3858, 0004-3591

Fortier LA, Miller BJ. (2006). Signaling through the small G-protein Cdc42 is involved in insulin-like growth factor-I resistance in aging articular chondrocytes. *J Orthop Res.*, 24(8), 1765–1772, 0736-0266

Fortier LA, Mohammed HO, Lust G, Nixon AJ. (2002). Insulin-like growth factor-I enhances cell-based repair of articular cartilage. *J Bone Joint Surg Br.*, 84(2), 276–288, 0301-620X

Goodrich LR, Hidaka C, Robbins PD, Evans CH, Nixon AJ. (2007). Genetic modification of chondrocytes with insulin-like growth factor-1 enhances cartilage healing in an equine model. *J Bone Joint Surg Br.*, 89(5), 672–685, 0301-620X

Loeser RF, Carlson CS, Del Carlo M, Cole A. (2002). Detection of nitrotyrosine in aging and osteoarthritic cartilage: correlation of oxidative damage with the presence of interleukin-1beta and with chondrocyte resistance to insulin-like growth factor 1. *Arthritis Rheum.*, 46(9), 2349–2357, 0004-3591

Longobardi L, O'Rear L, Aakula S, Johnstone B, Shimer K, Chytil A, Horton WA, Moses HL, Spagnoli A. (2006). Effect of IGF-I in the chondrogenesis of bone marrow mesenchymal stem cells in the presence or absence of TGF-beta signaling. *J Bone Miner Res.*, 21(4), 626–636, 0884-0431

Maehara H, Sotome S, Yoshii T, Torigoe I, Kawasaki Y, Sugata Y, Yuasa M, Hirano M, Mochizuki N, Kikuchi M, Shinomiya K, Okawa A. (2010). Repair of large osteochondral defects in rabbits using porous hydroxyapatite/collagen (HAp/Col) and fibroblast growth factor-2 (FGF-2). *J Orthop Res.*, 28(5), 677–686, 0736-0266

Martin JS, Ellerbrock SM, Buckwalter JA. (1997). Age-related decline in chondrocyte response to insulin-like growth factor-I: the role of growth factor binding proteins. *J Orthop Res.*, 15(4), 491–498, 0736-0266

McQuillan DJ, Handley CJ, Campbell MA, Bolis S, Milway VE, Herington AC. (1986). Stimulation of proteoglycan biosynthesis by serum and insulin-like growth factor-1 in cultured bovine articular cartilage. *Biochem J.*, 240(2), 423–430, 0264-6021

Middleton J, Manthey A, Tyler J. (1996). Insulin-like growth factor (IGF) receptor, IGF-I, interleukin-1b (IL-1b), and IL-6 mRNA expression in osteoarthritic and normal human cartilage. *J Histochem Cytochem.*, 44(2), 133–141, 0022-1554

Morales TI. (2008). The quantitative and functional relation between insulin-like growth factor-I (IGF) and IGF-binding proteins during human osteoarthritis. *J Orthop Res.*, 26(4), 465–474, 0736-0266

Posever J, Phillips FM, Pottenger LA. (1995). Effects of basic fibroblast growth factor, transforming growth factor-B1, insulin-like growth factor-1, and insulin on human osteoarthritic articular cartilage explants. *J Orthop Res.*, 13(6), 832–837, 0736-0266

Sah RL, Chen AC, Grodzinsky AJ, Trippel SB. (1994). Differential effects of bFGF and IGF-I on matrix metabolism in calf and adult bovine cartilage explants. *Archives Biochem Biophys.*, 308(1), 137–147, 0003-9861

Schalkwijk J, Joosten LAB, van den Berg WB, van de Putte LBA. (1989). Chondrocyte nonresponsiveness to insulin-like growth factor 1 in experimental arthritis. *Arthritis Rheum.*, 32(7), 894–900, 0004-3591

Tyler JA. (1989). Insulin-like growth factor 1 can decrease degradation and promote synthesis of proteoglycan in cartilage exposed to cytokines. *Biochem J.*, 260(2), 543–548, 0264-6021

Wang E, Wang J, Chin E, Zhou J, Bondy CA. (1995). Cellular patterns of insulin-like growth factor system gene expression in murine chondrogenesis and osteogenesis. *Endocrinology.*, 136(6), 2741–2751, 0013-7227

Worster AA, Brower-Toland BD, Fortier LA, Bent SJ, Williams J, Nixon AJ. (2001). Chondrocytic differentiation of mesenchymal stem cells sequentially exposed to transforming growth factor-beta1 in monolayer and insulin-like growth factor-I in a three-dimensional matrix. *J Orthop Res.*, 19(4), 738–749, 0736-0266

Martin JA, Ellerbroek SM, Buckwalter JA. (1997). Age-related decline in chondrocyte response to insulin-like growth factor-I: the role of growth factor binding proteins. *J Orthop Res.*, 15(4), 491-498, 0736-0266

Verschure PJ, Van Noorden CJ, Van Marle J, Van den Berg WB. (1996). Articular cartilage destruction in experimental inflammatory arthritis: insulin-like growth factor-1 regulation of proteoglycan metabolism in chondrocytes. *Histochem J.*, 28(12), 835-857, 0018-2214

Trippel SB. (1995). Growth factor actions on articular cartilage. *J Rheumatol Suppl.*, 43, 129-132, 0380-0903

van den Berg WB, van der Kraan PM, Scharstuhl A, van Beuningen HM. (2001). Growth factors and cartilage repair. *Clin Orthop.*, 391, S244-250, 0009-921X

Hickey DG, Frenkel SR, Di Cesare PE. (2003). Clinical applications of growth factors for articular cartilage repair. *Am J Orthop.*, 32(2), 70-76, 1078-4519

Lee SJ. (2000). Cytokine delivery and tissue engineering. *Yonsei Med J.*, 41(6), 704-719, 0513-5796

Spindler KP, Mayes CE, Miller RR, Imro AK, Davidson JM. (1995). Regional mitogenic response of the meniscus to platelet-derived growth factor (PDGF-AB). *J Orthop Res.*, 13(2), 201-207, 0736-0266

Smith RJ, Justen JM, Sam LM, Rohloff NA, Ruppel PL, Brunden MN, Chin JE. (1991). Platelet-derived growth factor potentiates cellular responses of articular chondrocytes to interleukin-1. *Arthritis Rheum.*, 34(6), 697-706, 0004-3591

Steadman JR, Rodkey WG, Rodrigo JJ. (2001). Microfracture: surgical technique and rehabilitation to treat chondral defects. *Clin Orthop.*, 391, S362-369, 0009-921X

Breinan HA, Martin SD, Hsu HP, Spector M. (2000). Healing of canine articular cartilage defects treated with microfracture, a type-II collagen matrix, or cultured autologous chondrocytes. *J Orthop Res.*, 18(5), 781-789, 0736-0266

Dorotka R, Windberger U, Macfelda K, Bindreiter U, Toma C, Nehrer S. (2005). Repair of articular cartilage defects treated by microfracture and a three-dimensional collagen matrix. *Biomaterials.*, 26(17), 3617-3629, 0142-9612

Schmidt MB, Chen EH, Lynch SE. (2006). A review of the effects of insulin-like growth factor and platelet derived growth factor on in vivo cartilage healing and repair. *Osteoarthritis Cartilage.*, 14(5), 403–412, 1063-4584

Hulth A, Johnell O, Miyazono K, Lindberg L, Heinegard D, Heldin C-H. (1996). Effect of transforming growth factor-B and plateletderived growth factor-BB on articular cartilage in rats. *J Orthop Res.*, 14(4), 547–553, 0736-0266

Nemirovskiy O, Zheng YJ, Tung D, Korniski B, Settle S, Skepner A, Yates M, Aggarwal P, Sunyer T, Aguiar DJ. (2010). Pharmacokinetic/pharmacodynamic (PK/PD) differentiation of native and PEGylated recombinant human growth hormone (rhGH and PEG-rhGH) in the rat model of osteoarthritis. *Xenobiotica.*, 40(8), 586-592, 0049-8254

Lis K. (2008). Insulin-like growth factor 1 (IGF-1) and growth hormone (hGH) as the markers of osteoarthritis. *Chir Narzadow Ruchu Ortop Pol.*, 73(1), 49-52, 0009-479X

Gaissmaier C, Koh JL, Weise K. (2008). Growth and differentiation factors for cartilage healing and repair. *Int. J. Care Injured.*, 39, S88-S96, 0020-1383

Adams ME, Atkinson MH, Lussier AJ, Schulz JI, Siminovitch KA, Wade JP, Zummer M. (1995). The role of viscosupplementation with hylan G-F 20 (Synvisc) in the treatment of osteoarthritis of the knee: a Canadian multicenter trial comparing hylan G-F 20 alone, hylan G-F 20 with non-steroidal anti-inflammatory drugs (NSAIDs) and NSAIDs alone. *Osteoarthritis Cartilage.*, 3(4), 213-225, 1063-4584

Bak B, Jørgensen PH, Andreassen TT. (1990). Increased mechanical strength of healing rat tibial fractures treated with biosynthetic human growth hormone. *Bone.*, 11(4), 233-239, 8756-3282

Kolbeck S, Bail H, Schmidmaier G, Alquiza M, Raun K, Kappelgard A, Flyvbjerg A, Haas N, Raschke M. (2003). Homologous growth hormone accelerates bone healing-a biomechanical and histological study. *Bone.*, 33(4), 628-637, 8756-3282

Carpenter JE, Hipp JA, Gerhart TN, Rudman CG, Hayes WC, Trippel SB. (1992). Failure of growth hormone to alter the biomechanics of fracture-healing in a rabbit model. *J Bone Joint Surg Am.*, 74(3), 359-367, 0021-9355

Dunn AR. (2002). Morphoangiogenesis: a unique action of growth hormone. *Microvasc Res.*, 63(3), 295-303, 0026-2862

Goldspink DF, Goldberg AL. (1975). Influence of pituitary growth hormone on DNA synthesis in rat tissues. *Am J Physiol.*, 228(1), 302-309, 0002-9513

Laursen T, Jørgensen JO, Jakobsen G, Hansen BL, Christiansen JS. (1995). Continuous infusion versus daily injections of growth hormone (GH) for 4 weeks in GH deficient patients. *J Clin Endocrinol Metab.*, 80(8), 2410-2418, 0021-972X

Fu K, Pack DW, Klibanov AM, Langer R. (2000). Visual evidence of acidic environment within degrading poly (lactic-co-glycolic acid) (PLGA) microspheres. *Pharm Res.*, 17(1), 100-106, 0724-8741

Anitua E, Sánchez M, Nurden AT, Nurden P, Orive G, Andía I. (2006). New insights into and novel applications for platelet-rich fibrin therapies. *Trends Biotechnol.*, 24(5), 227-234, 0167-7799

Samposon S, Gerhardt M, Mandelaum B. (2008). Platelet rich plasma injection grafts for musculoskeletal injuries: A review. *Curr Rew Musculoskeletal Med.*, 1(3 4), 165-174, 1935-973X

Saito M, Takahashi KA, Arai Y, Inoue A, Sakao K, Tonomura H, Honjo K, Nakagawa S, Inoue H, Tabata Y, Kubo T. (2009). Intraarticular administration of platelet-rich plasma with biodegradable gelatin hydrogel microspheres prevents osteoarthritis progression in the rabbit knee. *Clin Exp Rheumatol.*, 27(2), 201-207, 0392-856X

Wu W, Chen F, Liu Y, Ma Q, Mao T. (2007). Autologous injectable tissue-engineered cartilage by using platelet-rich plasma: experimental study in a rabbit model. *J oral Maxillofac Surg.*, 65(10), 1951-1957, 0278-2391

Tamoto K, Nochi H, Tada M, Shimada S, Mori Y, Kataoka S, Suzuki Y, Nakamura T. (1994). High-molecular weight hyaluronic acids inhibit chemotaxis and phagocytosis but not lysosomal enzyme release induced by receptor-mediated stimulations in guinea pig phagocytes. *Microbiol Immunol.*, 38(1), 73-80, 0385-5600

Kobayashi Y, Okamoto A, Nishinari K. (1994). Viscoelasticity of hyaluronic acid with different molecular weights. *Biorhelogy.*, 31(3), 235-244, 0006-355X

Larsen A, Dale K, Eek M. (1977). Radiographic evaluation of rheumatoid arthritis and related conditions by standard reference films. *Acta Radiol Diagnosis.*, 18(4), 481-491, 0567-8056

Nguyen RT, Borg-Stein J, McInnis K. (2011). Applications of platelet-rich plasma in musculoskeletal and sports medicine: an evidence-based approach. *PM R.*,3(3),226-250, 1934-1482

Kazemi M, Azma K, Tavana B, Reziee Moghaddam F, Panahi A. (2010). Autologous blood versus corticosteroid local injection in the short-term treatment of lateral elbow tendinopathy: a randomized clinical trial of efficacy. *Am J Phys Rehabil.*, 89(8), 660-667, 0894-9115

Wobig M, Dickhut A, Maier R, Vetter G. (1998). Viscosupplementation with hylan G-F 20: a 26-week controlled trial of efficacy and safety in the osteoarthritic knee. *Clin Ther.*, 20(3), 410-423, 0149-2918

Puhl W, Bernau A, Greiling H, Köpcke W, Pförringer W, Steck KJ, Zacher J, Scharf HP. (1993). Intra-articular sodium hyaluronate in osteoarthritis of the knee: a multicenter, double-blind study. *Osteoarthritis Cartilage.*, 1(4), 233-241, 1063-4584

Lohmander LS, Dalén N, Englund G, Hämäläinen M, Jensen EM, Karlsson K, Odensten M, Ryd L, Sernbo I, Suomalainen O, Tegnander A. (1996). Intra-articular hyaluronan injections in the treatment of osteoarthritis of the knee: a randomised, double blind, placebo controlled multicentre trial. Hyaluronan Multicentre Trial Group. *Ann Rheum Dis.*, 55(7), 424-431, 0003-4967

Jubb RW, Piva S, Beinat L, Dacre J, Gishen P. (2003). A one-year, randomised, placebo (saline) controlled clinical trial of 500-730 kDa sodium hyaluronate (Hyalgan) on the radiological change in osteoarthritis of the knee. *Int J Clin Pract.*, 57(6), 467-474, 1368-5031

Giusti I, Rughetti A, D'Ascenzo S, Millimaggi D, Pavan A, Dell'Orso L, Dolo V. (2009). Identification of an optimal concentration of platelet gel for promoting angiogenesis in human endothelial cells. *Transfusion.*, 49(4), 771-778, 0041-1132

Dohan Ehrenfest DM, Rasmusson L, Albrektsson T. (2009). Classification of platelet concentrates: from pure platelet-rich plasma (P-PRP) to leucocyte- and platelet-rich fibrin (L-PRF). *Trends Biotechnol.*, 27(3), 158-167, 0167-7799

Qureshi AH, Chaoji V, Maiguel D, Faridi MH, Barth CJ, Salem SM, Singhal M, Stoub D, Krastins B, Ogihara M, Zaki MJ, Gupta V. (2009). Proteomic and phospho-proteomic profile of human platelets in basal, resting state: insights into integrin signaling. *PLoS One.*, 4(10), e7627, 1932-6203

Banks A. A rationale for prolotherapy. *J Orthop Med.* 1991; 13: 54-59.

Reeves D, Fullerton B, Topol G. (2008). The sports medicine resource manual. 1st edition. Saunders Elsevier, 1-4160-3197-9, Philadelphia

Foster TE, Puskas BL, Mandelbaum BR, Gerhardt MB, Rodeo SA. (2009). Platelet-rich plasma: from basic science to clinical applications. *Am J Sports Med.*, 37(11), 2259-2272, 0363-5465

Mishra A, Woodall J Jr, Vieira A. (2009). Treatment of tendon and muscle using platelet-rich plasma. *Clin Sports Med.*, 28(1), 113-125, 0278-5919

Hall MP, Band PA, Meislin RJ, Jazrawi LM, Cardone DA. (2009). Platelet-rich plasma: current concepts and application in sports medicine. *J Am Acad Orthop Surg.*, 17(10), 602-608, 1067-151X

McQuillan DJ, Handley CJ, Campbell MA, Bolis S, Milway VE, Herington A. (1986). Stimulation of proteoglycan biosynthesis by serum and insulin-like growth factor-I in cultured bovine articular cartilage. *Biochem J.*, 240(2), 423e30, 0264-6021

Mankin HJ, Mow VC, Buckwalter JA. (2000). Orthopaedic Basic Science. American Academy of Orthopaedic Surgeons , 0892031778 9780892031771 089203176X 9780892031764, Chicago

Shi S, Mercer S, Eckert GJ, Trippel SB. (2009). Growth factor regulation of growth factors in articular chondrocytes. *J Biol Chem.*, 284(11), 6697-6704, 0021-9258

Sun Y, Feng Y, Zhang CQ, Chen SB, Cheng XG. (2010). The regenerative effect of platelet-rich plasma on healing in large osteochondral defects. *Int Orthop.*, 34(4), 589-597, 0341-2695

López-López J, Chimenos-Küstner E, Manzanares-Cespedes C, Muñoz-Sánchez J, Castañeda-Vega P, Jané-Salas E, Alvarez-López JM, Gimeno-Sanding A. (2009). Histomorphological study of the bone regeneration capacity of platelet-rich plasma, bone marrow and tricalcium phosphate: Experimental study on pigs. *Med Oral Patol Oral Cir Bucal.*, 14(12), e620-627, 1698-4447

Qi YY, Chen X, Jiang YZ, Cai HX, Wang LL, Song XH, Zou XH, Ouyang HW. (2009). Local delivery of autologous platelet in collagen matrix simulated in situ articular cartilage repair. *Cell Transplant.*, 18(10), 1161-1169, 0963-6897

Ranly DM, Lohmann CH, Andreacchio D, Boyan BD, Schwartz Z. (2007). Platelet-rich plasma inhibits demineralized bone matrix-induced bone formation in nude mice. *J Bone Joint Surg Am.*, 89(1), 139-147, 0021-9355

Li NY, Yuan RT, Chen T, Chen LQ, Jin XM. (2009). Effect of platelet-rich plasma and latissimus dorsi muscle flap on osteogenesis and vascularization of tissue-engineered bone in dogs. *J Oral Maxillofac Surg.*, 67(9), 1850-1858, 0278-2391

Nagata MJ, Melo LG, Messora MR, Bomfim SR, Fucini SE, Garcia VG, Bosco AF, Okamoto T. (2009). Effect of platelet-rich plasma on bone healing of autogenous bone grafts in critical-size defects. *J Clin Periodontol.*, 36(9), 775-783, 0303-6979

Gandhi A, Doumas C, O'Connor JP, Parsons JR, Lin SS. (2006). The effects of local platelet rich plasma delivery on diabetic fracture healing. Bone., 38(4), 540-546, 8756-3282

Hall MP, Band PA, Meislin RJ, Jazrawi LM, Cardone DA. (2009). Platelet-rich plasma: current concepts and application in sports medicine. *J Am Acad Orthop Surg.*, 17(10), 602-608, 1067-151X

Anitua E, Sánchez M, Nurden AT, Zalduendo MM, de la Fuente M, Azofra J, Andía I. (2007). Platelet-released growth factors enhance the secretion of hyaluronic acid and induce hepatocyte growth factor production by synovial fibroblasts from arthritic patients. *Rheumatology.*, 46(12), 1769-1772, 1462-0324

Saito M, Takahashi KA, Arai Y, Inoue A, Sakao K, Tonomura H, Honjo K, Nakagawa S, Inoue H, Tabata Y, Kubo T. (2009). Intraarticular administration of platelet-rich plasma with biodegradable gelatin hydrogel microspheres prevents osteoarthritis progression in the rabbit knee. *Clin Exp Rheumatol.*, 27(2), 201-207, 0392-856X

Sánchez M, Anitua E, Azofra J, Aguirre JJ, Andia I. (2008). Intraarticular injection of an autologous preparation rich in growth factors for the treatment of knee OA: a retrospective cohort study. Clin Exp Rheumatol., 26(5), 910-913, 0392-856X

Sánchez M, Anitua E, Orive G, Mujika I, Andia I. (2009). Platelet-rich plasma therapies in the treatment of orthopaedic sport injuries. *Sports Med.*, 39(5), 345-354, 0112-1642

Bellamy N, Buchanan WW, Goldsmith CH, Campbell J, Stitt LW. (1988). Validation study of WOMAC: a health status instrument for measuring clinically-important-platelet-relevant outcomes following total hip or knee arthroplasty in osteoarthritis. *J Rheumatol.*, 15(12), 1833-1840, 0315-162X

EuroQol Group. (1990). EuroQol-A New Facility for the Mesurement of Health-related Quality of Life. *Health Policy.*, 16(3), 199-208, 0168-8510

Irrgang JJ, Anderson AF, and Boland AL, Harner CD, Kurosaka M, Neyret P, Richmond JC, Shelborne KD. (2001). Development and validation of the International Knee Documentation Committee subjective knee form. *Am J Sports Med.*, 29(5), 600-613, 0363-5465

Filardo G, Kon E, Buda R, Timoncini A, Martino AD, Cenacchi A, Fornasari PM, Giannini S, Marcacci M. (2010). Platelet-rich plasma intra-articular knee injections for the treatment of degenerative cartilage lesions and osteoarthritis. *Knee Surg Sports Traumatol Arthrosc.*, 18(4), 472-479, 0942-2056

Nurden AT, Nurden P, Sanchez M, Andia I, Anitua E. (2008). Platelets and wound healing. *Front Biosci.*, 13, 3532-3548, 1093-9946

Kim SB, Kwon DR, Kwak H, Shin YB, Han HJ, Lee JH, Choi SH. (2010). Additive effects of intra-articular injection of growth hormone and hyaluronic acid in rabbit model of collagenase-induced osteoarthritis. *J Korean Med Sci.*, 25(5), 776-780, 1011-8934

5

Hyaluronic Acid in the Treatment of Osteoarthritis: What is New

Michele Abate and Vincenzo Salini
University "G. d' Annunzio" Chieti – Pescara
Italy

1. Introduction

Osteoarthritis is a very common disease, and its prevalence increases with age. According to the American College of Rheumatology, nearly 70 % of people over age 70 have X - ray evidence of osteoarthritis, although only half ever develop symptoms (Altman et al., 1991). Notwithstanding, due to the huge amount of persons affected, osteoarthritis is a frequent cause of disability (Lawrence et al., 1998).

Several pharmaceutical approaches, such as analgesics, non steroidal anti - inflammatory drugs, COX - 2 inhibitors and steroids (Hochberg et al., 1995), have been proposed, with the aim of reducing pain and maintaining and / or improving joint function. However, none of these options has shown to delay the progression of osteoarthritis or reverse joint damage.

In addition, the incidence of adverse reactions to these drugs increases with age. Data from epidemiological studies consistently show that the risk of gastro - intestinal complications is very high and largely dose - dependent (Griffin MR et al., 1991 ; Smalley & Griffin, 1996). It is well known that non steroidal anti - inflammatory drugs, as well as selective COX - 2 inhibitors, may cause renal failure, hypertension and water retention and have a thrombotic potential, especially for high doses and long term treatments (Roughead et al., 2008; Savage, 2005). Corticosteroids are burdened with relevant adverse reactions, when given systemically, and therefore are usually administered by intra - articular injection in patients who fail to respond to other conservative measures; in particular, patients with joint effusions and local tenderness may have greater benefit from this option (Flanagan et al., 1988).

Although it has been established that corticosteroid injections are relatively safe, there are concerns regarding their possible adverse effects, following repeated injections. These effects include local tissue atrophy, particularly when small joints are injected, long - term joint damage, due to reduced bone formation, and risk of infection, due to suppression of adrenocortical function (Mader et al., 2005; Weitoft et al., 2005).

Considering the limits of therapies at present available, drugs with minimal side effects are therefore warranted.

Viscosupplementation by intra - articular injections of hyaluronic acid has been proposed as useful therapeutic option in the treatment of osteoarthritis in different joints (Migliore et al., 2010).

Aim of the chapter is to summarize the more significant results of this therapeutic approach, reporting the recently published data and focusing attention on issues yet unsolved.

2. Synovial fluid

Synovial fluid is essential for the normal joint functioning : it acts both as a lubricant during slow movement (e.g. in walking), and as an elastic shock absorber during rapid movement (e.g. in running). It also serves as a medium for delivering nutrition, and transmitting cellular signals to articular cartilage.

Hyaluronic acid, produced by synoviocytes, fibroblasts and chondrocytes, is the major chemical component of synovial fluid. The native hyaluronic acid has a molecular weight of 4 - 10 millions Daltons, and is present in articular fluid in concentration about 0.35 gr / 100 ml (Weiss & Band, 1995). It is essential for the viscoelastic properties of the fluid because of high viscosity, and has a protective effect on articular cartilage and soft tissue surfaces of joints (O' Regan et al., 1994; Van den Bekerom et al., 2008).

In pathological conditions, the concentration and molecular weight of hyaluronic acid are reduced, resulting in synovial fluid of lower elasticity and viscosity : the factors which contribute to the low concentrations of hyaluronic acid are diluitional effects, reduced hyaluronan synthesis and free radical degradation (Van den Bekerom et al., 2006). When viscoelasticity of synovial fluid is reduced, the transmission of mechanical force to cartilage may increase its susceptibility to damage.

Therefore, the restoration of the normal articular homoeostasis is the rationale for hyaluronic acid administration into osteoarthritic joints. Moreover, being hyaluronic acid a physiological component, it is very likely that it may be deprived of adverse reactions, also after repeated administrations.

3. Therapeutic activities of hyaluronic acid

The direct injection of hyaluronic acid in the joint space allows to reach a proper concentration with low doses, favouring a longer permanence in the joint, and therefore the therapeutic response.

Hyaluronic acid preparations have a short half - life; therefore, the long term effects cannot solely be attributed to the substitution of molecule itself. The term viscosupplementation means restoration of visco - elastic properties, such as cushioning, lubrication, elasticity (Kikuchi et al., 2001), while the term biosupplementation is used to indicate the restoration of joint rheology, anti - inflammatory and anti - nociceptive effects, normalization of endogenous hyaluronic acid synthesis, and chondroprotection. These activities explain why the clinical efficacy is maintained for several months (Gigante & Callegari, 2010 ; Hiraoka et al., 2011; Julovi et al., 2011; Kumahashi et al., 2011).

In Table 1, the main beneficial effects of hyaluronic acid in osteoarthritis are summarized.

4. Hyaluronic acid preparations

At present, preparations with different molecular weight are available (Low and High Molecular Weight), which display distinct pharmaceutical effects (Ghosh & Guidolin, 2002).

The enhanced penetration of low molecular weight preparations (0.5 - 1.5 millions Dalton) through the extracellular matrix of the synovium is thought to maximize the concentration and to facilitate the interaction with target synovial cells, so reducing the synovial inflammation (Bagga H et al., 2006).

ACTION	TARGET	RESULTS
Inhibition	Lymphocyte transformation	**SLOW DOWN THE PROGRESSION OF JOINT DAMAGE** **ANTI - INFLAMMATORY ACTIVITY** **ANTI - NOCICEPTIVE EFFECTS** **MODIFIED STRUCTURAL ORGANIZATION TOWARDS NORMAL APPEARANCE**
	Phagocytic activity of macrophages and leukocytes	
	Adenosine triphosphate levels	
	Matrix Metalloproteinase (MMP)	
Promotion	Release of prostaglandins	
	Normalization of native hyaluronan synthesis	
	Production of tissue inhibitor of MMP - 1	
	Scavenging of free radicals	
	Proteoglycans synthesis by chondrocytes	
Protective	Effects on chondrocytes or cartilage explants from degradation by enzymes, Interleukin - 1, and oxygen - derived free radicals	

Table 1. Beneficial effects of hyaluronic acid (modified from Carpenter & Motley (2008))

However, because of the low elastoviscosity of these hyaluronan compounds, compared to native hyaluronan in the synovial fluid, interests were shifted to a viscosupplementation fluid similar to the native hyaluronic acid.
Recently, an hyaluronic acid cross - linked preparation (Hylan G - F 20), with high molecular weight (6 - 7 millions Dalton), has been developed (Migliore et al., 2010).
This formulation, by means of its hydrophilic properties, retains higher amounts of fluid in articular space; it is also provided by a greater anti - inflammatory activity, as shown by studies on migration of inflammatory cells in the joint and on reduced Prostaglandin E 2 and bradykinin concentration (Goto et al., 1999; Takahashi et al., 1999). Moreover, high molecular weight hyaluronic acid is considered more effective in relieving pain, compared to low molecular weight hyaluronic acid.
A novel hyaluronic acid preparation, non - animal stabilised hyaluronic acid (NASHA) (Berg & Olsson, 2004) has been manifactured by a two stage procedure : byosinthesis of hyaluronic acid by cultured bacteria, followed by a mild stabilization process. Stabilisation does not change the biochemical properties of hyaluronic acid, but creates bio - compatible gel with improved viscoelastic properties and a longer residence time in joint, compared with non - stabilised hyaluronic acid preparation.
Currently, with aim of favouring a longer presence of hyaluronic acid in the joint, long acting preparations are under study (Abate et al, 2010). Hopefully, these compounds, with better rheological and biological properties, could influence positively the natural history of osteoarthritic disease.

5. Indications to treatment

Viscosupplementation can be considered when the patient has not found pain relief from exercise, physical therapy, weight loss, use of orthotics and analgesics or non steroidal anti –

inflammatory drugs. Other indications may be the intolerance to drugs or the use of multiple systemic medications, as frequently happens in the elderly (Waddell, 2007).
The treatment, in general, is offered to patients with intermediate Kellgren - Lawrence score (mild osteoarthritis) (Kellgren & Lawrence, 1957), who report better results in term of function and pain reduction (Brzusek & Petron, 2005).
The administration of hyaluronic acid is contraindicated only in patients with known hypersensitivity to preparations components; patients with severe osteoarthritis (Kellgren - Lawrence score IV) or affected by inflammatory musculoskeletal diseases (rheumatoid arthritis, chondrocalcinosis, psoriasis, gout), may have limited benefit (Waddell, 2007).

6. Infiltration techniques

Intra - articular injection of hyaluronic acid must be performed in sterile conditions, to minimize the risk of inflammatory complications (i.e. septic arthritis).
Moreover, the use of "image - guided" infiltration techniques is mandatory; indeed, when joint infiltration is performed blindly, the failure rate is high, and the drug may be administered in the para - articular space. In this case, treatment loses its efficacy and side effects, mainly pain, frequently occur (Pourbagher et al., 2005; Zwar et al., 2004).
The ultrasound - guided injection, compared with fluoroscopy, has several advantages : it is simple, fast, economic and safe; it does not require the use of contrast media, allowing the infiltration in patients intolerant to iodized contrasts. It can be repeated without limits, allows an easy visualization of fluid in the articular recess (which may be aspirated) (Figure 1), and shows how narrow is the articular space.

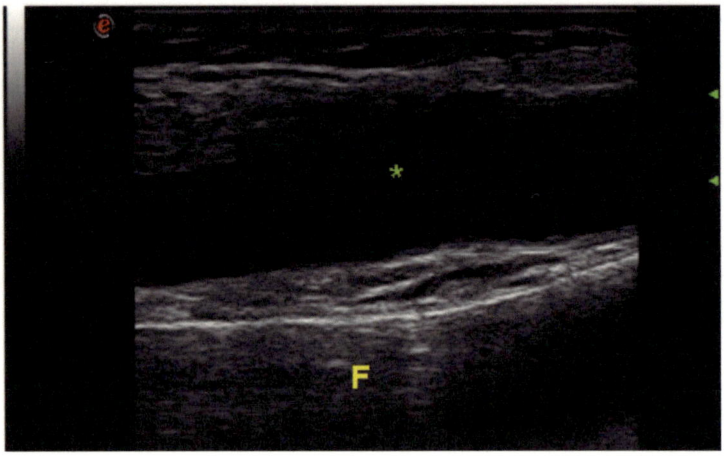

F = Femur

Fig. 1. Ultrasound imaging (longitudinal scan). An effusion (*) is present inside the articular space of knee joint.

Moreover, it is able to show the position of the needle, and, by means of continuous Color Doppler monitoring, to evaluate its distance from vessels. Finally, ultrasound technique allows the visualization of the viscous fluid injected inside the joint (Migliore et al., 2004).
In figure 2, an example of intra - articular injections of hip joint is presented.

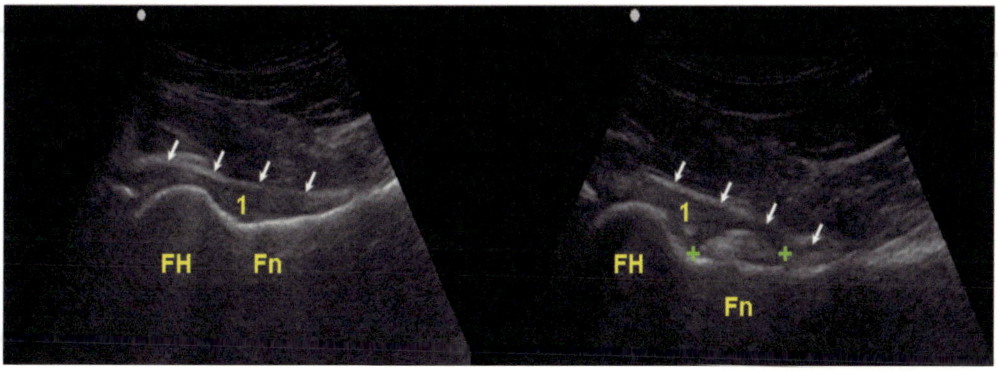

FH = Femoral head; Fn = Femoral neck; 1 = articular space; Arrows = articular capsule

Fig. 2. Ultrasound guided injection of hip joint (longitudinal scan). Before the injection, hip joint is evaluated (left panel). After the injection (right panel), the correct placement of hyaluronic acid (calipers) is confirmed by the presence of hyperechoic material inside the articular space.

7. Clinical results

In this section we report the main results obtained with hyaluronic acid in the treatment of osteoarthritis in different joints.

7.1 Knee osteoarthritis

Viscosupplementation with hyaluronic acid in knee osteoarthritis has been approved by Food and Drugs Administration (Hunter & Lo, 2008).

Recent guidelines are based on a meta - analysis, including 5257 participants to 40 Randomized Controlled Trials (Curran, 2010; National Collaborating Center for Chronic Conditions at the Royal College of Physicians, 2008). These studies were performed, single or double - blind, with different types of hyaluronic acid (low and high molecular weight) against placebo. The number of injections ranged from 3 to 5 weekly, with a maximum of 11 in 23 weeks, the doses from 15 to 60 mg and the trials length from 4 weeks to 18 months.

Pain was evaluated by means of Visual Analogic Scale and Western Ontario and McMaster Universities Osteoarthritis Index, at rest and under different load conditions. A minor number of studies evaluated the functional outcomes (Western Ontario and McMaster Universities Osteoarthritis Index [physical function], Lequesne Index, Range of motion), the subjective global assessment and the quality of life of the patients. The results of the majority of studies are in favour of hyaluronic acid, although in several randomized controlled trials no significant differences have been found in comparison with intra - articular placebo. The percentages of improvement from baseline, in all the outcomes measures, were 28 % to 54 % for pain, and 9 % to 32 % for function, and were similar in the trials where low molecular weight or high molecular weight hyaluronic acid were used (Aggarwal & Sempowski, 2004; Divine et al., 2007; Waddel 2007). However, the number of injection needed was in general lower for high molecular weight preparation and this is not a negligible advantage for the patients.

A recent systematic review has compared the post - intervention time course of the effects of hyaluronic acid and corticosteroid (the "therapeutic trajectory") (Bannuru et al., 2009).

This meta analysis highlights the therapeutic trajectory of hyaluronic acid for knee osteoarthritis pain over six months following the intervention. From baseline to week 4, intra - articular corticosteroid appear to be relatively more effective than hyaluronic acid. By week 4 the two approaches have equal efficacy, but beyond week 8 hyaluronic acid has greater efficacy.
It should be observed that the benefit is not equally distributed among patients, some of them being non - responders to therapy. The characteristics of responders, at present, have not been clearly identified, but some authors claim that a greater benefit may be obtained in patients with low grade osteoarthritis (Dagenais et al., 2006). On the contrary, age does not influence the therapeutic response (Abate et al., 2008).

7.2 Hip osteoarthritis

The number of studies about viscosupplementation of hip osteoarthritis is limited, when compared with studies in knee osteoarthritis. The reasons can be the deeper localization of this joint, and the proximity of femoral vessels and nerves.
Moreover, the level of evidence for most of these studies is low, because they are cohort studies and lack of a reference group (Abate et al., 2010), a score I (i.e. the highest level of evidence), according to the Center for Evidence Based Medicine criteria (Fletcher & Sackett, 1979), having been assigned only to Tikiz's (Tikiz et al., 2005) and Qvistgaard's (Qvistgaard et al., 2006) studies.
A new randomized controlled three - arm study, comparing intra - articular injection of hyaluronic acid, corticosteroid and bupivacaine, is in progress; this trial will hopefully provide robust information on the advantages of drugs towards the simple anaesthetic treatment (Colen et al., 2010).
In the published studies, several hyaluronic acid compounds were used. The number of injections ranged from 1 to 3 for each patients, and only in few cases 4 or 5 injections were performed. In general, the injections number was lower for high molecular weight preparations. The length of treatments and the outcome measures were similar to those used in knee randomized controlled trials.
All the trials have shown a reduction of pain, which, in general, becomes evident within 3 months and persists in the following months. Only few studies report a precocious reduction of the pain : within a week, according to Brocq (Brocq et al., 2002) (- 27 %), and within the first 2 - 4 weeks according to Qvistgaard (Qvistgaard et al., 2001) (- 14 % and - 32 %, respectively). The positive effects on pain after 1 - 3 months range from - 16.1 % to - 52.2 % (mean - 37.2 %), whereas, overall, the mean Visual Analogic Scale score decreases about 49 % after 3 - 6 months (range 31 - 80 %) (Abate et al., 2008).
Therefore, it seems that the benefit increases in the long term. However, it must be underlined that only few studies report longer follow - up periods : at 12 (Migliore et al., 2005) and at 18 months (Migliore et al., 2006a), with persistent benefit on the pain (VAS - 36.4 %). Besides the reduction of pain, also the articular function is improved. These positive effects have been observed using different evaluation scales : + 11 % in the Harris Hip Score, + 32 - 45 % in Western Ontario and McMaster Universities Osteoarthritis Index score, + 45 % in Lequesne Index, and + 95 % in American Academy of Orthopaedic Association Lower Limb Core Scale (Abate et al., 2008). A further observation, which confirms the previous data, is the reduction of non steroidal anti - inflammatory drugs consumption (Migliore et al., 2011).

7.3 Ankle osteoarthritis

Only few studies have been performed in ankle osteoarthritis and, among these, four were randomized / controlled trials (level of evidence 1) (Carpenter & Motley, 2008; Cohen et al., 2008; Karatosun et al., 2008; Salk et al., 2005, 2006), while seven studies (Hanson et al., 1999; Luciani et al., 2008; Mei - Dan et al., 2010; Sun et al., 2006; Valiveti et al., 2006; Witteveen et al., 2008, 2010) were case series (level of evidence 4).

In all these studies, patients suffering from post - traumatic Kellgreen - Lawrence grade II - IV ankle osteoarthritis were enrolled. Different hyluronic acid preparations were used, and patients received 1 up to 5 injections. Only in one study, the injections were performed by means of image guidance (fluoroscopy) (Cohen et al., 2008). Clinical benefit was evaluated by means of different scales (Visual Analogic Scale, Ankle Osteoarthritis Scale, American Orthopaedic Foot and Ankle Society, Short Form - 12, Short Form - 36, Western Ontario and McMaster Universities Osteoarthritis Index), and the follow - up period varied from 6 to 18 months.

In studies performed without control group (Hanson et al., 1999; Luciani et al., 2008; Mei - Dan et al., 2010; Sun et al., 2006; Valiveti et al., 2006; Witteveen et al., 2008, 2010) (Table 2), an improvement in all the outcome measures was reported, with the effect lasting for 18 months (Luciani et al., 2008). However, it is not clear from reports whether the pain reduction was clinically significant, or could be ascribed only to a placebo effect. In addition, the lack of controls does not allow definitive conclusions on the efficacy of hyaluronic acid.

Authors	Patients	Age	HA	Dose	Follow up	Results
Mei - Dan	15	43	LMW	1x5 wks	7 months	Positive
Sun	75	50	LMW	1x5 wks	6 monhts	Positive
Luciani	21	45	HMW	1x3 wks	3 monhts	Positive
Witteveen(2008)	55	41	HMW	1 or 2	6 - 9 months	Positive
Witteveen(2010)	26	43	HMW	1 or 2 or 3	6 months	Positive

HA = Hyaluronic acid; LMW = Low Molecular Weight; HMW = High Molecular Weight

Table 2. Case series studies on ankle osteoarthritis. Valiveti (2006) and Hanson (1999) studies' are not reported due to the small number of cases.

The level 1 evidence studies are more qualified to assess the therapeutic efficacy, but also these trials show several limitations (e.g., no information on the actual number of potential patients, no clear patients randomization, imbalance of baseline characteristics between intervention and control groups, statistical weakness), and therefore have to be considered as low quality studies.

In these studies (Carpenter & Motley, 2008; Cohen et al., 2008; Karatosun et al., 2008; Salk et al., 2005, 2006) (Table 3), the patients treated with hyaluronic acid showed a significant decrease in pain and disability at 6 months (Cohen et al., 2008; Salk et al., 2005, 2006), with the effects lasting 12 - 13 months (Carpenter & Motley, 2008; Karatosun et al., 2008). Besides the reduction of these parameters, an improvement in ankle sagittal range of motions, and gait quality was observed (Karatosun et al., 2008).

Authors	Patients	Age	HA	Dose	Control	Follow up	HA vs Controls
Carpenter	26	55	HMW	1x3 wks	Arthroscopy	13 months	> HA (moderate)
Cohen	30	49	LMW	1x5 wks	Saline	6 months	No difference
Karatosun	30	55	LMW	1x3 wks	Exercise	12 months	No difference
Salk	17	58	LMW	1x5 wks	Saline	6 months	No difference

Table 3. Randomized controlled trials on ankle osteoarthritis. Salk et al. (2006, 2005) presented their results in two different journals.

In any study the authors found difference between hyaluronic acid and controls groups. In particular, in the studies performed by Salk (Salk et al., 2005, 2006) and Cohen (Cohen et al., 2008), the patients, treated with a 1 - 2 ml phosphate - buffered saline solution injection, reported a similar improvement in all parameters evaluated. Analogously, positive results were observed in patients, who followed a 6 weeks exercise therapy (muscle strengthening and ankle range of motion exercises) (Karatosun et al., 2008), and after arthroscopic lavage of osteoarthritic ankle joint (Carpenter & Motley, 2008).

On the basis of these observations, no clear evidence on the efficacy of hyaluronic acid in reducing pain, and improving function, in ankle osteoarthritis, is provided.

Several factors can explain why viscosupplementation has limited efficacy in ankle osteoarthritis.

Ankle joint, anatomically and functionally, is more complex than other joints, which are usually treated with positive results with hyaluronic acid (hip, knee) (Saltzman et al., 2005).

Another possible reason of the limited benefit of hyaluronic acid can be related to its use mostly in post - traumatic osteoarthritis (Zhang & Jordan, 2010), which has a pathogenesis quite different from that of primary degenerative osteoarthritis.

Finally, it must be considered that all studies (Carpenter & Motley, 2008; Hanson et al., 1999; Karatosun et al., 2008; Luciani et al., 2008; Mei - Dan et al., 2010; Salk et al., 2005, 2006; Sun et al., 2006; Valiveti et al., 2006; Witteveen et al., 2008, 2010), but one (Cohen et al., 2008), were performed blindly, with any imaging guidance. This can be a valid explanation of several unsatisfactory results, because there is evidence that about one third of intra - articular injections are not delivered into the intra - articular cavity, when performed without a visual aid (Cunnington et al., 2010).

At this regard, ankle joint presents many technical difficulties of injecting intra - articularly, due to its complex anatomy, further complicated from the osteoarthritic joint changes (Woo et al., 2010).

7.4 Gleno – Humeral osteoarthritis

Hyaluronic acid is effective and well tolerated for the treatment of osteoarthritis and persistent shoulder pain refractory to other standard non operative interventions (Andrews, 2005).

Several authors (Blaine et al., 2008; Leardini et al., 1988) report that both 3 and 5 weekly intra - articular injections of low molecular weight hyaluronic acid provide significant improvement in terms of shoulder pain (Visual Analogic Scale score on movement), with the effects lasting 7 - 26 weeks (Blaine et al., 2008).

Similarly, in a 6 months follow - up studies (Merolla et al., 2011; Silverstain et al., 2007), a significant reduction in Visual Analogic Scale pain score was also provided with 3 weekly intra - articular high molecular weight hyaluronic acid (Hylan G - F 20) injections. In addition, most of the patients experienced an improvement in the shoulder function score and in the activities of daily living (Itokazu & Matsunaga, 1995; Merolla et al., 2011).
A recent study comparing Hylan G - F 20 versus 6 methylprednisolone acetate shows that hyaluronic acid is effective in reducing pain for up to 6 months, whereas corticosteroid injections result in improvement at 1 month only (Merolla et al., 2011).
Finally, the efficacy of hyaluronic acid has been demonstrated in the treatment of different shoulder diseases, such as subacromial bursitis, adhesive capsulitis and rotator cuff tear (Blaine et al., 2008; Calis et al., 2006; Fernandez - Palazzi et al., 2002; Rovetta & Monteforte, 1998; Tamai et al., 2004), with positive results on pain, joint mobility and shoulder function.

7.5 Carpo – Metacarpal osteoarthritis

Because carpo - metacarpal joint is essential for the closure of the first web, a loss of function causes an alteration of the thumb - index pinch, and therefore can lead to functional impairment (Spacek et al., 2004).
Several conservative treatments have been proposed (corticosteroids, non steroidal anti - inflammatory drugs, prolotherapy, splinting), but none of these has shown to delay the progression of osteoarthritis or reverse joint damage (Fuchs et al., 2006).
Recent studies have investigated the efficacy of hyaluronic acid in the treatment of carpo - metacarpal osteoarthritis (Figure 3) and positive results have been reported by most of the authors.

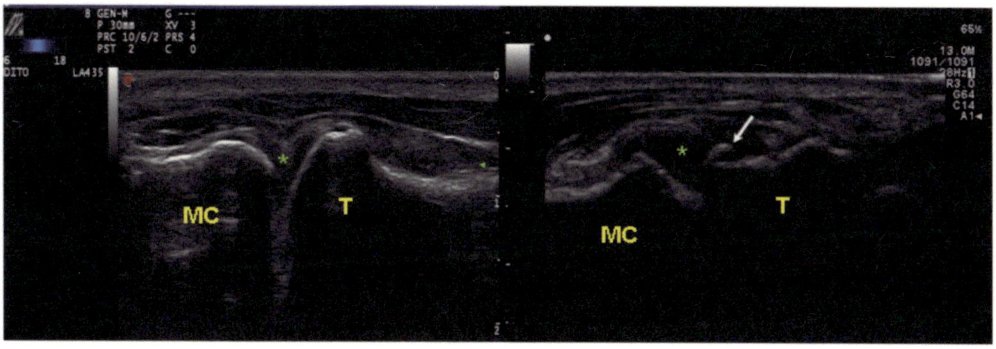

MC = Metacarpal bone

Fig. 3. Ultrasound features of carpo - metacarpal osteoarthritis (right panel) : the cortex of the trapezium bone (T) is irregular and an osteophyte is present (arrow); mild articular effusion (*) can be also appreciated. In left panel, normal features are reported.

In particular, an early improvement in Visual Analogic Scale score was observed after 2 weeks post treatment (Heyworth et al., 2008), with the effects lasting until 1 - 3 months (Coaccioli et al., 2006; Roux et al., 2007; Schumacher et al., 2004; Stahl et al., 2005). The long term effects of hyaluronan were demonstrated only in few studies (Fuchs et al., 2006; Heyworth et al., 2008;), in which the pain relief was reported at 6 months (Di Sante et al., 2011).

Beside pain reduction, also grip strength improved significantly in some studies (Migliore et al., 2010), although these effects were achieved slowly, with better results observed at 6 months (Fuchs et al., 2006; Heyworth et al., 2008; Stahl et al., 2005).
In our experience (Table 4), a single ultrasound guided injection of hyaluronic acid is effective in treatment of carpo - metacarpal osteoarthritis (Salini et al., 2009). After therapy the Visual Analogic Scale pain score, both at rest and during common daily activities, decreases, while the hand function and strength are improved. The best improvement is observed in the pulp pinch strength, because the carpo - metacarpal joint is strongly stressed in this movement (Spacek et al., 2004), and therefore a better mobility and a reduction of pain in the joint allow evident increase in performance.

	Baseline	**Follow - up**	**p**
VAS rest	1,8 ± 1	0,5 ± 0,6	< 0.001
VAS activities	8 ± 0,9	4,1 ± 1,4	< 0.001
Dreiser Index	18,5 ± 3,3	20,7 ± 2,7	< 0.004
Hand grip (Kg)	19,3 ± 16,5	19,6 ± 16,1	0.13
Lateral grip (Kg)	9,5 ± 4	10 ± 3,3	0.17
Pulp grip (Kg)	4,1 ± 1,4	5,4 ± 1,3	< 0.001
NSAIDs (n. of subjects)	16	7	
NSAIDs (tablets / week)	2,4 ± 1,9	1,1 ± 1,3	< 0.02

NSAID = Non Steroidal Anti - Inflammatory Drug; VAS = Visual Analogic Scale

Table 4. Positive results of hyaluronic acid on pain and hand function

7.6 Temporo-mandibular joint

At present, 19 studies have been published, and only 8 were randomized and controlled trials (Manfredini et al., 2010). All studies reported a decrease in pain levels independently by the patients' disorder and by the adopted injection protocol. Positive outcomes were maintained over the follow - up period, which ranged largely from 15 days to 24 months. The superiority of hyaluronic acid injections was shown only against placebo saline injections, but outcomes were comparable with those achieved with corticosteroid injections.
Interestingly, in an experimental model of arthropatic temporomandibular joint, El - Hakim and Elyamani (El - Hakim & Elyamani 2011) found, after repeated intra - articular injections of hyaluronic acid, an increase in the thickness of the cartilagineous layer, suggesting that hyaluronic acid can inhibit the progression of osteoarthritic changes.
A recent study, aiming to identify predictors for treatment efficacy, has shown that only unilateral temporomandibular joint osteoarthritis predicts better the benefit (Guarda - Nardini et al., 2011), while sex, age, pain duration are not provided of predictive power.

7.7 Other joints

Encouraging results have been reported in the treatment of painful hallux rigidus (Pons et al., 2007), of sacroiliac joint syndrome (Calvillo et al., 2000; Srejic et al., 1999), and of nerve root adhesion after lumbar intervertebral disco herniation (Wang et al., 2002).

In the treatment of elbow osteoarthritis the results are inconclusive. Positive effects have been observed only in two small studies (Fernandez - Palazzi et al., 2002; Hanson, 1999), while, in a larger study (18 patients), intra - articular hyaluronic acid was not effective in the treatment of post - traumatic osteoarthritis of the elbow (Van Brakel & Eygendaal, 2006).

Controversial results have been observed also in the treatment of spine osteoarthritis. Fuchs et al. (Fuchs et al., 2005) reported significant pain relief and improved quality of life, also in the long term, in patients affected from facet joints osteoarthritis with chronic non radicular pain in the lumbar spine. However, these results are not in agreement with a recent study by Cleary et al. (Cleary et al., 2008), who have not seen any benefit of viscosupplementation in the management of symptomatic lumbar facet osteoarthritis.

8. Side effects

Several factors may contribute to the occurrence of side effects : among them, the characteristics and amount of hyaluronic acid preparation injected, the number of injections, the skill of the operator, the technique used, the local and systemic tissues reactions.

In quite all the clinical trials, no general side effects were observed, and only few patients reported a sensation of heaviness and pain in their joint after injection (Abate M, 2009).

These effects were more frequent in studies performed in blind conditions compared to those performed under imaging guidance. No differences were observed in relation to hyaluronic acid preparation used or to the number of injections (Abate M, 2008).

Side effects usually disappeared after 2 - 7 days without any therapeutic intervention and did not limit basic or instrumental activities of daily living.

Vascular or nervous complications were never reported, neither gout, chondrocalcinosis, sometimes observed after viscosupplementation of the knee (Curran, 2010).

Septic arthritis or aseptic synovial effusion occurred in a very limited number of cases (Brocq et al., 2002; Chazerain et al., 1999).

9. Hyaluronic acid vs corticosteroids

Intra - articular corticosteroids are the alternative choice to hyaluronic acid for treatment of osteoarthritis. Therefore it is important to evaluate the studies, which compared these treatment modalities. The large majority of comparison studies has been performed between different hyaluronic acid preparations and steroids (methylprednisolone, triamcinolone) (Bellamy et al., 2006).

In several studies, better results were observed after hyaluronic acid injection (Cohen et al., 2008; Fuchs et al., 2005, 2006), in other no significant difference was found (Chazerain et al., 1999; Qvistgaard et al., 2006). Steroids however offered the best results on joints with inflammatory effusions (Atchia et al., 2011).

Only one study compared the clinical efficacy of hyaluronic acid versus corticosteroids and placebo in hip osteoarthritis. This very large trial, including 101 patients, did not show significant differences between the treatments in all the outcome measures, after 3 months

(Qvistgaard et al., 2006). However, within this time period, an improvement was found, which resulted clearly evident in the steroid group and moderate in hyaluronic acid group, compared to placebo (Qvistgaard et al., 2006).
A comparison study on the efficacy of Hylan G - F 20 versus 6 - methylprednisolone acetate in shoulder osteoarthritis shows that hyaluronic acid is effective in reducing pain for up to 6 months, whereas corticosteroids injections result in an improvement at 1 month only (Merolla et al., 2011).
Analogously, Bannuru et al. (Bannuru et al., 2009) have shown in the treatment of knee osteoarthritis that intra - articular corticosteroids appear to be relatively more effective for pain that hyaluronic acid in the first four weeks, but in the long term hyaluronic acid has greater efficacy.
In carpo - metacarpal joint osteoarthritis, a rapid pain relief was observed after triamcinolone or methylprednisolone injections (after 2 - 4 weeks), but disappeared soon after (Heyworth et al., 2008). Positive effects were achieved with hyaluronic acid more slowly, but were long - lasting and persisted 6 months after end of treatment period (Fuchs et al., 2006).
Also for the treatment of temporomandibular joint osteoarthritis, the comparison between corticosteroids and hyaluronic acid has shown that both compounds reduce pain and improve articular function (Manfredini et al., 2010).

10. Conclusions

On the basis of the published trials, we may affirm that viscosupplementation therapy with hyaluronic acid is a safe and effective method in the management of osteoarthritis resistant to conventional therapies. This treatment has been approved by Food and Drug Administration for knee osteoarthritis, whereas for the other osteoarthritic joints there are promising results but not conclusive evidence.
The use of hyaluronic acid is mainly recommended when non steroidal anti - inflammatory drugs are contraindicated or badly tolerated, when non steroidal anti - inflammatory drugs or corticosteroid are inefficacious, or in young patients candidate to prosthesis.
Viscosupplementation significantly reduces pain within 3 months and this beneficial effect is maintained in the long term (12 - 18 months). The articular function is improved and, therefore, patients can rapidly come back to work and to social activities.
Only few trials have shown a very early improvement, which has been related to the lubricating effect of hyaluronate in "dry" joints, as reported in studies of viscosupplementation in knee osteoarthritis, and / or to a short term placebo effect (Brocq et al., 2002).
The reduction in non steroidal anti - inflammatory drugs consumption is another important clinical achievement with significant health economic consideration (Sturkenboom et al., 2002). Not only direct costs (non steroidal anti - inflammatory drugs purchasing), but also the indirect costs associated with management of non steroidal anti - inflammatory drugs side effects, are saved. Cost - benefit analysis is difficult in comparison with corticosteroids. Corticosteroids doses are cheaper than hyaluronic acid preparation, but the efficacy of these drugs seems to last less longer than hyaluronic acid preparations, with more relevant side effects, which can offset the initial saving (Qvistgaard et al., 2006).

Patients with mild morphological alterations, and with preserved articular space, are more responsive to treatment (Brocq et al., 2002; Gaston et al., 2007; Van den Bekerom et al., 2006); the results are less encouraging in patients with severe osteoarthritis (Kellgreen - Lawrence IV), only few studies reporting a good therapeutic effects (Migliore et al., 2006b).

Articular effusion usually is associated to a reduced therapeutic efficacy due to the "dilution effect" of the drug (Qvistgaard et al., 2006). In this situation, a better therapeutic response is observed with intra - articular corticosteroids, probably linked to their anti - inflammatory activity (Qvistgaard et al., 2006).

The better biological activity, shown by high molecular weight hyaluronic acid preparations in vitro, has not been confirmed in clinical trials (Tikiz et al., 2005). In fact, the percentage of improvement in all the outcomes measures is similar with low molecular weight and high molecular weight hyaluronic acid preparations (Caglar - Yagchi et al., 2005). An advantage of high molecular weight hyaluronic acid may be the reduced number of the injections needed to obtain the therapeutic effect.

When the therapy is delivered by appropriately trained doctors, under strict imaging guidance, viscosupplementation is a safe procedure, without any systemic or local side effect, excluding the pain of the injection and a sensation of heaviness for few hours / days after treatment. It is likely that persistent pain and joint swelling or major complications, such as septic arthritis may occur when injection is not properly performed. Even experienced clinicians can miss intra - articular placement of the drug, especially in small joints (Gaffney et al., 1995; Jones et al., 1993). The very high tolerability of the preparation allows the contemporary use of other drugs, which is very important in elderly patients with comorbid conditions and poli - pharmaceutical treated.

Although these promising results, several questions are still opened.

Inclusion and exclusion criteria vary largely in different studies and therefore the characteristics of patients, who are better responsive to treatment, are not clearly defined. The identification of these patients is, therefore, strongly recommended.

No consensus exist about the doses of hyaluronic acid, the interval between doses and the number of injections, which are more effective in the different clinical situations. A 3 - 5 doses regimen is usually recommended, but studies which compare different treatment schedules are lacking (Tikiz et al., 2005).

It is also debated whether high molecular weight hyaluronic acid has to be preferred to low molecular weight hyaluronic acid. The better biological activity, showed by high molecular weight hyaluronic acid preparations in vitro, has not been confirmed in clinical trials (Tikiz et al., 2005). Some authors prefer to use high molecular weight hyaluronic acid because these preparations have a longer half - life time, so that the number of the injections needed to obtain the therapeutic effect may be reduced.

Interpretation of result is made difficult by the different degree of severity of osteoarthritis, genetic and biological characteristics of patients enrolled in the studies and by concurrent therapies with other drugs and rehabilitation treatments (Brocq et al., 2002; Conrozier et al., 2003; Migliore et al., 2003; Tikiz et al., 2005; Vad et al., 2003).

Finally, it must be remembered that there is a strong placebo effect from joint injection, which may cause a nearly 30 % reduction in pain relief during the first 2 weeks (Brocq et al., 2002; Egsmose et al., 1984; Kirwan, 2001; Ravaud et al., 1999; Tikiz et al., 2005).

11. References

Abate, M., Pulcini, D., Di Iorio, A. & Schiavone, C. (2010). Viscosupplementation with intra-articular hyaluronic acid for treatment of osteoarthritis in the elderly. *Curr Pharm Des,* Vol.16, No.6, pp. 631-640

Abate, M., Pelotti, P., De Amicis, D., Di Iorio, A., Galletti, S. & Salini, V. (2008). Viscosupplementation with hyaluronic acid in hip osteoarthritis (a review). *Ups J Med Sci,* Vol.113, No.3, pp. 261-277

Aggarwal, A. & Sempowski, IP. (2004). Hyaluronic acid injections for knee osteoarthritis. Systematic review of the literature. *Can Fam Physician,* Vol.50, pp. 249-256

Altman, R., Alarcon, G., Appelrouth, D., Bloch, D., Borenstein, D., Brandt, K., Brown, C., Cooke, TD., Daniel, W., Feldman, D. & et al. (1991). The American College of Rheumatology criteria for the classification and reporting of osteoarthritis of the hip. *Arthritis Rheum,* Vol.34, No.5, pp. 505-514

Andrews, JR. (2005). Diagnosis and treatment of chronic painful shoulder: review of nonsurgical interventions. *Arthroscopy,* Vol.21, No.3, pp. 333-347

Atchia I, Kane D, Reed MR, Isaacs JD, Birrell F. (2011). Efficacy of a single ultrasound-guided injection for the treatment of hip osteoarthritis. *Ann Rheum Dis,* Vol.70, No.1, pp. 110-116

Bagga, H., Burkhardt, D., Sambrook, P. & March, L. (2006). Longterm effects of intraarticular hyaluronan on synovial fluid in osteoarthritis of the knee. *J Rheumatol,* Vol. 33, No.5, pp. 946-950

Bannuru, RR., Natov, NS., Obadan, IE., Price, LL., Schmid, CH. & McAlindon, TE. (2009). Therapeutic trajectory of hyaluronic acid versus corticosteroids in the treatment of knee osteoarthritis: a systematic review and meta-analysis. *Arthritis Rheum,* Vol.61, No.12, pp. 1704-1711

Bellamy, N., Campbell, J., Robinson, V., Gee, T., Bourne, R. & Wells, G. (2006). Viscosupplementation for the treatment of osteoarthritis of the knee. *Cochrane Database of Systematic Revues,* Vol.19, No.2

Berg, P. & Olsson, U. (2004). Intra-articular injection of non-animal stabilised hyaluronic acid (NASHA) for osteoarthritis of the hip: a pilot study. *Clin Exp Rheumatol,* Vol.22, No.3, pp. 300-306

Blaine, T., Moskowitz, R., Udell, J., Skyhar, M., Levin, R., Friedlander, J., Daley, M. & Altman, R. (2008). Treatment of persistent shoulder pain with sodium hyaluronate: a randomized, controlled trial. A multicenter study. *J Bone Joint Surg Am,* Vol.90, No.5, pp. 970-979

Brocq, O., Tran, .G, Breuil, V., Grisot, C., Flory, P. & Euller-Ziegler, L. (2002). Hip osteoarthritis: short-term efficacy and safety of viscosupplementation by hylan G-F 20. An open-label study in 22 patients. *Joint Bone Spine,* Vol.69, No.4, pp. 388-391

Brzusek, D. & Petron, D. (2008).Treating knee osteoarthritis with intra-articular hyaluronans. *Curr Med Res Opin,* Vol.24, No.12, pp. 3307-3322

Caglar-Yagci, H., Unsal, S., Yagci, I., Dulgeroglu, D. & Ozel, S. (2005). Safety and efficacy of ultrasound-guided intra-articular hylan G-F 20 injection in osteoarthritis of the hip: a pilot study. *Rheumatol Int,* Vol.25, No.5, pp. 341-344

Calis, M., Demir, H., Ulker, S., Kirnap, M., Duygulu, F. & Calis, HT. (2006). Is intraarticular sodium hyaluronate injection an alternative treatment in patients with adhesive capsulitis? *Rheumatol Int,* Vol.26, No.6, pp. 536-540

Calvillo, O., Skaribas, I. & Turnipseed, J. (2000). Anatomy and pathophysiology of the sacroiliac joint. *Curr Rev Pain,* Vol.4, No.5, pp. 356-361

Carpenter, B. & Motley, T. (2008). The role of viscosupplementation in the ankle using hylan G - F 20. *Journal of Foot & Ankle Surgery,* Sep-Oct, Vol.47, No.5, pp. 377-384

Chazerain, P., Rolland, D., Cordonnier, C. & Ziza, JM. (1999). Septic hip arthritis after multiple injections into the joint of hyaluronate and glucocorticoid. *Rev Rhum Engl Ed,* Vol.66, No.7-9, pp. 436

Cleary, M., Keating, C. & Poynton, AR. (2008). Viscosupplementation in lumbar facet joint arthropathy: a pilot study. *J Spinal Disord Tech,* Vol.21, No.1, pp. 29-32

Coaccioli, S., Pinoca, F. & Puxeddu, A. (2006). Short term efficacy of intra-articular injection of hyaluronic acid in osteoarthritis of the first carpometacarpal joint in a preliminary open pilot study. *Clin Ter,* Vol.157, No.4, pp. 321-325

Cohen, MM., Altman, RD., Hollstrom, R., Hollstrom, C., Sun, C. & Gipson, B. (2008). Safety and efficacy of intra - articular sodium hyaluronate (Hyalgan) in a randomized, double - blind study for osteoarthritis of the ankle. *Foot and Ankle International,* Vol.29, No.7, pp. 657-663

Colen, S., van den Bekerom, MP., Bellemans, J. & Mulier, M. (2010). Comparison of intra-articular injections of hyaluronic acid and corticosteroid in the treatment of osteoarthritis of the hip in comparison with intra-articular injections of bupivacaine. Design of a prospective, randomized, controlled study with blinding of the patients and outcome assessors. *BMC Musculoskelet Disord,* Vol.11, pp. 264

Conrozier, T., Bertin, P., Mathieu, P., Charlot, J., Bailleul, F., Treves, R., Vignon, E. & Chevalier, X. (2003). Intra-articular injections of hylan G-F 20 in patients with symptomatic hip osteoarthritis: an open-label, multicentre, pilot study. *Clin Exp Rheumatol,* Vol.21, No.5, pp. 605-610

Cunnington, J., Marshall, N., Hide, G., Bracewell, C., Isaacs, J., Platt, P. & Kane, D. (2010). A randomized, double - blind, controlled study of ultrasound - guided corticosteroid injection into the joint of patients with inflammatory arthritis. *Arthritis Rheum,* Jul, Vol. 62, No.7, pp. 1862-1869

Curran, MP. (2010). Hyaluronic acid (Supartz®) : a review of its use in osteoarthritis of the knee. Drugs Aging, Vol.27, No.11, pp. 925-941

Dagenais, S. (2006). Intra-articular hyaluronic acid (viscosupplementation) for knee osteoarthritis. *Issues Emerg Health Technol,* Vol.94, pp. 1-4

Divine, JG., Zazulak, BT. & Hewett, TE. (2007). Viscosupplementation for knee osteoarthritis: a systematic review. *Clin Orthop Relat Res,* Vol.455, pp. 113-122

Di Sante, L., Cacchio, A., Scettri, P., Paoloni, M., Ioppolo, F. & Santilli, V. (2011). Ultrasound-guided procedure for the treatment of trapeziometacarpal osteoarthritis. *Clin Rheumatol,* Mar 22

Egsmose, C., Lund, B. & Bach, AR. (1984). Hip joint distension in osteoarthrosis. A triple-blind controlled study comparing the effect of intra-articular indoprofen with placebo. *Scand J Rheumatol,* Vol.13, No.3, pp. 238-242

El-Hakim, IE. & Elyamani, AO. (2011). Preliminary evaluation of histological changes found in a mechanical arthropatic temporomandibular joint (TMJ) exposed to an intra-articular Hyaluronic acid (HA) injection, in a rat model. *J Craniomaxillofac Surg,* Jan 7

Fernandez-Palazzi, F., Viso, R., Boadas, A., Ruiz-Saez, A., Caviglia, H. & De Bosch, NB. (2002). Intra-articular hyaluronic acid in the treatment of haemophilic chronic arthropathy. *Haemophilia,* Vol.8, No.3, pp. 375-381

Flanagan, J., Casale, FF., Thomas, TL. & Desai, KB. (1988). Intra-articular injection for pain relief in patients awaiting hip replacement. *Ann R Coll Surg Engl,* Vol.70, No.3, pp. 156-157

Fletcher, B. & Sackett, D. (1979). Canadian task force on the periodic health esamination: the Periodic Health Examination. *CMAJ,* Vol.121, pp. 1193-1254

Fuchs, S., Monikes, R., Wohlmeiner, A. & Heyse, T. (2006). Intra-articular hyaluronic acid compared with corticoid injections for the treatment of rhizarthrosis. *Osteoarthritis Cartilage,* Vol.14, No.1, pp. 82-88

Fuchs, S., Erbe, T., Fischer, HL. & Tibesku, CO. (2005). Intraarticular hyaluronic acid versus glucocorticoid injections for nonradicular pain in the lumbar spine. *J Vasc Interv Radiol,* Vol.16, No.11, pp. 1493-1498

Gaffney, K., Ledingham, J. & Perry, JD. (1995). Intra-articular triamcinolone hexacetonide in knee osteoarthritis: factors influencing the clinical response. *Ann Rheum Dis,* Vol.54, No.5, pp. 379-381

Gaston, MS., Tiemessen, CH. & Philips, JE. (2007). Intra-articular hip viscosupplementation with synthetic hyaluronic acid for osteoarthritis: efficacy, safety and relation to pre-injection radiographs. *Arch Orthop Trauma Surg,* Vol.127, No.10, pp. 899-903

Ghosh, P. & Guidolin, D. (2002). Potential mechanism of action of intra-articular hyaluronan therapy in osteoarthritis: are the effects molecular weight dependent? *Semin Arthritis Rheum,* Vol.32, No.1, pp. 10-37

Gigante, A. & Callegari, L. (2011). The role of intra-articular hyaluronan (Sinovial) in the treatment of osteoarthritis. *Rheumatol Int,* Vol. 31, No.4, pp. 427-444

Goto, H., Onodera, T., Hirano, H. & Shimamura, T. (1999). Hyaluronic acid suppresses the reduction of alpha2(VI) collagen gene expression caused by interleukin-1beta in cultured rabbit articular chondrocytes. *Tohoku J Exp Med,* Vol.187, No.1, pp. 1-13

Griffin, MR., Piper, JM., Daugherty, JR., Snowden, M. & Ray, WA. (1991). Non steroidal anti-inflammatory drug use and increased risk for peptic ulcer disease in elderly persons. *Ann Intern Med,* Vol.114, No.4, pp. 257-263

Guarda-Nardini, L., Ferronato, G., Favero, L. & Manfredini, D.(2011). Predictive factors of hyaluronic acid injections short-term effectiveness for TMJ degenerative joint disease. *J Oral Rehabil,* Vol.38, No.5, pp. 315-320

Hanson, EC. (1999). Sodium hyaluronate - application in a community practice. *American Journal of Orthopaedics,* Vol.28, Suppl.11, pp. 11-12

Heyworth, BE., Lee, JH., Kim, PD., Lipton, CB., Strauch, RJ. & Rosenwasser, MP. (2008). Hylan versus corticosteroid versus placebo for treatment of basal joint arthritis: a prospective, randomized, double-blinded clinical trial. *J Hand Surg [Am],* Vol.33, No.1, pp. 40-48

Hiraoka N, Takahashi KA, Arai Y, Sakao K, Mazda O, Kishida T, Honjo K, Tanaka S, Kubo T. (2011). Intra-articular injection of hyaluronan restores the aberrant expression of matrix metalloproteinase-13 in osteoarthritic subchondral bone. *J Orthop Res,* Vol.29, No.3, pp. 354-360

Hochberg, MC., Altman, RD., Brandt, KD., Clark, BM., Dieppe, PA., Griffin, MR., Moskowitz, RW. % Schnitzer, TJ. (1995). Guidelines for the medical management of osteoarthritis. Part II. Osteoarthritis of the knee. American College of Rheumatology. *Arthritis Rheum,* Vol.38, No.11, pp. 1541-1546

Hunter, DJ. & Lo, GH. (2008). The management of osteoarthritis: an overview and call to appropriate conservative treatment. *Rheum Dis Clin North Am,* Vol.34, No.3, pp. 689-712

Itokazu, M. & Matsunaga, T. (1995). Clinical evaluation of high-molecular-weight sodium hyaluronate for the treatment of patients with periarthritis of the shoulder. *Clin Ther,* Vol.17, No.5, pp. 946-955

Jones, A., Regan, M., Ledingham, J., Pattrick, M., Manhire, A. & Doherty, M. (1993). Importance of placement of intra-articular steroid injections. BMJ, Vol.307, No.6915, pp. 1329-1330

Julovi, SM., Ito, H., Nishitani, K., Jackson, CJ. & Nakamura, T. (2011). Hyaluronan inhibits matrix metalloproteinase-13 in human arthritic chondrocytes via CD44 and P38. J Orthop Res, Vol.29, No.2, pp. 258-264

Karatosun, V., Unver, B., Ozden, A., Ozay, Z. & Gunal, I. (2008). Intra - articular hyaluronic acid compared to exercise therapy in osteoarthritis of the ankle. A prospective randomized trial with long - term follow - up. *Clinical and experimental rheumatology,* Mar-Apr, Vol.26, No.2, pp. 288-294

Kellgren, JH. & Lawrence, JS. (1957). Radiological assessment of osteo-arthrosis. Ann Rheum Dis, Vol.16, No.4, pp. 494-502

Kikuchi, T., Yamada, H. & Fujikawa, K. (2001). Effects of high molecular weight hyaluronan on the distribution and movement of proteoglycan around chondrocytes cultured in alginate beads. Osteoarthritis Cartilage, Vol.9, No.4, pp. 351-356

Kirwan, J. (2001). Is there a place for intra-articular hyaluronate in osteoarthritis of the knee? *Knee,* Vol.8, No.2, pp. 93-101

Kumahashi, N., Naitou, K., Nishi, H., Oae, K., Watanabe, Y., Kuwata, S., Ochi, M., Ikeda, M. & Uchio, Y. (2011). Correlation of changes in pain intensity with synovial fluid adenosine triphosphate levels after treatment of patients with osteoarthritis of the knee with high-molecular-weight hyaluronic acid. *Knee,* Vol.18, No.3, pp. 160-164

Lawrence, RC., Helmick, CG., Arnett, FC., Deyo, RA., Felson, DT., Giannini, EH., Heyse, SP., Hirsch, R., Hochberg, MC., Hunder, GG., Liang, MH., Pillemer, SR., Steen, VD., & Wolfe, F. (1998). Estimates of the prevalence of arthritis and selected musculoskeletal disorders in the United States. *Arthritis Rheum,* Vol.41, No.5, pp. 778-799

Leardini, G., Perbellini, A., Franceschini, M. & Mattara, L. (1988). Intra-articular injections of hyaluronic acid in the treatment of painful shoulder. *Clin Ther,* Vol.10, No.5, pp. 521-526

Luciani, D., Cadossi, M., Tesei, F., Chiarello, E. & Giannini, S. (2008). Viscosupplementation for grade II osteoarthritis of the ankle : a prospective study at 18 months' follow - up. *Chir Organi Mov,* Dec, Vol.92, No.3, pp. 155-160

Mader, R., Lavi, I. & Luboshitzky, R. (2005). Evaluation of the pituitary-adrenal axis function following single intraarticular injection of methylprednisolone. *Arthritis Rheum,* Vol.52, No.3, pp. 924-928

Manfredini, D., Piccotti, F. & Guarda-Nardini, L. (2010). Hyaluronic acid in the treatment of TMJ disorders: a systematic review of the literature. *Cranio,* Vol.28, No.3, pp. 166-76

Mei - Dan, O., Kish, B., Shabat, S., Masarawa, S., Shteren, A., Mann, G. & Nyska, M. (2010). Treatment of osteoarthritis of the ankle by intra - articular injections of hyaluronic acid: a prospective study. *J Am Podiatr Med Assoc,* Mar-Apr, Vol.100, No.2, pp. 93-100

Merolla, G., Sperling, JW., Paladini, P. & Porcellini, G. (2011). Efficacy of Hylan G-F 20 versus 6-methylprednisolone acetate in painful shoulder osteoarthritis: a retrospective controlled trial. *Musculoskelet Surg,* May 13

Migliore, A., Granata, M., Tormenta, S., Laganà, B., Piscitelli, P., Bizzi, E., Massafra, U., Alimonti, A., Maggi, C., De Chiara, R., Iannessi, F., Sanfilippo, A., Sotera, R., Scapato, P., Carducci, S., Persod, P., Denaro, S., Camminiti, M., Pagano, MG., Bagnato, G. & Iolascon, G. (2011). Hip viscosupplementation under ultra-sound guidance riduces NSAID consumption in symptomatic hip osteoarthritis patients in a long follow-up. Data from Italian registry. *Eur Rev Med Pharmacol Sci,* Vol.15, No.1, pp. 25-34

Migliore, A., Giovannangeli, F., Granata, M. & Laganà, B. (2010). Hylan g-f 20: review of its safety and efficacy in the management of joint pain in osteoarthritis. *Clin Med Insights Arthritis Musculoskelet Disord,* Vol.20, No.3, pp. 55-68

Migliore, A., Tormenta, S., Massafra, U., Martin Martin, LS., Carloni, E., Padalino, C., Alimonti, A. & Granata, M. (2006a).[18-month observational study on efficacy of intraarticular hyaluronic acid (Hylan G-F 20) injections under ultrasound guidance in hip osteoarthritis]. *Reumatismo,* Vol.58, No.1, pp. 39-49

Migliore, A., Tormenta, S., Martin Martin, LS., Iannessi, F., Massafra, U., Carloni, E., Monno, D., Alimonti, A, Granata, M. (2006b). The symptomatic effects of intra-articular administration of hylan G-F 20 on osteoarthritis of the hip: clinical data of 6 months follow-up. *Clin Rheumatol,* Vol.25, No.3, pp. 389-393

Migliore, A., Tormenta, S., Valente, C., Massafra, U., Martin Martin, LS., Carmenini, E., Bernardini A & Alimonti, A. (2005). [Intra-articular treatment with Hylan G-F 20 under ultrasound guidance in hip osteoarthritis. Clinical results after 12 months follow-up]. *Reumatismo,* Vol.57, No.1, pp. 36-43

Migliore, A., Tormenta, S., Martin Martin, LS., Valente, C., Massafra, U., Latini, A. & Alimonti, A. (2004). [Safety profile of 185 ultrasound-guided intra-articular injections for treatment of rheumatic diseases of the hip]. *Reumatismo,* Vol.56, No.2, pp. 104-109

Migliore, A., Martin, LS., Alimonti, A., Valente, C. & Tormenta, S. (2003). Efficacy and safety of viscosupplementation by ultrasound-guided intra-articular injection in osteoarthritis of the hip. *Osteoarthritis Cartilage,* Vol.11, No.4, pp. 305-306

National Collaborating Centre for Chronic Conditions (UK). (2008). Osteoarthritis: National clinical guideline for care and management in adults. London: Royal College of Physicians (UK)

O'Regan, M., Martini, I., Crescenzi, F., De Luca, C. & Lansing, M. (1994). Molecular mechanisms and genetics of hyaluronan biosynthesis. *Int J Biol Macromol,* Vol.16, No.6, pp. 283-286

Pons, M., Alvarez, F., Solana, J., Viladot, R. & Varela, L. (2007). Sodium hyaluronate in the treatment of hallux rigidus. A single-blind, randomized study. *Foot Ankle Int,* Vol.28, No.1, pp. 38-42

Pourbagher, MA., Ozalay, M. & Pourbagher, A. (2005). Accuracy and outcome of sonographically guided intra-articular sodium hyaluronate injections in patients with osteoarthritis of the hip. *J Ultrasound Med,* Vol.24, No.10, pp. 1391-1395

Qvistgaard, E., Christensen, R., Torp-Pedersen, S. & Bliddal, H. (2006). Intra-articular treatment of hip osteoarthritis: a randomized trial of hyaluronic acid, corticosteroid, and isotonic saline. *Osteoarthritis Cartilage,* Vol.14, No.2, pp. 163-170

Qvistgaard, E., Kristoffersen, H., Terslev, L., Danneskiold-Samsoe, B., Torp-Pedersen, S. & Bliddal, H. (2001). Guidance by ultrasound of intra-articular injections in the knee and hip joints. *Osteoarthritis Cartilage,* Vol.9, No.6, pp. 512-517

Ravaud, P., Moulinier, L,, Giraudeau, B., Ayral, X., Guerin, C., Noel, E., Thomas, P., Fautrel, B., Mazieres, B. & Dougados, M. Effects of joint lavage and steroid injection in patients with osteoarthritis of the knee: results of a multicenter, randomized, controlled trial. *Arthritis Rheum,* Vol.42, No.3, pp. 475-482

Roughead, EE., Ramsay, E., Pratt, N. & Gilbert, AL. (2008). NSAID use in individuals at risk of renal adverse events: an observational study to investigate trends in Australian veterans. *Drug Saf,* Vol.31, No.11, pp. 997-1003

Roux, C., Fontas, E., Breuil, V., Brocq, O., Albert, C. & Euller-Ziegler, L. (2007). Injection of intra-articular sodium hyaluronidate (Sinovial) into the carpometacarpal joint of the thumb (CMC1) in osteoarthritis. A prospective evaluation of efficacy. *Joint Bone Spine,* Vol.74, No.4, pp. 368-372

Rovetta, G. & Monteforte, P. (1998). Intraarticular injection of sodium hyaluronate plus steroid versus steroid in adhesive capsulitis of the shoulder. *Int J Tissue React,* Vol.20, No.4, pp. 125-130

Salini, V., De Amicis, D., Abate, M., Natale, MA., Di Iorio, A. (2009). Ultrasound-guided hyaluronic acid injection in carpometacarpal osteoarthritis: short-term results. *Int J Immunopathol Pharmacol,* Vol.22, No.2, pp. 455-460

Salk, RS., Chang, TJ., D'Costa, WF., Soomekh, DJ. & Grogan, KA. (2006). Sodium hyaluronate in the treatment of osteoarthritis of the ankle : a controlled, randomized, double - blind pilot study. *J Bone Joint Surg Am,* Feb, Vol.88, No.2, pp. 295-302

Salk, R., Chang, T., D'Costa, W., Soomekh, D. & Grogan, K. (2005). Viscosupplementation (hyaluronans) in the treatment of ankle osteoarthritis. *Clin Podiatr Med Surg,* Oct, Vol.22, No.4, pp. 585-597

Saltzman, CL., Salamon, ML., Blanchard, GM., Huff, T., Hayes, A., Buckwalter, JA. & Amendola, A. (2005). Epidemiology of ankle arthritis : report of a consecutive series of 639 patients from a tertiary orthopaedic center. *Iowa Orthop J,* Vol.25, pp. 44-46

Savage, R. (2005). Cyclo-oxygenase-2 inhibitors: when should they be used in the elderly? *Drugs ageing,* Vol.22, No.3, pp. 185-200

Schumacher, HR., Meador, R., Sieck, M. & Mohammed, Y. (2004). Pilot Investigation of Hyaluronate Injections for First Metacarpal-Carpal (MC-C) Osteoarthritis. *J Clin Rheumatol,* Vol.10, No.2, pp. 59-62

Silverstein, E., Leger, R. & Shea, KP. (2007). The use of intra-articular hylan G-F 20 in the treatment of symptomatic osteoarthritis of the shoulder: a preliminary study. *Am J Sports Med,* Vol.35, No.6, pp. 979-985

Smalley, WE. & Griffin, MR. (1996). The risks and costs of upper gastrointestinal disease attributable to NSAIDs. *Gastroenterol Clin North Am,* Vol. 25, No.2, pp. 373-396

Spacek, E., Poiraudeau, S., Fayad, F., Lefèvre-Colau, MM., Beaudreuil, J., Rannou, F., Fermanian, J. & Revel, M. (2004). Disability induced by hand osteoarthritis: are patients with more symptoms at digits 2-5 interphalangeal joints different from those with more symptoms at the base of the thumb? *Osteoarthritis Cartilage,* Vol.12, No.5, pp. 366-373

Srejic, U., Calvillo, O. & Kabakibou, K. (1999). Viscosupplementation: a new concept in the treatment of sacroiliac joint syndrome: a preliminary report of four cases. *Reg Anesth Pain Med,* Vol.24, No.1, pp. 84-88

Stahl, S., Karsh-Zafrir, I., Ratzon, N. & Rosenberg, N. (2005). Comparison of intraarticular injection of depot corticosteroid and hyaluronic acid for treatment of degenerative trapeziometacarpal joints. *J Clin Rheumatol,* Vol.11, No.6, pp. 299-302

Sturkenboom, MC., Romano, F., Simon, G., Correa-Leite, ML., Villa, M., Nicolosi, A., Borgnolo, G., Bianchi-Porro, G. & Mannino, S. (2002). The iatrogenic costs of NSAID therapy: a population study. *Arthritis Rheum,* Vol.47, No.2, pp. 132-140

Sun, SF., Chou, YJ., Hsu, CW., Hwang, CW., Hsu, PT., Wang, JL., Hsu, YW. & Chou, MC. (2006). Efficacy of intra - articular hyaluronic acid in patients with osteoarthritis of the ankle : a prospective study. *Osteoarthritis & Cartilage,* Sep, Vol.14, No.9, pp. 867-874

Takahashi, K., Goomer, RS., Harwood, F., Kubo, T., Hirasawa, Y. & Amiel, D. (1999). The effects of hyaluronan on matrix metalloproteinase-3 (MMP-3), interleukin-1beta(IL-1beta), and tissue inhibitor of metalloproteinase-1 (TIMP-1) gene expression during the development of osteoarthritis. *Osteoarthritis Cartilage,* Vol.7, No.2, pp. 182-190

Tamai, K., Mashitori, H., Ohno, W., Hamada, J., Sakai, H. & Saotome, K. (2004). Synovial response to intraarticular injections of hyaluronate in frozen shoulder: a quantitative assessment with dynamic magnetic resonance imaging. *J Orthop Sci,* Vol.9, No.3, pp. 230-234

Tikiz, C., Unlu, Z., Sener, A., Efe, M. & Tuzun, C. (2005). Comparison of the efficacy of lower and higher molecular weight viscosupplementation in the treatment of hip osteoarthritis. *Clin Rheumatol,* Vol.24, No.3, pp. 244-250

Vad, VB., Sakalkale, D., Sculco, TP. & Wickiewicz, TL. (2003). Role of hylan G-F 20 in treatment of osteoarthritis of the hip joint. *Arch Phys Med Rehabil,* Vol.84, No.8, pp. 1224-1226

Valiveti, M., Reginato, AJ. & Falasca, GF. (2006). Viscosupplementation for degenerative joint disease of shoulder and ankle. *Journal of Clinical Rheumatology,* Vol.12, No.3, pp. 162- 163

Van Brakel, RW. & Eygendaal, D. (2006). Intra-articular injection of hyaluronic acid is not effective for the treatment of post-traumatic osteoarthritis of the elbow. *Arthroscopy,* Vol.22, No.11, pp. 1199-1203

Van den Bekerom, MP., Lamme, B., Sermon, A. & Mulier, M. (2008). What is the evidence for viscosupplementation in the treatment of patients with hip osteoarthritis? Systematic review of the literature. *Arch Orthop Trauma Surg,* Vol.128, No.8, pp. 815- 823

Van den Bekerom, MP., Mylle, G., Rys, B. & Mulier, M. (2006). Viscosupplementation in symptomatic severe hip osteoarthritis: a review of the literature and report on 60 patients. Acta Orthop Belg, Vol. 72, No.5, pp. 560-568

Waddell, DD. (2007). Viscosupplementation with hyaluronans for osteoarthritis of the knee: clinical efficacy and economic implications. *Drugs Aging,* Vol.24, No.8, pp. 629-642

Wang, W., Li, P., Zhang, YL., Yang, Y., Wang, FL. & Zhang, Y. (2002). [The clinical effects of percutaneous lumbar discectomy combined with sodium hyaluronate in the treatment of lumbar intervertebral disc herniation]. *Zhongguo Xiu Fu Chong Jian Wai Ke Za Zhi,* Vol.16, No.1, pp. 23-25

Weiss, C. & Band, P. (1995). Musculoskeletal applications of hyaluronan and hylan. Potential uses in the foot and ankle. *Clin Podiatr Med Surg,* Vol.12, No.3, pp. 497-517

Weitoft, T., Larsson, A., Saxne, T. & Ronnblom, L. (2005). Changes of cartilage and bone markers after intra-articular glucocorticoid treatment with and without postinjection rest in patients with rheumatoid arthritis. *Ann Rheum Dis* ,Vol.64, No.12, pp. 1750-1753

Witteveen, AGH., Sierevelt, IN., Blankevoort, L., Kerkhoffs, GM. & van Dijk, CN. (2010). Intra - articular sodium hyaluronate injections in the osteoarthritic ankle joint : effects, safety and dose dependency. *Foot Ankle Surg,* Dec, Vol.16, No.4, pp. 159-163

Witteveen, AGH., Giannini, S., Guido, G., Jerosch, J., Lohrer, H., Vannini, F., Donati, L., Schulz, A., Scholl, J., Sierevelt, IN. & van Dijk, CN. (2008). A prospective multi - centre, open study of the safety and efficacy of hylan G-F 20 (Synvisc) in patients with symptomatic ankle (talo - crural) osteoarthritis. *Foot and Ankle Surgery,* Vol.14, No.3, pp. 145-152

Woo, SB., Wong, TM., Chan, WL., Yen, CH., Wong, WC. & Mak, KL. (2010). Anatomic variations of neurovascular structures of the ankle in relation to arthroscopic portals: a cadaveric study of Chinese subjects. *J Orthop Surg (Hong Kong),* Apr, Vol.18, No.1, pp. 71-75

Zhang, Y. & Jordan, JM. (2010). Epidemiology of osteoarthritis. *Clin Geriatr Med,* Aug, Vol.26, No.3, pp. 355-369

Zwar, RB., Read, JW. & Noakes, JB. (2004). Sonographically guided glenohumeral joint injection. *AJR Am J Roentgenol,* Vol.183, No.1, pp. 48-50

6

Gene Therapy for Human Osteoarthritis

Magali Cucchiarini and Henning Madry
*Experimental Orthopaedics and Osteoarthritis Research,
Saarland University Medical Center, Homburg/Saar,
Germany*

1. Introduction

Articular cartilage has a reduced capacity for self-regeneration. Delivery of candidate genes to articular chondrocytes is an attractive strategy that has the potential to allow for a durable reestablishment of the structural integrity in osteoarthritic (OA) cartilage. Gene transfer approaches might be better suited to treat a slow and irreversible disorder such as OA over time instead of systems that are based on the application of recombinant factors with relatively short pharmacological half-lives. Current approaches that aim at re-equilibrating the metabolic balance in OA cartilage are based on the transfer of sequences coding for agents that either counteract the processes of matrix degradation or enhance the synthesis of matrix components. Importantly for the treatment of OA, the development of effective gene treatments will necessitate that the gene vehicle chosen allows for high and also sustained levels of expression of the sequence to be delivered due to the slow and irreversible progression of this disorder. The method elected to administer the therapeutic composition will be also important to achieve successful and long-term cartilage regeneration in OA patients.

2. Gene therapy

Gene therapy aims at treating human diseases via gene transfer techniques that introduce foreign genes or sequences in various cell types. The foreign material enters the cell where it is transferred towards the nucleus. Once there, it either integrates in the host genome or stays extrachromosomal under episomal forms that generally allows only for transient transgene expression. Gene transfer in sufficient number of cells is essential to allow for the production of therapeutically relevant concentrations of transgene products. The currently most employed vectors used in gene therapy trials include nonviral compounds (naked DNA, physical and chemical methods) and different viral gene carriers including adenoviral, herpes simplex virus-derived, retroviral, lentiviral, and recombinant adeno-associated viral vectors that utilize natural entry pathways in human cells (Cucchiarini et al., 2009a; Cucchiarini & Madry, 2005; Evans, 2004; Evans et al., 2004) (**Table 1**).

2.1 Nonviral vectors

Chemical methods of complexing DNA to various macromolecules include cationic lipids and liposomes, polymers, polyamines and polyethylenimines, and nanoparticles, besides the use of calcium phosphate coprecipitates. Nonviral methods avoid the risk of acquiring replication competence inherent to viral vectors. They can be repeatedly administered, have the capacity to deliver large therapeutic genes, and are easy to produce on a large scale. Also, they do not elicit immune responses in the host organism. Still, their efficacy is often much lower than those of viral vectors. In addition, as the transgenes remain as episomes in their targets, only short-term transgene expression is achievable. To overcome these shortcomings, nonviral gene transfer strategies *in vivo* are generally based on the use of *ex vivo*-modified cells for readministration in sites of damage.

		Benefits	Shortcomings	Integration
Nonviral vectors	Liposomes, others (chemical, electrical, mechanical methods)	Noninfectious, low toxicity, easy to produce, large capacity	Relatively low efficiency, short-term transgene expression	No
Viral vectors	Adenovirus	Very high efficiency	Potential replication competence, toxicity, immunogenicity, short-term transgene expression	No
	Retrovirus	High efficiency, long-term transgene expression	Potential replication competence, risk of insertional mutagenesis	Yes
	Herpes simplex virus	High efficiency, large capacity	Relative cytotoxicity, short-term transgene expression	No
	Adeno-associated virus	Very high efficiency, long-term transgene expression	Relative difficulty to produce	No

Table 1. Gene Transfer Vectors.

2.2 Adenoviral vectors

Adenoviruses have been among the most employed systems so far. They allow for high transduction efficiencies and transgene expression in a variety of cells, allowing for direct approaches *in vivo*. Yet, there are serious concerns about their safe use in the clinics due to the development of strong host immune responses to the remaining adenoviral gene products. Another problem is the limited period of transgene expression (1-2 weeks) as the sequences delivered remain as episomes that are cleared shortly after being introduced in the cells.

2.3 Retroviral vectors

An advantage of these viruses is their ability to integrate in the host genome, allowing for the maintenance of the transgene over extended periods of time. Nevertheless, this might lead to insertional mutagenesis and a potential to activate tumorigenic sequences. Also, such vectors transduce only dividing cells with a restricted host range (and a low efficacy) and are only produce at relatively low concentrations. Therefore, *ex vivo* approaches with pre-selection of transduced cells are usually employed. Interestingly, lentiviral vectors, a subclass of retroviruses derived from the human immunodeficiency virus (HIV) that integrate in the genome of nondividing cells avoid the need for cell division and show higher levels of transduction *in vivo*. Nevertheless, there are still concerns associated with their application, including the potential for insertional mutagenesis and the psychological problem of introducing genetic material carrying HIV sequences.

2.4 Herpes simplex viral vectors (HSV)

HSV-derived vectors are large vehicles that can deliver large transgenes to almost all known cell types, including nondividing cells. Although first-generation vectors induced high levels of cytoxicity, recent work has demonstrated that second-generation HSV were less deleterious, in particular for cartilage gene transfer. One problem remains the transient nature of transgene expression mediated by this family of vectors.

2.5 Recombinant adeno-associated viral vectors (rAAV)

Application of viral vectors raises additional safety concerns, as potentially infectious agents or sequences might be introduced *per se* in the body. This is particularly important for the treatment of OA as it is not a life-threatening disorder. In this regard, rAAV vectors based on the nonpathogenic, replication-defective human parvovirus AAV might be more adequate for gene therapy settings. rAAV are produced by complete removal of the viral gene coding sequences, making them less immunogenic than adenoviral vectors and less toxic than HSV. Also, rAAV can be transcribed in their targets at very high efficiencies for months to years due to the stabilization of the episomal transgene cassettes by concatemer formation, making them strong alternatives for direct gene transfer approaches *in vivo*. Cell division and integration are not required for expression of the foreign material delivered via rAAV, in marked contrast with retroviral vectors. Redosing of vectors is practicable with rAAV, based on the use of various serotypes of the virus. For these reasons, rAAV became a preferred gene transfer method for experimental settings *in vivo* and for clinical applications.

3. Osteoarthritis

3.1 Articular cartilage

Adult hyaline articular cartilage is an avascular and aneural tissue that does not possess a lymphatic drainage that allows for a smooth gliding of the articulating surfaces of a joint and protects the subchondral bone from mechanical stress. Hyaline articular cartilage has several laminar zones formed by chondrocytes surrounded by an intricate network of extracellular matrix rich in proteoglycans and collagen fibrils (mostly type-II collagen and also types type-VI, -IX, -XI, and -XIV collagens and additional macromolecules). Normal hyaline articular cartilage contains about 70-80% water bound to proteoglycans. The chondrocytes regulate the structural and functional properties of the cartilage according to the applied loads by producing and degrading the extracellular matrix.

3.2 Osteoarthritis

Osteoarthritis (OA) is the most disabling condition and prevalent form of arthritis (80%). OA is a chronic disorder of diarthrodial joints, mainly characterized by a slow, progressive, and irreversible deterioration of the articular cartilage, with changes in the subchondral bone. OA also affects to a minor degree the synovial lining, ligaments, tendons, and muscles.

OA is a complex disorder characterized by the activation of inflammatory cascades and alterations of the chondrocyte phenotype, leading ultimately to cartilage breakdown (loss of the major components of the cartilage matrix). Under mechanical or biochemical stress (interleukin-1, i.e. IL-1; tumor necrosis factor alpha, i.e. TNF-α; nitric oxide, i.e. NO, prostaglandins, matrix degradation products), the cells undergo pathological changes in gene expression patterns that impede the whole homeostasis: diminished production of matrix molecules, enhanced production of matrix-degrading enzymes (matrix metalloproteinases, i.e. MMPs; adamalysins), decreased responsiveness to reparative stimuli, degradation of the matrix, alteration of the cell viability, cell senescence with apoptosis (NO; Fas/FasL signaling).

Several nonsurgical options are available to manage the progression of OA, including pharmacological treatments such as nonsteroidal anti-inflammatory drugs (NSAIDs), slow-acting drugs in OA (SADOAs) like glucosamine, chondroitin sulfate, and diacerin, being either symptomatic slow-acting drugs in OA (SYSADOAs) or disease-modifying OA drugs (DMOADs). However, there is no convincing evidence yet that such drugs indeed modify or inhibit the progression of OA. Surgical interventions such as débridement, marrow stimulation, and osteotomy are specifically indicated in early stages of OA. Yet, restoration of a native cartilage that is identical in its structure to the normal cartilage and capable of withstanding mechanical stresses over time in OA has not been achieved to date. Causative treatment for OA therefore remains a problem, particularly troublesome for patients that are too young to undergo endoprosthetic joint replacement.

4. Osteoarthritis gene therapy

4.1 Target cells in OA – Gene transfer *in vitro*

Target cells in the OA joint include:

1. chondrocytes,
2. osteocytes,
3. cells of the synovial lining,
4. progenitor cells, or
5. cells of surrounding tissues (muscle, tendons, ligaments, meniscus).

Application of nonviral (Gerich et al., 1997b; Grossin et al., 2006; Kaul et al., 2006; Madry et al., 2004b; Madry et al., 2005; Madry et al., 2001; Nita et al., 1996; Tsuchiya et al., 2003; Zhang, H. N. et al., 2009), adenoviral (Baragi et al., 1995; Brower-Toland et al., 2001; Gelse et al., 2001; Gerich et al., 1997a; Gerich et al., 1996; Gerich et al., 1997b; Goto et al., 1999; Haupt et al., 2005; Ikeda et al., 2004; Li et al., 2004; Lou et al., 1997; Mehrara et al., 1999; Musgrave et al., 2002; Nita et al., 1996; Nixon et al., 2000; Nixon et al., 2005; Saxer et al.,

2001; Shuler et al., 2000; Smith et al., 2000; Steinert et al., 2007; Steinert et al., 2009; Steinert et al., 2008), or retroviral vectors (Baltzer et al., 1999; Gerich et al., 1997a; Gerich et al., 1996; Gerich et al., 1997b; Goto et al., 2000; Gouze, J. N. et al., 2003; Hildebrand et al., 1999; Li et al., 2004; Mason et al., 2000; Nita et al., 1996; Piera-Velazquez et al., 2002; Roessler et al., 1995; Tew et al., 2005) has been achieved in such cells with more or less success. rAAV are potent alternatives as they efficiently and durably transduce synoviocytes (Adriaansen et al., 2007; Apparailly et al., 2002; Goater et al., 2000; Goodrich et al., 2009; Hiraide et al., 2005; Traister et al., 2006; Zhang, H. G. et al., 2000), chondrocytes (Arai et al., 2000; Cucchiarini et al., 2005; Cucchiarini et al., 2009c; Cucchiarini et al., 2007; Dai & Rabie, 2007; Goodrich et al., 2009; Madry et al., 2003; Ulrich-Vinther et al., 2002; Ulrich-Vinther et al., 2005; Yokoo et al., 2005), mesenchymal stem cells (MSCs) (Chamberlain et al., 2008; Chamberlain et al., 2004; Chen, M. et al., 2011; Cucchiarini et al., 2011; Cucchiarini et al., 2005; Dai & Rabie, 2007; Ito et al., 2004; Kim, S. J. et al., 2007; Pagnotto et al., 2007; Shi & Wang, 2010; Stender et al., 2007), and other cell types relevant of the pathogenesis of OA (Arsic et al., 2004; Basile et al., 2008; Cucchiarini et al., 2009b; Gerich et al., 1997a; Gerich et al., 1997b; Ito et al., 2005; Kessler et al., 1996; Luk et al., 2003; Madry et al., 2004a; Tang et al., 2008; Wang et al., 2007; Wang et al., 2005).
Regeneration of a native (structural and functional) cartilage architecture might be achieved by:

1. inhibiting inflammatory and catabolic pathways,
2. stimulating anabolic pathways to rebuild the matrix,
3. impeding cell senescence,
4. avoiding the pathological formation of osteophytes,
5. prevention of apoptosis, and/or
6. influencing several of these processes.

Inhibition of catabolic pathways has been observed when expressing inhibitors of matrix-degrading enzymes (tissue inhibitor of MMPs, i.e. TIMP) (Kafienah et al., 2003), inhibitors of proinflammatory cytokines (IL-1Ra; the soluble receptors sIL-1R or sTNFR) (Attur et al., 2002; Baragi et al., 1995; Gouze, J. N. et al., 2003; Haupt et al., 2005; Roessler et al., 1995; Zhang, H. G. et al., 2000; Zhang, X. et al., 2006), and chondroprotective cytokines (IL-4; IL-10) (Kim, S. H. et al., 2001; Zhang, X. et al., 2006). Activation of anabolic processes has been noted by single or combined administration of components of the cartilage matrix or of the enzymes that synthesize them (Dharmavaram et al., 1999; Venkatesan et al., 2004), of growth factors and receptors (insulin-like growth factor I, i.e. IGF-I; fibroblast growth factor 2, i.e. FGF-2; bone morphogenetic proteins, i.e. BMPs; transforming growth factor beta, i.e. TGF-β) (Brower-Toland et al., 2001; Chen, B. et al., 2010; Cucchiarini et al., 2011; Cucchiarini et al., 2005; Cucchiarini et al., 2009c; Haupt et al., 2005; Lee et al., 2005; Madry et al., 2004b; Madry et al., 2001; Nixon et al., 2000; Nixon et al., 2005; Saxer et al., 2001; Schmal et al., 2005; Shuler et al., 2000; Smith et al., 2000; Ulrich-Vinther et al., 2005), and of transcription factors (SOX family of DNA-binding proteins, i.e. SOX5, SOX6, SOX9) (Cucchiarini et al., 2007; Ikeda et al., 2004; Li et al., 2004; Tew et al., 2005; Tsuchiya et al., 2003). Restoration of cell vitality and activation of proliferation have been achieved by application of IGF-I or FGF-2 (Cucchiarini et al., 2011; Cucchiarini et al., 2005; Cucchiarini et al., 2009c; Kaul et al., 2006; Madry et al., 2004b; Madry et al., 2001; Schmal et al., 2005), telomerase (hTERT) (Piera-Velazquez et al., 2002), of inhibitors of apoptosis (bcl-2) (Surendran et al., 2006), or of the heat shock protein 70 (HSP70) (Grossin et al., 2006). Remarkably, approaches that influence several of these processes have been also successfully attempted, like combining the transfer of inhibitors of catabolism pathways and of activators of anabolic events (IGF-I/IL-1Ra) (Haupt et al., 2005; Nixon et al., 2005), as well as that of activators of anabolic and proliferative processes (FGF-2/SOX9 or FGF-2/IGF-I) (Cucchiarini et al., 2009c; Orth et al., 2011).

4.2 Gene transfer *in vivo*

4.2.1 Direct gene transfer

The key issue in establishing an efficient therapy against OA is to access the targets of the treatment when the cells reside in the joint cavity. The following approaches have been therefore developed:

1. systemic delivery and
2. intraarticular administration:

2.1 by injection or

2.2 using arthrotomy

Systemic approaches are better suited to target diseases that are systemic in nature like rheumatoid arthritis (RA) (Evans et al., 2006b, 2009; Jorgensen & Apparailly, 2010).

Local administration of components might be preferable for OA that affects only a limited number of joints without major systemic manifestations. Intraarticular injection of most vector types preferentially transduce the synovium (Ghivizzani et al., 1997; Gouze, E. et al., 2002; Nita et al., 1996; Roessler et al., 1993), being rather suited for strategies aiming at inhibiting inflammatory and catabolic pathways (and a common approach employed against experimental RA). Direct application of gene vectors has been attempted in experimental OA using sequences coding for IL-1Ra (Fernandes et al., 1999; Frisbie et al., 2002; Frisbie & McIlwraith, 2000; Zhang, X. et al., 2006), IL-10 (Zhang, X. et al., 2006), HSP70 (Grossin et al., 2006), gene silencers (Chen, L. X. et al., 2008), or kallistatin and thrombospondin-1 (Hsieh et al., 2009; Hsieh et al., 2010). Yet, even if cartilage breakdown is contained, this may not be sufficient to fully compensate for the loss of matrix elements and cells noted during the disease progression. In this regard, synthesis of cartilage matrix components might be stimulated by providing vectors carrying genes for anabolic factors (FGF-2, IGF-I) (Chen, B. et al., 2010).

4.2.2 Indirect gene transfer

Ex vivo gene therapy is more complex but safer as no free vector particles are introduced in the body. Also, modified cells can be controlled, tested, and selected in culture. Administration of cells is also a means to increase the cellularity like needed for cases of severe OA.

Synoviocytes have been mostly employed to deliver inhibitors of inflammatory and catabolic processes (Pelletier et al., 1997; Zhang, X. et al., 2004). Such pathways were regulated by injecting cells overexpressing an IL-1Ra alone (Pelletier et al., 1997; Zhang, X. et al., 2004) or with IL-10 (Zhang, X. et al., 2004). Again, although OA was reduced in association with decreased cartilage breakdown, complete resurfacing was not reported. Nevertheless, the use of differentiated cells is impaired by the invasive methods of preparation from unaffected sites with a limited supply and by common changes in cell phenotype observed upon passaging in culture. Also, implantation of committed cells generally leads to the formation of a poorly differentiated (fibrous) cartilage. Progenitor cells might be better suited to generate a cartilage of enhanced quality in transplantation settings.

They can be easily isolated from multiple tissues (bone marrow, periosteum, perichondrium, muscle, fat, subdermis, cartilage, bone, synovial membrane, ligaments), even in OA patients, maintaining a multilineage potential with a reliability for differentiation and a capacity for expansion (Barry & Murphy, 2004; Yoo et al., 2000). Remarkably, injection of muscle-derived stem cells modified by combined gene transfer of BMP-4 with sFlt1 (an antagonist of the vascular endothelial growth factor, i.e. VEGF) allowed for cartilage repair in a rat model of OA (Matsumoto et al., 2009).

5. Clinical trials

Preclinical data, as those described above, have encouraged the initiation of human clinical trials mostly for RA. The first studies were based on retroviral gene transfer of human IL-1Ra in synoviocytes from RA patients and reinjection in the metacarpophalangeal joint (Evans et al., 2000a; Evans et al., 1996; Wehling et al., 2009). Transgene expression was noted locally without adverse events, leading to clinical improvements in some patients, encouraging the implementation of phase II studies (Evans, 2005; Evans et al., 2005a; Evans et al., 2000b; Evans et al., 2006a, 2008; Evans et al., 2004; Evans et al., 2005b; Robbins et al., 2003). Direct intraarticular injection of rAAV carrying an sTNFR-immunoglobulin in RA patients revealed that the treatment was safe and well tolerated (Evans, 2005; Evans et al., 2005a; Evans et al., 2006a, 2008; Mease et al., 2009), and a phase I/II trial was subsequently started. Regarding OA, a phase I protocol is ongoing, based on an *ex vivo* approach using the retroviral transfer of TGF-β (Evans et al., 2008).

6. Conclusions

Gene therapy holds great promise, but issues that need to be addressed include the duration of transgene expression, extended analyses in clinically relevant animal models, the benefit of *ex vivo* genetically modified cells versus direct approaches, and the identification of optimal therapeutic factors. Future studies will also have to shed light on the safety of these approaches regarding the nonlethal nature of OA. Successful application of gene therapy for OA requires a combined effort of surgeons and basic scientists in order to improve the currently available gene transfer systems.

7. Acknowledgments and funding

This work was supported by grants of the *Deutsche Forschungsgemeinschaft* (DFG CU 55/1-1, 1-2, 1-3) and of the *Deutsche Arthrose-Hilfe*.

8. Declaration of conflicting interests

The authors declare no potential conflicts of interest with respect to the authorship and/or publication of this article.

9. References

Adriaansen, J., Khoury, M., de Cortie, C. J., Fallaux, F. J., Bigey, P., Scherman, D., Gould, D. J., Chernajovsky, Y., Apparailly, F., Jorgensen, C., Vervoordeldonk, M. J.&Tak, P. P.

(2007). Reduction of arthritis following intra-articular administration of an adeno-associated virus serotype 5 expressing a disease-inducible TNF-blocking agent. *Ann Rheum Dis*, Vol. 66, No. 9, (Sep) pp. 1143-50, 0003-4967 (Print) 0003-4967 (Linking)

Apparailly, F., Millet, V., Noel, D., Jacquet, C., Sany, J.&Jorgensen, C. (2002). Tetracycline-inducible interleukin-10 gene transfer mediated by an adeno-associated virus: application to experimental arthritis. *Hum Gene Ther*, Vol. 13, No. 10, (Jul 1) pp. 1179-88, 1043-0342 (Print) 1043-0342 (Linking)

Arai, Y., Kubo, T., Fushiki, S., Mazda, O., Nakai, H., Iwaki, Y., Imanishi, J.&Hirasawa, Y. (2000). Gene delivery to human chondrocytes by an adeno associated virus vector. *J Rheumatol*, Vol. 27, No. 4, (Apr) pp. 979-82, 0315-162X (Print) 0315-162X (Linking)

Arsic, N., Zacchigna, S., Zentilin, L., Ramirez-Correa, G., Pattarini, L., Salvi, A., Sinagra, G.&Giacca, M. (2004). Vascular endothelial growth factor stimulates skeletal muscle regeneration in vivo. *Mol Ther*, Vol. 10, No. 5, (Nov) pp. 844-54, 1525-0016 (Print) 1525-0016 (Linking)

Attur, M. G., Dave, M. N., Leung, M. Y., Cipolletta, C., Meseck, M., Woo, S. L.&Amin, A. R. (2002). Functional genomic analysis of type II IL-1beta decoy receptor: potential for gene therapy in human arthritis and inflammation. *J Immunol*, Vol. 168, No. 4, (Feb 15) pp. 2001-10, 0022-1767 (Print) 0022-1767 (Linking)

Baltzer, A. W., Whalen, J. D., Muzzonegro, T., Georgescu, H. I., Robbins, P. D.&Evans, C. H. (1999). [In vitro transduction of human osteoblast cell populations with retroviral vectors]. *Z Rheumatol*, Vol. 58, No. 2, (Apr) pp. 88-94, 0340-1855 (Print) 0340-1855 (Linking)

Baragi, V. M., Renkiewicz, R. R., Jordan, H., Bonadio, J., Hartman, J. W.&Roessler, B. J. (1995). Transplantation of transduced chondrocytes protects articular cartilage from interleukin 1-induced extracellular matrix degradation. *J Clin Invest*, Vol. 96, No. 5, (Nov) pp. 2454-60, 0021-9738 (Print) 0021-9738 (Linking)

Barry, F. P.&Murphy, J. M. (2004). Mesenchymal stem cells: clinical applications and biological characterization. *Int J Biochem Cell Biol*, Vol. 36, No. 4, (Apr) pp. 568-84, 1357-2725 (Print) 1357-2725 (Linking)

Basile, P., Dadali, T., Jacobson, J., Hasslund, S., Ulrich-Vinther, M., Soballe, K., Nishio, Y., Drissi, M. H., Langstein, H. N., Mitten, D. J., O'Keefe, R. J., Schwarz, E. M.&Awad, H. A. (2008). Freeze-dried tendon allografts as tissue-engineering scaffolds for Gdf5 gene delivery. *Mol Ther*, Vol. 16, No. 3, (Mar) pp. 466-73, 1525-0024 (Electronic) 1525-0016 (Linking)

Brower-Toland, B. D., Saxer, R. A., Goodrich, L. R., Mi, Z., Robbins, P. D., Evans, C. H.&Nixon, A. J. (2001). Direct adenovirus-mediated insulin-like growth factor I gene transfer enhances transplant chondrocyte function. *Hum Gene Ther*, Vol. 12, No. 2, (Jan 20) pp. 117-29, 1043-0342 (Print) 1043-0342 (Linking)

Chamberlain, J. R., Deyle, D. R., Schwarze, U., Wang, P., Hirata, R. K., Li, Y., Byers, P. H.&Russell, D. W. (2008). Gene targeting of mutant COL1A2 alleles in mesenchymal stem cells from individuals with osteogenesis imperfecta. *Mol Ther*, Vol. 16, No. 1, (Jan) pp. 187-93, 1525-0024 (Electronic) 1525-0016 (Linking)

Chamberlain, J. R., Schwarze, U., Wang, P. R., Hirata, R. K., Hankenson, K. D., Pace, J. M., Underwood, R. A., Song, K. M., Sussman, M., Byers, P. H.&Russell, D. W. (2004). Gene targeting in stem cells from individuals with osteogenesis imperfecta. *Science*, Vol. 303, No. 5661, (Feb 20) pp. 1198-201, 1095-9203 (Electronic) 0036-8075 (Linking)

Chen, B., Qin, J., Wang, H., Magdalou, J.&Chen, L. (2010). Effects of adenovirus-mediated bFGF, IL-1Ra and IGF-1 gene transfer on human osteoarthritic chondrocytes and osteoarthritis in rabbits. *Exp Mol Med*, Vol. 42, No. 10, (Oct 31) pp. 684-95, 1226-3613 (Print) 1226-3613 (Linking)

Chen, L. X., Lin, L., Wang, H. J., Wei, X. L., Fu, X., Zhang, J. Y.&Yu, C. L. (2008). Suppression of early experimental osteoarthritis by in vivo delivery of the adenoviral vector-mediated NF-kappaBp65-specific siRNA. *Osteoarthritis Cartilage*, Vol. 16, No. 2, (Feb) pp. 174-84, 1063-4584 (Print) 1063-4584 (Linking)

Chen, M., Song, K., Rao, N., Huang, M., Huang, Z.&Cao, Y. (2011). Roles of exogenously regulated bFGF expression in angiogenesis and bone regeneration in rat calvarial defects. *Int J Mol Med*, Vol. 27, No. 4, (Apr) pp. 545-53, 1791-244X (Electronic) 1107-3756 (Linking)

Cucchiarini, M., Ekici, M., Schetting, S., Kohn, D.&Madry, H. (2011). Metabolic activities and chondrogenic differentiation of human mesenchymal stem cells following recombinant adeno-associated virus-mediated gene transfer and overexpression of fibroblast growth factor 2. *Tissue Eng Part A*, Vol. No. 17, (Aug) pp. 1921-33

Cucchiarini, M., Heiligenstein, S., Kohn, D.&Madry, H. (2009a). [Molecular tools to remodel osteoarthritic articular cartilage : growth, transcription, and signaling factors]. *Orthopade*, Vol. 38, No. 11, (Nov) pp. 1063-70, 1433-0431 (Electronic) 0085-4530 (Linking)

Cucchiarini, M.&Madry, H. (2005). Gene therapy for cartilage defects. *J Gene Med*, Vol. 7, No. 12, (Dec) pp. 1495-509, 1099-498X (Print) 1099-498X (Linking)

Cucchiarini, M., Madry, H., Ma, C., Thurn, T., Zurakowski, D., Menger, M. D., Kohn, D., Trippel, S. B.&Terwilliger, E. F. (2005). Improved tissue repair in articular cartilage defects in vivo by rAAV-mediated overexpression of human fibroblast growth factor 2. *Mol Ther*, Vol. 12, No. 2, (Aug) pp. 229-38, 1525-0016 (Print) 1525-0016 (Linking)

Cucchiarini, M., Schetting, S., Terwilliger, E. F., Kohn, D.&Madry, H. (2009b). rAAV-mediated overexpression of FGF-2 promotes cell proliferation, survival, and alpha-SMA expression in human meniscal lesions. *Gene Ther*, Vol. 16, No. 11, (Nov) pp. 1363-72, 1476-5462 (Electronic) 0969-7128 (Linking)

Cucchiarini, M., Terwilliger, E. F., Kohn, D.&Madry, H. (2009c). Remodelling of human osteoarthritic cartilage by FGF-2, alone or combined with Sox9 via rAAV gene transfer. *J Cell Mol Med*, Vol. 13, No. 8B, (Aug) pp. 2476-88, 1582-4934 (Electronic) 1582-1838 (Linking)

Cucchiarini, M., Thurn, T., Weimer, A., Kohn, D., Terwilliger, E. F.&Madry, H. (2007). Restoration of the extracellular matrix in human osteoarthritic articular cartilage by overexpression of the transcription factor SOX9. *Arthritis Rheum*, Vol. 56, No. 1, (Jan) pp. 158-67, 0004-3591 (Print) 0004-3591 (Linking)

Dai, J.&Rabie, A. B. (2007). Recombinant adeno-associated virus vector hybrids efficiently target different skeletal cells. *Front Biosci*, Vol. 12, No. pp. 4280-7, 1093-4715 (Electronic) 1093-4715 (Linking)

Dharmavaram, R. M., Liu, G., Tuan, R. S., Stokes, D. G.&Jimenez, S. A. (1999). Stable transfection of human fetal chondrocytes with a type II procollagen minigene: expression of the mutant protein and alterations in the structure of the extracellular matrix in vitro. *Arthritis Rheum*, Vol. 42, No. 7, (Jul) pp. 1433-42, 0004-3591 (Print) 0004-3591 (Linking)

Evans, C. H. (2004). Gene therapies for osteoarthritis. *Curr Rheumatol Rep*, Vol. 6, No. 1, (Feb) pp. 31-40, 1523-3774 (Print) 1523-3774 (Linking)

Evans, C. H. (2005). Gene therapy: what have we accomplished and where do we go from here? *J Rheumatol Suppl*, Vol. 72, No. (Jan) pp. 17-20, 0380-0903 (Print) 0380-0903 (Linking)

Evans, C. H., Ghivizzani, S. C., Herndon, J. H.&Robbins, P. D. (2005a). Gene therapy for the treatment of musculoskeletal diseases. *J Am Acad Orthop Surg*, Vol. 13, No. 4, (Jul-Aug) pp. 230-42, 1067-151X (Print) 1067-151X (Linking)

Evans, C. H., Ghivizzani, S. C., Herndon, J. H., Wasko, M. C., Reinecke, J., Wehling, P.&Robbins, P. D. (2000a). Clinical trials in the gene therapy of arthritis. *Clin Orthop Relat Res*, Vol. No. 379 Suppl, (Oct) pp. S300-7, 0009-921X (Print) 0009-921X (Linking)

Evans, C. H., Ghivizzani, S. C., Oligino, T. J.&Robbins, P. D. (2000b). Gene therapy for autoimmune disorders. *J Clin Immunol*, Vol. 20, No. 5, (Sep) pp. 334-46, 0271-9142 (Print) 0271-9142 (Linking)

Evans, C. H., Ghivizzani, S. C.&Robbins, P. D. (2006a). Gene therapy for arthritis: what next? *Arthritis Rheum*, Vol. 54, No. 6, (Jun) pp. 1714-29, 0004-3591 (Print) 0004-3591 (Linking)

Evans, C. H., Ghivizzani, S. C.&Robbins, P. D. (2006b). Will arthritis gene therapy become a clinical reality? *Nat Clin Pract Rheumatol*, Vol. 2, No. 7, (Jul) pp. 344-5, 1745-8382 (Print) 1745-8382 (Linking)

Evans, C. H., Ghivizzani, S. C.&Robbins, P. D. (2008). Arthritis gene therapy's first death. *Arthritis Res Ther*, Vol. 10, No. 3, pp. 110, 1478-6362 (Electronic) 1478-6354 (Linking)

Evans, C. H., Ghivizzani, S. C.&Robbins, P. D. (2009). Gene therapy of the rheumatic diseases: 1998 to 2008. *Arthritis Res Ther*, Vol. 11, No. 1, pp. 209, 1478-6362 (Electronic) 1478-6354 (Linking)

Evans, C. H., Gouze, J. N., Gouze, E., Robbins, P. D.&Ghivizzani, S. C. (2004). Osteoarthritis gene therapy. *Gene Ther*, Vol. 11, No. 4, (Feb) pp. 379-89, 0969-7128 (Print) 0969-7128 (Linking)

Evans, C. H., Robbins, P. D., Ghivizzani, S. C., Herndon, J. H., Kang, R., Bahnson, A. B., Barranger, J. A., Elders, E. M., Gay, S., Tomaino, M. M., Wasko, M. C., Watkins, S. C., Whiteside, T. L., Glorioso, J. C., Lotze, M. T.&Wright, T. M. (1996). Clinical trial to assess the safety, feasibility, and efficacy of transferring a potentially anti-arthritic cytokine gene to human joints with rheumatoid arthritis. *Hum Gene Ther*, Vol. 7, No. 10, (Jun 20) pp. 1261-80, 1043-0342 (Print) 1043-0342 (Linking)

Evans, C. H., Robbins, P. D., Ghivizzani, S. C., Wasko, M. C., Tomaino, M. M., Kang, R., Muzzonigro, T. A., Vogt, M., Elder, E. M., Whiteside, T. L., Watkins, S. C.&Herndon, J. H. (2005b). Gene transfer to human joints: progress toward a gene therapy of arthritis. *Proc Natl Acad Sci U S A*, Vol. 102, No. 24, (Jun 14) pp. 8698-703, 0027-8424 (Print) 0027-8424 (Linking)

Fernandes, J., Tardif, G., Martel-Pelletier, J., Lascau-Coman, V., Dupuis, M., Moldovan, F., Sheppard, M., Krishnan, B. R.&Pelletier, J. P. (1999). In vivo transfer of interleukin-1 receptor antagonist gene in osteoarthritic rabbit knee joints: prevention of osteoarthritis progression. *Am J Pathol*, Vol. 154, No. 4, (Apr) pp. 1159-69, 0002-9440 (Print) 0002-9440 (Linking)

Frisbie, D. D., Ghivizzani, S. C., Robbins, P. D., Evans, C. H.&McIlwraith, C. W. (2002). Treatment of experimental equine osteoarthritis by in vivo delivery of the equine interleukin-1 receptor antagonist gene. *Gene Ther*, Vol. 9, No. 1, (Jan) pp. 12-20, 0969-7128 (Print) 0969-7128 (Linking)

Frisbie, D. D.&McIlwraith, C. W. (2000). Evaluation of gene therapy as a treatment for equine traumatic arthritis and osteoarthritis. *Clin Orthop Relat Res*, Vol. No. 379 Suppl, (Oct) pp. S273-87, 0009-921X (Print) 0009-921X (Linking)

Gelse, K., Jiang, Q. J., Aigner, T., Ritter, T., Wagner, K., Poschl, E., von der Mark, K.&Schneider, H. (2001). Fibroblast-mediated delivery of growth factor complementary DNA into mouse joints induces chondrogenesis but avoids the disadvantages of direct viral gene transfer. *Arthritis Rheum*, Vol. 44, No. 8, (Aug) pp. 1943-53, 0004-3591 (Print) 0004-3591 (Linking)

Gerich, T. G., Ghivizani, S., Fu, F. H., Robbins, P. D.&Evans, C. H. (1997a). [Gene transfer into the patellar tendon of rabbits: a preliminary study of locoregional expression of growth factors]. *Wien Klin Wochenschr*, Vol. 109, No. 11, (Jun 6) pp. 384-9, 0043-5325 (Print) 0043-5325 (Linking)

Gerich, T. G., Kang, R., Fu, F. H., Robbins, P. D.&Evans, C. H. (1996). Gene transfer to the rabbit patellar tendon: potential for genetic enhancement of tendon and ligament healing. *Gene Ther*, Vol. 3, No. 12, (Dec) pp. 1089-93, 0969-7128 (Print) 0969-7128 (Linking)

Gerich, T. G., Lobenhoffer, H. P., Fu, F. H., Robbins, P. D.&Evans, C. H. (1997b). [Virally mediated gene transfer in the patellar tendon. An experimental study in rabbits]. *Unfallchirurg*, Vol. 100, No. 5, (May) pp. 354-62, 0177-5537 (Print) 0177-5537 (Linking)

Ghivizzani, S. C., Lechman, E. R., Tio, C., Mule, K. M., Chada, S., McCormack, J. E., Evans, C. H.&Robbins, P. D. (1997). Direct retrovirus-mediated gene transfer to the synovium of the rabbit knee: implications for arthritis gene therapy. *Gene Ther*, Vol. 4, No. 9, (Sep) pp. 977-82, 0969-7128 (Print) 0969-7128 (Linking)

Goater, J., Muller, R., Kollias, G., Firestein, G. S., Sanz, I., O'Keefe, R. J.&Schwarz, E. M. (2000). Empirical advantages of adeno associated viral vectors in vivo gene therapy for arthritis. *J Rheumatol*, Vol. 27, No. 4, (Apr) pp. 983-9, 0315-162X (Print) 0315-162X (Linking)

Goodrich, L. R., Choi, V. W., Carbone, B. A., McIlwraith, C. W.&Samulski, R. J. (2009). Ex vivo serotype-specific transduction of equine joint tissue by self-complementary adeno-associated viral vectors. *Hum Gene Ther*, Vol. 20, No. 12, (Dec) pp. 1697-702, 1557-7422 (Electronic) 1043-0342 (Linking)

Goto, H., Shuler, F. D., Lamsam, C., Moller, H. D., Niyibizi, C., Fu, F. H., Robbins, P. D.&Evans, C. H. (1999). Transfer of lacZ marker gene to the meniscus. *J Bone Joint Surg Am*, Vol. 81, No. 7, (Jul) pp. 918-25, 0021-9355 (Print)

Goto, H., Shuler, F. D., Niyibizi, C., Fu, F. H., Robbins, P. D.&Evans, C. H. (2000). Gene therapy for meniscal injury: enhanced synthesis of proteoglycan and collagen by meniscal cells transduced with a TGFbeta(1)gene. *Osteoarthritis Cartilage*, Vol. 8, No. 4, (Jul) pp. 266-71, 1063-4584 (Print) 1063-4584 (Linking)

Gouze, E., Pawliuk, R., Pilapil, C., Gouze, J. N., Fleet, C., Palmer, G. D., Evans, C. H., Leboulch, P.&Ghivizzani, S. C. (2002). In vivo gene delivery to synovium by lentiviral vectors. *Mol Ther*, Vol. 5, No. 4, (Apr) pp. 397-404, 1525-0016 (Print) 1525-0016 (Linking)

Gouze, J. N., Gouze, E., Palmer, G. D., Liew, V. S., Pascher, A., Betz, O. B., Thornhill, T. S., Evans, C. H., Grodzinsky, A. J.&Ghivizzani, S. C. (2003). A comparative study of the inhibitory effects of interleukin-1 receptor antagonist following administration as a recombinant protein or by gene transfer. *Arthritis Res Ther*, Vol. 5, No. 5, pp. R301-9, 1478-6362 (Electronic) 1478-6354 (Linking)

Grossin, L., Cournil-Henrionnet, C., Pinzano, A., Gaborit, N., Dumas, D., Etienne, S., Stoltz, J. F., Terlain, B., Netter, P., Mir, L. M.&Gillet, P. (2006). Gene transfer with HSP 70 in rat chondrocytes confers cytoprotection in vitro and during experimental osteoarthritis. *FASEB J*, Vol. 20, No. 1, (Jan) pp. 65-75, 1530-6860 (Electronic) 0892-6638 (Linking)

Haupt, J. L., Frisbie, D. D., McIlwraith, C. W., Robbins, P. D., Ghivizzani, S., Evans, C. H.&Nixon, A. J. (2005). Dual transduction of insulin-like growth factor-I and interleukin-1 receptor antagonist protein controls cartilage degradation in an osteoarthritic culture model. *J Orthop Res*, Vol. 23, No. 1, (Jan) pp. 118-26, 0736-0266 (Print) 0736-0266 (Linking)

Hildebrand, K. A., Deie, M., Allen, C. R., Smith, D. W., Georgescu, H. I., Evans, C. H., Robbins, P. D.&Woo, S. L. (1999). Early expression of marker genes in the rabbit medial collateral and anterior cruciate ligaments: the use of different viral vectors and the effects of injury. *J Orthop Res*, Vol. 17, No. 1, (Jan) pp. 37-42, 0736-0266 (Print) 0736-0266 (Linking)

Hiraide, A., Yokoo, N., Xin, K. Q., Okuda, K., Mizukami, H., Ozawa, K.&Saito, T. (2005). Repair of articular cartilage defect by intraarticular administration of basic fibroblast growth factor gene, using adeno-associated virus vector. *Hum Gene Ther*, Vol. 16, No. 12, (Dec) pp. 1413-21, 1043-0342 (Print) 1043-0342 (Linking)

Hsieh, J. L., Shen, P. C., Shiau, A. L., Jou, I. M., Lee, C. H., Teo, M. L., Wang, C. R., Chao, J., Chao, L.&Wu, C. L. (2009). Adenovirus-mediated kallistatin gene transfer ameliorates disease progression in a rat model of osteoarthritis induced by anterior cruciate ligament transection. *Hum Gene Ther*, Vol. 20, No. 2, (Feb) pp. 147-58, 1557-7422 (Electronic) 1043-0342 (Linking)

Hsieh, J. L., Shen, P. C., Shiau, A. L., Jou, I. M., Lee, C. H., Wang, C. R., Teo, M. L.&Wu, C. L. (2010). Intraarticular gene transfer of thrombospondin-1 suppresses the disease progression of experimental osteoarthritis. *J Orthop Res*, Vol. 28, No. 10, (Oct) pp. 1300-6, 1554-527X (Electronic) 0736-0266 (Linking)

Ikeda, T., Kamekura, S., Mabuchi, A., Kou, I., Seki, S., Takato, T., Nakamura, K., Kawaguchi, H., Ikegawa, S.&Chung, U. I. (2004). The combination of SOX5, SOX6, and SOX9 (the SOX trio) provides signals sufficient for induction of permanent cartilage. *Arthritis Rheum*, Vol. 50, No. 11, (Nov) pp. 3561-73, 0004-3591 (Print) 0004-3591 (Linking)

Ito, H., Goater, J. J., Tiyapatanaputi, P., Rubery, P. T., O'Keefe, R. J.&Schwarz, E. M. (2004). Light-activated gene transduction of recombinant adeno-associated virus in human mesenchymal stem cells. *Gene Ther*, Vol. 11, No. 1, (Jan) pp. 34-41, 0969-7128 (Print) 0969-7128 (Linking)

Ito, H., Koefoed, M., Tiyapatanaputi, P., Gromov, K., Goater, J. J., Carmouche, J., Zhang, X., Rubery, P. T., Rabinowitz, J., Samulski, R. J., Nakamura, T., Soballe, K., O'Keefe, R. J., Boyce, B. F.&Schwarz, E. M. (2005). Remodeling of cortical bone allografts mediated by adherent rAAV-RANKL and VEGF gene therapy. *Nat Med*, Vol. 11, No. 3, (Mar) pp. 291-7, 1078-8956 (Print) 1078-8956 (Linking)

Jorgensen, C.&Apparailly, F. (2010). Prospects for gene therapy in inflammatory arthritis. *Best Pract Res Clin Rheumatol*, Vol. 24, No. 4, (Aug) pp. 541-52, 1532-1770 (Electronic) 1521-6942 (Linking)

Kafienah, W., Al-Fayez, F., Hollander, A. P.&Barker, M. D. (2003). Inhibition of cartilage degradation: a combined tissue engineering and gene therapy approach. *Arthritis Rheum*, Vol. 48, No. 3, (Mar) pp. 709-18, 0004-3591 (Print) 0004-3591 (Linking)

Kaul, G., Cucchiarini, M., Arntzen, D., Zurakowski, D., Menger, M. D., Kohn, D., Trippel, S. B.&Madry, H. (2006). Local stimulation of articular cartilage repair by transplantation of encapsulated chondrocytes overexpressing human fibroblast growth factor 2 (FGF-2) in vivo. *J Gene Med*, Vol. 8, No. 1, (Jan) pp. 100-11, 1099-498X (Print) 1099-498X (Linking)

Kessler, P. D., Podsakoff, G. M., Chen, X., McQuiston, S. A., Colosi, P. C., Matelis, L. A., Kurtzman, G. J.&Byrne, B. J. (1996). Gene delivery to skeletal muscle results in sustained expression and systemic delivery of a therapeutic protein. *Proc Natl Acad Sci U S A*, Vol. 93, No. 24, (Nov 26) pp. 14082-7, 0027-8424 (Print) 0027-8424 (Linking)

Kim, S. H., Kim, S., Evans, C. H., Ghivizzani, S. C., Oligino, T.&Robbins, P. D. (2001). Effective treatment of established murine collagen-induced arthritis by systemic administration of dendritic cells genetically modified to express IL-4. *J Immunol*, Vol. 166, No. 5, (Mar 1) pp. 3499-505, 0022-1767 (Print) 0022-1767 (Linking)

Kim, S. J., Lee, W. I., Heo, H., Shin, O., Kwon, Y. K.&Lee, H. (2007). Stable gene expression by self-complementary adeno-associated viruses in human MSCs. *Biochem Biophys Res Commun*, Vol. 360, No. 3, (Aug 31) pp. 573-9, 0006-291X (Print) 0006-291X (Linking)

Lee, D. K., Choi, K. B., Oh, I. S., Song, S. U., Hwang, S., Lim, C. L., Hyun, J. P., Lee, H. Y., Chi, G. F., Yi, Y., Yip, V., Kim, J., Lee, E. B., Noh, M. J.&Lee, K. H. (2005). Continuous transforming growth factor beta1 secretion by cell-mediated gene therapy maintains chondrocyte redifferentiation. *Tissue Eng*, Vol. 11, No. 1-2, (Jan-Feb) pp. 310-8, 1076-3279 (Print) 1076-3279 (Linking)

Li, Y., Tew, S. R., Russell, A. M., Gonzalez, K. R., Hardingham, T. E.&Hawkins, R. E. (2004). Transduction of passaged human articular chondrocytes with adenoviral, retroviral, and lentiviral vectors and the effects of enhanced expression of SOX9. *Tissue Eng*, Vol. 10, No. 3-4, (Mar-Apr) pp. 575-84, 1076-3279 (Print) 1076-3279 (Linking)

Lou, J., Kubota, H., Hotokezaka, S., Ludwig, F. J.&Manske, P. R. (1997). In vivo gene transfer and overexpression of focal adhesion kinase (pp125 FAK) mediated by recombinant adenovirus-induced tendon adhesion formation and epitenon cell change. *J Orthop Res*, Vol. 15, No. 6, (Nov) pp. 911-8, 0736-0266 (Print) 0736-0266 (Linking)

Luk, K. D., Chen, Y., Cheung, K. M., Kung, H. F., Lu, W. W.&Leong, J. C. (2003). Adeno-associated virus-mediated bone morphogenetic protein-4 gene therapy for in vivo bone formation. *Biochem Biophys Res Commun*, Vol. 308, No. 3, (Aug 29) pp. 636-45, 0006-291X (Print) 0006-291X (Linking)

Madry, H., Cucchiarini, M., Kaul, G., Kohn, D., Terwilliger, E. F.&Trippel, S. B. (2004a). Menisci are efficiently transduced by recombinant adeno-associated virus vectors in vitro and in vivo. *Am J Sports Med*, Vol. 32, No. 8, (Dec) pp. 1860-5, 0363-5465 (Print) 0363-5465 (Linking)

Madry, H., Cucchiarini, M., Terwilliger, E. F.&Trippel, S. B. (2003). Recombinant adeno-associated virus vectors efficiently and persistently transduce chondrocytes in normal and osteoarthritic human articular cartilage. *Hum Gene Ther*, Vol. 14, No. 4, (Mar 1) pp. 393-402, 1043-0342 (Print) 1043-0342 (Linking)

Madry, H., Emkey, G., Zurakowski, D.&Trippel, S. B. (2004b). Overexpression of human fibroblast growth factor 2 stimulates cell proliferation in an ex vivo model of articular chondrocyte transplantation. *J Gene Med*, Vol. 6, No. 2, (Feb) pp. 238-45, 1099-498X (Print) 1099-498X (Linking)

Madry, H., Kaul, G., Cucchiarini, M., Stein, U., Zurakowski, D., Remberger, K., Menger, M. D., Kohn, D.&Trippel, S. B. (2005). Enhanced repair of articular cartilage defects in vivo by transplanted chondrocytes overexpressing insulin-like growth factor I (IGF-I). *Gene Ther*, Vol. 12, No. 15, (Aug) pp. 1171-9, 0969-7128 (Print) 0969-7128 (Linking)

Madry, H., Zurakowski, D.&Trippel, S. B. (2001). Overexpression of human insulin-like growth factor-I promotes new tissue formation in an ex vivo model of articular chondrocyte transplantation. *Gene Ther*, Vol. 8, No. 19, (Oct) pp. 1443-9, 0969-7128 (Print) 0969-7128 (Linking)

Mason, J. M., Breitbart, A. S., Barcia, M., Porti, D., Pergolizzi, R. G.&Grande, D. A. (2000). Cartilage and bone regeneration using gene-enhanced tissue engineering. *Clin Orthop Relat Res*, Vol. No. 379 Suppl, (Oct) pp. S171-8, 0009-921X (Print) 0009-921X (Linking)

Matsumoto, T., Cooper, G. M., Gharaibeh, B., Meszaros, L. B., Li, G., Usas, A., Fu, F. H.&Huard, J. (2009). Cartilage repair in a rat model of osteoarthritis through intraarticular transplantation of muscle-derived stem cells expressing bone morphogenetic protein 4 and soluble Flt-1. *Arthritis Rheum*, Vol. 60, No. 5, (May) pp. 1390-405, 0004-3591 (Print) 0004-3591 (Linking)

Mease, P. J., Hobbs, K., Chalmers, A., El-Gabalawy, H., Bookman, A., Keystone, E., Furst, D. E., Anklesaria, P.&Heald, A. E. (2009). Local delivery of a recombinant adenoassociated vector containing a tumour necrosis factor alpha antagonist gene in inflammatory arthritis: a phase 1 dose-escalation safety and tolerability study. *Ann Rheum Dis*, Vol. 68, No. 8, (Aug) pp. 1247-54, 1468-2060 (Electronic) 0003-4967 (Linking)

Mehrara, B. J., Saadeh, P. B., Steinbrech, D. S., Dudziak, M., Spector, J. A., Greenwald, J. A., Gittes, G. K.&Longaker, M. T. (1999). Adenovirus-mediated gene therapy of osteoblasts in vitro and in vivo. *J Bone Miner Res*, Vol. 14, No. 8, (Aug) pp. 1290-301, 0884-0431 (Print) 0884-0431 (Linking)

Musgrave, D. S., Pruchnic, R., Bosch, P., Ziran, B. H., Whalen, J.&Huard, J. (2002). Human skeletal muscle cells in ex vivo gene therapy to deliver bone morphogenetic protein-2. *J Bone Joint Surg Br*, Vol. 84, No. 1, (Jan) pp. 120-7, 0301-620X (Print)

Nita, I., Ghivizzani, S. C., Galea-Lauri, J., Bandara, G., Georgescu, H. I., Robbins, P. D.&Evans, C. H. (1996). Direct gene delivery to synovium. An evaluation of potential vectors in vitro and in vivo. *Arthritis Rheum*, Vol. 39, No. 5, (May) pp. 820-8, 0004-3591 (Print) 0004-3591 (Linking)

Nixon, A. J., Brower-Toland, B. D., Bent, S. J., Saxer, R. A., Wilke, M. J., Robbins, P. D.&Evans, C. H. (2000). Insulinlike growth factor-I gene therapy applications for cartilage repair. *Clin Orthop Relat Res*, Vol. No. 379 Suppl, (Oct) pp. S201-13, 0009-921X (Print) 0009-921X (Linking)

Nixon, A. J., Haupt, J. L., Frisbie, D. D., Morisset, S. S., McIlwraith, C. W., Robbins, P. D., Evans, C. H.&Ghivizzani, S. (2005). Gene-mediated restoration of cartilage matrix by combination insulin-like growth factor-I/interleukin-1 receptor antagonist therapy. *Gene Ther*, Vol. 12, No. 2, (Jan) pp. 177-86, 0969-7128 (Print) 0969-7128 (Linking)

Orth, P., Kaul, G., Cucchiarini, M., Zurakowski, D., Menger, M. D., Kohn, D.&Madry, H. (2011). Transplanted articular chondrocytes co-overexpressing IGF-I and FGF-2 stimulate cartilage repair in vivo. *Knee Surg Sports Traumatol Arthrosc*, Vol. No. (Feb 25) pp. 1433-7347 (Electronic) 0942-2056 (Linking)

Pagnotto, M. R., Wang, Z., Karpie, J. C., Ferretti, M., Xiao, X.&Chu, C. R. (2007). Adeno-associated viral gene transfer of transforming growth factor-beta1 to human mesenchymal stem cells improves cartilage repair. *Gene Ther*, Vol. 14, No. 10, (May) pp. 804-13, 0969-7128 (Print) 0969-7128 (Linking)

Pelletier, J. P., Caron, J. P., Evans, C., Robbins, P. D., Georgescu, H. I., Jovanovic, D., Fernandes, J. C.&Martel-Pelletier, J. (1997). In vivo suppression of early experimental osteoarthritis by interleukin-1 receptor antagonist using gene therapy. *Arthritis Rheum*, Vol. 40, No. 6, (Jun) pp. 1012-9, 0004-3591 (Print) 0004-3591 (Linking)

Piera-Velazquez, S., Jimenez, S. A.&Stokes, D. (2002). Increased life span of human osteoarthritic chondrocytes by exogenous expression of telomerase. *Arthritis Rheum*, Vol. 46, No. 3, (Mar) pp. 683-93, 0004-3591 (Print) 0004-3591 (Linking)

Robbins, P. D., Evans, C. H.&Chernajovsky, Y. (2003). Gene therapy for arthritis. *Gene Ther*, Vol. 10, No. 10, (May) pp. 902-11, 0969-7128 (Print) 0969-7128 (Linking)

Roessler, B. J., Allen, E. D., Wilson, J. M., Hartman, J. W.&Davidson, B. L. (1993). Adenoviral-mediated gene transfer to rabbit synovium in vivo. *J Clin Invest*, Vol. 92, No. 2, (Aug) pp. 1085-92, 0021-9738 (Print) 0021-9738 (Linking)

Roessler, B. J., Hartman, J. W., Vallance, D. K., Latta, J. M., Janich, S. L.&Davidson, B. L. (1995). Inhibition of interleukin-1-induced effects in synoviocytes transduced with the human IL-1 receptor antagonist cDNA using an adenoviral vector. *Hum Gene Ther*, Vol. 6, No. 3, (Mar) pp. 307-16, 1043-0342 (Print) 1043-0342 (Linking)

Saxer, R. A., Bent, S. J., Brower-Toland, B. D., Mi, Z., Robbins, P. D., Evans, C. H.&Nixon, A. J. (2001). Gene mediated insulin-like growth factor-I delivery to the synovium. *J Orthop Res*, Vol. 19, No. 5, (Sep) pp. 759-67, 0736-0266 (Print) 0736-0266 (Linking)

Schmal, H., Mehlhorn, A. T., Zwingmann, J., Muller, C. A., Stark, G. B.&Sudkamp, N. P. (2005). Stimulation of chondrocytes in vitro by gene transfer with plasmids coding for epidermal growth factor (hEGF) and basic fibroblast growth factor (bFGF). *Cytotherapy*, Vol. 7, No. 3, pp. 292-300, 1465-3249 (Print) 1465-3249 (Linking)

Shi, Z. B.&Wang, K. Z. (2010). Effects of recombinant adeno-associated viral vectors on angiopoiesis and osteogenesis in cultured rabbit bone marrow stem cells via co-expressing hVEGF and hBMP genes: a preliminary study in vitro. *Tissue Cell*, Vol. 42, No. 5, (Oct) pp. 314-21, 1532-3072 (Electronic) 0040-8166 (Linking)

Shuler, F. D., Georgescu, H. I., Niyibizi, C., Studer, R. K., Mi, Z., Johnstone, B., Robbins, R. D.&Evans, C. H. (2000). Increased matrix synthesis following adenoviral transfer of a transforming growth factor beta1 gene into articular chondrocytes. *J Orthop Res*, Vol. 18, No. 4, (Jul) pp. 585-92, 0736-0266 (Print) 0736-0266 (Linking)

Smith, P., Shuler, F. D., Georgescu, H. I., Ghivizzani, S. C., Johnstone, B., Niyibizi, C., Robbins, P. D.&Evans, C. H. (2000). Genetic enhancement of matrix synthesis by articular chondrocytes: comparison of different growth factor genes in the presence and absence of interleukin-1. *Arthritis Rheum*, Vol. 43, No. 5, (May) pp. 1156-64, 0004-3591 (Print) 0004-3591 (Linking)

Steinert, A. F., Palmer, G. D., Capito, R., Hofstaetter, J. G., Pilapil, C., Ghivizzani, S. C., Spector, M.&Evans, C. H. (2007). Genetically enhanced engineering of meniscus tissue using ex vivo delivery of transforming growth factor-beta 1 complementary deoxyribonucleic acid. *Tissue Eng*, Vol. 13, No. 9, (Sep) pp. 2227-37, 1076-3279 (Print) 1076-3279 (Linking)

Steinert, A. F., Proffen, B., Kunz, M., Hendrich, C., Ghivizzani, S. C., Noth, U., Rethwilm, A., Eulert, J.&Evans, C. H. (2009). Hypertrophy is induced during the in vitro chondrogenic differentiation of human mesenchymal stem cells by bone morphogenetic protein-2 and bone morphogenetic protein-4 gene transfer. *Arthritis Res Ther*, Vol. 11, No. 5, pp. R148, 1478-6362 (Electronic) 1478-6354 (Linking)

Steinert, A. F., Weber, M., Kunz, M., Palmer, G. D., Noth, U., Evans, C. H.&Murray, M. M. (2008). In situ IGF-1 gene delivery to cells emerging from the injured anterior cruciate ligament. *Biomaterials*, Vol. 29, No. 7, (Mar) pp. 904-16, 0142-9612 (Print) 0142-9612 (Linking)

Stender, S., Murphy, M., O'Brien, T., Stengaard, C., Ulrich-Vinther, M., Soballe, K.&Barry, F. (2007). Adeno-associated viral vector transduction of human mesenchymal stem cells. *Eur Cell Mater*, Vol. 13, No. pp. 93-9; discussion 99, 1473-2262 (Electronic) 1473-2262 (Linking)

Surendran, S., Kim, S. H., Jee, B. K., Ahn, S. H., Gopinathan, P.&Han, C. W. (2006). Anti-apoptotic Bcl-2 gene transfection of human articular chondrocytes protects against nitric oxide-induced apoptosis. *J Bone Joint Surg Br*, Vol. 88, No. 12, (Dec) pp. 1660-5, 0301-620X (Print)

Tang, J. B., Cao, Y., Zhu, B., Xin, K. Q., Wang, X. T.&Liu, P. Y. (2008). Adeno-associated virus-2-mediated bFGF gene transfer to digital flexor tendons significantly increases healing strength. an in vivo study. *J Bone Joint Surg Am*, Vol. 90, No. 5, (May) pp. 1078-89, 1535-1386 (Electronic)

Tew, S. R., Li, Y., Pothacharoen, P., Tweats, L. M., Hawkins, R. E.&Hardingham, T. E. (2005). Retroviral transduction with SOX9 enhances re-expression of the chondrocyte phenotype in passaged osteoarthritic human articular chondrocytes. *Osteoarthritis Cartilage*, Vol. 13, No. 1, (Jan) pp. 80-9, 1063-4584 (Print) 1063-4584 (Linking)

Traister, R. S., Fabre, S., Wang, Z., Xiao, X.&Hirsch, R. (2006). Inflammatory cytokine regulation of transgene expression in human fibroblast-like synoviocytes infected with adeno-associated virus. *Arthritis Rheum*, Vol. 54, No. 7, (Jul) pp. 2119-26, 0004-3591 (Print) 0004-3591 (Linking)

Tsuchiya, H., Kitoh, H., Sugiura, F.&Ishiguro, N. (2003). Chondrogenesis enhanced by overexpression of sox9 gene in mouse bone marrow-derived mesenchymal stem cells. *Biochem Biophys Res Commun*, Vol. 301, No. 2, (Feb 7) pp. 338-43, 0006-291X (Print) 0006-291X (Linking)

Ulrich-Vinther, M., Maloney, M. D., Goater, J. J., Soballe, K., Goldring, M. B., O'Keefe, R. J.&Schwarz, E. M. (2002). Light-activated gene transduction enhances adeno-associated virus vector-mediated gene expression in human articular chondrocytes. *Arthritis Rheum*, Vol. 46, No. 8, (Aug) pp. 2095-104, 0004-3591 (Print) 0004-3591 (Linking)

Ulrich-Vinther, M., Stengaard, C., Schwarz, E. M., Goldring, M. B.&Soballe, K. (2005). Adeno-associated vector mediated gene transfer of transforming growth factor-beta1 to normal and osteoarthritic human chondrocytes stimulates cartilage anabolism. *Eur Cell Mater*, Vol. 10, No. (Nov 14) pp. 40-50, 1473-2262 (Electronic) 1473-2262 (Linking)

Venkatesan, N., Barre, L., Benani, A., Netter, P., Magdalou, J., Fournel-Gigleux, S.&Ouzzine, M. (2004). Stimulation of proteoglycan synthesis by glucuronosyltransferase-I gene delivery: a strategy to promote cartilage repair. *Proc Natl Acad Sci U S A*, Vol. 101, No. 52, (Dec 28) pp. 18087-92, 0027-8424 (Print) 0027-8424 (Linking)

Wang, X. T., Liu, P. Y., Tang, J. B., Mizukami, H., Xin, K. Q., Ozawa, K.&Ushijima, H. (2007). Tendon healing in vitro: adeno-associated virus-2 effectively transduces intrasynovial tenocytes with persistent expression of the transgene, but other serotypes do not. *Plast Reconstr Surg*, Vol. 119, No. 1, (Jan) pp. 227-34, 1529-4242 (Electronic)

Wang, X. T., Liu, P. Y., Xin, K. Q.&Tang, J. B. (2005). Tendon healing in vitro: bFGF gene transfer to tenocytes by adeno-associated viral vectors promotes expression of collagen genes. *J Hand Surg Am*, Vol. 30, No. 6, (Nov) pp. 1255-61, 0363-5023 (Print) 0363-5023 (Linking)

Wehling, P., Reinecke, J., Baltzer, A. W., Granrath, M., Schulitz, K. P., Schultz, C., Krauspe, R., Whiteside, T. W., Elder, E., Ghivizzani, S. C., Robbins, P. D.&Evans, C. H. (2009). Clinical responses to gene therapy in joints of two subjects with rheumatoid arthritis. *Hum Gene Ther*, Vol. 20, No. 2, (Feb) pp. 97-101, 1557-7422 (Electronic) 1043-0342 (Linking)

Yokoo, N., Saito, T., Uesugi, M., Kobayashi, N., Xin, K. Q., Okuda, K., Mizukami, H., Ozawa, K.&Koshino, T. (2005). Repair of articular cartilage defect by autologous transplantation of basic fibroblast growth factor gene-transduced chondrocytes with adeno-associated virus vector. *Arthritis Rheum*, Vol. 52, No. 1, (Jan) pp. 164-70, 0004-3591 (Print) 0004-3591 (Linking)

Yoo, J. U., Mandell, I., Angele, P.&Johnstone, B. (2000). Chondrogenitor cells and gene therapy. *Clin Orthop Relat Res*, Vol. No. 379 Suppl, (Oct) pp. S164-70, 0009-921X (Print) 0009-921X (Linking)

Zhang, H. G., Xie, J., Yang, P., Wang, Y., Xu, L., Liu, D., Hsu, H. C., Zhou, T., Edwards, C. K., 3rd&Mountz, J. D. (2000). Adeno-associated virus production of soluble tumor necrosis factor receptor neutralizes tumor necrosis factor alpha and reduces arthritis. *Hum Gene Ther*, Vol. 11, No. 17, (Nov 20) pp. 2431-42, 1043-0342 (Print) 1043-0342 (Linking)

Zhang, H. N., Leng, P., Wang, Y. Z.&Zhang, J. (2009). Treating human meniscal fibrochondrocytes with hIGF-1 gene by liposome. *Clin Orthop Relat Res*, Vol. 467, No. 12, (Dec) pp. 3175-82, 1528-1132 (Electronic) 0009-921X (Linking)

Zhang, X., Mao, Z.&Yu, C. (2004). Suppression of early experimental osteoarthritis by gene transfer of interleukin-1 receptor antagonist and interleukin-10. *J Orthop Res*, Vol. 22, No. 4, (Jul) pp. 742-50, 0736-0266 (Print) 0736-0266 (Linking)

Zhang, X., Yu, C., Xushi, Zhang, C., Tang, T.&Dai, K. (2006). Direct chitosan-mediated gene delivery to the rabbit knee joints in vitro and in vivo. *Biochem Biophys Res Commun*, Vol. 341, No. 1, (Mar 3) pp. 202-8, 0006-291X (Print) 0006-291X (Linking)

Part 2

Alternative Treatment of OA

7

Peloidotherapy in Osteoarthritis-Modulation of Oxidative Stress

Viorica Marin[1], Olga Surdu[1,2], Daniela Profir[1] and Sibel Demirgian[1]
[1]*Balneal and Rehabilitation Sanatorium of Techirghiol, Constanta*
[2]*Ovidius" University Constanta, Faculty of Medicine, Constanta,*
Romania

1. Introduction

Osteoarthritis is a group of disorders with different etiologies, but similar pathophysiologic changes. In primary osteoarthritis, it is believed that excessive loading cause failure of an otherwise normal joint (Brandt, 1996). The changes eventually involve all of the previously named joint tissues. In particular, the cartilage undergoes breakdown early on, especially in its central areas. Histologically, small tears known as fibrillations and larger tears known as clefts both develop. These defects begin in the superficial zone of cartilage, extend into the transitional zone, and are also propagated by enzymatic breakdown of cartilage. Eventually, large areas of cartilage loss occur, thus essentially exposing the underlying subchondral bone. Other changes within the cartilage include an eventual decline in the ability of the chondrocytes to replicate, an initial increase in the water content of cartilage, a significant reduction in proteoglycan content, a reduction in the size of type II collagen fibers, a diminution of the keratin sulfate concentration, and an increase in the proportion of chondroitin-4-sulfate, consistent with immature cartilage being produced in an attempt to regenerate lost cartilage (Erlich at al, 1996).

Pathogenesis of OA is closely linked to pathogenesis of cartilage degradation. (Maddison, 1998)

Oxidative stress, defined as the imbalance between the production and degradation of ROS, is considered to play an important role in mechanism of cartilage degradation. Peroxidation of lipids, spontaneous or catalyzed by metals (iron, copper), and self-maintained by self-catalysis, generates the production of the reactive species of oxygen (ROS). The ROS are aggressive to cells and to macromolecules of cartilage. The ROS produce negative effects inducing oxidation, damage of membranes, modification of proteins and DNA. (Maddison, 1998)

It's well known that ROS have both positive effects - being involved in energy production, phagocytosis, regulation of cellular growth and intercellular signaling, synthesis of some biologically active compounds - and negative effects, initially altering membrane's lipids, tissues proteins, enzymes, carbohydrates and DNA, and finally having a determinant role in the aging process, which characterizes degenerative diseases. Prostaglandins generated by inflammatory reactions contribute to this aggressive phenomenon by hyper activation of macrophages, which generates ROS. (Curcă, 2003-2004)

The cytokines and growth factors produced as part of the changes that occur in OA can have profound effects on cartilage metabolism. The pro-degradative cytokines IL-1 and/or TNF α are prime candidates for intervention. How important they are in cartilage pathology remains to be more clearly established in human studies, although a mouse "knockout" approach points to the importance of IL-1α and IL-6 in cartilage and bone damage. A recent study using the Pond-Nuki dog model of OA has demonstrated that Tenidap (Pfizer Central Research, Groton, CT, USA), a cytokine-modulating drug, can significantly reduce cartilage damage and osteophyte formation, while simultaneously inhibiting the synthesis of IL-1 and the activity of collagenase-1 and stromelysin-1. (Pool and Webb as cited in Tsokos, 2000)

Certain factors are supposed to have a protective role in the mechanism of cartilage degradation. Superoxide dismutase (SOD), for example, is an enzyme which can be found in different tissues and in the vascular wall. SOD catalyzes superoxide radicals in a neutralization reaction and protects nitrogen monoxide (NO) against inactivation. In the presence of high concentrations of oxygen there is an acceleration of the SOD biosynthesis (Olinescu, 1994). SOD participates directly and indirectly to remove excess of superoxide ions, by inhibiting singlet oxygen and so prevents peroxidation of unsaturated free fatty acids (Salo, 1990). SOD controls the superoxide anions level, thus preventing initiation of the formation reaction of harmful hydroxyl radicals and peroxinitrite (as a result of the reaction between superoxide anions and NO) (Fredovich, 1978).

It was found that certain cytokines, as TNF, or certain lypocarbohydrates, known as stimulating agents of intracellular production of ROS, are also involved in some ROS inactivating mechanisms, from this resulting a fragile balance between production and destruction of ROS. Thus, through an induction mechanism, TNF can stimulate transcription of the Mn-SOD gene. (Pool et. al., 1995)

Gluthatione reductase (GR) is essential for redox cycle of glutathione, which maintains appropriate levels of cellular reduced glutathione. Oxidized glutathione is reduced through a sequence of reactions. (Goldberg & Spooner, 1983) G-SH is a capital factor in the detoxification of the free radicals, resulted from metabolism or from self-oxidation of polyunsaturated fatty acids in the cell membrane. Glutathione peroxidase reduces hydroperoxide (H_2O_2) in the presence of G-SH. (Roşoiu & Verman, 2008)

Reduced glutathione (G-SH) is one of the most important antioxidants from cells, a central component of adaptative system, very sofisticated. (Kidd, 1997) Glutathione exists in the cells both as reduced form (G-SH) and as oxidized form (GSSG), first one being predominant (oxidized form represents less than 10% from total glutathione). (Kosower, 1978)

G-SH is involved in multiple reactions and processes, is an ideal compound for mantaining intracellular redox potential (Meister, 1994). This involvement is due to the reactivity of -SH group. Unlike -SH groups of other enzymes, which are protected by a polypeptidic chain, those from G-SH or cysteine (thyols with low molecular weight) represent „first" target for free radicals.

G-SH can conjugate NO, forming S-nitroso-glutathione, which is cleaved by tioredoxine system, releasing G-SH and NO. Through its interaction with glutaredoxine and tioredoxine (thyol-proteins), G-SH is playing an important role in regulation of cellular redox homeostasis (Yun-Zhong Fang et al., 2002).

Inside the protective antioxidant mechanism (Wang et al., 1998), G-SH is the substrate for glutathione peroxidase (is used to reduce hydrogen and organic peroxides to water and alcohol), it combines with toxic exogenous and endogenous compounds, reducing disulfidic bridges of the proteins and other molecules and, thus, it mantains reduced state of antioxidative enzymes, glycolitic enzymes and redox status of cells (as a major source of thyols), depositing and functioning as transport mean for cysteine. G-SH-transhydrogenases are using reduced glutathione as cofactor for reconvert dehydroascorbate to ascorbate, ribonucleotides to deoxyribonucleotides, etc. G-SH is an efficient detoxifier of ROS (lipidic peroxil radicals, peroxinitrite and hydrogen peroxide), both on direct way and indirect through enzymatic reactions. (Meister, 1991)

Because of its significant reducing potential, G-SH probably contributes to recycle other antioxidants (which were oxidized), as α-tocopherol and carotenoids. (Meister, 1994, 1995)

In physiological conditions blood glucose can reduce molecular oxygen, releasing superoxide ions in the presence of traces of trasition metals (Fe, Cu) and forming cetoaldehides and intermediate oxidation products. Production of free radicals and H_2O_2 after self oxidation process of glucose can determine structural changes of proteins exposed to glucose *in vitro*.

It has been found that harmful effect due to glucose exposure of albumin is inhibited by catalase, antioxidant defense enzyme, and also by metals chelating agents. It has been suggested that glycosylation and oxidation of proteins are correlated processes, change of the proteins due to glycosylation being associated with peroxidation.

Uric acid is a substance easy to be oxidized and, due to its capacity to capture free radicals, is considered protective factor against continous oxidative aggression to which are exposed majority of body tissues.

"*In vitro*" experiments showed that uric acid and some purines capture ROS, playing a role in inhibition of peroxidation of polyunsaturated fatty acids, in protection of red blood cells against singlet oxygen attack, in protection of hemoglobin against oxidative stress, in protection of DNA etc. (Olinescu, 1994). The uric acid acts like an antioxidant in the prevention of lipids peroxidation. (Curcă, 2003-2004)

IL-1, although stimulates ROS production (especially NO and products of activated phagocitic cells), in certain conditions can manifest also an indirect antioxidant role, through stimulation of glucose-6-phosphate dehydrogenase activity, followed by an increased production of NADPH, which is essential in glutathion regeneration. (Mehraban, 1998)

Glucocorticoid hormones have indirect antioxidant activity by inhibation of A_2 phospholipase, which determines an increase of arahidonic acid available in cells and, therefore, they produce a decrease in quantity of endoperoxides which can attack cell membranes, inhibition of chemotactism for activated cells involved in phagocytosis, inhibition of immune complexes formation, thus reducing ROS formation in active cells during immune response.

Correlated with the activity of endocrine functional harmonization is, also, stimulation of activity of hypotalamic-hypophysis-suprarenalian shaft, resulting in optimisation of plasma levels of: β-endorphines, ACTH and cortisol.

Neuro-endocrine reactivity, enzymatic and metabolic changes from endocrine glands after mud therapy are different with secretor type of the gland, with functional stage of the gland and are connected with the type of therapeutical application. Under the action of mud there is a harmonical stimulation of all glands, in the direction of increasing enzymatic and synthesis activity, but maintaining each one specificity (Zirra et al., 1964).

The endocrine mechanism is, also, involved in induction of anti-inflammatory effects of mud therapy, due to modulation of activity of hypotalamic-hypophysis-suprarenalian shaft and to endocrine balance, effects which can be seen even after the cure (Modval et al., 1972).

2. Techirghiol mud

Non-conventional therapies using natural factors (as mineral salted water and peloid/sapropelic mud from Techirghiol Lake) are used on empiric basis from ancient times and have unchallenged benefits in rheumatic pathology, but the intimate biological mechanisms of action are yet not known.

Techirghiol therapeutic mud consists in black deposits, rich in colloidal iron hydro sulfur, from the bottom of the salty lake, formed under the action of micro-organisms, from the inorganic substance of the soil, the flora and fauna of the aquatic basin, as the consequence of some biological and chemical transformations, during the biological ages (Ţuculescu I., 1965).

2.1 Peloidogenesis

The peloidogenesis, as a complex process involving geological , physical, chemical, climatic and biological factors, it is based on organic material which forms tanatozoocenosis and tanatofitocenosis, with an anaerobic evolution, being generated mainly by the *Artemia salina* crustacean, together with *Haliella taurica* and the *Cladophora vagabunda* algae, distributed unequally on the bottom of the lake. In the second phase the iron sulphur is born, the black component of the mud, formed through the activity of the sulphur reduction bacteria, from the combination of the iron with the hydrogen sulphide resulted from the decomposition of the organic materials or, as the case of the iron, from the meteoric waters.

Peloidogenesis runs in three stages:

1. the phase of accumulation and alteration of organic and mineral components. In this stage the origin of mud is established;
2. the sedimentation stage in which the elements are deposited on the bottom of the basin;
3. the physical, chemical and microbiological transformation phase of the flora, fauna and micro-organisms - so called pelogen active agents - convert organic material and minerals in successive stages in the final product. Natural conditions of the lake - density, degree of mineralization, biogenic elements content, gas system - all influence the evolution, the dynamics and the microbiological population component. The dying phytoplankton and zooplankton generate organic substances rich in protein and fat. Almost every bacterium participate in this process with enzymatic equipment: dehydrogenase, carboxylase, catalase. The organic remains, the minerals from the bottom of the lake, together with the material transported by water erosion from the lake are transformed into peloidogen material and then peloid. Micro-organisms break down organic substances and mineralize them and enrich mud with their waste products: vitamins (C, B1, B2, B12), biostimuline, auxinic, biotin, nicotinic acid, carotenoids, substances such estrogenic phenols group. In the liquid phase carbohydrates are oxidized, proteins are decomposed, the fatty acids are desaturated resulting the acetic, formic and valerian acid. Bacteria are present and involved in the "life" of mud, not only in the training forming stage, but also afterwards when they help maintain the biological balance and self-purification of mud and and water basins - a phenomenon called bacteriophagy. (Teleki, 1984; Banciu, 1996) Micro-organisms grow in an environment represented by protein substances, pectin, soluble carbohydrates, soluble proteins, etc. The fauna and flora, as well as the microfauna and microflora present in the mud are: protozoa, copepods, cladocers, hemipters, diptych, beetles, hydrofilids, rotifers, diatomaceous, chlorofycee, cyanophycee. Peloidogenesis is a

complex phenomenon that takes thousands of years and never stops, being conditioned by the hydro-geological characteristics of the area and elements influenced by physico-chemical, biological and microbiological (enzymatic micro equipment: catalasis, oxidasis, reductasis, gelatinasis), each ecosystem and each mud peloidogen resulted is unique. (Diaconescu, 1973) The rhythm, the amount and evolution of peloidogenesis at a certain time may be determined by placement and periodic control of sedimentation on the bottom platform in selected areas for this purpose. It is in fact an analysis of current status of deposit. The mud is mineralizing slowly in time, aging, a phenomenon called diagenesis. (Teleki, 1974). Peloids formation and maturation are slow and permanent processes reflected in their chemical composition. Comparison of some chemical compounds of peloids at different intervals and in certain circumstances allows the assessment of the evolution and maturation of the mud. Ratio of the crystal structure and structure of calcium-magnesian clay is the coefficient incarbonization of peloid, showing maturation stage. Its value ranges between 0.003 and 2.1. Ratio of sulphates and carbonates from the mud reflects its age: increased sulfate content is characteristic to "young" peloids, while carbonates characterise "mature, old" peloids. The peat age is appreciated by the ratio of humic acids / cellulose, an increased value - at around 2.8 - indicating a mature peat.

The mud from the Techirghiol lake is very well hydrated, with a high content of mineral substances and a lower content of organic substances. It has a great capacity of absorption of the ions Ca, Ng, K and Fe, which is very important for therapeutic effects, because of the mobilization of these ions in the organism.

The specificity of the therapeutic mud is given by the primary factor (H_2O of the lacustrine basin), and by the mineral and organic substances.

In time the mud quality depends on the balance of the three elements and on the uniformity of the peloidogenesis process.

2.2 Physical characteristics of Techirghiol mud

Techirghiol mud is an alkaline mud, pH is 8,2.

Density value is 1,283 g/cm^3 and is determined by the nature of the elements which compose it.

Thermopexy is the capacity of absorption, retention/storage and release caloric energy (gives therapeutic value to the mud), and is the most important feature, along with spreading capacity; it is determined by the Denade.

Plasticity is the feature of the mud to change its form under the action of an external force in time. The coefficient of flowing is 43-56% (medium). (Ţuculescu I., 1965)

The spreading capacity depends on the size of the mud granules and for Techirghiol mud is 99.57%. The spreading of the mud is the capacity of fine particles (0,1 mm) to spread uniformly in the tube water and to adhere tightly to the tegument (Teleki et al, 1984).

2.3 Chemical characteristics of Techirghiol mud

The chemical composition of Techirghiol mud consists in: water, mineral substances, organic substances.

The water represents over 70% from the mud's components and it is found as hydrating and colloidal water.

Mineral substances: insoluble salts (calcium sulfates and carbonates, silicates); clay component: SiO_2 and small quantities of oxides; the colloidal component: iron hydro-sulfur, iron and aluminum silicates, organic-mineral complexes.
Organic substances: from the fito-zooplakton of the aquatic basin, from vegetal remains and decomposed animals are represented by carbonhydrates (cellulose and hemicelluloses), humic and humic acids, lipids, proteins and amino-acids, the B group vitamins, nicotinic acid, a bituminous component which contains estrogen-like active substances. According to the standards of National Research Institute of Rehabilitation and Physical Medicine and following the procedure of Romanian Farmacopee for natural products analysis, the report on Techirghiol sapropelic mud is shown in table 1. (Surdu, 2006)

2.4 Methods of mud application

Known and used from the antiquity, mud's ways of applications are still the same: cold ointment (following the antique egyptian method), thermoneutral mud bath and hyperthermic mud wrapping/pack.
Warm salted bath can be performed on a daily basis, as a single major procedure of hydrotherapy, or every other day alternatively with mud application or with warm bath containing herbal extracts. Prescribed temperature for salted bath must belong to the neutral field; it means around 37, 5°-38°C. For hydro-kineto-therapy the water is heated up to 35°C (Lupu, 1956; Surdu, 2006).
Cold mud ointment is a therapeutic complex, which consists from hot-cold contrast. Cold mud ointment is performed in the summer time, on a specially designed beach, where fresh extracted mud is brought daily or every other day. After a 15-20 minutes sun exposure, the patient applies on the whole body surface a mud layer of 1-1. 5 cm thick. Drying of the mud on the skin takes 15-30 minutes, depending of the environment temperature. The patient enters into the lake water in order to remove dried mud, and then performs active movements of all body segments. In the end of the procedure the patient takes a tap water shower. Duration of sun exposure is increasing daily (from 5-10 minutes first day up to 30-40 minutes in the end of the cure), as well as the number of lake immersions. The number of mud applications per day is constant. Meanwhile the cure one must take only one mud application per day. (Teleki et al., 1984)
Thermoneutral mud bath is prepared using 10 kg of mud in 120-150 L of salted water from the lake. Application temperature is around 37. 5°C -38°C, thermoneutrality point for mud being at 38°C. The mud bath takes 20-25 minutes and temperature is maintained almost constant adding warm water after half the time. Once the time expired, the patient takes a warm shower in order to remove the mud from the skin and a quick cold shower in order to avoid systemic vasodilatation. General mud bath is indicated once every two days, alternatively with salted warm bath (in the swimming pool or in the tube) or herbal extracts warm bath. (Onose, 2000)
Hot mud general packing is prepared using 10-15 kg of mud heated at 42°C – 45°C. The mud is smeared all over the body surface, from neck to toes. The patient is covered with a sheet and a blanket, gets a cold compress on his forehead in order to avoid a strong vasodilatation of cerebral vessels and remains like that for 30 minutes. After time expires, the mud is washed with a warm shower. The procedure ends with a short cold shower, in order to prevent irreversible dilatation produced by heat. Mud packing is performed once two days, alternative with a warm salted bath or with a bath containing herbal extracts. (Surdu, 2006; Onose, 2000)

CRT. NR.	PHYSICAL CHEMICAL PARAMETERS	VALUES	OBSERVATIONS
GLOBAL CHEMICAL COMPOSITION (G %)			
1.	Humidity (water)	71,24 g %	Reported in whole humid mud
2.	Volatile substances	8,4 g %	
3	Total mineralisation	20,36 g %	
TOTAL =		100,00 g %	
ORGANIC SUBSTANCES (G%)			
1	Total humic substances	0,9551 g %	Reported in whole humid mud
2	Proteins	1,112 g %	
3	Total waxes + resins	1,612 g % (ether extract)	
4	cellulose	0,4834 g %	
5	bituminous	3,209 g % (benzene-alcohol extract)	
6	Pectins + carbohydrates	2,213 g % (water extract)	
MINERAL CONTENT (PPM / G%)			
1	Iron	3448,332 / *0,3449* ppm / g%	Reported in whole dry mud
2	Calcium	32205,91 / *3,2206* ppm / g%	
3	Sodium	44608,94/ *4,4609* ppm / g%	
4	Kalium	18771,12 / *1,8771* ppm / g%	
5	Manganese	270,022 / *0,027* ppm / g%	
6	Magnesium	39544,64 / *3,9545* ppm / g%	
7	Silicates	/ *13,82* ppm / g%	
INDICATORS OF PELOIDOGENESIS (G%)			
1	Organic carbon (C)	1,313 g %	Reported in whole humid mud
2	Organic azoth (N)	0,129 g %	
3	Ratio C / N	10,18 g %	
SULFUR COMPOUNDS (G%)			
1	Total H_2S from wich	0,1257 g %	Reported in whole humid mud
2	H_2S free	0,0449 g %	
3	H_2S linked	0,0808 g %	
GLOBAL PHYSICAL CHARACTERISATION			
1	pH	8,2	determined in whole humid mud
2	Density ρ_{20}	1,283 g/ cm^3	
3	Dry substance (DS)	28,73 g %	
4	Changeable basis	47,6 mEq / 100 g mud	Reported in whole humid mud
5	Spread index of mud Particules` diameter (mm)	mm / % 0,315 / 0,16 0,200 / 0,30 0,100 / 1,68 0,090 / 0,60 0,080 / 3,88 0,063 / 19,6 0,056 / 7,28 0,050 / 5,90 0,045 / 40,80 0,040 / 9,92 Less than 0,040 / 9,86	Determined in whole dry mud

Table 1. Physical-chemical characterisation report on Techirghiol sapropelic mud

Mud collection is performed from the central area of the lake, where there are three deposits ("islands") of therapeutic mud. Here the mud is settled uniformly, without any foreign material, having a characteristic aspect: black, shiny, unctuous, very plastic, with a very fine granular structure and a specific smell. This is the area from where mud is extracted for over one hundred years and used in all sanatoriums on the seaside (Diaconescu et al., 1973; Ţuculescu, 1965). For mud collection is necessary a claw bucket mounted on a boat. From the boat mud is absorbed with a pump and loaded into a tank, which transports it inside the treatment area, where is deposited in special boilers provided with electric heating and mixing systems. Mud shelf life in the bunker is 4-6 days. From here is provided also the mud for cold ointments in the summer time. After collection from the lake, mud is transported to the solarium, where is stored in the recipients outside (Surdu et al., 2005).

2.5 Physical mechanisms of mud action

The thermal factor: effects are according to the temperature of the mud - the warm application (38° C) determines pain relief, decrease of muscles contracture and has anti-inflammatory effects; higher temperature application has immune-stimulating, tonic, cardiovascular overwork effects.

The physical component of the action of mud on the human body refers to the existing mechanical and thermal conditions during application. Mud thermotherapy is possible due to mud's properties to maintain temperature. This capability of mud allows its application at higher temperatures than body's temperature. There is a slow transfer of heat stored in the mud, allowing the body to take over an amount of this heat. Temperature affects living systems starting with the fundamental biophysics and molecular energy levels up to the most complex systems functionally speaking. The temperature influences the structure of cell membranes and protoplasmatic parts - non-covalent bonds (ionic, van der Waals, hydrogen bridges), the number of hydrogen bridges from the helix structure of nucleic acids and proteins, the phospholipids mezomorphysm, the state of lamellar or hexagonal phase of membranes, the state of oil and fatty acid chains. The temperature continues to be the one that influences functions and biochemical reactions in the membrane and cytosol - the mobility of membrane receptors (with implications in the defense processes as for instance, the formation of lymphocyte cap), plasmalemma vesicles formation, hydrophobic binding of insulin receptors, activitation of adenilcyclasis, enzymes synthesis, the presence / appearance or not of isoenzymes, the rate of diffusion, the Donnan equilibrium, oxygen consumption, etc. The temperature influences the bioenergetic cellular activity, multiplication, defense, various functional control and protection systems. For all biological processes, the temperature is one of the most important conditions for ideal development. For the vast majority of warm-blooded organisms the optimal functional thermal point is located around the temperature of 39°C +/- 1°C, but most organisms live below this heat value. The environmental temperature to which the request of thermoregulatory mechanisms is minimum represents the neutral area, that is to say the individual has no heat needs. The thermal field of peloidotherapy begins with cold application and goes to hyperthermia, each type of application having typical therapeutic effects and consequences. The application of cold mud is a complex heat treatment which consists of successive contrast hot-cold, developed in two phases: the first phase includes sun exposure on the solarium hot sand / beach for about 20 minutes and anointing with mud, and the second phase involves sun exposure for about 30 minutes in order to install a mild hyperthermia, followed by a lake bath/cold shower. Under the direct influence of thermal contrast and indirect influence of the information from thermal receptors, the effector function of peripheral variable heat flow is enhanced by modulating local, partial and finally general circulation and by optimizing the release of self-amplification cell eicosanoids factors. Recent studies on the thermodynamics of soft tissue during cold applications reveal hemodynamic changes as a substrate of thermal changes occurring during application. The muscle tissue is the source of skin reheating after cold application and, even it does not suffer significant decreases in temperature during application, 40 minutes after the end of application it cools, along with the increasing of skin and subcutaneous tissue temperature. (Enwemeka et al., 2002). Thermogenesis and thermolysis reactions are obtained through contrasting therapy, optimizing thus the thermal homeostatic balance. The activation of these programs, their hierarchy, the increasing of the anticipation and reply capacity (feed before) lead to increased performance of adaptive response of the body as a result of an improvement in balance and finally warm-blooded overall body homeostasis. (Andrieş, 1994) Thermal neutrality is the temperature which gives no termoestesic sensation and reduces / maintains the minimizes heat setting processes. This temperature is around 34-35°C for water and 38°C for mud. During the thermoneutral mud bath the body is subject to mechanical forces according the laws of physics stated by Archimedes (body weight loss equal to the weight of displaced liquid) and Pascal (the reduction of chest, abdomen and limbs circumferences in relation to the immersion due to pressure transmission in a liquid in all directions with the same intensity). So, besides from the thermal factor there is also a mechanical acting. During the immersion in mud bath gravity and termoestesic information are reduced, and therefore cortical activation is minimal, allowing stabilization of humoral and neuro-endocrine homeostasis stability in neuropsychological and biological parameters of comfort. While reducing the gravitational and thermal information, information from interoceptors begin to grow, especially from the baroreceptors stimulated by the new hemodynamic conditions and therefore neuroendocrine cardiac depressant processes activate (Bainbridge effect), the Henry-Gauer reflex of inhibiting secretion of vasopressin sets in with its natural consequence of lowering blood pressure. The prolongation of the immersion in the bath over 20 minutes leads to thermoneutrality, mostly because of some endocrine-regulating processes, which secrete a humoral natriuretic and diuretic factor ANF (Atrial natriuretic factor), related with a feedback loop by vasopressin. The vasopressin stimulates the secretion of ANF, which in turn inhibits the secretion of vasopressin. Thus, a thermoneutral bath lasting for 30-40 minutes can lead to blood pressure decrease with about 30%. (Andrieş, 1994) Because its thermoregulatory qualities, mud can be used in the treatment of hyperthermia. Hyperthermia appears when core temperature increases over 37.3ºC by passive heat input. Increased temperature in central area and further in peripheral thermoregulatory area - the poikiloterm area (extremities) - has the following consequences: increased migration of leukocyte inhibitory factor (LIF), macrophag inhibitory factor (MIF), the activation of lymphoblastic transformation, the stimulation of platelet activity of fibrinolytic system, the increase in interferon synthesis. Not only functional, but also structural changes take place under the influence of temperature increase, such as formation of lymphocyte caps (capping) of plasmalemma vesicles, etc. Cellular defense and immunity are two areas with particular benefits from hyperthermia. The central serotonin core system is activated at a temperature of 38-39°C (which inhibits the activity of the sympathetic nervous system at central level), so it stimulates hypothalamic-pituitary system (with ACTH, endorphins, melanotropin release) and synthesis of prolactin.

However, under the action of mud baths, the whole body temperature is "baffled", all devices and systems "work transitory" in a regime requiring all means of antientropic control for maintaining homeostasis of internal environment (Andrieş, 1994). In conclusion, we should bare in mind that there are few effects under the action of the heat factor of mud application.

2.6 Chemical mechanisms of mud action

The humic acid and the humic salts are ions changeable substances, influencing ions` passage between skin and bath medium. They also modify the status of some skin enzymes such as: cytochrome-oxidase, ATP-ase, and alkaline phosphatase, that become active within skin.
The skin pH modification increase the permeability at this level. (Teleki et al., 1984).
Among the chemical components with proven and / or recognized action there are: the humic component, the estrogen bitumen component, the hydrogen sulfide, various ions, biologically active substances produced by microbiological flora and fauna, etc. Because of their chemical composition, peloids acts pharmacodynamically by ion exchange with skin or mucous membranes that come into contact with. Ion exchange capacity is determined mainly by colloidal substances: humic acids, hydrosulfuric colloidal iron. Sorption peloids capacity was calculated using the Mehlich-Dowexhil method, which expresses the ion exchange degree in mEq%. For example at 20°C, 1 kg of Techirghiol mud retains 5.48 g / l calcium, 11.50 g / l magnesium and 9.34 g / l iron. Ions in mud bath selectively penetrate the skin, depending on the electrical charge of the skin and the permeability of skin is increased by the environmental temperature. Soluble elements from the mud's soluble phase participate in the exchange between the skin and mucous membranes, and more intense is the exchange, more diluted is mud. In addition, a comparative study was made in order to compare effects of concentrated mud baths (70-150 kg mud / water in a bath tube with 300 l chlorosodic water from lake Techirghiol) versus diluted mud baths (1 kg mud in a valve with the same amount of water). The overall effects of treatment with diluted mud baths were superior to those obtained with concentrated mud baths and confirmed statistically. The soluble elements transfer from the liquid components of mud, through epithelial cells, is activated by an "enzymatic barrier" represented by cytochrome, alkaline phosphatase and ATPase. In addition, if salted water (such as the water from Techirghiol lake), is combined with mud to prepare mud bath, crystals and salts remain on the skin as a "salt sheath", and along with the hygroscopic action of NaCl stimulate the nerve endings. The crystals on the skin surface retain water from atmosphere, thus making possible different osmotic exchanges at the skin level compared with basal needs. Skin acid pH gives permeability only for cations. A change in pH increases the permeability of skin also for anions. The alkaline hot mud baths change the skin electronegatively, while the acid mud baths - the only acid mud found in Romania is in Stobor - change the skin electropositively. Some of the ions leave the skin and pass into the bath water. Thus, there is a double passage of ions that alter the excitability of skin and skin reflexes starting points. The chemical composition of environment influences mud bath and hydro-mineral balance of the body by various ions which can either accumulate (K^+, Br^+, Mg^{2+}), or they can favour the retention / removal of elements such as chlorides and carbonates of sodium, by increased Ca and P retention in the body, or by established inter-relationships between Cl^-, Br^-,K^+, Na^+, Ca^{2+}, Mg^{2+}. The action of ions can be seen as qualitative exchanges in the body's mineral composition by replacing certain elements with others that are in excess and by accumulation those with low level. The humic substances have antihyaluronidasic

activity, while variations in fibrinogen and fibrinolytic activity are neither parallel nor significant. Antihialuronidazic activity of humic acids from mud has been demonstrated *in vitro*. (Pizzoferrato, 2000) The thermal bath at 35°C does not have this action, which led to the conclusion that inhibitory action is due to mud and not to its thermal effect. Histoenzymatic studies at various levels (skin, internal organs, endocrine glands) revealed differences of enzyme substrates in relation to different type of mud application. In this context, it is insufficient to mention only the enzymatic activity of mud. We can rather talk about the modulating role upon enzymatic that some of mud's components exercise. We have already mentioned the activation of enzyme systems as well as the effects of skin temperature on metabolic reactions. Hydrogen sulfide produces skin hyperthermia even in lower temperatures of mud, it enhances the activity in histaminasis tissue and increases histaminopexic serum activity with the effect of desensitizing the body. Estrogen-active elements from the bitumen component are highlighted through biological tests that revealed the estrogenic action of mud. The microbiological component of mud produces besides vitamins, growth factors, auxine - biogenic stimulators - biotine - a sulphoglicolipid with anti-inflammatory action. (Tolomino et al., 1999) The list of the substances / active ingredients in mud is not complete and can not be completed. Each mud and its aquatic environment of formation and existence are like living organisms in a continuous dynamics. Chemical composition of mud is a "puzzle", that can have all the pieces but not yet arranged for us to create the image of the possibilities of action.

The peloidotherapy produces an harmonic stimulation in all the glands, namely increasing the enzymatic activity and the glandular synthesis, and keeping the specificity of each gland, a persistent and post-cura stimulation. There is a persistent after treatment stimulation the hypothalamus -hypofisal -suprarenalian shaft, emphasized by the increasing of A.C.T.H. secretion, an improvement of vasomotor reactions and of the thermo regulation process.

3. Conclusion

Evaluation of anti-inflammatory potential of sapropelic mud from Techirghiol in patients with osteoarthritis, through assessment of oxidative stress markers, was confirmed by a statistically significant increase of SOD level and by a decrease of reduced glutathione level under the action of mud treatment. The increase of SOD level after mud treatment suggests a positive response of the body, considering the positive role of enzyme in ROS neutralization and NO inactivation. The levels of glutathione reductase, uric acid or blood glucose, protective factors in oxidative stress balance, haven't been influenced by mud treatment. This conclusion emphasizes the protective character of mud therapy on oxidative stress, the enzymes with positive effect on this metabolism increasing, as in SOD case, or maintaining in normal range, as in GR and TAS case (Marin et al., 2009)

Assessment of stress hormones activity showed an optimization of plasma cortisol level and revealed, also, a stimulation of hypotalamic-hypophysis-suprarenalian shaft, sustained by significant increase of tyroid stimulating hormone (TSH) level. The increase of TSH level, for both warm and cold mud applications, shows a stimulation of hypotalamic-hypophysis-suprarenalian shaft under the action of mud. So, the endocrine mechanism is involved, also, in induction of anti-inflammatory effects of mud therapy, by modulating of activity of hypotalamic-hypophysis-suprarenalian shaft and by general balancing of endocrine system, effects that last probably even after cure (Marin et al., 2007).

Assessment of anti-inflammatory potential of sapropelic mud from Techirghiol in patients with osteoarthritis, by measuring inflammatory cytokines levels, has confirmed this effect through an important decrease of TNF-α and IL-6 values in patients which had initially peak values. Also, it has decreased statistically significant the level of receptors for TNF-α, sCD27, fact that sustains the decrease of TNF-α level. (Marin et al., 2011).

Increase of oxygen intake in peripheral blood by opening arterial-venous shunts and improving circulation to peripheral tissues, and osteoarticular tissue also. It was demonstrated the strong growth and consistent within 24 hours of oxygen saturation in the peripheral blood SO_2%, partial pressure of oxygen at this level pO_2 , the oxygen-binding capacity of the hemoglobin O_2CAP and oxygen content of hemoglobin O_2CT. A lower amount of lactate in the peripheral blood and a constant blood pH and carbon dioxide partial pressure suggests an improvement in peripheral tissue metabolism through increased intake of oxygen and nutrients. (Marin et al., 2011).

The obtained results, confirming anti-inflammatory action of mud, should recommend mud as a therapeutic solution for osteoarthritis treatment.

4. References

[1] Andrieş, V. (1994). *Note de curs, Medicina Fizică, Balneoclimatică şi Kinetoterapie*, Universitatea Carol Davila Bucureşti, Editura medicală, Partea I, 37-38, 65-66, 72, 75-77.

[2] Banciu, M. (1996). Balneofizioterapie generala si concepte moderne de recuperare, Editura Mirton, Timisoara,.5-12.

[3] Curcă, D. (2003-2004). Efectele benefice şi cele malefice ale speciilor de oxigen reactive şi radicalilor liberi la animale, *Lucrări ştiinţifice U.Ş.A.M.V.B. Seria C*, vol. XLVI-XLVII.

[4] Diaconescu, L. E.; Anghelopol, C.; Dumitrescu, C. (1973). Studiul comparativ al microelementelor: Zn, Cu, Co, Ni, Ţi, V, Mo şi Cr din apa Mării Negre a litoralului românesc pe patru niveluri; apa lacului şi extrasului de Techirghiol, în *Apele minerale şi nămolurile terapeutice din Republica Socialistă România* , Editura Medicală Bucureşti, 11, 517-526.

[5] Enwemeka, C.S.; Allen. C.; Avila, P.; Bina, J.; Konrade, J.; Munns, S. (2002). Soft tissue thermodynamics before, during, and after cold pack therapy; *Med Sci Sports Exerc.* January, 34(1), 45-50.

[6] Fredovich, I. (1978). Superoxide dismutases: defence against endogenous superoxide radical,. *Ciba Foundation Symposium.* 65, 77-93J

[7] Goldberg, D.; Spooner, R. (1983). Glutathione reductase, *In Bergmeyer H.U.*, Ed. Methods in enzymology , Vol 3, 258-265, isbn 3-527-26041-2, Basel: Verlag Chemie.

[8] Kidd, M., (1997). Glutathione: Systemic Protectant against Oxidative and Free Radical Damage, *Alternative Medicine Review*, Vol.2, nr.3, 155-156.

[9] Kosower, N.; Kosower, E. (1978). The glutathione status of cells, *International Review of Cytology*, 54, 109-156.

[10] Lupu N. Gh. (1956), Medicină internă, volumul I, *Semiologie şi terapeutică generală*, Editura Medicală Bucureşti, Capitolul balneologie - prof. Dr. E. Moraru., 378.

[11] Maddison, P., Isenberg, D., Woo, P., Blass, D., (1998). *Oxford text book of Rheumatology*, isbn 978-019-850-948-6, Ed. Oxford University Press 2 edition.

[12] Marin, V.; Profir, D.; Surdu, O.; Rosoiu, N. (2007), Therapeutically effects of Techirghiol sapropelic mud in oxidative stress at patients with osteoartritis, *FEBS Journal*, Volume 274, Supplement 1, Julay 2007, pp.1-378, 32nd FEBS Congress, "Molecular Machines", Vienna, Austria, C4-76, 213.

[13] Marin, V.; Profir, D.; Ionescu, E. V.; Başa, M.; Roşoiu, N.; (2009). Effects of Techirghiol mud in oxidative stress at patients with osteoarthritis, Archives of the Balkan Medical union, 44, 3, 196-200.
[14] Marin, V.; Profir, D.; Surdu, T. V.; Roşoiu, N. (2011). Variation of Serum Level of Proinflammatory Cytokines after Mud Therapy in Patients with Osteoarthritis, *Archives of the Balkan Medical Union*, 45, 1, 69-74.
[15] Marin, V.; Profir, D.; Roşoiu, N.; Petcu, L. (2011). Evaluation of Blood Gases Pressure in Patients Treated with Sapropelic Mud of Techirghiol, Archives of the Balkan Medical Union, 45, 1, 69-74.
[16] Mehraban, F.; Lark, M.; Ahmed, F.; Xu, F.; Moskowitz, R. (1998). Increased secretion and activity of matrix metalloproteinase-3 in synovial tissues and chondrocytes from experimental osteoarthritis, *Osteoarthritis Cartilage*, 1, 286-294.
[17] Meister, A., (1991). Glutathione deficiency produced by inhibition of its synthesis, and its reversal; applications in research and therapy, *Pharmacology and Therapeutics*, 51, 155-194.
[18] Meister, A. (1994). Minireview: Glutathione-ascorbic acid antioxidant system in animals, *Journal of Biology and Chemistry*, 269(13), 9397-9400.
[19] Meister, A. (1994). Glutathione, ascorbate, and cellular protection, *Cancer Research (Suppl)*, 54, 1969S-1975S.
[20] Meister, A. (1995). Glutathione metabolism, Methods in Enzymology, 251, 3-7, 61.
[21] Modval, M.; Benetato, V.; Constantinescu, I.; Popescu ,V.; Popa, M.; Bălăceanu, V. (1972). Acţiunea aerohelioterapiei asociata cu ungeri de nămol rece asupra funcţiei hipotalamo-hipofizare şi suprarenalelor la bolnavii artrozici, *Studii şi cercetări de balneologie şi fizioterapie*, vol. XI, Ed. Medicală Bucureşti. pag. 148 -149.
[22] Olinescu R., 1994, Radicali liberi în fiziopatologia umană, Ed. Tehnică Bucureşti.
[23] Onose G. (2000). Aspecte conceptuale actuale ale prescripţiilor balneare hidro-termo-terapeutice la vârstnici, *Raport la Conferinţa Naţională cu participare internaţională Actualităţi şi perspective în gerontologie şi geriatrie la cumpăna dintre milenii,* 31 mai-2 iunie, Otopeni, Bucureşti
[24] Pizzoferrato, A.; Garzia, I.; Cenni, E.; Pratelli, L.; Tarabusi, C. (2000). Beta - endorfinele si hormonii de stres la pacientii artrozici tratati cu impachetari calde cu namol; Minerva Med Oct; 91 (10), 239-45.
[25] Poole, A.R.; Rizkalla, G.; Ionescu, M.; Reiner A.; Brooke, E.; Rorabeck, C. (1995). Osteoarthritis în the human knee: dynamic process of cartilage matrix degradation, synthesis and reorganization in *Joint Destruction, in Arthritis and Osteoarthritis*, Birkhaeuser, Basel, 10, 3–13.
[26] Roşoiu, N.; Verman, G.I. (2008). *Biochimie clinică*, Editura Muntenia, Constanţa.
[27] Salo, D.C.; Pacifici, R.E.; Lin, S.W.; Giuilivi, C.; Davies, K.J. (1990). Superoxide dismutase undergoes proteolysis and fragmentation following oxidative modification and inactivation, *Journal of Biological Chemistry*, 15, 265, 11919-27
[28] Surdu, O.; Ţebrencu, C.; Marin, V.; Profir, D. (2005). Studiul variaţiei în timp a compoziţiei chimice a nămolului sapropelic de Techirghiol de la extracţie până la finalul aplicaţiei terapeutice, *Revista de Recuperare, Medicina Fizica si de Balneologie,* nr. 3 –4, pp. 52
[29] Surdu, O. (2006). Evaluarea factorului chimic de acţiune al nămolului sapropelic de Techirghiol, 18-19, isbn 978-973-591-520-9, Ed. Gramar, Bucureşti
[30] Teleki, N.; Munteanu, L., Stoicescu, C.; Teodoreanu, E.; Grigore, L.; (1984). *Cura balneoclimatica în România,* 50-52, 76-82, Editura Sport-Turism, Bucureşti
[31] Tolomino C, Ceschi-Berrini C, Moschin E, Galzigna I. (1999). Colonization by diatoms and antirheumatic activity of thermal mud, *Cell Biochem Funct.* Mar; 17(1), 29-33.

[32] Tsokos, G.C. (2000). *Principles of molecular rheumatology*, Ed. Humana Press Inc., New Jersey.
[33] Ţuculescu, I. (1965). *Biodinamica lacului Techirghiol; Biocenozele şi Geneza nămolului*, Ed. Academiei Republicii Socialiste România, 120.
[34] Wang, L.; Yeh, C.; Hou, M.; Tsai, S.; Lin, S.; Hsiao, J.; Huang, J.; Wu, S.; Hou, L.; Ma, H.; Tsai, L. (1998). Superoxide anion radical, lipid peroxides and antioxidant status in the blood of patients with breast cancer, *Clinica Chimica Acta*, 361(1-2), 104-111.
[35] Yun-Zhong, F.; Sheng, Y.; Guoyao, W. (2002). Free radicals, Antioxidants and Nutrition, *Nutrition*, Elsevier Science Inc., 18, 872-879.
[36] Zirra, A. M.; Voicu, A.; Comnoiu, M.; Stratulat, L.; (1964). Modificări histochimice în glandele endocrine sub acţiunea nămolului sapropelic de Techirghiol şi a extractelor sale, *Studii şi Cercetări de Balneologie*, vol VII, Ed. Medicală Bucureşti, 147-15329.
[37] Marin V., Profir D., Surdu O., Demergian S., Rosoiu N., (2010), Dynamic variation of blood ions during treatment with therapeutic mud, Archives of the Balkan Medical Union, 45, 1, 69-74.

8

Ginger and Osteoarthritis

Tessa Therkleson
Edith Cowan University
Australia

1. Introduction

Ginger has been used for 1000s of years as a food and medicine; it is likely one of the most ancient remedies valued by humans. Ancient Indian and Chinese cultures reportedly used ginger for a wide variety of conditions and modern day research has found it effective as an anti-emetic and anti-inflammatory agent, when taken internally. Random controlled trials using ginger extract have been found effective in relieving symptoms of osteoarthritis. Osteoarthritis is the primary cause of musculoskeletal pain and disability in Western cultures. Current management is primarily through the use of anti-inflammatory and analgesic medication, with cortisone injections and joint replacements a final resort. There is a need for a self-administered, non-toxic, natural therapy that relieves osteoarthritis symptoms, with none of the disadvantages of conventional medication or surgical procedures. A treatment is needed to control symptoms that are: easy to administer, using minimal materials, comfortable to receive, with no known side effects. People with osteoarthritis require a simple treatment that supports the management of chronic pain, relieves their anxiety and improves mobility.

This chapter introduces the significant effect on osteoarthritis symptoms, when ginger is applied externally rather than ingested internally. Four aspects are discussed: 1) ginger for arthritis, 2) ginger qualities and characteristics, 3) ginger for osteoarthritis and, 4) management and ginger therapy.

2. Ginger for arthritis

2.1 Indian medicine

Ginger is one of the significant medicinal plants used in ancient Indian Medicine. It is found effective internally, when used in food preparation and herbal extracts and externally as a ginger compress or mixed with oil to massage around the joints (Chopra, Saluja et al., 2010; Ernst, Pittler et al., 2006). Ayurveda is the term given to indigenous Indian medicine that uses the concepts of prana, prakriti and dosha to understand illness. Prana manifests as movement and energy, it is the source of all existence. Prana healing is a re-vitalising of the body, mind and soul, the basis of ayurveda. Prakriti relates to the constitutional type, while dosha to the bodies elemental forces or energies. There are three dosha: 1) vata dosha relating to space and air, 2) pitta dosha to fire and, 3) kapha dosha to a combination of water and earth. When all three dosha are in balance the body is in good health. Ayurveda medicine refers to osteoarthritis as sandhivata from the Sanskrit 'sandhi' for joint and vata for vata dosha. People with osteoarthritis are understood to have an imbalance of vata dosha that often leads to worry and anxiety, insomnia and cramping in the body, with a decrease of fluidity and increase of catabolic activities in the joints. In osteoarthritis there is a striving to rebalance the tired body and strengthen the digestive and metabolic systems. Ginger is considered to be a plant with qualities to rebalance symptoms of osteoarthritis. Ayurveda treatments are holistic using natural remedies from medicinal plants and minerals accompanied by changes in diet and life style.

2.2 Chinese medicine

Traditional Chinese Medicine (TCM) is a unique medical system using distinct terminology and understanding alongside the use of herbs, acupuncture and moxibustion. TCM involves differentiating the causes such as; emotions, climate, diet and injuries as well as selecting the most effective medicinal herb for a given condition. Since ancient times, ginger has been taken internally and used externally in China, often as a compress, patch or in combination with moxibustion (Lai, Chen et al., 2007; Wu, 2002; Xinangcai, 1998). '*The yellow emperor's classic of internal medicine*' written about 1000BC by a number of authors referred to as Huangdi, provides the first description of ginger rhizome's medicinal use as a warming, stimulating agent. TCM refers to Chi, prana in ayurveda, the universal life force that is the source of all warmth and energy. Chi's continual movement and variation in the natural world, including medicinal plants and the human body leads to the two opposing and interdependent poles of yin and yang; yin relating to the cold, dark, contracting forces and yang to the warm, light, expanding forces. The kidneys are the root of Chi, and the yin and yang of the body. In illness Chi becomes blocked and needs to be bought back into balance. Ginger' qualities are considered to activate stagnating Chi, dispel cold and strengthen yang, where there is a predominance of yin activity as in osteoarthritis. Excessive cold and fear drives Chi downwards in the body leading to kidney/bladder weakness and bone atrophy. People with osteoarthritis tend to have an aversion to cold and suffer from injured and atrophied joints. Ginger is often the herb of choice and is used in combination with moxibustion or other warming herbs, as a compress and/or taken internally as a herbal extract for osteoarthritis.

2.3 Macrobiotics

Traditional Chinese medicine was bought to the West as macrobiotic healing by George Ohsawa in the late 1940's. Ohsawa's students travelled to France, Spain and Germany. In 1950, Mischio Kushi went to the U.S.A., where his books introducing macrobiotics were published (Kushi, 1978, 1985). In Europe and the USA, the East West Foundation is committed to introducing macrobiotic medicine that requires understanding of oriental medicine, with treatments involving diet, life style, exercise and medicinal plants. Macrobiotic medicine classifies arthritis according to the cause, which dictates the treatment approach. Yin arthritis is caused by excessive intake of yin forces for example through the intake of certain foods, such as fruits, sugars and plants from the nitrate family, while yang arthritis is caused by excessive intake of yang foods, such as meat, eggs, salt and dairy products. Both yin and yang arthritis are understood to be aggravated by excessive oil and fat from both animal and vegetable sources, with ice cream being claimed as one of the major contributing causes of arthritis (Kushi, 1978). Ginger is often taken internally for yin arthritis because of its strong yang qualities, while ginger compresses are used both on the abdomen and back to warm the body and stimulate the metabolism in both forms of arthritis. Arthritis is understood to be related to metabolic disturbances and when chronic intestinal stagnation is a contributing cause the ginger compress is often applied over the abdomen (Beere, 2000).

2.4 Anthroposophic medicine

Anthroposophic medicine was founded in the Ita Wegman Clinic, Switzerland in 1923 under the guidance of Dr Ita Wegman (1876-1943) and inspired by the ideas of Rudolf Steiner (1861-1925), an Austrian scientist, philosopher and mystic (Steiner & Wegman, 1925/1967). In 2010, in Europe there were at least 25 hospitals and clinics specialising in Anthroposophic medicine. Anthroposophic medicine takes cognisance of Ayurvedic, Traditional Chinese, herbal and allopathic medicine, with spiritual insights from the ancient esoteric and Christian religions. It is an integrative healing approach that encompasses the understanding there is an interrelation between the physical, life and emotional/sense being of people, which is interwoven by an individual inner organisation and life biography (Evans & Rodger, 1992; Therkleson, 2007). The physical is associated with the mineralising processes of the bone and cartilage, the life with the moving fluids that are most evident in the posture, the emotional with nervous and sensory perception, and the individual inner organisation, with the warm blood. This theoretical understanding finds expression in imbalances of different health conditions. For example, osteoarthritis develops, when the physical and life being is weakened in the joint(s), the sense being increases its activity causing additional tension and pain, while the individual organisation deteriorates and withdraws allowing excessive degeneration to continue unmanaged. The kidneys are considered very important metabolic organs in managing arthritis symptoms primarily due to their involvement in the movement of the blood and the assimilation and excretion of minerals in the body fluids. Typically in osteoarthritis, external treatments are selected to re-enliven and stimulate the metabolic region, such as warm sulphur baths and ginger compresses over the kidneys.

In Ayurveda, Traditional Chinese, Macrobiotic and Anthroposophic Medicine the relationship between a therapeutic plant substance and that of a potential recipient is significant. Ginger is regularly chosen as the herb of choice for people with osteoarthritis due to its warming and stimulating qualities. The qualities and characteristics of ginger are discussed in the following section.

3. Ginger qualities and characteristics

Zingiber officinale (ginger) comes from the zingiberacae family, which has 1300 species of which about 90 comprise the zingiber species. Zingiber officinale is the only medicinal plant in the zingiber species. Ginger's rhizome has been used since ancient times as a food and a medicine. It is taken both internally and externally for a variety of effects including carminative, anti-spasmodic and anti-inflammatory (Blumenthal, 1998; Castleman, 2001/2003; Ferry-Swainson, 2000; Newall, Anderson et al., 1996). The rhizome is the medicinal part of ginger and it contains: 4 - 7.5% oleoresin such as gingerols and their related dehydration products known as shogaols, 1 - 3.5% of volatile oils primarily sesquiterpenes such as bisabolene, zingi-benene, camphene and acurcumene, 6 - 10% lipids comprising triglycerides, phosphatidic acid, lecithins and free fatty acids, 9 - 10% proteins and 40 - 60% carbohydrates in the form of silicate starches. Pharmacological and experimental studies have found the active principle of gingerols and shogaols have anti-inflammatory and anti-emetic qualities (Chrubasik, Pittler et al., 2005). Ginger rhizome is cultivated widely for commercial use in the warm, moist, tropical areas of Africa, Australia, China, Fiji, India, Indonesia and Sri Lanka. People purchasing and using ginger rarely have the opportunity to observe its cultivation and even more uncommon is the sighting of zingiber officinale flowers. The following description of the ginger plant, with a brief summary of its specific features in relation to its therapeutic use is an introduction to this unique healing plant. The photos were taken, whilst on an organic ginger farm in Northern Queensland, Australia.

3.1 Rhizome

The ginger rhizome is a spreading bulbous, stem that develops horizontally close to the soil surface. It forms regularly spaced buds that grow to either shoots or new rhizomes. The rounded fresh buds are about the size of a knuckle, and coloured soft lemon-green, with a fleck of pink. A freshly prepared rhizome reflects these colours in Fig 1.

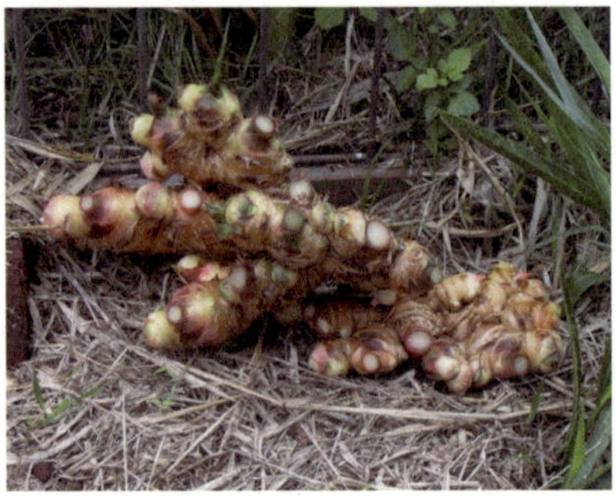

Fig. 1. Fresh rhizome

The ginger rhizome has a pungent aroma, smelling fresh and sweet, and tastes hot, with a sharp and awakening effect. The rhizomes are harvested, when the leaves start to dry and contract in the winter period as shown in Fig 2. It is the rhizome that concentrates ginger's nourishing, healing and reproductive qualities. Ginger is propagated in spring from stored rhizome stock of the previous year.

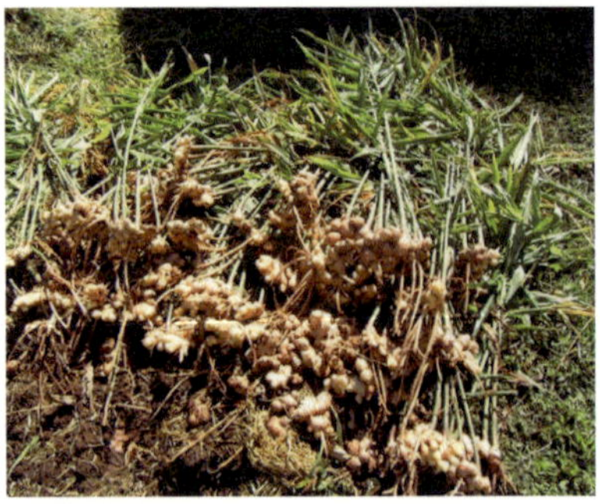

Fig. 2. Ginger harvest

3.2 Root

Long tap roots grow from the seams of the lower buds and anchor the plant deep in the earth. These tap roots reach to about 80cm and are milky-white, strong and juicy; tasting rather like ginger radishes. The tap roots have few hairs and no lateral shoots. Thin, short fibrous roots also grow from the seams of the fresh buds and these are coated in loose soil and minute micro-organisms.

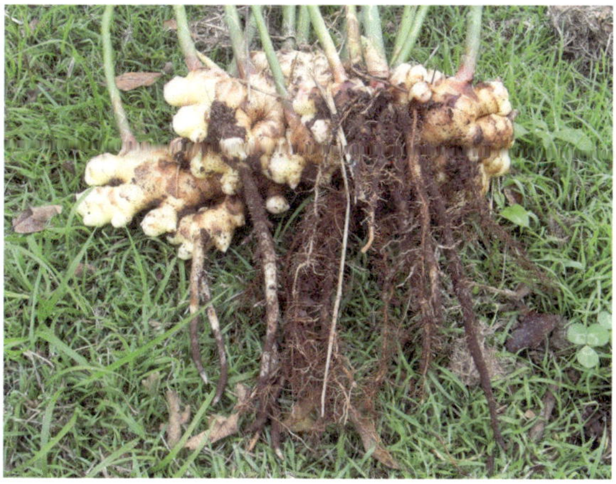

Fig. 3. Ginger roots

3.3 Leaf

As the shoots emerge from the rhizome buds they are their full diameter and grow upwards about 4cms a day until the stalk reaches full height at about 1.5 metres after 30 days. This growth is phenomenal and similar to that of young hollow bamboo stalks. Each mother rhizome develops between 10 - 14 stalks that are slender and erect with between 10 to 14 leaf buds on each. The lower leaf buds appear as contracted leaves, while the upper buds develop single stems that slowly unfurl into large spreading leaves. About 8 - 10 leaves rhythmically alternate up each stem and only open fully once the stalks have reached full height. The lower contracted leaf buds are a dark emerald green, while the upper buds are a soft lemon green. The upper buds open into ovate leaves that are light filled yellow-green, soft and smooth. Each leaf is between 18 - 20cm long and 3 - 4cm wide, with marked longitudinal veins running from the base to the leaf tip.

3.4 Flower

In the plant's autumn, when conditions are dry and cool the flowering buds appear. These buds are positioned on stalks that grow to about 30cms. Each mother rhizome may form between 4 - 6 flower stalks that are dwarfed by the canopy of large drying leaves. At the end of each flower stalk is a green, oval, cone-like flower bud, as in Fig. 4.

Daily in autumn, the cones relax a petal to release a small, cream coloured flower that opens at dusk. The flowers are delicate, 1cm across, orchid-like, with a distinct maroon red or purple speckled tongue, as seen in Fig. 5. It is small wonder that these flowers are rarely seen, not only are they inconspicuous being shrouded by the leaves, they also open as the sun is going down and are spent by dawn.

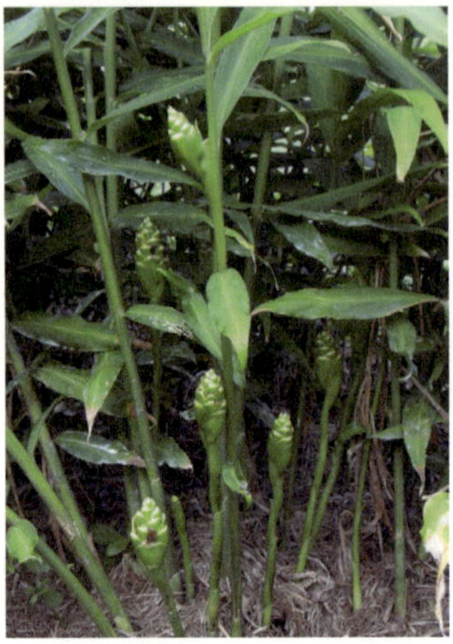

Fig. 4. Ginger flower cones

Ginger has specific features that relate to its selection in the therapeutic treatment of osteoarthritis. The ginger plant is robust, upright and balanced, with strong life giving forces of warmth and energy focused in the swollen stem base or rhizome. Ginger is a unique plant that stores all its reproductive, nourishing and medicinal forces in a rhizome, with the flowers and seeds being inconspicuous and often absent. Both Eastern and Western alternative medical approaches utilise the heat and vitality of the ginger rhizome in managing osteoarthritis symptoms.

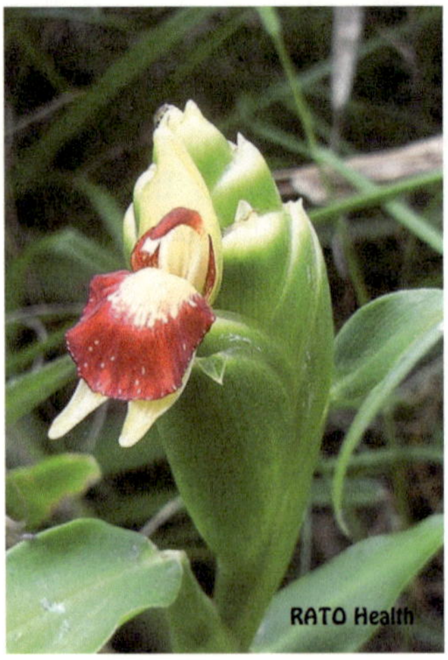

Fig. 5. Ginger flower

4. Ginger for osteoarthritis

The use of ginger externally and internally for osteoarthritis likely had its origins in traditional herbal medicine. Ginger has been applied externally to relieve painful joints for over a 1000 years in India and China, often in combination with other hot herbs (Xinangcai, 1998). In

Guangzhou, China in 2006, I observed raw, grated ginger being applied to swollen ankle joints of travellers in street clinics. In TCM hospitals ginger slices were combined with moxibustion or ginger combined with other heat inducing herbs to remove blockages in the flow of chi, relieve sore joints and assist chronic chest conditions (Therkleson, 2009). For decades, ginger has been used in external therapies in specialised Anthroposophic hospitals in Europe. More recently, anecdotal experiences among groups of nurses have found the ginger footbath an effective adjunct treatment for tired, aching muscles and joints. Modern research reports random controlled trials show oral ginger extract is effective in managing osteoarthritis symptoms (Altman & Marcussen, 2001; Bliddal, Rosetzsky et al., 2000; Haghighi, Khalvat et al., 2005; Marcus & Suarez-Almazor, 2001). However, these studies claim that the high doses of ginger extract required to relieve symptoms often lead to gastrointestinal complaints. The external topical anti-inflammatory activity of dry ginger extracts from solutions and plasters looks promising, with ginger's active ingredient gingerol permeating the epidermis (Minghetti, Sosa et al., 2007). It is posited that transdermal delivery of ginger is likely as effective as internal ginger extracts in achieving an anti- inflammatory response.

4.1 Transdermal delivery of zingiber officinale

Herbs were first recorded as being delivered through the skin around 1550 BC in the Egyptian medical text *Ebers Papyrus*, where the crushed castor oil plant in water is applied externally to treat an aching head. Chinese sources provide directions for using ginger in combination with other medicinal herbs in a wide variety of external applications for a number of different conditions ranging from chronic chest infections, musculoskeletal conditions and metabolic disorders (Xinangcai, 1998). Transdermal delivery is defined as, 'a term that should be restricted to the situation in which a solute diffuses through various layers of the skin and into the systemic circulation for a therapeutic effect to be exerted'(Brown, Martin et al., 2006). This definition is relevant to the use of the external application of ginger in which the active ingredients, gingerols and/or shogaols have the potential to pass through the skin, enter the systemic circulation and provide a therapeutic effect. There are a number of limitations and some significant enhancers to transdermal delivery, which are relevant in the consideration of the therapeutic effect of the external application of ginger.

The primary limitation is the skin barrier. The uppermost membrane of the skin known as the stratum corneum is a thousand times less permeable to water than all the other membranes of the body. To penetrate the stratum corneum a substance must be soluble in oil and water and contain fatty acids that enhance skin penetration (Potts & Lobo, 2005). Penetration of the skin barrier is influenced by the molecular size and the quality of fat solubility of a substance. When a substance has a molecular weight <500 Daltons (Da) and lipophilicity log P range 1 - 3 it has the potential to pass through the skin (Finnin & Morgan, 1999; Guy & Hadgraft, 2003). Gingerols and shogaols, the active principles of ginger, have a molecular weight 150 - 190 Da, a lipophilicity log P range 3.5 and moderate solubility in water and oil, which suggest good potential for skin penetration (Jolad, Lantz et al., 2004; Minghetti, Sosa et al., 2007). There are three significant factors that enhance skin absorption; 1) thermal activity, 2) hydration and, 3) occlusion. Firstly, normal skin temperature is about 32 ^{0}C and, when the temperature is increased to 40 - 45 ^{0}C the closely packed lipids in the stratum corneum become more permeable. Secondly, the application of warm fluid increases the fluidity of the stratum corneum lipids, with a corresponding expansion in the intracellular spaces. Thirdly, occlusion additionally leads to increased hydration and permeability. When the skin has a warm external compress or patch firmly pressed against it, moisture and heat become trapped and increase the swelling and opening of the intracellular spaces. Permeability of the stratum corneum by the active principles of zingiber officinale is likely enhanced by the use of a hot moist ginger compress or patch.

4.2 Ginger compress

European Anthroposophic hospitals report external ginger applications are effective for chest, metabolic, arthritic and psychiatric conditions, especially when applied to the kidney region (Schurholz, Vogele et al., 1992/2002). Ginger applications to the kidney region in the form of ginger compresses are found to warm and reactivate the metabolic forces of the body, which has a corresponding positive effect on the will to be active and mobile. The external application of ginger to the kidney region combines both heat and relaxation therapy and is found especially effective for people with osteoarthritis (Therkleson, 2010; 2004).

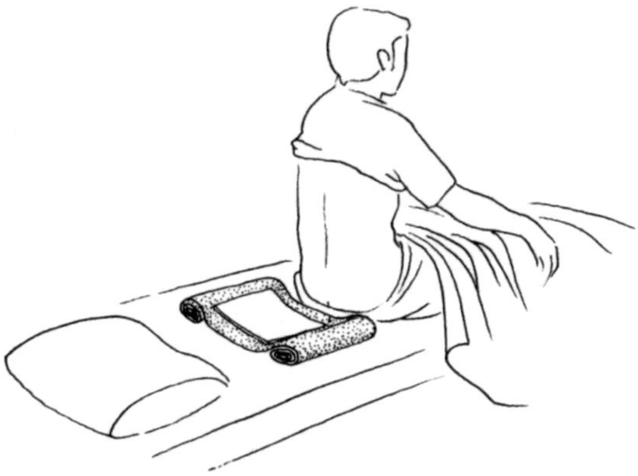

Fig. 6. Ginger kidney compress (Fingado, 2001)

The external application of ginger in the form of a compress to the kidney region was given for 7 consecutive days to 10 people with osteoarthritis. This treatment was termed ginger therapy and it involves having a warm footbath, resting 30 minutes supine, with a ginger compress in place on the kidney region (mid back), followed by a rest of 15 minutes. The ginger compress is a cotton cloth soaked in a hot ginger infusion, squeezed well so just moist and applied to the mid back. The ginger infusion comprises 10 g of ground dry ginger to 200 ml of very hot water. The recipient rests comfortably warm and quiet, on top of the compress that is held firmly in position by a thick cotton binder/towel encasing both the back and front.

Warm ginger compresses applied to the back in this manner activate the movement of body fluids and stimulate the circulation of blood, which has a corresponding positive effect on the weakened joint(s) and surrounding tissues. Following a course of ginger therapy, people with osteoarthritis describe feeling warm and relaxed. In TCM and Anthroposophic medicine, the typical person selected for an external ginger application tends to react negatively to cold, both externally and internally. The likely characteristics of a person being considered for external ginger therapy are that they experience: cold impacting negatively on symptoms, general body tension and a lack of coping skills in times of stress

(Therkleson, 2009). People with osteoarthritis often have very cold extremities, of which they are oblivious. For this reason prior to ginger therapy, a footbath using warm water is generally given to activate the body's natural warmth forces.

4.3 Ginger footbath

A ginger footbath is a fresh approach to applying ginger externally for musculoskeletal tension. This is a simple, convenient and very effective therapy. Anecdotal experiences of groups of nurses describe warmth penetrating through the body, activating a deep relaxation that enables release of mental and physical tension.

The method involves filling a deep basin with warm water and adding 10g of ground dry ginger. The ginger is mixed into the water for about 30 seconds. The recipient sits in a relaxed position for the footbath, encompassed in a warm soft blanket/sheet that is large enough to wrap around the shoulders and reach to the floor. The feet are placed in the footbath 10 minutes, as long as the footbath is experienced as warm and comfortable then dried well and warm socks put on. The recipient can rest a further 15 minutes if required.

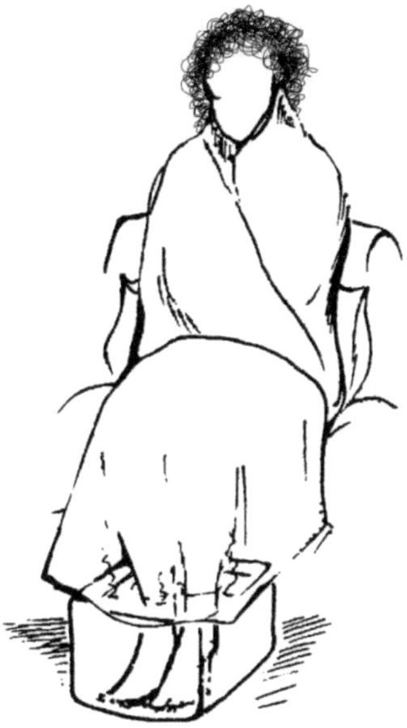

Fig. 7. Ginger footbath

The use of ginger externally is largely unexplored and, with current interest in alternative ways of managing osteoarthritis, it offers hope to those with a condition that has hitherto led to declining health and quality of life.

5. Management and ginger therapy

Osteoarthritis is a health condition that accounts for the majority of hip and knee joint replacements and lost efficacy at work and is the most common cause of musculoskeletal pain and disability in older adults in Western society (Grainger & Cicuttini, 2004). It is a condition that could be better managed, with increased understanding of human motivation and movement. The wisdom of Eastern herbal medicine combined with Anthroposophic insights may well provide the answer towards a more effective approach. Conventional management of osteoarthritis is typically through the use of non-steroidal anti-inflammatory drugs and analgesics (Hunt, Lanas et al., 2009). These medications are often rejected by people, either due to side effects from long-term use or personal preference (Fendrick & Greenberg, 2009). Gastro-intestinal, renal, liver and cardio-vascular risk factors restrict the use of non-steroidal anti-inflammatory drugs and analgesics resulting in osteoarthritis sufferers using a variety of non-pharmacological treatments, such as exercise, heat and hydrotherapy (Grainger & Cicuttini, 2004). Rheumatologists have developed guidelines for the management of osteoarthritis after finding there is no statistically significant difference between pharmacological and non-pharmacological treatments (Zhang, Moskowitz et al., 2008). Considering non-pharmacological treatments are found so effective, more attention needs to be given to alternatives. Ginger therapy is one such non-pharmacological treatment that is worthy of further attention.

5.1 Ginger therapy

Ginger therapy involves a warm footbath, resting 30 minutes supine, with a ginger compress in place on the kidney region, followed by a rest of 15 minutes. Current phenomenological research indicates it is a potentially significant treatment in osteoarthritis. Further research is needed to assess its efficacy, with larger numbers of elderly people. In 2011, a pilot study as preparation for a full trial is commencing in New Zealand. This pilot study is evaluating the feasibility of the most suitable methods and procedures to extend ginger therapy research. Whilst there are no known side, this study will be interested in any potential adverse effects. Additionally, there is a secondary interest in the feasibility and effectiveness of using a manufactured ginger patch that can be self-applied in the home or residential setting over an extended period. A prospective study is following the pilot study and evaluate the efficacy of self-applied ginger therapy using the ginger patch for people with osteoarthritis. The ginger patch has the potential to replace the ginger compress, with the advantage of it being manufactured for convenient application both in the research and clinical situation. The ginger patch would be consistently reliable and appropriately encased in a waterproof package that is hygienically sealed from air and light.

Developing the research of ginger therapy for osteoarthritis will extend the possibility of researching its use for other relevant health conditions. Hospitals in Europe use external ginger applications to manage a number of different conditions such as: chronic chest problems, metabolic disturbances, arthritis and psychiatric conditions. Schurholz et al (1992/2002) is the only European research available and it is limited by the numbers of people involved and lack of a clearly defined methodology. Unfortunately this research has not been published in a recognised peer reviewed journal.

6. Conclusion

Ginger's therapeutic qualities in osteoarthritis are well grounded in the experiences of Eastern medicine and modern research trials. Evidence suggests the high doses required for a positive effect in osteoarthritis often result in digestive disturbances. The external application of ginger avoids this negative, with ginger therapy and the ginger footbath as good alternatives. Ginger is a medicinal plant with strong heat activating and anti-inflammatory qualities, when applied to the skin in ginger therapy these qualities seem to magnify for people with osteoarthritis. Current research on the experiences of ginger therapy indicates this is a novel approach to osteoarthritis management. Further research on larger numbers of people receiving ginger therapy is necessary to advance the existing knowledge base and extend this treatment to increased numbers of osteoarthritis sufferers. Ginger therapy needs to be considered as a viable, non-invasive treatment option in caring for people with osteoarthritis symptoms. The potential socio-economic benefits are considerable and include a decrease in medication, surgical procedures and loss of working potential accompanied by improved quality of life and increased independence.

7. References

Altman, R. D., & Marcussen, K. C. (2001). Effects of a Ginger Extract on Knee Pain in Patients with Osteoarthritis. *Arthritis & Rheumatism,* Vol. 44, No. 11, pp. 2461-2462

Beere, K. (2000). *The End of Medicine,* Transtana Alchemysts, Albany, California

Bliddal, H., Rosetzsky, A., Schlichting, P., Weidner, M. S., Andersen, L. A., Ibfelt, H. H., Christensen, K., Jensen, O. N., & Barslev, J. (2000). A Randomized, Placebo-Controlled, Cross-over Study of Ginger Extracts and Ibuprofen in Osteoarthritis. *Osteoarthritis Cartilage,* Vol. 8, No. 1, pp. 9-12

Blumenthal, M. (1998). *The Complete German Commission E Monographs: Therapeutic Guide to Herbal Medicines.* Texas, U.S.A.: American Botanical Council.

Brown, M. B., Martin, G. P., Jones, S. A., & Akomeah, F. K. (2006). Dermal and Transdermal Drug Delivery Systems: Current and Future Prospects. *Drug Deliv,* Vol. 13, No. 3, pp. 175-187

Castleman, M. (2001/2003). *The New Healing Herbs,* Hinkler Books, Australia

Chopra, A., Saluja, M., & Tillu, G. (2010). Ayurveda-Modern Medicine Interface: A Critical Appraisal of Studies of Ayurvedic Medicines to Treat Osteoarthritis and Rheumatoid Arthritis. *Journal Ayurveda and Integrative Medicine,* Vol. 1, No. 3, pp. 190-198

Chrubasik, S., Pittler, M. H., & Roufogalis, B. D. (2005). Zingiberis Rhizoma: A Comprehensive Review on the Ginger Effect and Efficacy Profiles. *Phytomedicine,* Vol. 12, No. 9, pp. 684-701

Ernst, E., Pittler, M., & Wider, B. (2006). *Desktop Guide to Alternative and Complementary Medicine,* Mosby Elsevier, St Louis, USA

Evans, M., & Rodger, I. (1992). *Anthroposophical Medicine,* Thorsons, London

Fendrick, A., & Greenberg, B. (2009). A Review of the Benefits and Risks of Nonsteroidal Anti-Inflammatory Drugs in the Management of Mild-to-Moderate Osteoarthritis. *Osteopathic medicine and primary care,* Vol. 3, No. 1, pp. 1-7, ISSN 1750-4732

Ferry-Swainson, K. (2000). *Ginger,* Tuttle Publishing, Massachusetts, USA

Fingado, M. (2012) *Compresses and therapeutic applications,* translator Tessa Therkleson and Sarah Therkleson, Floris Books, Edinburgh, United Kingdom

Finnin, B. C., & Morgan, T. M. (1999). Transdermal Penetration Enhancers: Applications, Limitations, and Potential. *J Pharm Sci,* Vol. 88, No. 10, pp. 955-958

Grainger, R., & Cicuttini, F. M. (2004). Medical Management of Osteoarthritis of the Knee and Hip Joints. *Medical Journal Australia,* Vol. 180, No. 5, pp. 232-236

Guy, R. H., & Hadgraft, J. (2003). *Transdermal Drug Delivery* (2nd ed.), Marcel Dekker, New York

Haghighi, M., Khalvat, A., Toliat, T., & Jallaei, S. (2005). Comparing the Effects of Ginger (Zingiber Officinale) Extract and Ibuprofen on Patients with Osteoarthritis. *Archives of Iranian medicine,* Vol. 8, No. 4, pp. 267-271, ISSN 1029-2977

Hunt, R., Lanas, A., & Stichtenoth, D. (2009). Myths and Facts in the Use of Anti-Inflammatory Drugs. *Annals of Medicine,* No. 8, pp. 1-16

Jolad, S. D., Lantz, R. C., Solyom, A. M., Chen, G. J., Bates, R. B., & Timmermann, B. N. (2004). Fresh Organically Grown Ginger (Zingiber Officinale): Composition and Effects on Lps-Induced Pge2 Production. *Phytochemistry,* Vol. 65, No. 13, pp. 1937-1954

Kushi, M. (1978). *Natural Healing through Macrobiotics,* Japan Publications, New York

Kushi, M. (1985). *Macrobiotics and Home Remedies,* Japan Publications, New York

Lai, J. N., Chen, H. J., Chen, C. C., Lin, J. H., Hwang, J. S., & Wang, J. D. (2007). Duhuo Jisheng Tang for Treating Osteoarthritis of the Knee: A Prospective Clinical Observation. *Chin Med,* Vol. 2, pp. 4, ISSN 1749-8546 (Electronic)

Marcus, D. M., & Suarez-Almazor, M. E. (2001). Is There a Role for Ginger in the Treatment of Osteoarthritis? *Arthritis and Rheumatisim,* Vol. 44, No. 11, pp. 2461-2462

Minghetti, P., Sosa, S., Cilurzo, F., Casiraghi, A., Alberti, E., Tubaro, A., Loggia, R., & Montanari, L. (2007). Evaluation of the Topical Anti-Inflammatory Activity of Ginger Dry Extracts from Solutions and Plasters. *Planta medica,* Vol. 73, No. 15, pp. 1525-1530, ISSN 0032-0943

Newall, C., Anderson, L., & Phillipson, J. (1996). *Herbal Medicines: A Guide for Health-Care Professionals,* The Pharmaceutical Press, London

Potts, R. O., & Lobo, R. A. (2005). Transdermal Drug Delivery: Clinical Considerations for the Obstetrician-Gynecologist. *Obstet Gynecol,* Vol. 105, No. 5 Pt 1, pp. 953-961

Schurholz, J., Vogele, M., Heine, R., Muck, H., Sauer, M., Simon, L., & et al. (1992/2002). *Study of the External Application of Ginger,* Rato Health, Lower Hutt, New Zealand

Steiner, R., & Wegman, I. (1925/1967). *Fundamentals of Therapy,* Rudolf Steiner Press, London

Therkleson, T. (2007). *Nursing the Human Being: An Anthroposophic Perspective,* Mercury Press, New York

Therkleson, T. (2009). *The Experience of Receiving Ginger Compresses in Persons with Osteoarthritis - a Phenomenological Study.* Unpublished PhD, Edith Cowan University, Perth, Western Australia

Therkleson, T. (2010). Ginger Compress Therapy for Adults with Osteoarthritis. *Journal Advanced Nursing,* Vol. 66, No. 10, pp. 2225 - 2233

Therkleson, T., & Sherwood, P. (2004). Patients Experience of the External Therapeutic Application of Ginger by Anthroposophically Trained Nurses. *Indo-Pacific Journal of Phenomenology,* Vol. 4, No. 1, pp. 86-97

Wu, C. (2002). *Basic Theory of Traditional Chinese Medicine,* Publishing House of Shanghai University TCM, Peoples Republic of China

Xinangcai, X. (1998). *Complete External Therapies of Chinese Drugs,* Foreign Languages Press, Beijing, Peoples Republic of China

Zhang, W., Moskowitz, R., Nuki, G., Abramson, S., Altman, R., Arden, N., Bierma-Zeinstra, S., Brandt, K., Croft, P., Doherty, M., Dougados, M., Hochberg, M., Hunter, D., Kwoh, K., Lohmander, L., & Tugwell, P. (2008). Oarsi Recommendations for the Management of Hip and Knee Osteoarthritis, Part Ii: Oarsi Evidence-Based, Expert Consensus Guidelines. *Osteoarthritis Cartilage,* Vol. 16, No. 2, pp. 137-162

Part 3

OA in Upper Extremity (Hand, Wrist, Shoulder, and Elbow)

9

Osteoarthritis of the Wrist

Nimit Patel, Glenn Russo and Craig Rodner
University of Connecticut
United States of America

1. Introduction

Our hands are a uniquely human characteristic. They have helped us throughout our evolution and even today they help us to live, work, and play. While osteoarthritis can cause great pain wherever it presents, it is a particularly crippling disease when it affects the wrist and the hands. Unfortunately, osteoarthritis of the wrist can result from a multitude of causes. One can divide these causes into two major categories: traumatic and non-traumatic. Trauma leading to osteoarthritis often occurs because of ligament and bone injury that causes instability, dyskinesis, and altered loading forces that can lead to joint degeneration. Intra- or extra-articular fractures can also produce abnormal joint loading and arthritis. For example, some prototypical patters of injury include the common scapholunate advanced collapse (SLAC) and the closely related scaphoid fracture and non-union (SNAC).
When conducting a general exam on a patient with suspected wrist osteoarthritis, it is essential to begin with a broad differential diagnosis to avoid falling into the trap of premature closure. Congenital, inflammatory, vascular, post-traumatic and idiopathic etiologies have all been known to cause wrist pain. The goal of the history and physical (H&P), therefore, is to articulate the precise cause of this pain in order to design the best treatment plan. The patient's age, hand dominance, aggravating and alleviating pain factors, prior trauma, family history, occupation, hobbies and limb functionality are all essential parts of a good history. The physical exam, given the close proximity and complexity of the intercarpal joints, is particularly important in isolating the exact source of pain. A general inspection should note any swelling, erythema or atrophy. Passive and active range of motion should be assessed with full flexion, extension, pronation and supination as well as radial and ulnar deviation. Physical examination should also comment on any tenderness in the joint in addition to the patient's vascular and neurologic status. Additionally, other joints like the elbow, shoulder and neck should be inspected for injury or symptomatology. All tests should be bilateral. Functional measures like the Disabilities of the Arm, Shoulder and Hand, the Patient Evaluation Measure and the Michigan Hand Outcome Questionnaire have also been used to establish one's functional status (Dias, Rajan et al. 2008).
Joint palpation is the most useful technique in localizing articulations that produce pain. In addition to general palpation, there is an array of pain-producing maneuvers that can be used to isolate particular joints. The thumb grind can be used to show thumb carpometacarpal (CMC) arthritis. The scaphoid shift test will point towards a scapholunate instability (Watson, Ashmead et al. 1988). The shear or ballottment test indicates lunotriquestral instability (Reagan, Linscheid et al. 1984). The catch-up-clunk test indentifies midcarpal joint instability

(Lichtman, Schneider et al. 1981). Pisiform tracking can be used to isolate pisotriquetral osteoarthritis. (Nagle 2000) (Friedman and Palmer 1991). Pain on pronosupination during elbow flexion will help isolate a distal radioulnar joint arthritis. Pre- and post-operative pain scales, like the Nagy and Buchler system can also be used (Nagy and Buchler 1997).

Strength should be evaluated and is most useful when objectively quantified with a goniometer. Abnormalities in grip strength can indicate pathology and its testing is most accurate when used with the rapid exchange grip strength technique which is best at determining submaximal effort (Hildreth, Breidenbach et al. 1989). In addition to the initial patient visit, this is a useful measure for pre-operative and post-operative comparison.

A patient's laboratory evaluation should include, when appropriate, plasma ESR, CRP, white blood cell count, uric acid, ANA and rheumatoid factor to rule out any infections or likely rheumatologic conditions.

Imaging studies are another valuable tool at the physician's disposal that allows him or her to better determine which joints are affected by the degenerative processes. The standard x-ray series should include a posteroanterior (PA), oblique, and lateral view.. A wrist with normal anatomic relationships will show that the radial shaft, capitate, and third metacarpal will line up along the same vertical axis in the PA wrist x-ray. The physican's initial evaluation should focus on the radioscaphoid, radioluate and capitolunate joints. A secondary evaluation should include assessment of the Carpometacarpal, scapho-trapezium-trapezoid (STT), ulnocarpal and distal radioulnar joint (Weiss and Rodner 2007). The articular surface of the radiocarpal joints can sometimes be better seen with a tangeiental view. Radioscaphoid and STT joints can be seen best with radial and ulnar deviation views. Carpal tunnel and oblique supination views are excellent for the evaluation of the pisotriquetral joint (Peterson and Szabo 2006). As always, to control for normal anatomic variation, all findings should be compared with the contralateral wrist.

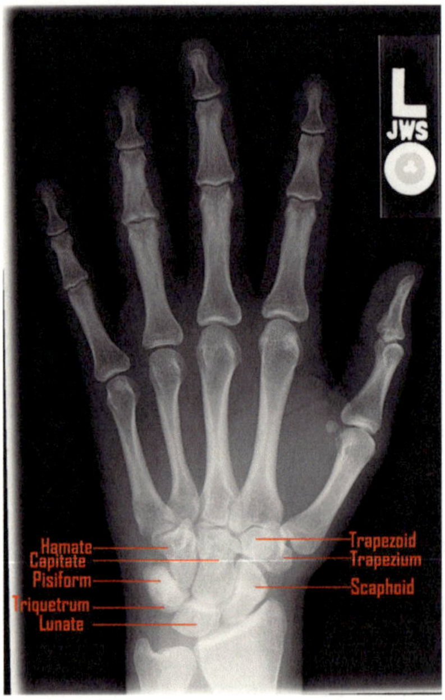

Fig. 1. PA Radiograph of Normal Wrist

Sonographic imaging can be a useful tool when used by a radiologist with sufficient training in its application to hand anatomy. A CT scan may be useful for the evaluation of the smaller intra-carpal articulations as well as the pisotriquetral joint. Less obvious distal radioulnar joint malalignment can also be picked up with CT views in neutral, supination, and pronation positions. However, the CT scan is inferior when compared to the MRI for the evaluation of soft tissue defects (Mutimer, Green et al. 2008). An MRI is therefore better than a CT to evaluate for cartilage injury. Bone scintigraphy is a nonspecific scan that is best used to supplement inconclusive findings. A three-phase scan can be useful in determining the chronicity of a pathological condition; a chronic condition is indicated when technetium uptake is only seen in delayed images. Finally, a diagnostic injection with corticosteroid or anesthetic can be used to confirm the pain-generating joint in the hand. If injection of the suspected joint alleviates the patient's pain, then it is highly likely that you have isolated the source of the problem. This technique is particularly useful in differentiating radiocarpal, midcarpal, and DRUJ insults. It can also confirm pisotriquetral, STT or basilar thumb arthritis. Injection can also distinguish an extra- versus intra-articular pain source.

Treatment is only effective when correctly paired to an accurate diagnosis. Given the wide array of wrist pathologies, the exam and work up of a patient with wrist pain is crucial. All other causes of wrist pain must be ruled out before a diagnosis of osteoarthritis is reached. Moreover, the surgical treatments discussed below are only to be considered after a patient has failed other forms of non-pharmacologic and medical therapies. Some of the more common causes of wrist osteoarthritis, their pathogenesis, diagnostic workup and treatment are discussed below.

2. Osteoarthritis of the radioscaphoid joint

2.1 Scapholunate advanced collapse

Scapholunate advanced collapse (SLAC) represents the most common pattern of degenerative wrist arthritis and accounts for 72% of the cases of wrist arthritis seen today (Watson and Weinzweig 1999). This pattern was first described by Watson and Ballet who reviewed four thousand wrist x-ray films for sequential degenerative changes and determined that arthritis between the scaphoid, lunate, and radius represented 57% of cases surveyed (Watson and Ballet 1984).

In this disease process, the initial insult is a trauma to the scapholuate (SL) ligament which allows for a rotary subluxation of the distal scaphoid, resulting in progressive intercarpal instability and joint degeneration. Degenerative changes first affect the radial styloid and distal pole of the scaphoid (stage I). Arthritic changes then occur in the radioscaphoid joint (stage II), further progress to the capitolunate articulation (stage III), and can culminate with pancarpal involvement (Weiss and Rodner 2007).

In addition to SL ligament trauma, calcium pyrophosphate dehydrate (CPPD) crystal deposition can also produce a SLAC wrist pattern of arthritic change (Chen, Chandnani et al. 1990). Also, a recent study suggested that SLAC wrist could result independently of trauma or CPPD. Studies suggest that congenital SL laxity may predispose certain individuals to develop SLAC wrist. (Pollock, Giachino et al. 2010). Other conditions like avascular necrosis of the scaphoid (Kienbock disease), Preiser's disease, intra-articular fractures affecting the radioscaphoid or capitolunate joints, perilunate dislocation, malunion of a distal radius fracture and carpal instability can also produce a SLAC pattern of degeneration in the wrist (Vender, Watson et al. 1987).

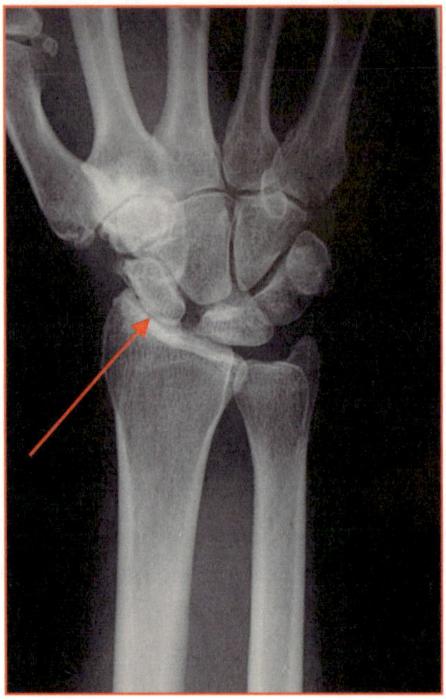

Fig. 2. PA Radiograph SLAC Wrist

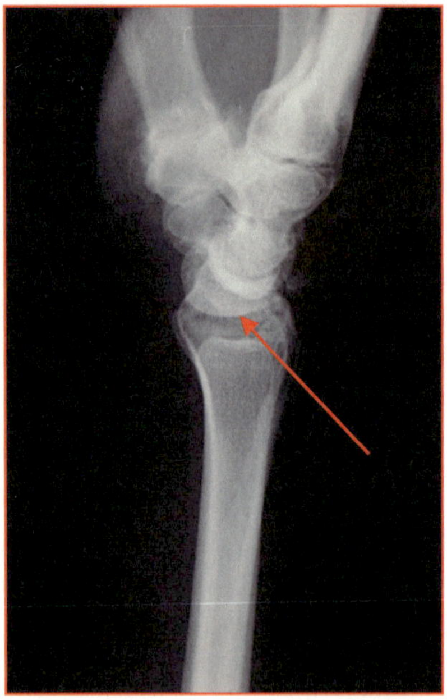

Fig. 3. Lateral Radiograph of SLAC Wrist

As with much of orthopaedics, the anatomy of this system is implicit to its pathology. The proximal pole of the scaphoid is elliptical in shape and it articulates in a corresponding elliptical surface in the distal radius. With scaphoid instability due to SL ligament injury, the scaphoid will rotate causing it to sublux and articulate only on the edges of its joint diathasis. As a result, unequal loading forces can cause degenerative change and joint destruction. Imagine two nested spoons; if one were to rotate by 90 degrees, they would articulate on smaller contact points instead of their entire surface (Mastella, Ashmead et al. 2009). This subluxation and rotation results in the radioscaphoid pain that designates stage II of SLAC. Conversely, the radiolunate joint is spherical, so that rotation of the lunate will not cause a change in the force distribution across the joint. It is for this reason that the radiolunate joint is preserved in a SLAC wrist pattern of degeneration. This concept is important because it serves as the basis for surgical intervention.

The presentation of the SLAC wrist typically involves dorsal wrist swelling and tenderness in a periscaphoid distribution. The patient may complain of restricted mobility of their wrist. Patients will demonstrate a positive "shift test" which has been described as the definitive test for scaphoid instability. Pain while applying pressure to the scaphoid during radial deviation of the wrist is a positive test result. (Watson, Ashmead et al. 1988). Wrist ganglia have also been known to develop in the presence of carpal instability. However, in the case of a SLAC wrist, as the disease becomes more advanced the structures needed to form ganglia are abolished. Therefore, this complication may be appreciated early on in the disease process, but is less apparent with advanced pathology. As always, these clinical symptoms should be evaluated in comparison to the contralateral wrist. Also, there have been reports of SLAC wrist that are not associated with pain. These are typically isolated to older, low-demand patients who's arthritic disease is discovered during investigation of another complaint (Fassler, Stern et al. 1993). Other diagnoses to rule out include thumb CMC arthritis, carpal tunnel syndrome, and trigger finger. The diagnosis of SLAC wrist is confirmed with bilateral plain x-rays with evidence of degeneration in the affected hand.

Nonsurgical management of a SLAC wrist or its related conditions currently lacks long term data. This therapy consists of non-steroidal anti-inflammatory drugs (NSAIDS), splints, and injections for symptomatic treatment. By decreasing inflammation with NSAIDS and corticosteroids, and decreasing mobility with splinting we are able to provide some pain relief. Anti-inflammatory medications may need to be tailored to each individual patient as some respond better to some medications than others. Corticosteroid injections can be particularly beneficial in patients who show swelling and synovitis. Moreover, intermittent injections can have less side effects than those associated with chronic anti-inflammatory use. Splints are to be worn intermittently throughout the day and during the night. One study determined that if pain is not limiting and grip strength is greater than or equal to 80%, managing these symptoms non-surgically is a reasonable option (Pilny, Kubes et al. 2006).

Surgical contraindications are due to any pathology that affects the radiolunate joint. A SLAC wrist pattern represents a final common pathway in a variety of disease processes but a defining feature remains to be the preservation of the radiolunate joint. This joint's integrity is critical because it serves as the main point of force translation through the wrist after several of the surgical options. Therefore, any significant degeneration of the radiolunate joint would qualify as a contraindication for surgery. Similarly, any ulnar translation of the carpus on the radius will alter the radiolunate relationship and also serve as a contraindication for surgery (Pellegrini, Parentis et al. 1996).

Surgical therapy can be accomplished through a variety of approaches. Historically, this consisted of scaphoid excision and replacement with a silicone arthroplasty along with fusion of the capitate, lunate, hamate and triquetrum by using Kirschner-wires (K-wires). Use of the silicone scaphoid replacement has fallen out of favor due to the fact that silicone wear resulted in particulate formation, synovitis, and joint collapse (Ashmead, Watson et al. 1994). Despite the failure of the silicone scaphoid replacement, the technique of fusing the four aforementioned carpal bones along with scaphoid excision remains to be a popular surgical option for patients suffering from a SLAC wrist; this procedure is referred to as a scaphoid excision with a four-corner arthrodesis. This is a reliable and effective procedure that provides a stable column for force transfer through the radiolunate joint. Dacho has shown encouraging results with this technique on long-term follow-up in the treatment of both SLAC and SNAC wrist injury (Dacho, Grundel et al. 2006). Mid-term results using K-wires specifically have also enjoyed similar success (Winkler, Borisch et al. 2010).

Alternatively, a proximal row carpectomy (PRC) can be used in lieu of a four-corner arthrodesis. This technique calls for the removal of the proximal row of carpal bones and allows the distal row to collapse proximally. In this scenario, the capitate articulates with the lunate facet of the radius. This surgery preserves a fair amount of wrist mobility and requires no arthrodesis. PRC is a viable alternative to four-corner arthrodesis as it has shown success in long-term follow-up (Liu, Zhou et al. 2009).

Controversy exists in determining which procedure is superior; four-corner arthrodesis with scaphoid excision or PRC. Studies suggest no difference in outcomes when comparing these two procedures. However, some patients may prefer the PRC procedure as it allows for greater wrist mobility. In a high demand wrist the loss of stability could become problematic and the four-corner arthrodesis may be the preferred technique in this patient. (Mulford, Ceulemans et al. 2009) (Cohen and Kozin 2001; Dacho, Baumeister et al. 2008; Bisneto, Freitas et al. 2011).

Other surgical techniques include denervation, total wrist fusion, wrist arthroplasty and variations of intercarpal arthrodeses. Denervation can be accomplished through transection of all articular nerve branches or it can be limited to the anterior or posterior interosseous nerves proximal to the carpus. One study showed long-term data supporting the use of dennervation as a treatment for SLAC/SNAC wrist injury (Rothe, Rudolf et al. 2006).

Any symptoms of complex regional pain syndrome (intense burning pain that gets worse over time and spreads to adjacent or contralateral limbs) should be treated with a stress loading program (active exercise with minimal joint motion). Also, the patient should be monitored for triquetral impingement ligament tear syndrome (TILT). This syndrome occurs secondary to ulnar translation of the carpus due to the increased laxity of the radiocarpal ligaments (Watson and Weinzweig 1999). TILT will manifest as pain and tenderness on the ulnar aspect of the wrist. When occurring after a reconstructive surgery, TILT will often resolve spontaneously, however, if it persists it can be corrected by resecting the impinging portion of the ulnar sling. Radiolunate degeneration is a rare complication of reconstruction and is always seen in the context of ulnar translation of the carpus. When this occurs, it can be successfully repaired with total wrist arthrodesis.

Overall, the treatment of SLAC wrist enjoys encouraging outcomes. Post operative follow up shows that patients generally have improved pain levels while maintaining ROM and grip strength. (Malerich, Clifford et al. 1999)Although controversy remains with regard to the "best" procedure with which to treat a SLAC wrist, we are able to take solace in the fact that regardless of operative technique, patient satisfaction remains very high.

2.2 Scaphoid nonunion advanced collapse

It has become clear that scaphoid nonunion advanced collapse (SNAC) is a clinical entity similar to SLAC wrist in that it is identified by a series of predictable degenerative changes. In a SNAC wrist, however, the initial injury is a fracture and nonunion of the scaphoid rather than an SL ligament injury. A scaphoid malunion can also cause a SNAC injury. Interestingly, in a SNAC injury, because the SL ligament is preserved, the proximal scaphoid fragment is not involved in the degenerative changes and it is the scaphocapitate that tends to be affected (Vender, Watson et al. 1987).

Because of its close similarity to the SLAC wrist, a SNAC injury shares a similar disease progression with comparable stages of joint degeneration. Stage I is associated with arthritis localized to the distal scaphoid and radial styloid. Stage II shows radioscaphoid and scaphocapitate arthritis with a preserved lunocapitate joint. Once the lunocapitate joint becomes involved, a stage III designation is warranted.

Much like the presentation and evaluation of SLAC wrist, a patient with a SNAC wrist injury will present with wrist pain at the radioscaphoid joint and dorsal swelling. Diagnosis will be based on the history and physical but confirmed with an x-ray and its comparison to the contralateral wrist. Treatments for SNAC wrist also overlap with the SLAC wrist and are comprised of nonsurgical management with splinting and injections, as well as surgical options like arthrodesis, proximal row carpectomy, denervation, and radial styloidectomy. One notable difference in between the treatment plans for SLAC and SNAC wrists is that the SNAC wrist can be treated with the excision of the distal scaphoid fragment. One study noted that 13 out of 19 patients showed significant pain relief as well as improved ROM and grip strength with this procedure (Malerich, Clifford et al. 1999).

In summary, a SNAC wrist injury shares a great deal with a SLAC wrist and is discerned through a careful history, physical, and radiographic evaluation. Treatment options are almost identical for the two pathologies with a notable distinction that a SNAC wrist can be treated with a distal scaphoid excision.

3. Osteoarthritis of the distal radioulnar joint

The distal radioulnar joint (DRUJ) is essential to painless pronation and supination of the wrist. A DRUJ that is plagued by osteoarthritis will show restriction and pain with these motions as well as a significantly decreased grip strength. Arthritis in this joint, therefore, severely limits the function of one's entire hand. Injury can occur secondary to intra-articular fractures involving the DRUJ or malunion of forearm fractures which result in altered biomechanics. The Colles' fractures in particular can create carpal instability and subsequent arthritis (Cooney, Dobyns et al. 1980).

The radius and ulna are connected by both a proximal and distal radioulnar joint which allow for forearm pronation and supination. Stability of the joints is conferred by a series of ligamentous supports. The DRUJ specifically is supported by the triangular fibrocartilage complex (TFCC). The TFCC is composed of the articular disc, the dorsal and volar radioulnar ligaments, the meniscus homologue, the ulnar collateral ligament, and the sheath of the extensor carpi ulnaris (Palmer and Werner 1981). The articular disc is largely an avascular structure. The main stabilizers of the DRUJ are dorsal and palmar radioulnar ligaments (af Ekenstam, Palmer et al. 1984). The blood supply is provided by the anterior interosseous artery, the ulnar artery, and the medullary interosseous arteries. Understandably, those structures with ample blood supply, like the TFCC, are able to heal readily while the avascular structures, like the articular disc, are less able to do so. The annular ligament supports the proximal radioulnar joint and the interosseous membrane serves as a connection between the diathasis of the radius and ulna.

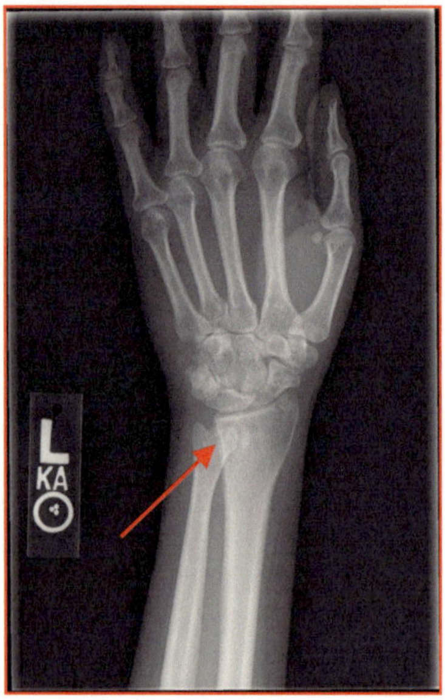

Fig. 4. PA Radiograph of Osteoarthritis of the DRUJ

The natural history of DRUJ arthritis begins with a pre-arthritic condition, usually a radial fracture malunion or instability of the DRUJ, which can develop into a degenerative arthritis over time. DRUJ instability is defined as the inability of the DRUJ to maintain its normal anatomic relationship under physiologic loading. Instability can be classified as either acute or chronic. In a case of acute DRUJ instability, the cause is often a fall on an outstretched hand resulting in an acute dislocation, fracture of the radial head or either bones of the forearm (Edwards and Jupiter 1988). This may result in injury to the joint surface, its supporting ligaments, or both (Bruckner, Alexander et al. 1996). In this scenario, ulna volar dislocation occurs secondary to hypersupination while ulna dorsal dislocations occur secondary to hyperpronation. Dislocations can be classified as either simple (reduced spontaneously or with minimal effort) or complex (irreducible or easily dislocated), the latter of which is usually due to a tear in the TFCC (Bruckner, Alexander et al. 1996). Chronic DRUJ instability can also be the result of a particular injury or it can result from a fracture of the radius and/or ulna, malunion or ligament injury. If left untreated, acute or chronic instability can progress into an arthritic degeneration of the DRUJ and can be associated with ulnar impaction (Kakar, Carlsen et al. 2010).
Most patients will present with painful wrist motions and restricted mobility. If there is a grossly apparent acute fracture, complete radiologic evaluation is warranted (Braun 1992). However, with an injury of a more insidious onset (like subluxation or dislocation) then swelling may be the only physical finding. A volar dislocation of the DRUJ will not allow pronation while a dorsal dislocation will not allow supination (Hauck, Skahen et al. 1996).

The differential diagnosis includes piso-triquetral and triquetro-hamate arthritis. The presence of a piano-key sign should be assessed in patients complaining of DRUJ pain (Scheker, 2009). The patient places their palms down on the examination table and pushes. The sign is present if the head of the ulna can be seen moving up and down. Such a finding is indicative of damage to the triangular fibrocartilage and is more common in rheumatoid arthritis as opposed to osteoarthritis. A second maneuver begins with the patient placing their elbows on the examination table with their forearms positioned perpendicular to the table's surface. Shear force is applied to the DRUJ. Any pain or displacement between the radius and ulna will indicate DRUJ instability. A third maneuver to be performed would be to apply shear force by pushing down on the patient's forearms while the patient pronates and supinates. Pain may be indicative of DRUJ incongruity and/or arthritis.

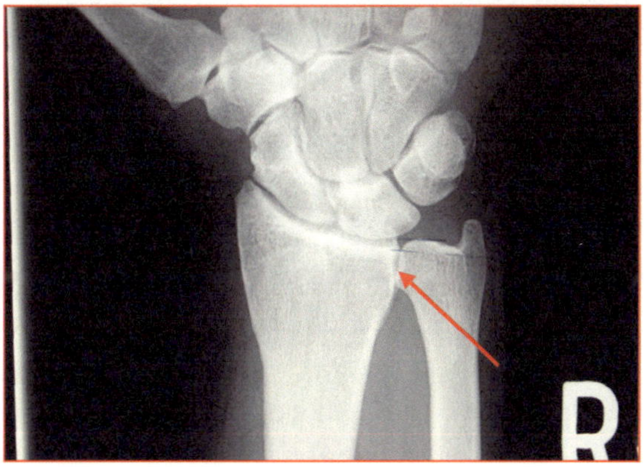

Fig. 5. PA Radiograph of Ulnar Impaction with an Ulnar -sided Lunate Cyst in Setting of DRUJ Arthritis

Radiographic assessment of the DRUJ is important in diagnosis and treatment planning. Typically, plain radiographs are used to survey the joint for any deterioration. A PA x-rays should be taken with the shoulder abducted to 90 degrees, with the elbow flexed at 90 degrees and the wrist in neutral position. The PA view is important in evaluating DRUJ congruency. Typically, the sigmoid notch slants towards the ulnar styloid with a 20 degree angle (af Ekenstam and Hagert 1985). However, evaluation of this angle is important because it has significant implications in ulnar shortening osteotomy as well as some of the other surgical treatment modalities. The lateral x-ray is also essential in determining DRUJ congruency. One can confirm that their scan is a true lateral view when the pisiform is in line with the distal third of the scaphoid. A true lateral view of the carpus will be required to evaluate for DRUJ subluxation. The pisotriquetral joint and hook of hamate can be evaluated from an oblique view with the wrist in a semipronanted and semisupinated position. All radiography should be compared with the contralateral side. CT scans can be useful when x-ray findings are unequivocal and may identify joint surface defects and subluxation. (Staron, Feldman et al. 1994). (Pirela-Cruz, Goll et al. 1991). An MRI is more useful if there is clinical suspicion of a triangular fibrocartilage tear or other cartilage defects (Golimbu, Firooznia et al. 1989). A bone scan is warranted in patients with a high clinical suspicion of DRUJ pathology who have a negative plain radiograph (Shewring, Savage et al. 1994). While this is a very sensitive technique, unfortunately, it lacks in specificity. Infection, bruising, and inflammation can be readily detected with scintigraphy.

Treatment will obviously vary greatly depending on the presentation of either a pre-arthritic or arthritic joint. In the case of a simple subluxation or dislocation, treatment consists of immobilization in a reduced position with an above-elbow cast for 6 weeks. A closed reduction, if needed, should be performed under regional anesthesia. If the DRUJ remains unstable after reduction, surgery may be necessary to repair the torn TFCC. Open reduction is only indicated when a closed reduction is impossible or unsatisfactory. Fractures are to be evaluated individually as there are many unique patterns with an ever changing array of plates and screws available for repair. With regard to more chronic DRUJ instability, soft tissue reconstruction is usually satisfactory. Ligamentous injuries can be repaired by either extra-articular or intra-acricular approaches. The extra-articular approach is technicnically an easier surgery and is achieved by a direct radioulnar tether (Fulkerson and Watson 1978) or an indirect radioulnar link (with the use of a ulnocarpal sling or tenodesis) (Breen and Jupiter 1989). An intra-articular repair, though a more demanding procedure, can reconstitute the original ligamentous anatomy and can yield very satisfactory results (Scheker, Belliappa et al. 1994).

In patients with evidence of joint misalignment without the presence of arthritis, treatment can be centered on realignment procedures through a variety of approaches, osteotomy or ulnar shortening osteotomy. An ulnar shortening procedure is another technique that can be used to re-establish stability in an otherwise lax TFCC (Nishiwaki, Nakamura et al. 2005). With this technique, more extensive surgery is avoided and early pre-arthritic conditions can be corrected before they progress further. However, it should be noted that Jupiter and his group determined that shortening by 6mm was enough to produce painful symptoms in the DRUJ (Jupiter and Masem 1988). This evidence of altered kinematics in a cadaver model corroborate this finding (Adams 1993). It was determined that a possible remedy for this cause of DRUJ arthritis is dependent on the status of the articular cartilage of the sigmoid notch and the ulnar seat (Hunt, Hastings et al. 1998). This study also concluded that for less advanced disease, where the DRUJ showed only mild arthosis, the joint stability could be regained with ulnar shortening osteotomy (Hunt, Hastings et al. 1998).

Once arthritis has developed in the DRUJ, a different armamentarium is available for use. The Darrach resection is the oldest of these procedures and it refers to the resection of the distal end of the ulna; effectively eliminating the pain-generating grinding that would otherwise occur at the DRUJ (Darrach 1992). However, this particular technique is not without post-operative complications which are related to the de-stabilizing nature of the procedure (snapping the ulnar stump and ulnar translocation with tendon rupture). When compared to the Sauve-Kapandji and hemiresection-interposition arthroplastic procedures, the Darrach procedure is less favorable and was only preferred in elderly patients with severe osteoarthritic changes (Minami, Iwasaki et al. 2005). The Sauve-Kapandji technique involves the fusion of the head of the ulna to the radius. In such a surgery, the TFCC will be preserved and the ulnar carpus will remain adequately supported. A recent study suggest that for moderate, but not more complex disease, the Sauve-Kapandji procedure showed good improvement in forearm rotation, grip strength, and pain reduction (Czermak, Wittemann et al. 2007).

While the aforementioned techniques are all useful in relieving pain by removing the grinding contact forces responsible for that pain, they also inherently result in some destabilization. This may be acceptable in a patient with a low-demand lifestyle but it can also be problematic in someone in need of a more durable solution. Recently, prosthetic replacements have been developed and have outcomes as varied as their designs. Advantages and disadvantages of each particular device is best managed by the operating surgeon. Arthrodesis of the wrist remains a viable final alternative and is usually reserved for malunited fractures of the carpal scapohoid and other complex pathology. However, the fact remains that a thorough H&P and early intervention with a skilled physician will allow a patient the greatest chance of a successful outcome by preventing more advanced disease.

4. Osteoarthritis of the carpometacarpal joint

Though the thumb carpometacarpal (CMC) joint is technically located in the hand, its close proximity to the carpal bone often implicates it as a pain generator when differentiating different causes of chronic wrist pain. Osteoarthritis(OA) of the thumb carpometacarpal (CMC) joint can cause debilitating pain and decreased strength and range of motion, making it difficult to do even the most common household tasks such as turning door-knobs or opening jars. CMC arthritis is the 2nd most common arthritic condition of the hand and in incidence, is the second only to arthritis of the distal interphalngeal joint (DIP).(Wilder, Barrett et al. 2006) Furthermore, it is the most common upper extremity arthritis requiring surgical intervention. It commonly affects women in their 5th to 6th decade of life. Epidemiologic studies have shown that post menopausal women are more likely to develop this condition; radiographic CMC arthritis is present in 25% of men and 40% of women over the age of 75. (Van Heest and Kallemeier 2008)

The thumb CMC is a biconcave-convex "saddle" joint that consists of the articular surfaces of the distal trapezium and the proximal thumb metacarpal. The unique nature of the joint allows for flexion, extension, abduction, adduction, and oppositional movements. Stability of the joint is provided primarily by the bony structures and several key ligaments: anterior oblique, posterior oblique, dorosoradial, palmar oblique, ulnar collateral, and intermetacarpal ligaments. The dorsoradial ligament, one of the thickest CMC ligaments, prevents excessive dorsoradial translation while the intermetacapal prevents radial translation. Excess pronation, abduction, and extension of the thumb are prevented by the palmar obique or "beak" ligament which has been regarded as the most important stabilizing structure.(Sung and Akelman 2009) Interestingly, this unique ability and movement of the thumb has been implicated in the pathophysiology of thumb CMC osteoarthritis.

However, the specific etiology of CMC arthritis has yet to be published. Currently, experts believe that the pathogenesis is multifactorial. Genetic and environmental factors, hypermobility of the joint, ligament laxity, anatomic variations, and extrinsic trauma have all been implicated. It has been suggested that genetic influences play a role in the development of CMC arthritis, but its exact pathway has yet to be determined.(MacGregor, Li et al. 2009) Increased joint laxity has been associated as studies have shown that radial subluxation of the base of the thumb CMC joint from the trapezium predisposes patients to developing osteoarthritis of the joint.(Hunter, Zhang et al. 2005) Women have higher incidence of thumb CMC osteoarthritis, possibly suggesting hormonal influences (prolactin, relaxin, and estrogen) as mechanisms for hypermobility and increased joint laxity. (Sung and Akelman 2009). In addition to this, cadaveric studies have shown that women also have a smaller, less congruous trapezium that along with hypermobility and joint laxity contribute to increased stress on the joint.(North and Rutledge 1983; Ateshian, Rosenwasser et al. 1992) It is this increased focal and loading stress on joint cartilage which is believed to be the instigating event. Furthermore, pinching and gripping generate large loads across the CMC joint and may explain why people who actively sew and knit develop arthritis at a higher rate. (Cooney and Chao 1977) Increased body mass index (BMI) has also been associated with higher rates of CMC arthritis as it is believed increased BMI generates a higher biomechanical load.(Haara, Heliovaara et al. 2004) Finally, prior extrinsic trauma such as a Bennett fracture can predispose an individual to developing OA of the CMC joint and contribute to increased joint laxity and altered biomechanics.(Sung and Akelman 2009) Overall, it is difficult to ascertain one specific cause or risk factor for developing osteoarthritis of the CMC joint; rather, it is important to view the pathophysiology as multifactorial as ongoing research continues to develop and clarify the picture.

Symptomatic patients typically present with diffuse pain around the thenar eminence and perhaps on the dorsum of the thumb base which is exacerbated by pinching and grasping activities. Including the previously mentioned examples, turning the key or holding onto a large jar are often activities that illicit pain. Early in the disease, stiffness and loss of motion are not the primary complaints. As the disease progresses, both symptoms can occur as osteophytes limit motion resulting in a subluxed joint that is adducted, dorsally fixed, and has limited palmar abduction. Chronic stiffness can lead to changes in the metacarpophalangeal (MCP) joint resulting in hyperextension to compensate for the proximal loss of motion and loss of the thumb index web space.(Sung and Akelman 2009) Advanced disease may have dorsoradial subluxation of the first metacarpal on the trapezium termed the "shoulder sign".

Physical examination demonstrates tenderness to palpation over the dorsal or dorsoradial aspect of the thumb. Erythema, edema, and calor may be present but is not a prerequisite for diagnosis. The "grind test" is performed by rotation the thumb metacarpal while applying axial compression. It is considered positive if there pain with or without crepitus. The test has a high specificity (80-93%) and moderate sensitivity (42-53%) making it useful in confirming the diagnosis of CMC osteoarthritis.(Merritt, Roddey et al. 2010)

Radiographic imaging is the most useful initial study to evaluate and stage CMC osteoarthritis. In the majority of cases posterioranterior, lateral, and oblique views are all that are necessary. A stress view of both thumb CMC joints taken together as the patient pushes their thumb tips together can help assess the degree of joint space loss, but is not required.(Eaton and Littler 1973) The contralateral hand should also be imaged for comparative purposes. There are two major classification systems used for staging. The Eaton staging system is the most widely used and is based on degenerative changes noted on the radiographs. Stage 1 has normal articular cartilage with possible mild narrowing of the joint space secondary to joint effusion or ligament laxity. Stage 2 disease has narrowing of the joint space associated with subchondral sclerotic changes and the possibility of ostephyte formation <2 mm. Mild to moderate subluxation of the thumb on the trapezium radially and dorsally may also be present. Stage 3 involves significant joint space narrowing with cystic and sclerotic changes with osteophytes larger than 2 mm. Stage 4 represents advanced degenerative changes of the CMC joint along with clear evidence scapho-trapezio-trapizoidal (STT) joint destruction. It has also been shown that pain and stiffness do not exactly correlate with radiographic findings.(Eaton and Glickel 1987) The Burton system uses clinical signs, symptoms, and radiographic evidence of disease and can also be used.

The differential diagnosis for pain around the base of the thumb also includes de Quervain tenosynovitis, flexor carpi radialis (FCR) tendonitis, radioscaphoid pathology, and carpal tunnel syndrome. Patients with de Quervain tenosynovitis will have tenderness at the tip of the radial styloid and 1st extensor compartment and may have a positive Finkelstein's test. FCR tendonitis would elicit pain with flexion of the wrist and tend to be more ulnar compared to CMC osteoarthritis. Fracture or arthritis of the scaphoid bone can present similarly and a detailed history and physical investigating for recent trauma is essential in differentiating the diagnosis. Finally, close to 40% of patients with CMC arthritis had concomitant carpal tunnel syndrome, making it important to diagnose to eliminate additional operations as both conditions can be repaired simultaneously.(Florack, Miller et al. 1992) Likewise, this condition is associated with concomitant arthritis of other carpal joints in the hand such as STT joint. Many times, corticosteroid intra-articular injections can help differentiate between different potential conditions based on subsequent pain relief.

Initial treatment should focus on behavior modification, NSAIDS, and rest. Also, all patients should undergo a trial of conservative management including occupational therapy, splinting, and steroid injections. Occupational therapy should focus on strengthening the surrounding muscles to support the joint while stretching to maximize range of motion. Splinting can reduce the focal and load stress on the joint. The effectiveness of corticosteroid injections is widely debated with several studies demonstrating conflicting conclusions.(Day, Gelberman et al. 2004; Meenagh, Patton et al. 2004; Khan, Waseem et al. 2009; Swindells, Logan et al. 2010) A combination of these two treatments has shown to be effective in stage I and stage II disease.(Swigart, Eaton et al. 1999) As the disease progresses and the joint undergoes further degenerative changes the results of this treatment modality becomes less predictable. A recent study in 2009 also demonstrated hylan injections as an alternative to corticosteroid with equal efficacy.(Heyworth, Lee et al. 2008)

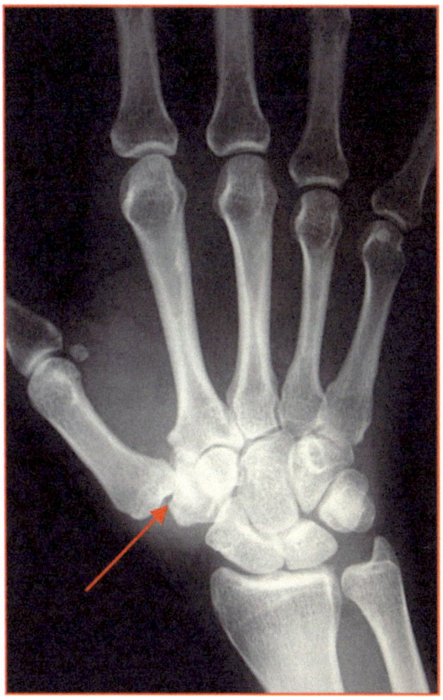

Fig. 6. PA Radiograph of Thumb CMC Arthritis

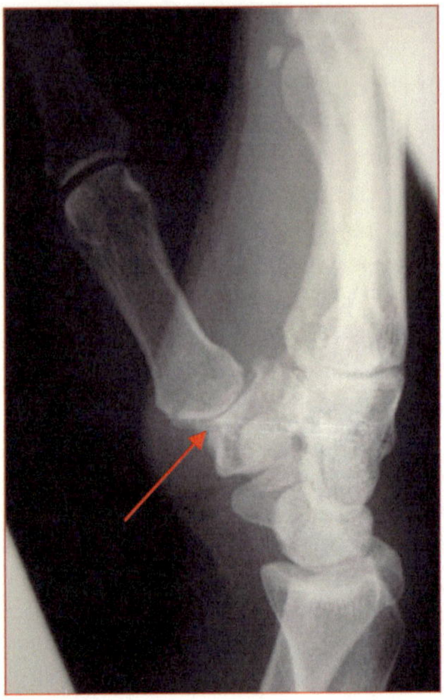

Fig. 7. Lateral Radiograph of Thumb CMC Arthritis

Surgical treatment should be considered when conservative measures have failed to relieve pain and improve day to day thumb function. Various options exist and it is therefore essential to engage the patient in an informed two-way discussion regarding the relative merits and drawbacks of each alternative. Patients with stage 1 or 2 disease have shown good outcomes with arthroscopy, metacarpal extension osteotomy, and volar ligament reconstruction. Arthroscopy is minimally invasive and allows for direct visualization of the articular surface and has been shown to be effective for the treatment of early osteoarthritis of the thumb CMC(Badia and Khanchandani 2007). Likewise, metacarpal extension osteotomy can correct the alignment of the thumb and transfer the load from the diseased palmar compartment to the normal dorsal compartment of the trapezium.(Pellegrini, Parentis et al. 1996) Eaton and Littler have well described a volar ligament reconstruction using part of the FCR tendon and have shown excellent results in 100% of patients with stage 1 and 82%-91% of patients with stage 2 disease.(Eaton, Lane et al. 1984; Freedman, Eaton et al. 2000).

For advanced disease, many surgical options exist: arthrodesis, implant arthroplasty, or resection arthroplasty with or without ligament reconstruction and tendon interposition. Arthrodesis of the thumb CMC joint provides pain relief and a strong and stable thumb for pinch and grasp activities. Disadvantages of the procedure include the risk of nonunion and altered biomechanics (Carroll and Hill 1973) Historically, surgeons have recommended this procedure to younger patients with high demanding jobs post traumatic injury; however, due to the recent success or arthroplasty this procedure may be falling out of favor. All the arthroplasty procedures involve either a full or partial trapeziectomy. Implant arthoplasty have used materials such as silicone, zircon, circonia, and titanium. All have their respective disadvantages from efficacy to side effects.(Sung and Akelman 2009) Total prosthetic joint arthroplasty is a promising field and further research need to assess reproducibility and long term risks and benefits.(Ulrich-Vinther,

Puggaard et al. 2008) Currently, the gold standard is resection arthroplasty with or without ligament reconstruction and tendon interposition. This procedure requires a complete trapeziectomy.(Tomaino 2006; Mathoulin, Moreel et al. 2008; Sammer and Amadio 2010) On the other hand, there are studies that show that ligament recreation provides no further benefit and that trapeziectomy alone is the best and safest operation. (Wajon, Ada et al. 2005; Field and Buchanan 2007) Further studies need to be conducted to clarify this promising therapeutic modality.

In addition to the thumb CMC joint, osteoarthritis of the second or third CMC joint can also cause significant wrist pain. Osteoarthritis of these joints is less common than thumb CMC arthritis. Typically, patients present with dorsal wrist pain and a bony prominence over the CMC joint that is often misdiagnosed as an isolated dorsal ganglion. Generally, repeated subacute trauma from extensive radial or ulnar deviation causes degenerative changes and carpal bossing of the CMC joint. Nonsurgical options consist of rest, NSAIDS, splitting, and intra-articular corticosteroid injections. Surgical options include boss excision and arthrodesis.

Thumb carpometocarpal osteoarthritis is one of the most common orthopaedic conditions a hand surgeon will face. The Eaton classification aids in stratifying the treatment regimen. Patients with early degenerative disease may benefit greatly from a regimen combining intra-articular corticosteroid injections and splinting. Several procedures exist for advanced disease and currently no one particular procedure has shown to be efficacious compared to another.(Wajon, Carr et al. 2009)

5. Osteoarthritis of the scaphotrapeziotrapezoid joint

Scaphotrapeziotrapezoid (STT) arthritis is the second most common degenerative disease of the wrist and often is linked with thumb CMC arthritis due to its close anatomical location. Isolated STT arthritis can also exist and it has been reported in 15% of wrist radiographs and 21% of cadaveric wrists.(Watson and Ballet 1984; Viegas, Patterson et al. 1993). Higher incidence rates have also been published and it is believed that the age of the cadavers may explain the differences in values. (Bhatia, Pisoh et al. 1996; Wollstein and Carlson 2009) Therefore, due to differences between radiographic findings and clinical symptoms, the exact incidence of isolated STT arthritis is unknown. There appears to be a gender bias as it commonly affects postmenopausal women after the age of 50.(Moritomo, Viegas et al. 2000; Kapoutsis, Dardas et al. 2011)

The scaphoid is the largest bone in the proximal carpal row and is an important link between the proximal and distal wrist. It articulates with the distal radius, the lunate, the capitate, the trapezium, and the trapezoid. The trapezium articulates with the scaphoid and first metacarpal via the CMC joint. The trapezoid articulates with the trapezium, scaphoid, capitate, and second metacarpal. Moritomo et al. described the ligaments and biomechanics of the STT joint.(Moritomo, Viegas et al. 2000). The capitate-trapezium ligament originates from the trapezium and inserts into the volar waist of the capitates and deepens the socket of the STT joint acting as a labrum for the distal pole of the scaphoid while reinforcing the volar aspect of the joint capsule as well. The scaphotrapezial and trapeziotrapezoid ligament are two other volar ligaments that stabilize the joint. Dorsally, the dorsolateral STT ligament stabilizes and links the joint to the rest of the midcarpus. The function of the joint is to allow transfer of load from the thumb and radial hand to the scaphoid, capitate, and other carpal bones.

The exact etiology of STT arthritis is unknown; however, there are numerous studies investigating the biomechanics and bony morphology as the underlying mechanism for degenerative change. Moritomo et al. demonstrated that underdevelopment of the capitate-trapezium ligament has been associated with increased prevalence of STT arthritis. The trapezium trapezoid (TT) inclination measures the degree of bone coverage by the facets of each bone over the distal pole of the scaphoid. Degenerative changes of the STT joint were associated with a higher TT inclincation suggesting that the trapezium and trapezoid are more palmar relative to the scaphoid in patients with STT arthritis.(Moritomo, Viegas et al. 2000) Interestingly, the morphology of other carpal bones, specifically the lunate, and its effects on wrist kinematics has also been associated with STT arthritis. Type I lunate morphology consist of lunates with a single distal articulation for the capitates, no articulation for the hamate, and a capitates to triquetrum (CT) distance of <2mm. Type II lunates had radial articulation for the capitates and a ulnar articulation for the hamate with a CT distance of ≥4mm. McLean et al. demonstrated that patients with type II lunate morphology had significantly higher incidences of STT arthritis compared to type I lunates and hypothesized that the difference in morphology make type II lunates have comparatively restricted range of motion creating an environment for degenerative change.(McLean, Turner et al. 2009) Carpal instability such as dorsal intercalated segment instability (DISI) has also been associated with increased prevalence of STT arthritis.(Tay, Moran et al. 2007) Finally, STT arthritis has been associated with prior trauma to the joint and surrounding structures.

The patient typically presents with diffuse pain around the base of the thumb and thenar eminence. Generally, isolated STT arthritic pain tends to be more midline (ulnar) compared to CMC arthritis and has been reported as a deep aching pain that may not be associated with thumb motion.(Cannon, Pincus et al. 2008) The pain can be exacerbated by radial extension and flexion of the wrist.

Physical examination generally demonstrates tenderness to palpation of the STT joint. Erythema, edema, and calor rarely are present unless there is significant disease of the thumb CMC joint as well. There is often difficulty differentiating the two clinically even with the use of the grind test.(Tomaino, Vogt et al. 1999) Due to the difficulty in accurate assessment from the history and physical exam, radiography is essential in making the proper diagnosis.

Bilateral PA, lateral, and oblique views should be routinely obtained. Due to the plane of the STT joint, the oblique view appears to be the best study to evaluate the STT joint. Degenerative changes such as narrowing of the joint space between any of the scaphoid, trapezium, and trapezoid or presence of osteophytes signifies STT arthritis. Stress views of the thumb described earlier may also be beneficial. There have been several views that have been developed to specifically target the STT joint but have been difficult to readily obtain in practice.(Wollstein, Wandzy et al. 2005) Comparison should be made to the contra-lateral wrist. There have been some thoughts of using CT or MRI scan for evaluation of the STT joint, but there are no published studies or guidelines regarding their utility. Currently, there is no universal staging system. However, one such system has been proposed that describes the progression of the disease based on radiographic findings. In this categorization, stage I disease has joint space narrowing as compared to other intercarpal joints in the same hand with or without periarticular sclerosis. Stage II disease has the defining characteristics of stage I disease along with the presence of cysts and/or osteophytes. Finally, stage III disease demonstrates complete collapse of the joint.(Wollstein and Carlson 2009)

As previously mentioned, the differential diagnosis must include thumb CMC arthritis. In a cadaveric study, 46 % of patients with STT arthritis had concomitant thumb CMC arthritis.(North and Rutledge 1983) Many hand surgeons term concomitant STT and thumb CMC arthritis as pantrapezial arthritis. As result of its shared prevalence and clinical presentation, it is important to combine clinical exam with radiographic findings for the definitive diagnosis. De Quervain tenosynovitis can present similarly, but the tenderness would be at the tip of the radial styloid and along the 1st extensor compartment with a positive Finkelstein's test. Direct trauma to the STT joint as the primary pain generator should be investigated with a thorough and detailed history. Arthroscopy of the STT joint can be performed as a diagnostic procedure and palmar portal has been described as safe and efficacious.(Bare, Graham et al. 2003)

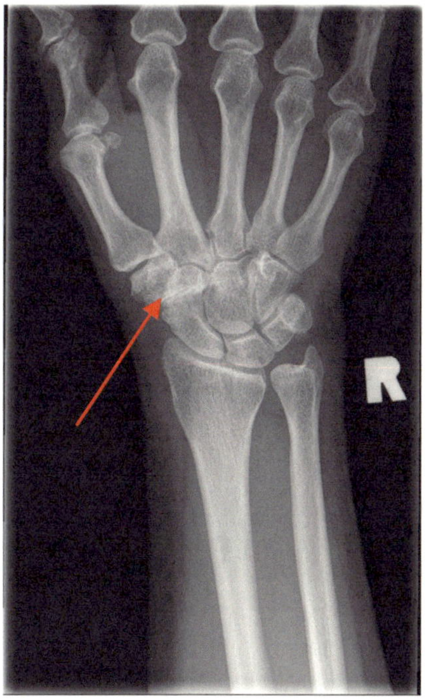

Fig. 8. PA Radiograph of STT Arthritis

Treatment of STT osteoarthritis should begin with nonoperative therapy. Behavior modification, NSAIDS, and rest are mainstay primary therapies. Splinting can especially be effective if there is concomitant thumb CMC arthritis. Intra-articular corticosteroids have been shown to be effective along with splinting for thumb CMC arthritis but there is paucity of data regarding its utility specifically for isolated STT arthritis.

Several operative techniques for management of STT arthritis exist including arthrodesis, resurfacing, and arthroplasty with or without implant. Historically, fusion of the STT joint has been the most common progression of treatment after failed conservative management. STT arthrodesis has been indicated for the treatment of isolated STT arthritis, scapholunate instability, and Kienbock disease. Nonunion complications are generally a concern with arthrodesis and Watson et al reported overall nonunion rate of 4% for STT arthrodesis and specifically 2% for patients whose primary indication was STT arthritis. They also report good functionality in terms of wrist mobility, grip, key, and tip pinch strength compared to the unaffected side.(Wollstein and Watson 2005) Several technical aspects of the procedure have been shown to be associated with optimal results. The surgeon must thoroughly denude the articular surfaces of cartilage. As the joint is decorticated, the original joint height must be maintained and packed with bone graft from iliac crest or distal radius. The fusing of the scaphoid should be at an angle of 55 to 60 degrees of palmar flexion relative to the long axis of the radius as seen in a lateral radiograph. A radial styloidectomy is necessary and the postoperative protocol consists of long arm cast for 3 weeks followed by a short arm thumb spica cast for an additional 3 weeks. In addition to nonunion other reported complications include reflex sympathetic dystrophy and radial styloid impingment.(Wolf 2008)

Resection arthroplasty refers to excision of 3 to 4 mm of the distal articulation of the scaphoid with or without interposition via the flexor carpi radialis (FCR) tendon. (Garcia-Elias, Lluch et al. 1999) This procedure is an alternative to STT arthrodesis and allows for pain control, improvement of symptoms, and requires less postoperative immobilization.(Weiss and Rodner 2007) The concern with this surgical procedure is the risk of creating carpal instability that can lead to arthritis of other joints in the hand and wrist. Arthroscopic techniques have also been described.(Bare, Graham et al. 2003)

Implant arthroplasty is another option for surgical treatment of the STT joint. Silicone implants have been used in the past and shown to be effective, especially for the treatment of the PIP joint. It is believed that silicone cannot withstand the same amount of compressive forces as bone and therefore prone to fragmentation and development of silicone synovitis.(Swindells, Logan et al. 2010) As a result, different implants such as pyrocarbon and degradable polyurethanurea spacers have been used. Pyrocarbon implants have elastic properties similar to cortical bone and therefore may allow for better transfer of stress load.(Cook, Klawitter et al. 1981) Preliminary studies have shown significant promise for the use of pyrocarbon implants for the treatment of STT arthritis; however, these studies have been limited for sample size and length of follow up.(Pequignot, D'Asnieres de Veigy et al. 2005; Low and Edmunds 2007). Studies for arthroplasty with a polyurethanurea spacer (Artelon) are undergoing and perhaps a promising avenue for future treatment.

STT arthritis is the second most common degenerative disease of the wrist and often coexists with thumb CMC arthritis. Patients present with deep pain along the base of the thumb and medial wrist that is exacerbated by flexion and extension. Radiographic imaging is essential in determining the diagnosis. Conservative management should being with activity modification, NSAIDS, are rest. Splinting and inrta-articular corticosteroid injections may also be of benefit to some patients. Surgical management includes arthrodesis, resection arthroplasty, and implant arthroplasty with or without interposition.

6. Osteoarthritis of the radiolunate and radioscaphoid joint

Arthritis at the radiolunate and radioscahpoid joints is a rare phenomenon; however, three common causes are avascular necrosis (including Kienbock and Preiser's disease), post traumatic, and inflammatory. Inflammatory arthritis of the radiolunate and radioscaphoid joint can occur; however, this discussion focuses on degenerative osteoarthritis of the wrist.

6.1 Kienbock disease

Kienbock disease, also known as avascular necrosis of the lunate, is another rare cause of osteoarthritis of the wrist. The classical disorder was first described in 1910 by the radiologist Robert Kienbock who, after a series of clinical and radiographic studies, defined a distinct symptomatology of volar wrist pain with isolated degeneration of the lunate that he termed lunatomalcia.(Kienbock 1910) Despite a century of research, the exact etiology and pathophysiology of this disease is unknown.

Currently, there are many factors implicated in the pathophysiology of Kienbock disease and it is likely a combination of these factors that lead to its progression. Primary causes are generally divided into mechanical and vascular factors. Mechanical factors may be due to the local anatomy of the lunate and wrist and uneven distribution of stress and loading forces. Vascular factors imply that a primary disruption in circulation leads to secondary bony pathology.

Historically, negative ulnar variance has been implicated as a mechanical cause of Kienbock disease. Negative ulnar variance refers to the presence of a shortened ulna compared to the radius in terms of distal articular surface. It is believed that a short ulna cannot share axial loads with the radius and therefore increases the amount of stress across the lunate.(Hulten 1928) However, there are studies that also report no association between negative ulnar variance and Kienbock disease. (Gelberman, Bauman et al. 1980; Chen and Shih 1990; D'Hoore, De Smet et al. 1994) A meta-analysis in 2001 demonstrated that many of these previous studies were under powered and had flawed study designs. They concluded that patients with negative ulnar variance were 3.1 times more likely to develop Kienbock disease; however there was no statistical significance. Other mechanical factors associated with the development of Kienbock disease include: the size and shape of the lunate, "radiolunate coverage index", and persistent trauma. Smaller sized lunates and type II shaped lunates are associated with the disease. Patients with a smaller contact area between the radius and lunate have a smaller "radiolunate coverage index" and a higher association with Kienbock disease. Finally, patients with repeated trauma or fracture to the joint may have a higher association to the disease, possibly due to compromise of the vasculature. (Tsuge and Nakamura 1993; Irisarri 2004; Lluch and Garcia-Elias 2011)

Vascular impairment can be either at the external vascular net that supplies the lunate or at the small vessels that penetrate the subchondral bone. Studies have shown that lunates typically have two nutrient supplying vessels. It has been postulated that patients with Kienbock disease have either 1 supplying vessel or a decreased amount of penetrating interosseous branches.(Lluch and Garcia-Elias 2011) The mechanism of injury to these vessels is not known. Lack of blood supply causes necrosis of the bone with subsequent remodeling by osteoclasts and osteoblasts. This remodeling can cause degenerative change and ultimately collapse of the lunate.(Lluch and Garcia-Elias 2011) Other potential causes associated with Kienbock disease include coagulation disorders such as sickle cell disease, long term steroid use, and venous congestion.(Nagasawa, Ishii et al. 1989; Glueck, Freiberg et al. 2008; Lluch and Garcia-Elias 2011)

Patient will typically present with dorsal wrist pain, decreased flexion-extension range of motion, and poor grip strength. Local swelling and tenderness of the lunate may be present, especially as the disease progresses. Radiographic imaging is necessary for the definitive diagnosis. MRI has shown to be more useful in diagnosis and the monitoring of treatment while plain radiographs are best used for staging.

Stage I disease demonstrates mild pain, normal radiographs, and early degenerative changes on MRI. Stage II disease presents with increased pain, edema, and radiographs show increased lunate density Stage III is divided into IIIA and IIIB. In stage IIIA radiographs show lunate collapse without scapholunate instability while stage IIIB disease shows lunate collapse with scapholuante instability. Stage IV is characteristic of pancarpal arthrosis.(Saunders and Lichtman 2011)

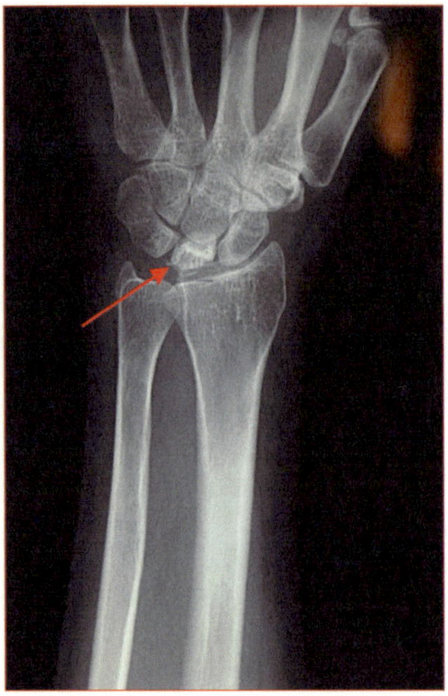

Fig. 9. PA Radiograph of Kienbock Disease

Current treatment recommendations are based on the classification system. Stage I disease is treated with rest, NSAIDS, and possible 3-6 month periods of immobilization. Stage II can be managed conservatively or surgically via radial and capitate osteotomies and lunate revascularization procedures. Radial and capitate osteotomies can change loading forces across the joint and lunate revascularization by transferring a vascularized pedicle with bone from the pisiform or distal radius has shown to be effective.(Shin and Bishop 2002) Stage IIIA is managed with oseotomies and revascularization procedures similar to surgical options for stage II disease. Stage IIIB disease requires procedures that result in increased stability of the joint and therefore scaphocapitate and STT fusion techniques are preferred. Stage IV disease requires salvage procedures such as total wrist arthrodesis, arthroplasty, or proximal row carpectomy.(Saunders and Lichtman 2011) Patients with negative ulnar variance can undergo radial shortening and ulnar lengthening procedures. Currently, no single surgical procedure has shown to be superior.(Delaere, Dury et al. 1998)

Early diagnosis of Kienbock disease may help prevent progression as we continue to investigate the utility of bisphosphonates, stem cells, and prophylactic surgical intervention. The use of gadolinium infused MRI and "lunate stress tests" are techniques that may allow diagnosis at "stage 0" similar to that of osteonecrosis of the femoral head.(Saunders and

Lichtman 2011) Kienbock disease remains a partial enigma to physicians despite being known for over a century. However, as researchers continue to investigate its etiology and develop treatment modalities, the future looks promising.

6.2 Preiser's disease

Similar to Kienbock disease, avascular necrosis of the scaphoid is termed Preiser's disease. The exact epidemiology of Preiser's disease is unknown, but it is considered even rarer than Kienbock disease. Furthermore, the exact etiology is unknown; however, physicians often imply a shared pathophysiology similar to Kienbock disease. Patients generally present with dorsoradial wrist pain, limited range of motion, and possible joint swelling and erythema. Patients may have tenderness to palpation along the anatomic "snuff" box. Diagnosis is confirmed with radiographs or MRI. Currently, a classification does not exist, perhaps due to the low incidence of the disease. Treatment options are similar to Kienbock disease and begins with conservative therapy of immobilization, NSAIDS, splinting, and intra articular injections. Surgical options include revascularization procedures, proximal row carpectomy, and four corner's fusion with scaphoid resection(Amillo-Garayoa, Romero-Munoz et al. 2011).

6.3 Post distal radius fracture

Fracture of the distal radius is one of the most common fractures in orthopaedics and can often cause joint instability and subsequent osteoarthritis. There are various surgical and nonsurgical options for the treatment of a distal radius fracture. Complications may arise from the traumatic injury and/or method of treatment, leading to osteoarthritis of the radiolunate and radioscaphoid joint.

Osteoarthritis generally develops due to incongruity between joint surfaces. Furthermore, there is a potential for abnormal loading forces across a misaligned and unstable joint causing joint step off. Over time, this wear and tear can cause degenerative changes and osteophyte formation. Post traumatic chondromalacia has also been implicated as a potential cause of osteoarthritis status post distal radius fracture due to compression of the articular cartilage.

Patients typical with pain and tenderness near the radioscaphoid and radioulnar joint. Previous history of distal radial fracture, clinical presentation, and radiographs help confirm the diagnosis. Pathology of the radiolunate joint differentiates this disorder from a SLAC/SNAC wrist where the radiolunate joint is preserved. Treatment options include conservative management with NSAIDs, splinting, physical therapy, and intra articular injections. Surgical options include denervation, total wrist fusion, wrist arthroplasty and variations of intercarpal arthrodesis. (Nagy 2005; Handoll, Huntley et al. 2008)

7. Osteoarthritis of the pisotriquetral joint

Pisotriquetral (PT) arthritis is a relatively uncommon diagnosis. It is thought to be the result of PT joint instability which can occur after injury to the pisiform ligament complex (PLC) which serves to stabilize the PT joint. Injury to these PT joint stabilizers are what could predispose a patient to degenerative joint disease (Rayan, Jameson et al. 2005). Such a ligament injury is either found in the acute setting after a fall onto an outstretched hand, or is associated with a more chronic repetitive motion-type injury.

The pisiform is a sesamoid bone, nearly spherical in shape, which can be found within the fibers of the flexor carpi ulnaris tendon and articulates with the triquetrum. The pisiform forms the medial wall to Guyon's canal and is itself bordered medially by the dorsal retinaculum. The pisiform ligament complex is composed of those ligaments that stabilize the pisiform, namely the pisometacarpal, pisohamate, radial pisotriquetral, ulnar pisotriquetral and transverse carpal ligaments (Rayan, Jameson et al. 2005). Its blood supply is obtained via the proximal and distal poles which contain branches from the ulnar artery. The ulnar nerve lies just radially to the pisiform in most instances. The PT joint is ensheathed by a joint capsule that sometimes communicates with the proximal wrist joint (Viegas, Patterson et al. 1993).

The pathogenesis of PT joint pain can originate from several sources. In a study by Paley et al, it was noted that out of 216 cases of PT pain, primary osteoarthritis only contributed to a minority of the findings (2.3%) while secondary osteoarthritis and flexor carpi ulnaris enthesopathy contributed 48.4% and 44.6% respectively (other arthridities comprised the remaining 4.7%) (Paley, McMurtry et al. 1987). Fractures, tumors, ganglions and congenital malformations have also been noted to contribute to ulnar volar pain (Kernohan, Beacon et al. 1985) (Chen, Barnwell et al. 2011) (El-Morshidy, Rabia et al. 2000). Loose bodies as well as PT arthrosis secondary to a triquetral fracture malunion have also been documented (Steinmann and Linscheid 1997) (Aiki, Wada et al. 2006). Finally, a recent case series has also made the suggestion that PT arthritis can develop after an intercarpal arthodesis (Gaston, Lourie et al. 2007). These clinical entities should be considered in a patient's work-up because they each require a distinct treatment plan to alleviate pain.

It has been hypothesized that injury to the PLC results in PT joint instability and a subsequent arthritis (Rayan, Jameson et al. 2005). Trauma is a likely cause of injury and there are multiple studies that describe a carpal injury that specifically resulted in the dislocation of the pisiform (Goriainov, Bayne et al. 2010) (Matsumoto, Tsunoda et al. 2005). Direct force to the volar hand is the most likely culprit resulting in ligament injury and pisiform subluxation. The insult can be an acute fall on an outstretched hand or it can be the result of a chronic occupational exposure or racket-sport activity. Regardless of the cause, instability begets incongruity and abnormal wearing of the PT joint takes place and causes arthritis.

Presentation of a patient with PT joint pathology typically takes the form of either a chondromalacia, osteoarthritis or flexor carpi ulnaris tendinopathy. Patients will present with a palmar ulnar wrist pain. Exam findings of tenderness in the soft tissues distal and radial to the pisiform as well an ulnar volar pain that is provoked by passive wrist extension are all consistent with a diagnosis of PT instability. The pisiform tracking test is a useful to elicit PT instability: with the wrist in a fully flexed position, the examiner applies pressure to the pisiform in both a radial and ulnar direction (Hoepfner 2009). Crepitance and pain during this maneuver indicate PT pathology. Also, flexor carpi ulnaris tendinopathy (indicated by tenderness to palpation along the FCU tendon) may or may not coexist with PT dysfunction. In fact, there have been documented cases of FCU rupture in the setting of PT osteoarthritis (Corten, van den Broecke et al. 2004). It is thought that the PT arthritis resulted in impingement and attenuation of the FCU, causing its rupture.

Radiographic analysis can be useful to supplement the physical exam findings. Several semilateral wrist views including (1) full wrist extension and forearm supination of 30 degrees, (2) neutral wrist position with 30 degrees of forearm supination, (3) active and (4) passive full wrist flexion, and (5) a 45 degree of forearm supination with thumb fully abducted will all be needed to isolate this joint (Jameson, Rayan et al. 2002). Dynamic fluoroscopy can also be a useful tool to isolate the PT joint radiographically and determine its "normal" position. A diagnosis of PT pathology may be confirmed with PT joint injection. Other diagnoses to consider should include triangular fibrocartilage complex tears, ulnar impingement, lunotriquetral dysfunction, distal radioulnar joint subluxation, fracture/nonunion of the hook of hamate and ulnar artery thrombosis.

Like many of the arthritic joint conditions, PT pathology can be treated medically with wrist splints that maintain a neutral position, NSAIDS, and intra-articular steroid injections. Only when a patient's pain is refractory to these therapies, should surgery be considered. Although PT instability is what leads to the joint degeneration, clinically, we do not attempt to stabilize the pisiform by repairing the ligaments of the PLC. Instead, excision of the pisiform has been used to treat this condition for many years (Carroll and Coyle 1985) (Gomez, Renart et al. 2005) and has consistently provided pain relief without any functional limitations. There have been case reports, however, that promote the use of PT arthodesis in patients who have more high demand wrists (Abrams and Tontz 2006) (Singer, Eberl et al. 2011). Although this does not represent the current trend in treating PT pathology, with further study, it could serve as a promising alternative to pisiform excision.

In short, PT arthritis may not be a very common cause of ulnar-sided wrist pain, but it can be a very debilitating condition when present. It likely results from an instability due to an imbalance in the complex ligamentous attachments that keep the pisiform suspended in its proper orientation. When evaluating a patient for PT arthritis, the astute physician will keep a high clinical suspicion for the array of conditions that could mimic this type of wrist pain. Pisiform excision remains a very successful surgery for those patients who fail splinting, anti-inflammatories, and injection treatments.

8. Summary

Osteoarthritis of the wrist and hand can be a painful and debilitating disease. This chapter focused on the various causes, clinical presentations, and treatment options of wrist osteoarthritis. Many times evaluation of a patient with wrist pain reveals an extensive differential diagnosis. While obtaining the history, special attention should be focused on the patient's age, hand dominance, location and quality of the pain, aggravating and relieving factors, prior trauma history, occupation, hobbies, and limb function. Physical exam and palpation of the carpus and hand is essential to identify and localize the pain source. Special maneuvers such as the grind and shift test can help navigate the differential diagnosis and identify the pathologic joint. Ultimately, radiographic imaging can be used for definitive diagnosis and staging the progression of the disease.

SLAC and SNAC wrists are common degenerative patterns seen in osteoarthritis of the wrist and typically present with dorsal wrist swelling and periscaphoid tenderness. Pain and decreased range of motion with pronation and supination is typically indicative of arthritis of the DRUJ joint. Patients with arthritis of the thumb CMC and STT joint present with pain over the thenar eminence that is exacerbated by pinching and grasping activities. Kienbock disease can also present with dorsal wrist pain similar to SLAC wrist; however, the swelling and tenderness is along the lunate. In our discussion of wrist arthritis, degenerative change of the PT joint is the final cause of wrist pain and patients typically present with palmar ulnar pain.

Conservative management should be tried on all patients with wrist pain, especially if the disease is identified early in its progression. Rest, NSAIDS, behavior modification, occupational therapy, splinting, and intra-articular corticosteroid injections are all options that have shown different degrees of efficacy. Furthermore, intra-articular injections can be used as a final tool in differentiating the diagnosis.

Many different surgical options exist for the treatment of advanced degenerative disease. The common goal of surgical treatment is to remove the pain source when possible and stabilize the joint and its surrounding structures. Osteotomies, revascularization techniques, arthroscopy, resection arthroplasty, implant arthroplasty, and arthrodesis are some of the more common procedures used to treat the various arthropathies of the wrist. Physicians and patients must have an interactive discussion regarding the individual merits and drawbacks of each alternative to determine which procedures maximize recovery potential.

Surgeons continue to refine and develop new techniques as arthroscopy and total joint arthroplasty of the small joints in the hand and wrist become more common. As long term data regarding the efficacy of each procedure becomes more available, the "best" procedure for each disease may be determined. Research in the 21st century is currently focused on novel treatment methods including gene therapy, cartilage regeneration, and identification of specific etiologic factors that cause osteoarthritis of the wrist. With time, this may allow the physician to prevent the development and progression of the disease altogether.

9. References

Abrams, R. and W. Tontz (2006). "Pisotriquetral arthrodesis as an alternative to excision for pisotriquetral instability in high-demand patients: a case report in a gymnast." The Journal of hand surgery 31(4): 611-614.

Adams, B. D. (1993). "Effects of radial deformity on distal radioulnar joint mechanics." The Journal of hand surgery 18(3): 492-498.

af Ekenstam, F. and C. G. Hagert (1985). "Anatomical studies on the geometry and stability of the distal radio ulnar joint." Scandinavian journal of plastic and reconstructive surgery 19(1): 17-25.

af Ekenstam, F. W., A. K. Palmer, et al. (1984). "The load on the radius and ulna in different positions of the wrist and forearm. A cadaver study." Acta orthopaedica Scandinavica 55(3): 363-365.

Aiki, H., T. Wada, et al. (2006). "Pisotriquetral arthrosis after triquetral malunion: a case report." The Journal of hand surgery 31(7): 1157-1159.

Amillo-Garayoa, S., L. M. Romero-Munoz, et al. (2011). "Bilateral Preiser's disease: a case report and review of the literature." Musculoskeletal surgery.

Ashmead, D. t., H. K. Watson, et al. (1994). "Scapholunate advanced collapse wrist salvage." The Journal of hand surgery 19(5): 741-750.

Ateshian, G. A., M. P. Rosenwasser, et al. (1992). "Curvature characteristics and congruence of the thumb carpometacarpal joint: differences between female and male joints." Journal of biomechanics 25(6): 591-607.

Badia, A. and P. Khanchandani (2007). "Treatment of early basal joint arthritis using a combined arthroscopic debridement and metacarpal osteotomy." Techniques in hand & upper extremity surgery 11(2): 168-173.

Bare, J., A. J. Graham, et al. (2003). "Scaphotrapezial joint arthroscopy: a palmar portal." The Journal of hand surgery 28(4): 605-609.

Bhatia, A., T. Pisoh, et al. (1996). "Incidence and distribution of scaphotrapezotrapezoidal arthritis in 73 fresh cadaveric wrists." Annales de chirurgie de la main et du membre superieur : organe officiel des societes de chirurgie de la main = Annals of hand and upper limb surgery 15(4): 220-225.

Bisneto, E. N., M. C. Freitas, et al. (2011). "Comparison between proximal row carpectomy and four-corner fusion for treating osteoarthrosis following carpal trauma: a prospective randomized study." Clinics 66(1): 51-55.

Braun, R. M. (1992). "The distal joint of the radius and ulna. Diagnostic studies and treatment rationale." Clinical orthopaedics and related research(275): 74-78.

Breen, T. F. and J. B. Jupiter (1989). "Extensor carpi ulnaris and flexor carpi ulnaris tenodesis of the unstable distal ulna." The Journal of hand surgery 14(4): 612-617.

Bruckner, J. D., A. H. Alexander, et al. (1996). "Acute dislocations of the distal radioulnar joint." Instructional course lectures 45: 27-36.

Cannon, G. W., S. H. Pincus, et al. (2008). "Double-blind trial of recombinant gamma-interferon versus placebo in the treatment of rheumatoid arthritis. 1989." Arthritis and Rheumatism 58(2 Suppl): S79-88.

Carroll, R. E. and M. P. Coyle, Jr. (1985). "Dysfunction of the pisotriquetral joint: treatment by excision of the pisiform." The Journal of hand surgery 10(5): 703-707.

Carroll, R. E. and N. A. Hill (1973). "Arthrodesis of the carpo-metacarpal joint of the thumb." The Journal of bone and joint surgery. British volume 55(2): 292-294.

Chen, C., V. P. Chandnani, et al. (1990). "Scapholunate advanced collapse: a common wrist abnormality in calcium pyrophosphate dihydrate crystal deposition disease." Radiology 177(2): 459-461.

Chen, W. A., J. C. Barnwell, et al. (2011). "An ulnar intraneural ganglion arising from the pisotriquetral joint: case report." The Journal of hand surgery 36(1): 65-67.

Chen, W. S. and C. H. Shih (1990). "Ulnar variance and Kienbock's disease. An investigation in Taiwan." Clinical orthopaedics and related research(255): 124-127.

Cohen, M. S. and S. H. Kozin (2001). "Degenerative arthritis of the wrist: proximal row carpectomy versus scaphoid excision and four-corner arthrodesis." The Journal of hand surgery 26(1): 94-104.

Cook, S. D., J. J. Klawitter, et al. (1981). "The influence of implant elastic modulus on the stress distribution around LTI carbon and aluminum oxide dental implants." Journal of biomedical materials research 15(6): 879-887.

Cooney, W. P., 3rd and E. Y. Chao (1977). "Biomechanical analysis of static forces in the thumb during hand function." The Journal of bone and joint surgery. American volume 59(1): 27-36.

Cooney, W. P., 3rd, J. H. Dobyns, et al. (1980). "Complications of Colles' fractures." The Journal of bone and joint surgery. American volume 62(4): 613-619.

Corten, E. M., D. G. van den Broecke, et al. (2004). "Pisotriquetral instability causing an unusual flexor tendon rupture." The Journal of hand surgery 29(2): 236-239.

Czermak, C., M. Wittemann, et al. (2007). "[Functional results after the Kapandji-Sauve operation for salvage of the distal radioulnar joint]." Handchirurgie, Mikrochirurgie, plastische Chirurgie : Organ der Deutschsprachigen

Arbeitsgemeinschaft fur Handchirurgie : Organ der Deutschsprachigen Arbeitsgemeinschaft fur Mikrochirurgie der Peripheren Nerven und Gefasse : Organ der Vereinigung der Deutschen Plastischen Chirurgen 39(6): 403-408.

D'Hoore, K., L. De Smet, et al. (1994). "Negative ulnar variance is not a risk factor for Kienbock's disease." The Journal of hand surgery 19(2): 229-231.

Dacho, A., J. Grundel, et al. (2006). "Long-term results of midcarpal arthrodesis in the treatment of scaphoid nonunion advanced collapse (SNAC-Wrist) and scapholunate advanced collapse (SLAC-Wrist)." Annals of plastic surgery 56(2): 139-144.

Dacho, A. K., S. Baumeister, et al. (2008). "Comparison of proximal row carpectomy and midcarpal arthrodesis for the treatment of scaphoid nonunion advanced collapse (SNAC-wrist) and scapholunate advanced collapse (SLAC-wrist) in stage II." Journal of plastic, reconstructive & aesthetic surgery : JPRAS 61(10): 1210-1218.

Darrach, W. (1992). "Partial excision of lower shaft of ulna for deformity following Colles's fracture. 1913." Clinical orthopaedics and related research(275): 3-4.

Day, C. S., R. Gelberman, et al. (2004). "Basal joint osteoarthritis of the thumb: a prospective trial of steroid injection and splinting." The Journal of hand surgery 29(2): 247-251.

Delaere, O., M. Dury, et al. (1998). "Conservative versus operative treatment for Kienbock's disease. A retrospective study." Journal of hand surgery 23(1): 33-36.

Dias, J. J., R. A. Rajan, et al. (2008). "Which questionnaire is best? The reliability, validity and ease of use of the Patient Evaluation Measure, the Disabilities of the Arm, Shoulder and Hand and the Michigan Hand Outcome Measure." The Journal of hand surgery, European volume 33(1): 9-17.

Eaton, R. G. and S. Z. Glickel (1987). "Trapeziometacarpal osteoarthritis. Staging as a rationale for treatment." Hand clinics 3(4): 455-471.

Eaton, R. G., L. B. Lane, et al. (1984). "Ligament reconstruction for the painful thumb carpometacarpal joint: a long-term assessment." The Journal of hand surgery 9(5): 692-699.

Eaton, R. G. and J. W. Littler (1973). "Ligament reconstruction for the painful thumb carpometacarpal joint." The Journal of bone and joint surgery. American volume 55(8): 1655-1666.

Edwards, G. S., Jr. and J. B. Jupiter (1988). "Radial head fractures with acute distal radioulnar dislocation. Essex-Lopresti revisited." Clinical orthopaedics and related research(234): 61-69.

El-Morshidy, A. F., F. Rabia, et al. (2000). "Bilateral asymptomatic pisiform and hamate coalition--a case report." Hand surgery : an international journal devoted to hand and upper limb surgery and related research : journal of the Asia-Pacific Federation of Societies for Surgery of the Hand 5(1): 57-60.

Fassler, P. R., P. J. Stern, et al. (1993). "Asymptomatic SLAC wrist: does it exist?" The Journal of hand surgery 18(4): 682-686.

Field, J. and D. Buchanan (2007). "To suspend or not to suspend: a randomised single blind trial of simple trapeziectomy versus trapeziectomy and flexor carpi radialis suspension." The Journal of hand surgery, European volume 32(4): 462-466.

Florack, T. M., R. J. Miller, et al. (1992). "The prevalence of carpal tunnel syndrome in patients with basal joint arthritis of the thumb." The Journal of hand surgery 17(4): 624-630.

Freedman, D. M., R. G. Eaton, et al. (2000). "Long-term results of volar ligament reconstruction for symptomatic basal joint laxity." The Journal of hand surgery 25(2): 297-304.

Friedman, S. L. and A. K. Palmer (1991). "The ulnar impaction syndrome." Hand clinics 7(2): 295-310.

Fulkerson, J. P. and H. K. Watson (1978). "Congenital anterior subluxation of the distal ulna. A case report." Clinical orthopaedics and related research(131): 179-182.

Garcia-Elias, M., A. L. Lluch, et al. (1999). "Resection of the distal scaphoid for scaphotrapeziotrapezoid osteoarthritis." Journal of hand surgery 24(4): 448-452.

Gaston, R. G., G. M. Lourie, et al. (2007). "Pisotriquetral dysfunction following limited and total wrist arthrodesis." The Journal of hand surgery 32(9): 1348-1355.

Gelberman, R. H., T. D. Bauman, et al. (1980). "The vascularity of the lunate bone and Kienbock's disease." The Journal of hand surgery 5(3): 272-278.

Glueck, C. J., R. A. Freiberg, et al. (2008). "Heritable thrombophilia-hypofibrinolysis and osteonecrosis of the femoral head." Clinical orthopaedics and related research 466(5): 1034-1040.

Golimbu, C. N., H. Firooznia, et al. (1989). "Tears of the triangular fibrocartilage of the wrist: MR imaging." Radiology 173(3): 731-733.

Gomez, C. L., I. P. Renart, et al. (2005). "Dysfunction of the pisotriquetral joint: degenerative arthritis treated by excision of the pisiform." Orthopedics 28(4): 405-408.

Goriainov, V., G. Bayne, et al. (2010). "Traumatic dislocation of the pisiform: a case report." Journal of orthopaedic surgery 18(3): 389-390.

Haara, M. M., M. Heliovaara, et al. (2004). "Osteoarthritis in the carpometacarpal joint of the thumb. Prevalence and associations with disability and mortality." The Journal of bone and joint surgery. American volume 86-A(7): 1452-1457.

Handoll, H. H., J. S. Huntley, et al. (2008). "Different methods of external fixation for treating distal radial fractures in adults." Cochrane Database Syst Rev(1): CD006522.

Hauck, R. M., J. Skahen, 3rd, et al. (1996). "Classification and treatment of ulnar styloid nonunion." The Journal of hand surgery 21(3): 418-422.

Heyworth, B. E., J. H. Lee, et al. (2008). "Hylan versus corticosteroid versus placebo for treatment of basal joint arthritis: a prospective, randomized, double-blinded clinical trial." The Journal of hand surgery 33(1): 40-48.

Hildreth, D. H., W. C. Breidenbach, et al. (1989). "Detection of submaximal effort by use of the rapid exchange grip." The Journal of hand surgery 14(4): 742-745.

Hulten, O. (1928). "Concerning anatomical variations of the carpal bones." Acta Radiologica 9: 155-168.

Hunt, T. R., H. Hastings, 2nd, et al. (1998). "A systematic approach to handling the distal radio-ulnar joint in cases of malunited distal radius fractures." Hand clinics 14(2): 239-249.

Hunter, D. J., Y. Zhang, et al. (2005). "Trapeziometacarpal subluxation predisposes to incident trapeziometacarpal osteoarthritis (OA): the Framingham Study."

Osteoarthritis and cartilage / OARS, Osteoarthritis Research Society 13(11): 953-957.
Irisarri, C. (2004). "Aetiology of Kienbock's disease." Journal of hand surgery 29(3): 281-287.
Jameson, B. H., G. M. Rayan, et al. (2002). "Radiographic analysis of pisotriquetral joint and pisiform motion." The Journal of hand surgery 27(5): 863-869.
Jupiter, J. B. and M. Masem (1988). "Reconstruction of post-traumatic deformity of the distal radius and ulna." Hand clinics 4(3): 377-390.
Kakar, S., B. T. Carlsen, et al. (2010). "The management of chronic distal radioulnar instability." Hand clinics 26(4): 517-528.
Kapoutsis, D. V., A. Dardas, et al. (2011). "Carpometacarpal and scaphotrapeziotrapezoid arthritis: arthroscopy, arthroplasty, and arthrodesis." The Journal of hand surgery 36(2): 354-366.
Kernohan, J., J. P. Beacon, et al. (1985). "Osteoid osteoma of the pisiform." Journal of hand surgery 10(3): 411-414.
Khan, M., M. Waseem, et al. (2009). "Quantitative Assessment of Improvement with Single Corticosteroid Injection in Thumb CMC Joint Osteoarthritis?" The open orthopaedics journal 3: 48-51.
Kienbock, R. (1910). "Concerning traumatic malacia of the lunate and its consequences: joint degeneration and compression." Fortsch Geb Roentgen 16: 77-103.
Lichtman, D. M., J. R. Schneider, et al. (1981). "Ulnar midcarpal instability-clinical and laboratory analysis." The Journal of hand surgery 6(5): 515-523.
Liu, M., H. Zhou, et al. (2009). "Clinical evaluation of proximal row carpectomy revealed by follow-up for 10-29 years." International orthopaedics 33(5): 1315-1321.
Lluch, A. and M. Garcia-Elias (2011). "Etiology of Kienbock disease." Techniques in hand & upper extremity surgery 15(1): 33-37.
Low, A. K. and I. A. Edmunds (2007). "Isolated scaphotrapeziotrapezoid osteoarthritis: preliminary results of treatment using a pyrocarbon implant." Hand surgery : an international journal devoted to hand and upper limb surgery and related research : journal of the Asia-Pacific Federation of Societies for Surgery of the Hand 12(2): 73-77.
MacGregor, A. J., Q. Li, et al. (2009). "The genetic influence on radiographic osteoarthritis is site specific at the hand, hip and knee." Rheumatology 48(3): 277-280.
Malerich, M. M., J. Clifford, et al. (1999). "Distal scaphoid resection arthroplasty for the treatment of degenerative arthritis secondary to scaphoid nonunion." The Journal of hand surgery 24(6): 1196-1205.
Mathoulin, C., P. Moreel, et al. (2008). "Abductor pollicis longus "hammock" ligamentoplasty for treatment of first carpometacarpal arthritis." The Journal of hand surgery, European volume 33(3): 292-297.
Matsumoto, T., M. Tsunoda, et al. (2005). "Traumatic dislocation of the hamate and pisiform: a case report and review of the literature." Journal of orthopaedic trauma 19(4): 282-285.
McLean, J. M., P. C. Turner, et al. (2009). "An association between lunate morphology and scaphoid-trapezium-trapezoid arthritis." The Journal of hand surgery, European volume 34(6): 778-782.

Meenagh, G. K., J. Patton, et al. (2004). "A randomised controlled trial of intra-articular corticosteroid injection of the carpometacarpal joint of the thumb in osteoarthritis." Annals of the rheumatic diseases 63(10): 1260-1263.

Merritt, M. M., T. S. Roddey, et al. (2010). "Diagnostic value of clinical grind test for carpometacarpal osteoarthritis of the thumb." Journal of hand therapy : official journal of the American Society of Hand Therapists 23(3): 261-267; quiz 268.

Minami, A., N. Iwasaki, et al. (2005). "Treatments of osteoarthritis of the distal radioulnar joint: long-term results of three procedures." Hand surgery : an international journal devoted to hand and upper limb surgery and related research : journal of the Asia-Pacific Federation of Societies for Surgery of the Hand 10(2-3): 243-248.

Moritomo, H., S. F. Viegas, et al. (2000). "The scaphotrapezio-trapezoidal joint. Part 2: A kinematic study." The Journal of hand surgery 25(5): 911-920.

Moritomo, H., S. F. Viegas, et al. (2000). "The scaphotrapezio-trapezoidal joint. Part 1: An anatomic and radiographic study." The Journal of hand surgery 25(5): 899-910.

Mulford, J. S., L. J. Ceulemans, et al. (2009). "Proximal row carpectomy vs four corner fusion for scapholunate (Slac) or scaphoid nonunion advanced collapse (Snac) wrists: a systematic review of outcomes." The Journal of hand surgery, European volume 34(2): 256-263.

Mutimer, J., J. Green, et al. (2008). "Comparison of MRI and wrist arthroscopy for assessment of wrist cartilage." The Journal of hand surgery, European volume 33(3): 380-382.

Nagasawa, K., Y. Ishii, et al. (1989). "Avascular necrosis of bone in systemic lupus erythematosus: possible role of haemostatic abnormalities." Annals of the rheumatic diseases 48(8): 672-676.

Nagy, L. (2005). "Salvage of post-traumatic arthritis following distal radius fracture." Hand Clin 21(3): 489-498.

Nagy, L. and U. Buchler (1997). "Long-term results of radioscapholunate fusion following fractures of the distal radius." Journal of hand surgery 22(6): 705-710.

Nishiwaki, M., T. Nakamura, et al. (2005). "Ulnar shortening effect on distal radioulnar joint stability: a biomechanical study." The Journal of hand surgery 30(4): 719-726.

North, E. R. and W. M. Rutledge (1983). "The trapezium-thumb metacarpal joint: the relationship of joint shape and degenerative joint disease." The Hand 15(2): 201-206.

Paley, D., R. Y. McMurtry, et al. (1987). "Pathologic conditions of the pisiform and pisotriquetral joint." The Journal of hand surgery 12(1): 110-119.

Palmer, A. K. and F. W. Werner (1981). "The triangular fibrocartilage complex of the wrist--anatomy and function." The Journal of hand surgery 6(2): 153-162.

Pellegrini, V. D., Jr., M. Parentis, et al. (1996). "Extension metacarpal osteotomy in the treatment of trapeziometacarpal osteoarthritis: a biomechanical study." The Journal of hand surgery 21(1): 16-23.

Pequignot, J. P., L. D'Asnieres de Veigy, et al. (2005). "[Arthroplasty for scaphotrapeziotrapezoidal arthrosis using a pyrolytic carbon implant. Preliminary results]." Chirurgie de la main 24(3-4): 148-152.

Peterson, B. and R. M. Szabo (2006). "Carpal osteoarthrosis." Hand clinics 22(4): 517-528; abstract vii.

Pilny, J., J. Kubes, et al. (2006). "[Consequennce of nontreatment scapholunate instability of the wrist]." Rozhledy v chirurgii : mesicnik Ceskoslovenske chirurgicke spolecnosti 85(12): 637-640.

Pirela-Cruz, M. A., S. R. Goll, et al. (1991). "Stress computed tomography analysis of the distal radioulnar joint: a diagnostic tool for determining translational motion." The Journal of hand surgery 16(1): 75-82.

Pollock, J., A. A. Giachino, et al. (2010). "SLAC wrist in the absence of recognised trauma and CPPD." Hand surgery : an international journal devoted to hand and upper limb surgery and related research : journal of the Asia-Pacific Federation of Societies for Surgery of the Hand 15(3): 193-201.

Rayan, G. M., B. H. Jameson, et al. (2005). "The pisotriquetral joint: anatomic, biomechanical, and radiographic analysis." The Journal of hand surgery 30(3): 596-602.

Reagan, D. S., R. L. Linscheid, et al. (1984). "Lunotriquetral sprains." The Journal of hand surgery 9(4): 502-514.

Rothe, M., K. D. Rudolf, et al. (2006). "[Long-term results following denervation of the wrist in patients with stages II and III SLAC-/SNAC-wrist]." Handchirurgie, Mikrochirurgie, plastische Chirurgie: Organ der Deutschsprachigen Arbeitsgemeinschaft fur Handchirurgie: Organ der Deutschsprachigen Arbeitsgemeinschaft fur Mikrochirurgie der Peripheren Nerven und Gefasse : Organ der Vereinigung der Deutschen Plastischen Chirurgen 38(4): 261-266.

Sammer, D. M. and P. C. Amadio (2010). "Description and outcomes of a new technique for thumb Basal joint arthroplasty." The Journal of hand surgery 35(7): 1198-1205.

Saunders, B. M. and D. Lichtman (2011). "A classification-based treatment algorithm for Kienbock disease: current and future considerations." Techniques in hand & upper extremity surgery 15(1): 38-40.

Scheker, L. R., P. P. Belliappa, et al. (1994). "Reconstruction of the dorsal ligament of the triangular fibrocartilage complex." Journal of hand surgery 19(3): 310-318.

Shewring, D. J., R. Savage, et al. (1994). "Experience of the early use of technetium 99 bone scintigraphy in wrist injury." Journal of hand surgery 19(1): 114-117.

Shin, A. Y. and A. T. Bishop (2002). "Pedicled vascularized bone grafts for disorders of the carpus: scaphoid nonunion and Kienbock's disease." The Journal of the American Academy of Orthopaedic Surgeons 10(3): 210-216.

Singer, G., R. Eberl, et al. (2011). "Pisotriquetral arthrodesis for pisotriquetral instability: case report." The Journal of hand surgery 36(2): 299-303.

Staron, R. B., F. Feldman, et al. (1994). "Abnormal geometry of the distal radioulnar joint: MR findings." Skeletal radiology 23(5): 369-372.

Steinmann, S. P. and R. L. Linscheid (1997). "Pisotriquetral loose bodies." The Journal of hand surgery 22(5): 918-921.

Sung, J. K. and E. Akelman (2009). "Thumb Carpometacarpal Arthritis." Techniques in Orthopaedics 24(1): 23-26.

Swigart, C. R., R. G. Eaton, et al. (1999). "Splinting in the treatment of arthritis of the first carpometacarpal joint." The Journal of hand surgery 24(1): 86-91.

Swindells, M. G., A. J. Logan, et al. (2010). "The benefit of radiologically-guided steroid injections for trapeziometacarpal osteoarthritis." Annals of the Royal College of Surgeons of England 92(8): 680-684.

Tay, S. C., S. L. Moran, et al. (2007). "The clinical implications of scaphotrapezium-trapezoidal arthritis with associated carpal instability." The Journal of hand surgery 32(1): 47-54.

Tomaino, M. M. (2006). "Suspensionplasty for basal joint arthritis: why and how." Hand clinics 22(2): 171-175.

Tomaino, M. M., M. Vogt, et al. (1999). "Scaphotrapezoid arthritis: prevalence in thumbs undergoing trapezium excision arthroplasty and efficacy of proximal trapezoid excision." The Journal of hand surgery 24(6): 1220-1224.

Tsuge, S. and R. Nakamura (1993). "Anatomical risk factors for Kienbock's disease." Journal of hand surgery 18(1): 70-75.

Ulrich-Vinther, M., H. Puggaard, et al. (2008). "Prospective 1-year follow-up study comparing joint prosthesis with tendon interposition arthroplasty in treatment of trapeziometacarpal osteoarthritis." The Journal of hand surgery 33(8): 1369-1377.

Van Heest, A. E. and P. Kallemeier (2008). "Thumb carpal metacarpal arthritis." The Journal of the American Academy of Orthopaedic Surgeons 16(3): 140-151.

Vender, M. I., H. K. Watson, et al. (1987). "Degenerative change in symptomatic scaphoid nonunion." The Journal of hand surgery 12(4): 514-519.

Viegas, S. F., R. M. Patterson, et al. (1993). "Wrist anatomy: incidence, distribution, and correlation of anatomic variations, tears, and arthrosis." The Journal of hand surgery 18(3): 463-475.

Wajon, A., L. Ada, et al. (2005). "Surgery for thumb (trapeziometacarpal joint) osteoarthritis." Cochrane database of systematic reviews(4): CD004631.

Wajon, A., E. Carr, et al. (2009). "Surgery for thumb (trapeziometacarpal joint) osteoarthritis." Cochrane database of systematic reviews(4): CD004631.

Watson, H. K., D. t. Ashmead, et al. (1988). "Examination of the scaphoid." The Journal of hand surgery 13(5): 657-660.

Watson, H. K. and F. L. Ballet (1984). "The SLAC wrist: scapholunate advanced collapse pattern of degenerative arthritis." The Journal of hand surgery 9(3): 358-365.

Watson, H. K. and J. Weinzweig (1999). "Triquetral impingement ligament tear (tilt)." Journal of hand surgery 24(3): 321-324.

Weiss, K. E. and C. M. Rodner (2007). "Osteoarthritis of the wrist." The Journal of hand surgery 32(5): 725-746.

Wilder, F. V., J. P. Barrett, et al. (2006). "Joint-specific prevalence of osteoarthritis of the hand." Osteoarthritis and cartilage / OARS, Osteoarthritis Research Society 14(9): 953-957.

Winkler, F. J., N. Borisch, et al. (2010). "[Mid-term results after scaphoid excision and four-corner wrist arthrodesis using K-wires for advanced carpal collapse]." Zeitschrift fur Orthopadie und Unfallchirurgie 148(3): 332-337.

Wolf, J. M. (2008). "Treatment of scaphotrapezio-trapezoid arthritis." Hand clinics 24(3): 301-306, vii.

Wollstein, R. and L. Carlson (2009). "STT (Scapho-Trapezium-Trapezoid) Arhritis." Techniques in Orthopaedics 24(1): 19-21.

Wollstein, R., N. Wandzy, et al. (2005). "A radiographic view of the scaphotrapezium-trapezoid joint." The Journal of hand surgery 30(6): 1161-1163.

Wollstein, R. and H. K. Watson (2005). "Scaphotrapeziotrapezoid arthrodesis for arthritis." Hand clinics 21(4): 539-543, vi.

10

Osteoarthritis of the Trapeziometacarpal Joint (TMJ): A Review of the Literature

Oliver Boughton and Hugh Mackenzie
Department of Trauma and Orthopaedics, Kingston Hospital
United Kingdom

1. Introduction

Osteoarthritis (OA) of the base of the thumb is a common, painful and debilitating condition. It is more common in women and most commonly presents in Caucasian women in their late forties (Wilson and Bossley, 1983). It affects approximately 16-20% of women over 45 years old and 6% of men over this age (Bettinger et al., 2001). It is the site most frequently operated on in the upper extremity for primary osteoarthritis. (Pellegrini, 2005). Pain is the main presenting symptom. It is often brought on by writing, by opening jars and using the hand for a long time, particularly in pinching movements and there is difficulty in performing these activities. The patients often have weakness due to the pain that may affect their ability to work, perform activities of daily living and follow leisure pursuits. They may also have an adduction deformity of their thumb. Signs include tenderness over the carpometacarpal joint at the base of the thumb, thenar wasting, reduced pinch grip strength and crepitus on moving the thumb (Wilson and Bossley, 1983; Gwynne-Jones et al., 2006).

The severity of basal thumb osteoarthritis can be graded according to the Eaton stages. Eaton Stage I basal thumb osteoarthritis indicates joint pain and symptoms but no joint space-narrowing or cartilage degeneration shown on X-ray. Eaton stage II is classified as joint space narrowing seen on X-ray with osteophytes present of less than 2mm in size. An osteophyte is a small outgrowth of bone which occurs at joints in association with degeneration of joint cartilage. Eaton Stage III osteoarthritis is characterised by osteophytes of greater than 2mm in size being present on x-ray and significant destruction of the joint. In stage IV basal thumb OA there is significant degeneration of the scaphotrapezial joint in addition to the trapeziometacarpal joint (Eaton at al., 1985).

2. The anatomy of the basal joint of the thumb

The basal joint of the thumb is formed by the articulation between the trapezium bone proximally and the first metacarpal bone distally. It is therefore called the trapeziometacarpal joint or the carpometacarpal joint of the thumb. The trapezium, a bone of the second carpal row, articulates with the scaphoid bone proximally, the trapezoid medially and the bases of the first and second metacarpal bones distally. The trapezium is on the palmar and radial side of the wrist. It is angled such that it projects towards the palmar side. It angles the first metacarpal bone (the most proximal bone of the thumb) radially and in a palmar direction. The articular facet of the trapezium with the first metacarpal is angled 35 degrees towards the palmar direction and 20 degrees radially. This results in the neutral position of the thumb being 35 degrees in a palmar direction and 20 degrees in a radial direction (Zancolli, 1979).

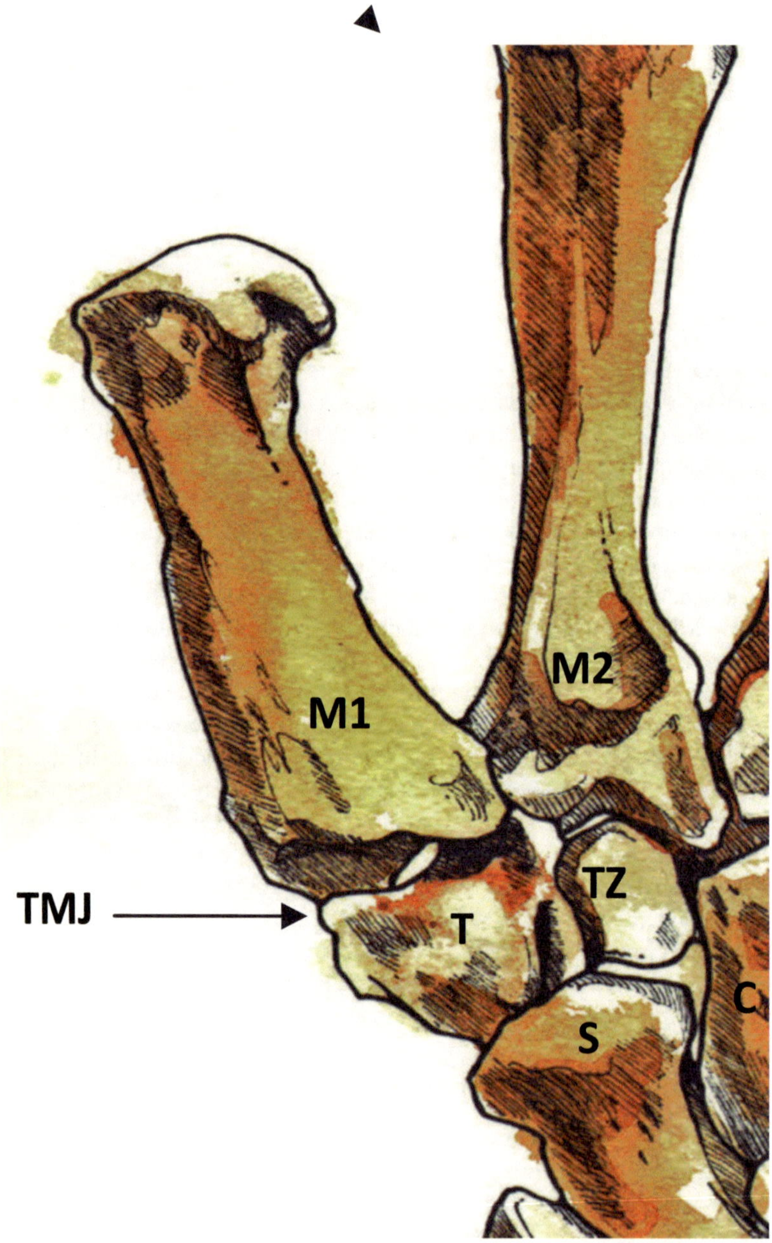

Fig. 1. Illustration of the trapeziometacarpal joint (TMJ) of the left thumb. The first (M1) and second (M2) metacarpals, the trapezium (T), the trapezoid (TZ), the scaphoid (S) and the capitate (C) bones are illustrated. Illustration courtesy of Mr Donald Sammut, Consultant Hand Surgeon, The Hand Clinic, Windsor.

The trapeziometacarpal joint is a saddle joint with wide mobility due to extensive articular surfaces. It is called a saddle joint because the trapezial articular surface is concave in a dorsopalmar direction and convex in the radioulnar direction. The first metacarpal base is complimentary to the trapezial articular surface. The trapezium is compared to the saddle of a horse and the base of the first metacarpal bone may be compared to the horse rider as it is mobile. It is a synovial joint and is surrounded by a joint capsule that is strengthened by three ligaments. The most important of these is the ulnar beak ligament. This is a very thick and wide ligament that runs from the crest of the trapezium and attaches to the ulnar side of the base of the first metacarpal. This ligament maintains the stability of the thumb and is tense in abduction of the first metacarpal. The other two ligaments are less widely described as they are believed to be less important in the stability of the thumb. The radial ligament originates from the radial side of the trapezium and travels dorsally and medially to attach to the dorsal tubercle of the first metacarpal. A palmar wide ligament is also sometimes described (Zancolli, 1979; Zancolli and Cozzi, 1992; Standring, 2008). A wide range of movement is permitted at the trapeziometacarpal joint: flexion, extension, abduction, adduction, opposition and retroposition.

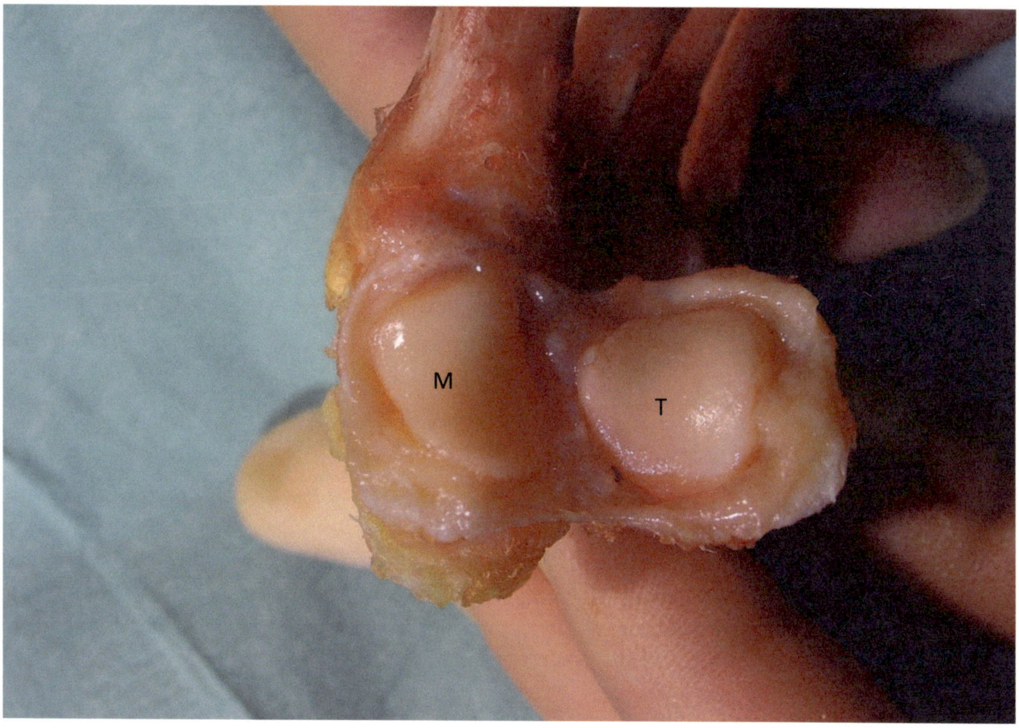

Fig. 2. Dissection of the trapeziometacarpal joint showing, on the left, the base of the first metacarpal (M) and, on the right, the articular surface of the trapezium (T). Dissection courtesy of Mr Donald Sammut, Consultant Hand Surgeon, The Hand Clinic, Windsor.

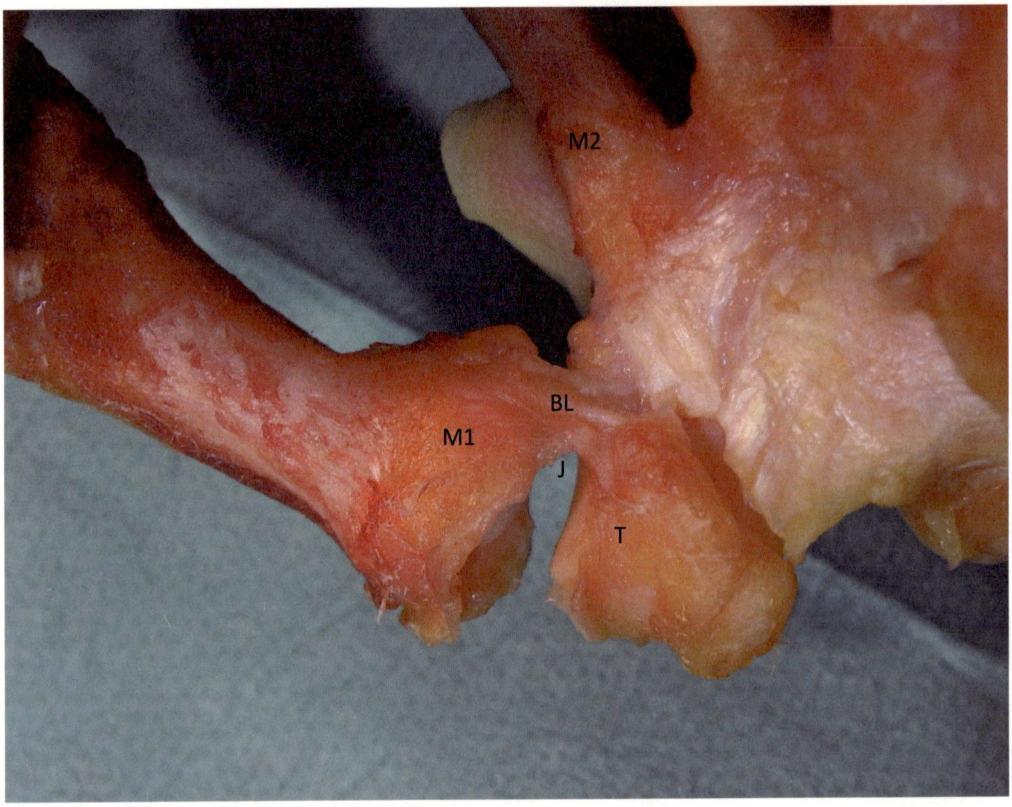

Fig. 3. Dissection displaying the strong ulnar beak ligament (BL) of the trapeziometacarpal joint. Traction is applied to the first metacarpal to open and display the joint (J). The base of the first metacarpal (M1) is on the left side of the joint. The articular surface of the trapezium (T) is on the right side of the joint in this image. The base of the second metacarpal is also seen (M2). Dissection image courtesy of Mr Donald Sammut, Consultant Hand Surgeon, The Hand Clinic, Windsor.

3. Pathophysiology of osteoarthritis of the base of the thumb

Many authors have described theories on how osteoarthritis of the base of the thumb occurs. There is often degeneration of the ulnar beak ligament due to recurrent stress and overuse which leads to ligament and joint instability. With increased laxity there may be abnormal translation of the first metacarpal on the trapezium. This can result in excessive shear forces between the joint surfaces (Tomaino, 2000; Kapandji TG and Kapandji AI, 1993). In addition there is articular degeneration. This may be secondary to instability which leads to joint surface incongruity. The incongruity may result in areas of high contact stress developing in the joint. This then causes cartilage erosion and the symptoms and signs of osteoarthritis (Bettinger et al., 2001). It has been shown that articular degeneration occurs on the palmar side first and gradually progresses to dorsoradial cartilage degeneration in the later stages of osteoarthritis of the joint (Pellegrini, 2005; Hobby et al., 1998). Radiological studies looking at the angle of the trapezium compared to the second metacarpal have shown that there is an increased radial trapezial tilt in Eaton stages III and IV compared to Eaton stages

I and II osteoarthritis of the base of the thumb (Bettinger et al., 2001; Kapandji AI and Heim, 2002). Studies have also shown accessory tendons of abductor pollicis longus inserting into the radial side of the metacarpal base in some people. These pull the metacarpal base radially and hence have a tendency to cause joint instability and may contribute to the development of osteoarthritis (Zancolli and Cozzi, 1992).

4. Treatment of trapeziometacarpal osteoarthritis

Trapeziometacarpal osteoarthritis may be treated conservatively with non-steroidal anti-inflammatory drugs (NSAIDs) first. If these are ineffective at symptom control a splint can be used which holds the thumb in abduction preventing the movements of adduction and retroposition. This ensures that the metacarpal base is covered by the trapezium and joint stability is increased, reducing metacarpal subluxation and wear of the joint cartilage (Zancolli and Cozzi, 1992). Depending on the severity of the symptoms the splint may be effective if just worn nocturnally (Goubau et al., 2007; Hobby et al., 1998).

For temporary relief of symptoms, lignocaine and steroid injections into the joint are effective. However, repeated injections into the joint are harmful to the joint itself and surrounding tissue. As well as accelerating joint damage, if the steroid leaks into the surrounding tissue it can lead to subcutaneous fat necrosis. This loss of the fatty tissue around the thumb leads to an undesirable cosmetic outcome.

If, despite conservative measures, pain or deformity interferes with daily activities such as holding a key or gripping an object, surgical treatment is advocated. As already mentioned, the trapeziometacarpal joint is the most commonly surgically reconstructed joint for osteoarthritis in the upper limb (Pellegrini, 2005; Tomaino, 2000). The first operation which can be considered for early osteoarthritis is reconstruction of the ulnar beak ligament. This is achieved using a tendon slip from the flexor carpi radialis tendon. As it does not involve any of the articular surfaces it is reserved for patients with joint laxity without appreciable degenerative changes. Thumb metacarpal osteotomy is another operation which can be effective in early disease. It transfers load bearing from the worn volar cartilage to the more intact dorsal articular surface. As well as giving symptom relief it also slows the progression to more severe osteoarthritis (Hobby et al., 1998). Another more experimental method of reconfiguring the joint alignment is wedge osteotomy of the trapezium. This realigns the trapezial saddle reducing metacarpal subluxation. However, studies are in their early stages and evidence for this procedure is limited (Kapandji AI and Heim, 2002).

For more severe disease with significant degenerative changes the surgical options include trapeziectomy, arthrodesis and total joint arthroplasty. Trapeziectomy is associated with good pain relief but can lead to weakness and instability lasting several months so is often reserved for Eaton Stages III and IV osteoarthritis (Hobby et al., 1998; Gwynne-Jones et al., 2006; Wilson and Bossley, 1983). Trapeziectomy may be performed in isolation or in combination with tendon sling interposition or ligament reconstruction. However, the outcome of these operations appears to be equivalent (Davis et al 2004).

Arthrodesis is a less frequently performed procedure in the trapeziometacarpal joint than other joints in the hand. It is associated with increased joint stability but longer immobilisation and an incidence of non-union (Hobby et al., 1998). It leaves a strong but rather immobile thumb.

Total joint arthroplasty has been a less successful procedure in this joint. There is frequent loosening of the components, implant fracture and an increased infection rate. Revision

procedures of total joint replacements of this joint are common (Lanzetta and Foucher, 1995; Wilson and Bossley, 1983).
The choice of surgical procedure for trapeziometacarpal arthritis is still controversial. There is limited evidence as to which procedure produces optimal results whilst limiting complications. Therefore, randomised clinical trials are awaited comparing these surgical techniques (Vermeulen et al, 2011).

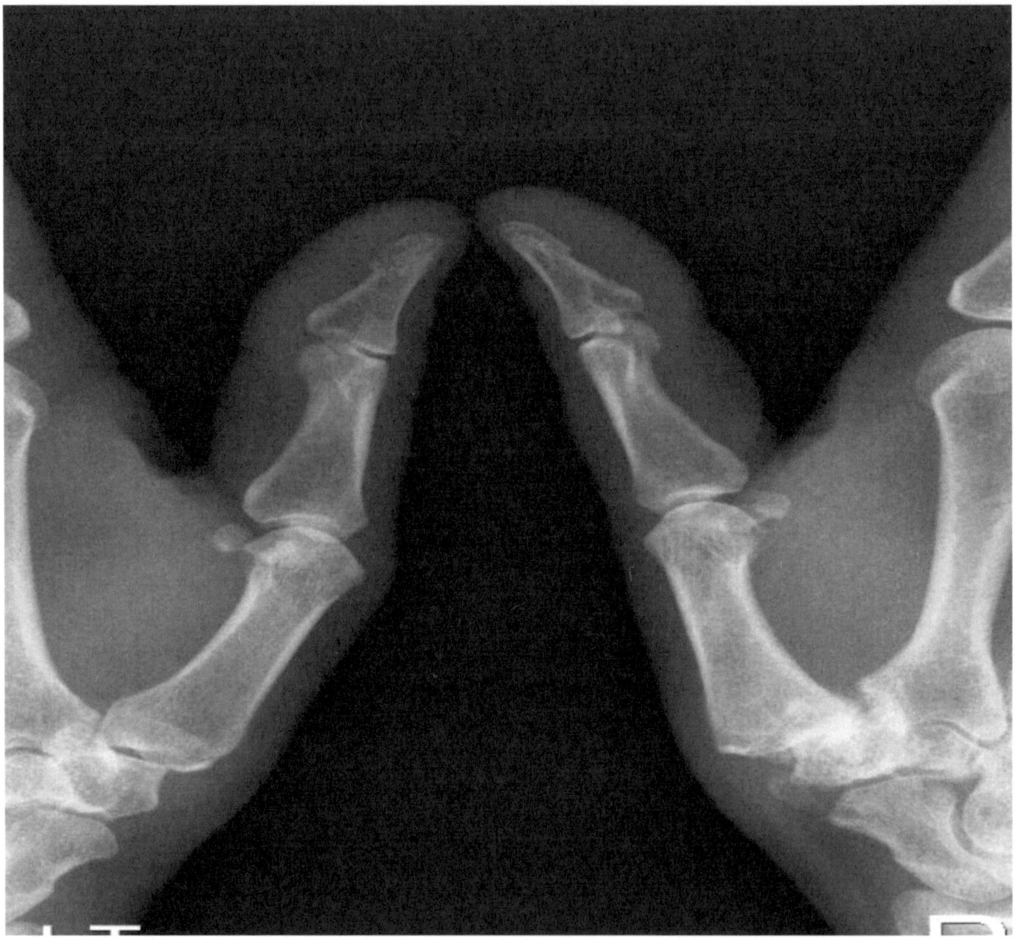

Fig. 4. Plain radiograph showing Eaton Stage III osteoarthritis of the trapeziometacarpal joint of the right thumb

5. Conclusion

Trapeziometacarpal arthritis is a common, painful and debilitating condition. The complex anatomy allows for an extensive range of movement. However, it is this inherent instability within the joint that leads to wear of the articular cartilage and osteoarthritis.
Once conservative measures have failed there are a wide variety of surgical treatment options.

6. References

Bettinger PC, Linscheid RL, Cooney WP 3rd, An KN (2001). Trapezial tilt: a radiographic correlation with advanced trapeziometacarpal joint arthritis. Journal of Hand Surgery - American Volume. 26(4):692-7

Davis TR, Brady O, Dias JJ (2004). Excision of the trapezium for osteoarthritis of the trapeziometacarpal joint: a study of the benefit of ligament reconstruction or tendon interposition. J Hand Surg [Am]. Volume 29(6):1069-77

Eaton RG, Glickel SZ, Littler JW (1985). Tendon interposition arthroplasty for degenerative arthritis of the trapeziometacarpal joint of the thumb. Journal of Hand Surgery - American Volume. 10(5):645-54

Eaton RG, Glickel SZ (1987). Trapeziometacarpal osteoarthritis. Staging as a rationale for treatment. Hand Clinics. 3(4):455-71

Goubau JF, Kerckhove D, Berghs B (2007). [Addition-subtraction osteotomy combined with ligamentoplasty for symptomatic trapezial dysplasia with instability]. [French] Traitement des dysplasies trapeziennes symptomatiques instables par osteotomie d'addition-soustraction et ligamentoplastie. Chirurgie de la Main. 26(1):26-30

Gwynne-Jones DP, Penny ID, Sewell SA, Hughes TH (2006). Basal thumb metacarpal osteotomy for trapeziometacarpal osteoarthritis. Journal of Orthopaedic Surgery. 14(1):58-63

Hobby JL, Lyall HA, Meggitt BF (1998). First metacarpal osteotomy for trapeziometacarpal osteoarthritis. Journal of Bone & Joint Surgery - British Volume. 80(3):508-12

Holmberg J, Lundborg G (1996). Osteotomy of the first metacarpal for osteoarthrosis of the basal joints of the thumb. Scandinavian Journal of Plastic & Reconstructive Surgery & Hand Surgery. 30(1):67-70

Kapandji AI, Heim UF (2002). [Reorientation osteotomy of the trapezial saddle]. [French] L'osteotomie de reorientation de la selle trapezienne. Chirurgie de la Main. 21(2):124-33

Kapandji TG, Kapandji AI (1993). [New radiologic data on the trapezo-metacarpal joint. The results of 330 cases]. [French] Nouvelles donnees radiologiques sur la trapezo-metacarpienne. Resultats sur 330 dossiers. Annales de Chirurgie de la Main et du Membre Superieur. 12(4):263-74

Lanzetta M, Foucher G (1995). A comparison of different surgical techniques in treating degenerative arthrosis of the carpometacarpal joint of the thumb. A retrospective study of 98 cases. Journal of Hand Surgery - British Volume. 20(1):105-10

Pellegrini VD Jr (2005). The ABJS 2005 Nicolas Andry Award: osteoarthritis and injury at the base of the human thumb: survival of the fittest? Clinical Orthopaedics & Related Research. 438:266-76

Standring S (2008). Gray's Anatomy: The Anatomical Basis of Clinical Practice, 40th Edition. Churchill Livingstone Elsevier. p 857-898

Tomaino MM (2000). Treatment of Eaton stage I trapeziometacarpal disease with thumb metacarpal extension osteotomy. Journal of Hand Surgery - American Volume. 25(6):1100-6

Vermeulen GM, Slijper H, Feitz R, Hovius SE, Moojen TM, Selles RW (2011). Surgical management of primary thumb carpometacarpal osteoarthritis: a systematic review. J Hand Surg Am. 36(1):157-69.

Wilson JN (1973). Basal osteotomy of the first metacarpal in the treatment of arthritis of the carpometacarpal of the thumb. The British Journal of Surgery. 60:854-858

Wilson JN, Bossley CJ (1983). Osteotomy in the treatment of osteoarthritis of the first carpometacarpal joint. Journal of Bone & Joint Surgery - British Volume. 65(2):179-81

Zancolli E (1979). Structural and Dynamic Bases of Hand Surgery, 2nd Edition. J.B. Lippincott Company

Zancolli EA, Cozzi EP (1992). Atlas of Surgical Anatomy of the Hand. Churchill Livingstone.

11

Low Level Laser Therapy in the Treatment of Temporomandibular Joint Arthritis: Questions and Answers

Marini Ida and Gatto Maria Rosaria
Department of Oral Sciences, School of Dentistry, "Alma Mater Studiorum", University of Bologna Italy

1. Introduction

Temporomandibular disorder (TMD) is a collective term for a number of clinical signs and symptoms involving masticatory muscles, temporomandibular joint (TMJ) and associated structures (De Leeuw, 2008)
Some studies show that 3-7% of the adult population seek care for TMJ pain and dysfunction (Carlsson, 1999) and the range of symptom occurrence to be between 16%and 59% and the range of clinical signs to be between 33% and 86%. Among individuals with TMJ disorders 11% had symptoms of TMJ arthritis. (Mejersjo & Hollender, 1984; Tanaka, Detamore et al., 2008) There is disagreement between the classification of degenerative joint disease as presented by the American Association of Orofacial Pain and the RCD/TMD(Research Diagnostic Criteria of Temporomandibular Disorders) (LeResche, 1997)

1.1 Anatomy of TMJ

Before we start discussing TMD treatments, it is important to review anatomy.

Is the TMJ similar to other synovial joints in the human body?

No. TMJ is the only synovial joint whose surface is not covered with hyaline cartilage but with fibrocartilage. One more difference is the fact that in the TMJ teeth are present as an intermediate structure (Schwartz & Marbach, 1965). The masticatory system is dynamic, not static, and it continuously changes due to the abrasion of dental surfaces

Position of the TMJ

Typically, the mandible has been considered to be connected to the skull by means of two synergically acting joints: the right and left TMJs. Both these joints are condylar synovial joints (diarthroses) that enable the characteristic anterior displacement (Testut, 1971).
Because of this displacement, the TMJ has been regarded to as an atypical joint.

Composition of the TMJ

The TMJ is a ginglymoarthrodial synovial joint. The joint is encapsulated and immersed in synovial fluid, and is stress bearing and capable of both rotational and translatory movements. The mandibular condyle can move in a variety of directions within the mandibular fossa. Condylar movements are protected from direct contact with the bony architecture of the fossa through an intricate system of fibrocartilage and synovial structures. The TMJ is structurally unique, consisting of only two joint in the body with vascularised tissue within the capsular ligament. Since the disc is a vascular and not innervated, pain from within the joint is in all probability due to inflammation or injury of the highly vascularised and innervated retrodiscal tissue or inflammation of the synovial tissues. (Loughner, Miller et al., 1997)

Movement of the TMJ

When the TMJ is in motion, the interarticular disc is always positioned between the fossa/eminence and condyle by the action of the superior lateral pterygoid muscle and the uppermost elastic portion of the posterior attachment known as the postero-superior retrodiscal lamina of the retrodiscal tissue. During function, the lateral and medial discal collateral ligaments attach the disc to the condyle on the inferior surface of the disc (fig. 1).

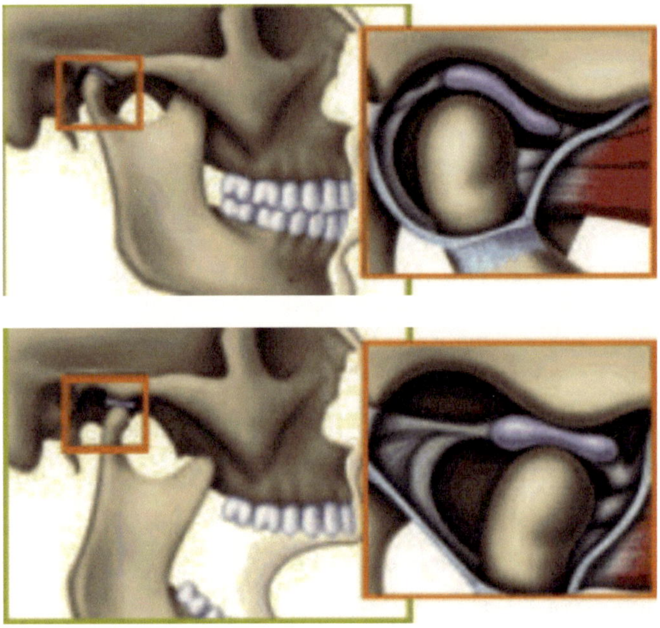

Fig. 1. Functional anatomy of TMJ.

The superior surface of the disc translates or slides along the posterior aspect of the articular eminence during full mouth opening. Translation of the condyle occurs as a result of the action of the inferior lateral pterygoid muscle, which protrudes from the mandible, in concert with other mandibular depressors the infra- and suprahyoid musculature. The posterosuperior retrodiscal lamina acts passively to pull the disc posteriorly during opening as the condyle translates anteriorly. The superior lateral pterygoid muscle contracts eccentrically during closure, stabilizing the disc against the distal slope of the articular eminence. (Laskin, 1994) The two synovial membrane layers line the joint capsule and disc, except on the articulating surface, and produce synovial fluid, fulfilling the nutritional needs of the joint. (Dijkgraaf, de Bont et al., 1996)

Composition of the synovial fluid

The joint space is filled by the highly viscous synovial fluid, containing hyaluronic acid and glycoprotein lubricant. Hyaluronic acid is a polymer of D-glucuronic acid and D-N-acetylglucosamine, which is highly unstable and degrades in the presence of inflammation.(Nitzan, Nitzan et al., 2001)

In synovial joints is shared by the articular cartilage, the subchondral bone, and the disc. In synovial joints the subchondral bone shares loading with articular cartilage. Only 1-3% of load forces are attenuated by cartilage while the normal subchondral bone is able to attenuate about 30% of the load through the joints.(Imhof, Sulzbacher et al., 2000) The subchondral bone protects the articlar cartilage from damage caused by excessive loading. The condylar ear and the articular fossa receive their blood supply from arteries supplying the underlying bone. In the TMJ, the disc, through its viscoelastic properties, functions as a stress absorber and stress distributor. It contributes to prevent stress concentration and excessive stress in the cartilage and bone components of the joint, thus protecting the joint. (Tanaka & van Eijden, 2003) Articular surface remodelling potential persists having the proliferative layer in the articular cartilage that can resume the proliferative activity if the occasion demands.

Blood supply to the TMJ

The articulating surfaces are free of blood vessels, but the synovial membrane is usually well supplied with minute vessels. The most significant blood supply enters the posterior aspect of the joint through the retrodiscal pad. A less significant quantity of the blood supply to this plexus comes from vessels within the mandible or temporal bone, which enter the joint at the peripheral attachment of the joint capsule. (Charles, Boyer et al., 1964)

2. Initiating events in TMJ arthritis

The term arthritis refers to an inflammatory condition affecting an articulation that results in erosion and fibrillation of articular cartilage and degeneration of adjacent sub-condral bone. Over recent years the term arthritis has evolved to distinguish a non inflammatory condition producing similar degenerative changes.

Initiation of TMJ OA

Wilkes (Wilkes, 1989) has suggested that TMJ arthritis is the last stage in the process of TMJ internal derangement, to explain the process is that as a result of joint intrinsic or extrinsic overloading, the lubrication system is compromised, the disc lags behind, and the condyle is pulled forward, away from the lagging disc. The normally firm attachment of the disc to the condyle becomes loose. The loose disc does not stay in its normal position but falls, usually anteriorly, starting the process of disc displacement (Nitzan, 2001) When the retrodiscal area is inadaptable, it perforates on loading, thus leading to arthritis. Conversely, it has been suggested that TMJ arthritis may precede disc displacement (de Bont , Boering et al., 1986) Joint degeneration is associated with disintegration of the joint constituents. Many studies have shown arthritis changes prior to disc displacement. (de Bont & Stegenga, 1993)

Is arthritis a reparative or a disruptive process?

Arthritis is a reparative process in the first place, with the purpose of recovering joint cartilage lesions.

When the loading is controlled, the retrodiscal area is adaptable and becomes disk-like (Manfredini, 2010)

This process of compensation unfortunately fails most of the times and a degradation takes place, which leads to losing normal functions in the affected joints. Early signs of TMJ arthritis are cellular proliferation and increased condrocytes metabolic activity. Said phenomena, when observed with SEM, present with a very developed wrinkled endoplasmatic reticle, a luxuriant Golgi apparatus and numerous secretory vescicles (de Bont & Liem, 1985). That leads to active reparative processes so that arthritis can remain asymptomatic for years. Next, an increase in the cartilage volume is observed, caused by a higher water absorption, and the cartilage surface becomes irregular (de Bont , Liem et al., 1985).

Condrocytes multiply and present with an increased metabolic activity. Collagene begins to lose its organization presumably following the liberation of proteolitic enzymes (de Bont & Liem, 1985).

After that follows a phase in which TMJ presents at first with deep surface cracks and then with progressive loss of the cartilage due to mechanical abrasion (de Bont , Liem et al., 1985).

In this phase proliferated condrocytes can be observed next to the deeper cracks of the cartilage (de Bont , Boering et al., 1986).

At a final stage, cracks in the cartilage appear more and more deep and the cartilage gradually disappears as a consequence of total destruction of collagene and proteoglycans. The last condrocytes die and the underlining bone becomes exposed.

TMJ arthritis is clinically present with clicks and, less often, with limited mobility of the mandible.

These descriptions, as observed with optical microscopy and SEM, are perfectly coincident with clinical and histological findings in great joints. Although enzymatic processes have not been studied in the TMJ, it can be thought that an analogy exists with the mechanisms described in this chapter.

Is TMJ arthritis a rare event?

It is not a rare event. It is not typical of the adult age and it can present in both adults and young subjects.

2.1 Local and systemic risk factors of arthritis

The TMJ function will remain normal as long as its adaptive capacity is not compromised. The changes in the joint associated with the adaptation process are considered as asymptomatic arthritis. The failure of the joint to adjust may cause symptoms such as pain and/or limitation depending on the presence of risk factors, thus confirming the cyclic nature of arthritis. Local and systemic risk factors (micro- and macro-trauma, parafunction, joint laxity, abnormal alignment, occlusal changes etc.) may results in overloading and/or immobilization, thus jeopardizing TMJ integrity.

Which are the risks factors of TMJ overloading?

Causes that lead to loading of the joint include clenching, occlusal changes (eg premature contact, teeth extractions, posterior bite collapse, teeth inclination) etc. These may set off abnormal compressive and shear forces.

On the other hand, it has an intra-articular origin, eg inflammation, infection, and hemarthritis, in which there is an increase in intra-articular pressure that consequently increases the joint loading.

Macro-trauma such as whiplash, for example, involves both extrinsic and intrinsic joint overloading. By stretching the joint ligaments, the joint's stability to withstand extrinsic loading is affected, and the initiation of an inflammatory reaction within the joint increases the intrinsic loading (Manfredini, 2010). Abnormal alignment, joint laxity, and disc displacement all decrease the joint's ability to cope with increased joint loading.

Which are the risks factors of TMJ immobilization?

TMJ immobilization is considered to be one of the principal causes of joint deterioration, mainly due to inability of the body to eliminate the harmful effects of inflammation. Immobilization might be caused by extrinsic or intrinsic factors and rehabilitation is possible only when the correct diagnosis is made. Extrinsic or extra-articular causes included myofascial pain disorder, extra-articular infection, coronoid hyperplasia, or other pathologies. Intra-articular inflammatory perfusion, infection, and hemarthritis are all intrinsic causes of immobilization. Advancing age, sex, hormonal factors, genetics, nutrition, obesity, and systemic illnesses such as atherosclerosis, diabetes, or osteoporosis may affect the host's adaptive capacity. These factors may contribute to dysfunctional remodelling of the TMJ, even when the biomechanical stresses are within a normal physiologic range. (Laskin , 1994; Arnett, Miliam , Miliam et al., 1996)

3. TMJ diagnosis

TMJ arthritis is a disorder represented by variable combinations of signs and symptoms including pain, limitation in movements, joint noises, malocclusion etc that may be uncovered by means of several type of examination.

The TMJ diagnosis

3.1 Clinical extraoral and intraoral examination

Pain may not necessarily be present, when it occurs, it might be severe and localized to the joint. Mouth opening may not be limited or may present limitation originating in the affected joint. Noise such as cliking and or crepitus may or may not be present. Lateral movements, protrusive mandibular movements, existence of deviation, and the exact location of pain during each movement are considered. Intraorally, occlusal findings, such as deviation of dental midline, crossbites, ipsi or controlateral open bite, missing teeth, and posterior bite collapse are recorded.

Auscultation for joint noises (cliking, crepitus) and eliciting pain on palpation of TMJ, head and neck muscles are recommended.

3.2 Imaging

Imaging has played an important role in the diagnosis of TMJ arthritis, however there is only a limited correlation between clinical and radiographic findings. Severe symptoms may be associated with imaging changes or, alternatively severe changes on radiographs may be associated with an asymptomatic joint.

For radiologic evaluation panoramic radiographs can be obtained for initial screening purposes. Computed tomography (CT) provides a three dimensional view of the morphologic changes in the TMJ and bone mineral density in the mandibular condyle. Imaging of an osteoarthritic joint in the advanced stages typically shows erosion of the cortical outline, osteophytes, subcortical cysts, reduced joint space, and the presence of condylar deformities and osteophytes (Fig. 2, 3).

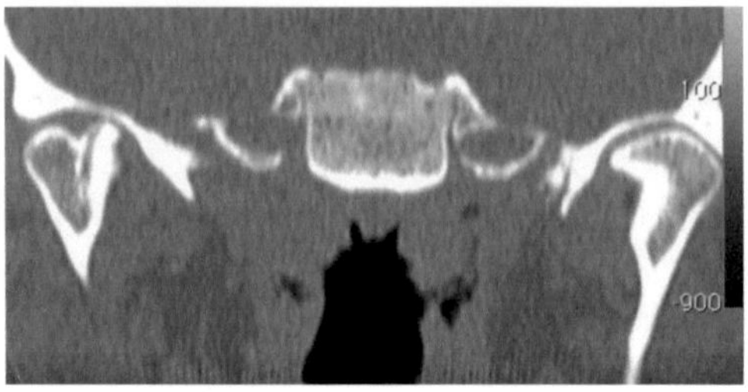

Fig. 2. CT of TMJ arthritis (coronal section)

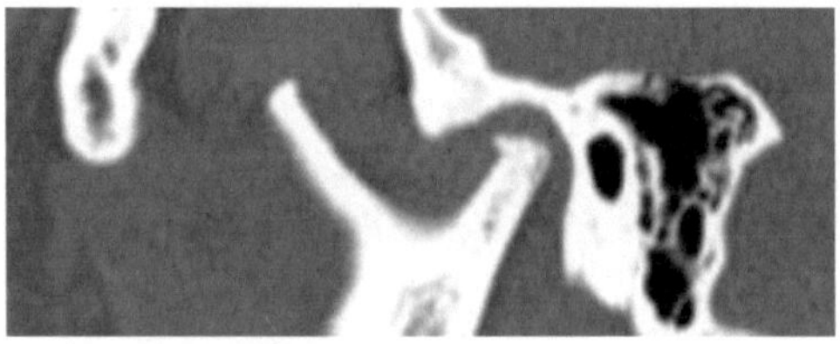

Fig. 3. CT of TMJ arthritis (sagittal section)

MRI imaging shows TMJ soft tissue abnormalities such as disc displacement, join perfusion and bone marrow signal changes related to TMJ arthritis (fig. 4).

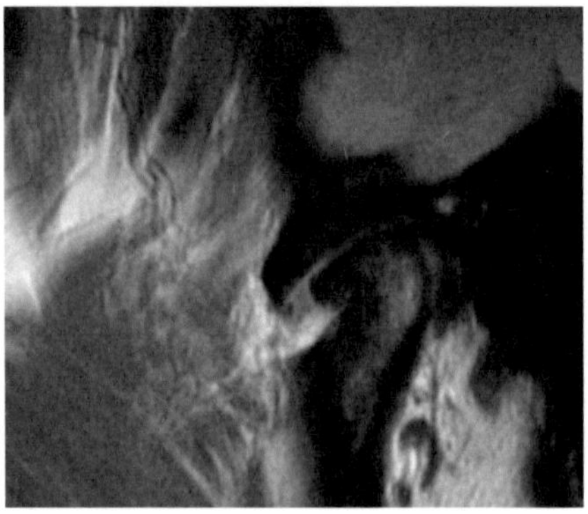

Fig. 4. MRI of TMJ arthritis (sagittal section)

4. Treatment of TMJ arthritis

A correct evaluation of the patient is the key for appropriate treatment. The prognosis of arthritis following conservative management has been shown to be good and stable. Although, radiologically, bone may show deterioration, clinical sign and symptoms tend to improve.

Treatment, in general, should address the rehabilitation of the joint defence mechanisms such as blood supply, movements, shock absorbance, and remodelling potential by coping with the patient's risk factors.

4.1 Non surgical treatment

A large variety of non-steroidal anti-inflammatory drugs (NSAIDs) can be used to reduce TMJ inflammation and the associated pain. They should be used at an early stage before any other treatment. However, they are not a long-term remedy for TMJ arthritis.

4.1.1 Local treatments

Physical therapy for the TMJ

Reduced mandibular mobility is caused by intra-articular restriction or by muscular dysfunction, physical exercises are beneficial to prevent formation of intra-articular adhesions and to increase the blood flow and strength of the jaw muscles. Physical therapy is a valuable adjunct to other treatments for TMJ arthritis aimed at normalizing the functional capability of temporomandibular system

In difficult cases or when cooperation is not achieved, it is the physician's responsibility to refer the patient to a professional physical therapist; exercises include passive and active symmetric movements in all directions, further stretching on maximal movement exercises, as well as movements against resistence.

4.1.2 Acupuncture

Acupuncture has been used as an adjunct to other therapy for pain relief in patients with OA. Furthermore, acupuncture has not effect on joint pain and tenderness or on the acute phase reactants and disease activity (Casimiro ,Barnsley et al., 2004).

Iontophoresis and Phonophoresi

Iontophoresis and Phonophoresi are techniques to enhance the transport of drug ions across a tissue barrier. The effects of iontophoretically-applied dexamethasone in combination with lidocaine were evaluated in patients with painful TMJ disc displacement, with or without reduction and in patients with OA. Iontophoretically-applied dexamethasone was effective in improving mandibular function, mobility but not in reducing pain.

4.1.3 Bite appliances

Muscular hyperfunction or occlusal trauma can be a primary cause of OA, and these factors might also be detrimental and accelerate tissue destruction in the case of systemic inflammatory joint disease involving the TMJ. Treatment with occlusal bite appliances has been advocated mainly in patients with pain of muscular origin due to muscle hyperfunction or tension (Major & Nebbe, 1997; Ekberg , Vallon et al., 2003).

But there is no evidence of the efficacy of treating TMJ OA with occlusal appliance (Al -Ani , Davies et al., 2004).

4.1.4 Low-level laser therapy

Superpulsed low-level laser therapy (LLLT) seems to be a good choice as a non-invasive treatment for tempomandibular joint pain while exhibiting a low cost for the patient. Many authors have reported significant pain reduction with low-level laser therapy in acute and chronic musculoskeletal pain conditions (Bjordal, Couppè et al., 2003; Ninomiya, Hosoya et al., 2007).

The results of many works show no statistical improvements for any of following: localized swelling, muscle strength, functional status, or global assessments with laser treatment. The major limitation of the systematic meta-analyses about LLLT is the heterogeneity of clinical application, including different dosages, wavelengths and types of LLLT.

Which are the evidence-based proves of the efficacy of LLLT in the treatment of TMJ ARTHRITIS?

Our superiority randomized double-blind clinical trial in parallel arms was carried out with the aim to investigate the efficacy of the new superpulsed low-level laser therapy versus anti-inflammatory and placebo therapy in the treatment of TMD, and to determine the optimal time and exposure application to LLLT for treating arthritis with pain. (Marini, Gatto et al., 2010)

How was the trial designed?

A total of 99 patients with temporomandibular joint disorders, secondary to disc displacement without reduction (Fig. 5) or arthritis with articular effusion (Fig. 6) were randomly divided into 3 groups. Thirty-nine patients received LLLT in 10 sessions over 2 weeks, 30 patients received ibuprofen 800 mg twice a day for 10 days, and 30 patients received sham laser as placebo in 10 sessions over 2 weeks. Pain intensity was measured by visual analogue scale at baseline, 2, 5, 10, and 15 days of treatment. Mandibular function was evaluated by monitoring active and passive mouth openings and right and left lateral motions at baseline, 15 days, and 1 month of treatment. Magnetic resonance imaging was performed at baseline and the end of therapy.

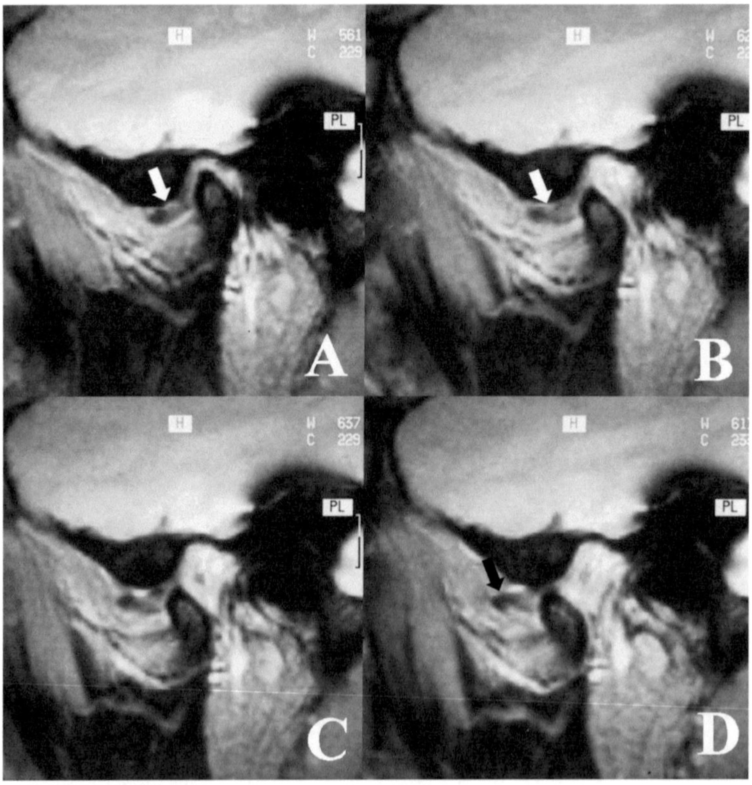

Fig. 5. MRI of TMJ disc displacement without reduction

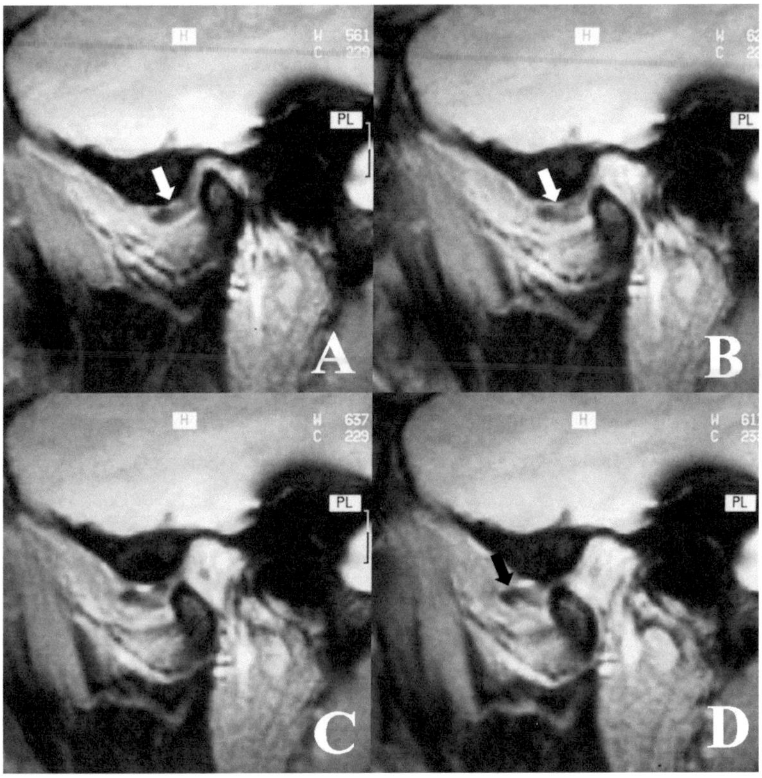

Fig. 6. MRI of TMJ arthritis with articular effusion (sagittal section)

Which were the results?

Mean visual analogue scale pain scores in LLLT group was significantly lower than in non-steroidal anti-inflammatory drug group and control group (P=0.0001) from fifth day up to the end of the observation period. As for active and passive mouth openings and right and left lateral motions, superiority of LLLT was evident 1 month after treatment (interaction time treatment, P=0.0001).

Therefore mandibular function improved in all LLLT patients proving the effectiveness in the treatment of pain, as demonstrated by a significant improvement in clinical signs and symptoms of temporomandibular joint disc displacement without reduction and arthritis at the end of treatment and stability over a period of 1 month.

Which were doses and times of LLLT?

Each patient received laser therapy, gallium-arsenide diode superpulsed laser, (LUMIX 2 HFPL Fisioline, Verduno, Italy) with time pulsation<200 ns; frequency range 1 to 50 kHz, wave length 910 nm, mean power 400 mW, and peak power 45W. The affected TMJ areas of these patients were treated daily in 3 steps:

1. 20 kHz for 10 minutes
2. 18 kHz for 5 minutes
3. 16 kHz for 5 minutes

All patients were treated for 10 consecutive days (5 d/wk) in right and left TMJ,. Laser test was performed at the end of every application to measure the laser output. The laser parameters selected were based pragmatically on those used in everyday practice by a principal author, which had been formally piloted in previous studies. (Marini , Scala et al., 2003)

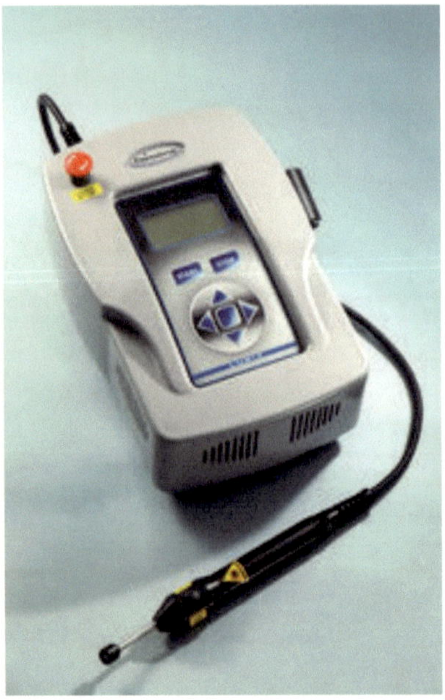

Fig. 7. Low-Level Laser device.

Which were the main differences between LLLT and NSAIDs treatment, observed in our study?

The laser group showed an increase in pain, which then disappeared for a long time; the increased pain could be explained with an increased local hyperemia.
Patients treated with NSAIDs showed an improvement in pain and mandibular function during the time of treatment but returned to more or less the same level as pretreatment conditions after treatment terminated. It is hard to compare our outcomes with those of other studies that obtained similar results despite differences in design, dosage, intensity, and frequency. In Italy, administration of NSAIDs is suggested for not more than 7 to 10 days, except for rheumatoid arthritis, whereas in many countries this therapy can be prolonged from 4 to 6 weeks.
Real hazards of long-term administration of NSAIDs have been recognized lately as involving renal disease and serious toxicity to the gastrointestinal tract, as well as increasing the risks of adverse cardiovascular events. A comprehensive review of the primary literature reveals modest scientific support for the assertion that the daily use of NSAIDs offers benefits for patients with chronic TMD pain. (List , Axellson et al., 2003)

Does laser treatment influence active and passive mouth opening and right and left lateral motion?

These parameters are always significantly different between patients treated with laser and patients treated with NSAIDs (Table 1 and 2). Superiority of laser is mostly evident one month after treatment (interaction time-treatment p=0.0001)

Comparison	Active mouth opening p-values at Baseline 15 days 1 month			Passive mouth opening p-values at Baseline 15 days 1 month		
Laser vs NSAIDs	0.001	0.001	0.001	0.001	0.001	0.001
Laser vs Control	0.031	0.001	0.001	0.012	0.001	0.001
NSAIDs vs Control	0.026	0.083	0.003	0.041	0.069	0.001

(1) Marini, Ida MD, DDS; Gatto, Maria Rosaria PhD; Bonetti, Giulio Alessandri MD, DDS* Effects of Superpulsed Low-level Laser Therapy on Temporomandibular Joint Pain The Clinical Journal of Pain Issue: Volume 26(7), September 2010, pp 611-616 (http://lww.com)

Table 1. Comparisons of the difference of active and passive mouth opening, right and left lateral motion between the groups . α = 0.02

Comparison	Right lateral motion p-values at Baseline 15 days 1 month			Left lateral motion p-values at Baseline 15days 1 month		
Laser vs NSAIDs	0.013	0.001	0.001	0.001	0.001	0.0010
Laser vs Control	0.683	0.228	0.001	0.631	0.001	0.001
NSAIDs vs Control	0.296	0.232	0.741	0.411	0.123	0.412

(1)α = 0.02

Table 2. Comparisons of the difference of right and left lateral motion between the groups.

Does time influence active and passive mouth opening and right and left lateral motion in patients treated with laser and patients treated with NSAIDs ?

Mean values of these parameters remain stable across the times (Table 3).

	Baseline	After treatment	1 month after treatment
Active mouth opening(mm)	L 36,28 ± 3.44 A 39.85 ± 2.89 C 38.06 ± 3.19	L 43.24 ± 2.71 A 41,27 ± 2.49 C 39.77 ± 3.96	L 45.89 ± 2.13 A 40.90 ± 3.37 C 37.46 ± 4.94
Passive mouth opening (mm)	L 37.97 ± 3.22 A 41.68 ± 3.01 C 40.00 ± 3.21	L 45.28 ± 2.37 A 42.43 ± 2.77 C 40.77 ± 4.06	L 47.22 ± 2.31 A 42.54 ± 2.20 C 38.28 ± 4.67
Right lateral motion (mm)	L 6,37 ± 1.08 A 7.10 ± 1.28 C 6.57 ± 2.43	L 8.54 ± 1.41 A 8.63 ± 1.97 C 7,98 ± 2.20	L 12.20 ± 1.08 A 8.22 ± 1.92 C 8.04 ± 2.26
Left lateral Motion (mm)	L 6.67 ± 1.14 A 6.87 ± 1.57 C 6.44 ± 2.39	L 13.01 ± 1.57 A 8.82 ± 1.78 C 8.01 ± 2.19	L 13.19 ± 1.54 A 8.43 ± 1.97 C 7.98 ± 2.21

Table 3. Active and passive mouth opening, right and left lateral motion at baseline, after treatment and one month after treatment (mean±SD) (1)

May be hypothesized the mechanism of action of LLLT?

It is interesting to observe that patients examined with MRI at the end of treatment showed a more or less abundant effusion within the intra-articular, which disappeared after laser therapy, whereas it remained stable in the other 2 groups, control and patients treated with NSAIDs. This reabsorption could explain the disappearance of pain through a wash out of the algogenic metabolites and the functional improvement through the elimination of the mechanical obstacle created by the liquid. In the case of arthritis, a series of pathologic phenomenon is present, which results in a synovial inflammation inducing a cascade of reactions and, in particular, prostaglandins and leukotrienes. LLLT might act on the synovia and stimulate cellular energy processes that appear. It could be hypothesized that in the condyle-meniscus coordination a synovitis could arise, even without the evident signs of arthritis, which could result in arthritis as indicated by an author (Stegenga , de Bont et al., 1991)

Which are the main advantages in using LLLT?

Our therapeutic protocol and the characteristics of LLLT (highest peak power for a few seconds) are suggested in the treatment of painful TMD. An important adjunctive factor is the low cost of the therapy.

4.2 Surgical treatment

Surgical procedure is available for the treatment of TMD, ranging from simple arthrocentesis and lavage to more complex open joint surgical procedures.

The general indication for TMJ arthritis surgery is significant TMJ pain and or dysfunction that originates in the joint and worsens during jaw functions, such as talking or clewing on the contralateral side and is refractory to non surgical treatment.

Arthrocentesis and arthroscopy should resolve limited mouth opening, and pain associated with OA .

Condylotomy should be used for high intensity of pain with restriction of opening the mouth. Whereas TMJ surgery should be reserved for advances cases of TMJ arthritis.

5. References

Al -Ani MZ, Davies SJ, Gray RJM, Sloan P, Glenny AM. Stabilisation splint therapy for temporomandibular pain disfunction syndrome. The Cochrane Database of Systematic Reviews(website). In: The Cochrane Library , Issue 2, 2004. Oxford, England: Update Software. Available at: http://www.mrw.interscience.wiley.com/cochrane/clysrev/articles/CD002778/frame.html. Accessed 16 Sept 2004

Arnett GW, Miliam SB, Gottesman L. Progressive mandibular retrusiom - idiopathic condylar resorption. Part. I. Am J Orthodo Dentofacial Orthop 1996;110:8-15.

Bjordal JM, Couppè C, , Chow RT, et al. A systematic review of low level laser therapy with location- specific doses for pain from chronic joint disorders . Aust J Phisiother. 2003;49:107-116.

Carlsson GE Epidemiology and treatment need for temporomandibular disorders. J Orofac Pain 1999;13:232-237.

Casimiro L,Barnsley L,Brosseau L, et all.Acupuncture and electroacupuncture for the treatment of RA. The Cochrane Database of Systematic Reviews[web-site]In the Cochrane Library, Issue 3,2003.Oxford,England: Update Software.Available at://www.mrw.interscience.wiley.com /Cochrane/ clsysrev/ articles/ CD003788/ frame.html. Accessed 16 Sept 2004

Charles C, Boyer CC, Williams TW, Stevens FH. Blood supply of the temporomandibular joint. J Dent res 1964;43:224-228

de Bont LG, Liem RS, Boering G. Ultrastructure of the articular cartilage of the mandibular condyle: aging and degeneration Oral Surg Med Pathos 1985; 60: 631-641.

de Bont LG, Liem RS, Boering G., et al. Arthritis of the temporamandibular joint: a light microscopic and scannino electron microscopic study of the articular cartilage of the mandibular condyle. J Oral Maxillofac Surg 1985, 43. 401-400

de Bont LG, Boering G, Liem RS, Eulderink F,, Westesson P-L. Arthritis and internal derangement of the temporomandibular joint: a light microscopic study. J Oral Maxillofac Surg 1986;44:634-643.

de Bont LG, Stegenga B. Pathology of temporomandibular joint internal derangement and arthritis. Int J Oral Maxillofac Surg 1993;22:71-74.

De Leeuw R,ed Orofacial Pain: guidelines for assessment, diagnosis, and management.4th.ed.Chicago:Quintessence;2008.

Dijkgraaf LC, de Bont LG, Boerning G, Liem RS. Structure of the normal synovial membrane of the temporomandibular joint: a review of the literature. J Oral Maxillofac Surg 1996;64:332-338.

Ekberg E, Vallon D, Nilner M. The efficacy of appliance therapy in patients with temporomandibular disorders of mainly myogenous origin. A randomized, controlled, shortterm trial. J Orofac Pain 2003;17:133-139.

Imhof H, Sulzbacher I, Grampp S, Czerny C, Youssefzadeh S, Kainberger F. Subchondral bone and cartilage disease: a rediscovered functional unit. Invest Radiol 2000;35:581-588.

Laskin DM. Etiology and pathogenesis of internal derangement of the temporomandibular joint: current controversies in surgery for internal derangements of the temporomandibular joint. Oral Maxillofac Surg Clin North Am 1994;6:217.

LeResche L. Epidemiology of temporomandibular disorders: implications for the investigation of etiologic factors. Crit Rev Oral Biol Med 1997;8:291-305.

List T, Axellson S, Leijon G. Pharmacological interventions in the treatment of temporomandibular disorders, atypical facial pain, and burning mouth syndrome. A qualitative systematic review. J Orofac Pain. 2003;17:301–310

Loughner B, Miller J, Broumand V, Cooper B. The development of strains, forces and nociceptor activity in retrodiscal tissues of the temporomandibular joint: current controversies in surgery for internal derangements of the temporomandibular joint of male and female goats. Exp Brain Res 1997;113:311-326.

Major PW, Nebbe B. Use and effectiveness of splint appliance theray: Review of literature. Cranio 1997;15:159-166.

Marini I, Scala A, Russo A, et al. Diode laser therapy is an effective tool for the treatment of temporomandibular joint arthritis. J.Dent Res. 2003;82:C–544

Marini, Ida MD, DDS; Gatto, Maria Rosaria PhD; Bonetti, Giulio Alessandri MD, DDS* Effects of Superpulsed Low-level Laser Therapy on Temporomandibular Joint Pain The Clinical Journal of Pain Issue: Volume 26(7), September 2010, pp 611-616

Mejersjo C, Hollender L. TMJ pain and dysfunction: relation between clinical and radiofraphic findings in the short and long term. Scand J Dent Res 1984;92:241-248.

Ninomiya T, Hosoya A, Nakaura H, et al. Increase of bone volume by a nanosecond pulsed laser irradiation is caused by decreased osteoclast number and an actived osteoblasts. Bone 2007;40:140-148.

Nitzan DW. The process of lubrication impairment and its involvement temporomandibular joint disc displacement: a theoretical concept. J Oral Maxillofac Surg 2001;59:36-45.

Nitzan DW, Nitzan U, DanP, Yedgar S. The role of hyaluronic acid in protecting surface-active phospholipids from lysis by exogenous phospolipase A(2). Rheumatology (Oxford) 2001;40:336-340

Nitzan D,Roisentul Temporomandibular joint arthritis 111-134 in Manfredini D. Current concepts on temporomandibular disorders Quintessence Publishing Co.Ltd print in Germany 2010

Schwartz L, Marbach JJ, Changes in the temporomandibular joints with age. Periodontics 1965; 3: 184-189 .

Stegenga B, de Bont LG, Boering G. Tissue response to degenerative changes in the temporomandibular joint: a review. J Oral Maxillofac Surg. 1991;49:1079–1088.

Tanaka E, van Eijden T. Biomechanical behaviour of the temporomandibular joint disc. Crit Rev Oral Biol Med 2003;14:138-150.

Tanaka E, Detamore MS, Mercuri LG. Degenerative disorders of the temporomandibular joint: etiology, diagnosis, and treatment, J Dent Res 2008;87:296-307.

Testut L,Trattato di anatomia V ed., UTET, Torino.1971 Vol 1 .

Wilkes C. Internal derangement of the TMJ. Arch Otolaryngol Head Neck Surg 1989;115-469.

Part 4

Diagnosis of OA in Lower Extremity (Hip, Knee, and Ankle)

12

Treatment Preferences in Patients with Knee or Hip Osteoarthritis: An Overview

Amado Rivero-Santana[1], Lilisbeth Perestelo-Perez[2,3], Jeanette Perez-Ramos[1], Marien Gonzalez-Lorenzo[1] and Pedro Serrano-Aguilar[2,3]
[1]*Canarian Foundation of Health and Research (FUNCIS), Tenerife,*
[2]*Evaluation Unit of the Canary Islands Health Service (SESCS), Tenerife,*
[3]*CIBER en Epidemiologia y Salud Publica (CIBERESP), Tenerife,*
Spain

1. Introduction

Osteoarthritis (OA) is a degenerative chronic condition that involves degradation of joints—primarily articular cartilage, synovium, and subchondral bones, producing joint pain, tenderness and stiffness. It can occur in any joint but knees, hips and small hand joints are the most commonly affected. Although OA can occur in any age group, its prevalence increases with age especially after the 4th or 5th decades of life (Jordan et al., 2007; Lawrence et al., 2008). OA is one of the most prevalent chronic conditions in Western countries, although prevalence rates vary depending on whether symptomatic or radiographic criteria were used (Busija et al., 2010; Comas et al., 2010), as it is well known that the severity of a patient's symptoms often is not correlated to the degree of disease progression evaluated on radiographs (Hannan et al., 2000). Women show, in general, a greater risk of prevalent OA and more severe symptoms, particularly after menopausal age (Srikanth et al., 2005).

OA is a leading cause of disability and decreased quality of life, as it produces important functional limitations in daily activities (Elliot et al., 2007; van Dijk et al., 2008; Salaffi et al., 2005). The socioeconomic burden of the condition is immense and is not only the leading cause of disability in Western countries but is also responsible for a large number of physician visits, hospitalisations, and time lost from work (Kotlarz et al., 2009; Bitton, 2009).

There is no known cure for OA, so available treatments aim to relieve symptoms and improve or maintain functional capacity. Therapeutic options include nonpharmacologic, pharmacologic, and surgical interventions. Nonpharmacologic therapies, such as exercise, weight loss, physiotherapy, heat and cold application, or assistive devices entail no inherent risks and therefore they are recommended at all levels of severity, although they have revealed a modest effect in reducing symptoms (Scott & Kowalczyk, 2006).

Acetaminophen is also a safe core treatment recommended as a first line option for pain relief. At more severe levels of symptoms, oral non-steroidal anti-inflammatory drugs (NSAIDs) should be considered, although they have shown a higher risk of adverse effects (gastrointestinal, liver and cardio-renal) than acetaminophen or topical NSAIDs. Therefore, when selecting the agent and dose, healthcare professionals must take into account individual patient risk factors, including age, and they should be used at the lowest effective dose for the shortest possible period of time.

When nonsurgical treatments are ineffective at relieving symptoms and there is prolonged and established functional limitation and severe pain, referral for joint replacement surgery is recommended. This is a highly efficacious and cost-effective procedure for the treatment of advanced OA in its capability to relieve pain, increase mobility, and improve the quality of life (Losina et al., 2009).

In the last two decades there has been increasing interest in shared decision-making (SDM) as a collaborative model of health care (Charles et al., 1997; Edwards & Elwyn, 2009). SDM, as opposed to a more traditional authoritative and paternalistic patient-practitioner relationship, requires information exchange between patients and professionals, where the latter offer technical information about the disease and available treatments, while patients offer their personal knowledge about their concerns, expectations and preferences about treatments, their efficacy and potential risks, in order to reach a consensus about medical decisions. SDM is especially applicable in those situations where there is uncertainty about the probability of outcomes, or when there are two or more treatment options that offer a similar balance between benefits and risks. From this perspective, taking into account patients' preferences is increasingly advocated as an optimal model of collaborative care.

In the case of OA, as commented above, clinical recommendations vary depending on symptoms severity and prior experience with other treatments. In spite of this, OA is a clinical condition that is highly sensitive to patient preferences at all stages of severity. Treatments recommended for mild symptoms (exercise, physiotherapy, acetanomiphen, etc) have modest efficacy but no inherent risks of adverse effects, while more effective options which reduce pain and increase functionality, such as NSAIDs or opioid analgesics, present a higher risk of side effects. Even a highly effective procedure such as total joint replacement (TJR) is subjected to relevant trade-offs between its demonstrated benefits and risks associated with every surgical intervention, or other factors such as convalescence or costs, in those societies without universal healthcare systems. Therefore, patients with OA are continually faced with decisions that imply relevant trade-offs between benefits and the risk of undesired outcomes, so their personal preferences should be incorporated during deliberations and decisions about treatment of their condition.

Although research and implementation of SDM in OA remains scarce (Weng et al., 2007; Fraenkel et al., 2007), in the last decade an increasing number of studies have been performed that assessed patients' preferences about treatment options for OA and its characteristics. The aim of this article is to present an overview about the research on preferences and use of treatments by patients with hip and/or knee OA.

2. Patients' awareness, use and satisfaction with treatments

Several studies have analyzed patient awareness, prior utilization and/or satisfaction with treatments for OA, using survey measures. With some exceptions, results show that medications represent the most frequently used option in the treatment of OA. For instance, Juby et al. (2005) observed patients with clinical and radiographic evidence of OA (either hip or knee), and found a good awareness of 12 treatments, with diet modification and viscosupplementation being the less known (and used) options, with approximately 40% of the sample. Medications (non-narcotic and narcotic analgesics, NSAIDs, cyclooxygenase inhibitors COXIBs, steroid injections) were the most frequently known (more than 85% of the sample) and used treatments (50% to 75%), and between half and two-thirds of the patients who have taken them reported to be satisfied with their efficacy. Tallon et al. (2000) also found medications to be the most frequently used treatment among knee OA patients, with more than 70% of participants considering them moderately or extremely helpful. In both the studies commented, nonpharmacological treatment options such as physical therapy or aids/adaptations were used by 40% to 60% of participants, and of these, a similar percentage considered them satisfactory. Joint replacement surgery was the least frequently used treatment, as it is recommended only for those with high severity, but among those who have undergone this procedure it was the most valuated.

Mitchell & Hurley (2008), with 415 patients who consulted a primary care physician for knee pain of more than 6 months duration also found drugs (analgesic or NSAIDs) to be the treatment most frequently received (83%), followed by physiotherapy (41%), with other therapies showing rates of use lower than 10%. Sixty per cent of participants reported their preferences, and among these, physiotherapy was the most preferred treatment (41%), while only 4% reported drugs as their primary option.

Blake et al. (2002) obtained quite a different result, with rates of treatments tried more equally distributed, exercise being the most frequently used (35%), while oral medications were tried by approximately 25% of respondents (only over-the-counter-medication was included in the survey). This study was population-based and data on treatment use refer to those participants who reported knee or hip pain (37% of the sample) and therefore, although a small subsample was required to present verifiable radiographic evidence of OA, it cannot be assured that other rheumatic conditions were not present in the sample. The fact that only use of over-the-counter medication was assessed was possibly responsible for the discrepancies with the studies previously commented.

Other studies have analyzed patients' preferences when two specific treatments are compared. For instance, Wolfe et al. (2000) studied a cohort of patients with OA, rheumatoid arthritis and fibromyalgia, assessing their preferences for acetaminophen versus NSAIDs. Among OA patients, 56% of them considered acetaminophen significantly or somewhat less effective than NSAIDs, and 30% stated that the efficacy of both drugs was about the same. When considering overall satisfaction with the drugs also taking into account their side effects, results were almost identical. In the context of a randomised trial comparing treatments for knee OA, three studies reported patients' preferences for the treatments implemented. Underwood et al. (2007) offered patients the possibility of participating in a randomised trial or a preference study comparing topical versus oral ibuprofen for chronic knee pain. Among those who decided to participate in the preference study, 74% opted for the topical modality of the drug. Denegar et al. (2010) randomised 34 patients, in a crossover design, to heat, cold or contrast therapy, and after trial termination 47% of participants stated a preference for warm treatment, while equal preferences were observed for cold and contrast (24% in both cases). Foster et al. (2010), in a trial comparing physiotherapy advice and exercise versus the same condition plus acupuncture, assessed treatment preferences (not only for those implemented in the trial) before treatment was commenced, and found that only 20% of the participants stated a treatment preference; of these, 10% stated advice and exercise, 13% acupuncture and 44% both.

3. Studies that use preferences elicitation techniques

A number of studies have used different techniques to elicit patients' preferences about treatments or its characteristics. The most frequently used technique has been Conjoint

Analysis (CA), a task where patients construct their treatment preferences by making trade-offs between competing treatment characteristics (e.g., efficacy, risks or route of administration) in a series of rating tasks. Preferences are then predicted based on trade-offs between specific treatment characteristics and not the treatment itself. CA enables both health-related and nonhealth-related attributes, taking into account a wider range of outcomes.

Byrne et al. (2006) used CA to assess racial differences in preferences for TJR in a sample that includes general population and patients with knee OA. Participants were faced with different hypothetical scenarios of surgical and nonsurgical states for OA, developed from combinations of several attributes with different levels: pain, walking, costs, death, complications and failure of the surgical procedure. Results showed that all attributes except failure of TJR significantly predicts participants' choices: as differences between surgical and nonsurgical scenarios were smaller for pain and walking ability, and when the attribute of surgery (costs, death, complications) is larger participants were less likely to opt for surgery. Regarding participant characteristics, women, African-American and older individuals were less likely to choose surgery, while income level or kind of sample (public or patient) did not have a significant effect on choice.

Fraenkel et al. (2004) also used CA to assess knee patients' preferences for medications commonly prescribed for OA when an inadequate response for acetaminophen is obtained (nonselective NSAIDs, COXIBs, opioid analgesics) as well as other agents such as glucosamine and/or chondroitin sulphate, and capsaicine. Seven characteristics (with different levels) of medication were combined in the CA tasks: label, administration route, time to benefit, response rate, common adverse effects, risk of ulcer and monthly copayments. Results showed that the risk of adverse effects had the greatest impact on patient preferences; nonselective NSAIDs were almost never preferred, while topical capsaicine was the most preferred option even when it was reported as much less effective than the other alternatives. No significant associations between patients' demographic or clinical characteristics and treatment preferences were obtained.

In a more recent article, Fraenkel et al. (2008) also used CA to compare knee patient preferences for characteristics corresponding to four treatment options: topical capsaicin, oral medications (acetanomiphen, NSAIDs), intra-articular injections and exercise. Once again, patients' preferences were more strongly influenced by the risk of side effects compared to the chance of benefit. Exercise and NSAIDs were the most and least preferred options respectively, whether this latter option was described as 20% (base case) or 50% (benefits maximized) more effective compared to the other options.

In Ratcliffe et al. (2004), however, physical mobility was the most important attribute influencing patients' preferences, although risk of serious adverse effects and level of joint aches were also significant predictors (level of joint pains and risk of mild to moderate side effects did not attain statistical significance in the prediction of patients' choices). These results were moderated by factors such as symptoms severity, age or income; for instance, the importance attached to the level of mobility achieved decreased as the severity of symptoms increased. Chang et al. (2005), when combining health states for OA with different gastrointestinal side effects profiles (using a visual analogue scale, VAS), also found that the influence of side effects depends on the severity of the disease: it is lower when OA pain is severe and higher when OA pain is milder.

Kopec et al. (2007) analyzed patients' maximum acceptable risk increments (MARI) for different adverse effects from OA medication, using a probabilistic threshold technique. In this task, patients are presented with two treatment options that only differ in one attribute (e.g., pain relief), so most patients would logically opt for the more effective one. Then, the task proceeds by increasing (in the most favourable option) by small units the probability of one of the side effects presented, until the respondent switches to accepting the alternative option. Results showed that the lowest MARI was observed for heart attack/stroke (3% to 5%, depending on the level of pain relief and initial risk) and highest for dyspepsia (23% to 35%). Higher initial-risk levels correlated with greater subsequent willingness to run additional risk to obtain a benefit in pain relief.

4. Willingness and use of total joint replacement

Total joint arthroplasty has been revealed to be an effective procedure for the management of end-stage hip and knee OA (Losina el at., 2009). Ninety per cent of those who undergo TJR experience relief of pain and functional improvement, and the probability of associated risks is lower than 1%. In spite of this, significant variations in the rates of utilisation of TJR have been found (Jones et al., 2005; Skinner et al., 2003). Race was the most frequently studied variable to explain these disparities, as numerous studies have shown that white patients are more likely than Afro-American patients to have TJR, results that can be extrapolated to other ethnic minorities (Escalante et al., 2000; Oishi et al., 1998). These disparities cannot be accounted for by differences in disease prevalence or in access to healthcare, since most of the candidates for these procedures are older persons with access to public health insurance, and studies in universal health care systems have also found ethnic disparities in utilisation. Haussman et al. (2010) have found that TJR recommendations were lower for Afro-American than white patients of similar age and disease severity, but after adjusting for patients' preference for TJR this difference was no longer significant. Therefore, it seems that patient-level factors may be responsible, at least in part, for these disparities.

Several studies have analyzed which variables, both at system and patient level, predict willingness to undergo TJR. Hawker et al. (2001, 2002, 2004) have demonstrated that some sociodemographic, clinical and psychological variables (patients' beliefs and/or expectations about TJR) significantly predict their willingness for surgery: younger age, having spoken to the physician about having surgery, higher perceived severity, less comorbidities, considering friends as the best information source, perceiving the risk of TJR revision acceptable, or some perceived indications for treatments. Income and educational level are significantly related to the potential need for TJR, but not with willingness to undergo the procedure. Suarez-Almanzor et al. (2005) observed that when patients were asked whether they had considered knee replacement in the past, the most powerful predictor of an affirmative response was to have a previous recommendation by their physicians, followed by not being Afro-American, being male, higher perceived efficacy, and more confidence in the physician. When the question referred to considering TJR in the future if it was recommended by the physician, only ethnicity and perceived efficacy were significant predictors. To date, studies strongly suggest that less willingness of Afro-Americans to undergo TJR compared with white patients is accounted for by several psychological factors: they have worse expectations about TJR outcomes (Ibrahim et al., 2002a), expect a longer hospital stay (Ibrahim et al., 2002b), are more likely to perceive

various traditional and complementary care modalities as efficacious (Ibrahim et al., 2001), and consider that prayer is a helpful option to face up to OA disability (Ang et al., 2002). These beliefs and expectations may have important historical roots; discrimination against African Americans, for example, may have created cultural expectations of avoiding medical interventions in favour of home remedies. In any case, these data reflect the importance of taking patients' preferences into account when making decisions about treatment, and the necessity of implementing interventions that could correct erroneous perceptions about the efficacy of medical procedures.
It seems logical that physician recommendation of surgery was the most powerful predictor to undergo TJR, as found by Hawker et al. (2006). This study only reported unadjusted analyses in the prediction of undergoing TJR and also found that age between 62-82, higher education level, higher body mass index, worse perceived severity, and a better perceived general health significantly predict the use of TJR. In Hamel et al. (2008), age was a significant predictor in unadjusted analyses, but not when the remaining predictors were introduced in the regression model. Independent significant predictors of receiving the procedure were higher income level, higher perceived severity and less concern about dying or having complications from surgery.

5. Qualitative studies

Qualitative studies may help to obtain a more in depth viewpoint on the experiences of patients with the disease, in addition to their beliefs, perceptions and concerns about therapies to follow and in general their relationship with the health system. In the case of OA, a considerable number of studies have been performed which analyse various issues related to living with the disease and the treatment options.
As for sociodemographic variables which might have an influence on patients' preferences and decisions, in accordance with the results obtained in some of these studies, sex is one of the variables which may lead to differences in the way to live with OA and its possible treatments. Chang et al. (2004), observed that in general women generate more topics of interest than men (while in the sample there were twice as many women as men); some were exclusive to women: anatomy of OA, disadvantages of surgery, pain following surgery and methods to relieve this pain. In the case of intra-operative issues, women focused more on anaesthesia, and men on surgical technique. The study by Karlsson et al. (1997) focused specifically on sex-based differences. The results highlighted that women were more concerned about their function in basic activities, and tended to attain a worse functional level prior to considering surgery; they prefer to endure the suffering instigated by OA. They were more sceptical regarding the results of the arthroplasty and had less confidence in the doctor. The reasons provided for having more reservations towards surgery refer to expecting better technology to exist, their responsibilities as carers or concerns on becoming a burden to others.
Just as for the quantitative studies, race also seems to differentially affect living with OA and treatment preferences. In Chang et al. (2004), Afro-American patients generated less topics (especially men), and these dealt with more issues related to financial aspects, the ideal nature of the treatment or lack of trust in the doctor and health system in general. In Kroll et al. (2007), racial differences focused especially on four categories: causes of the disease (Afro-Americans tended to offer internal explanations, related to wear of the body and ageing, whilst Caucasians and Hispanics referred more frequently to external variables,

such as lesions or accidents), lifestyle changes (Afro-Americans report the disease as more debilitating, while white people and Hispanics, although they recognise the functional impairment, more frequently name the ways in which they try to overcome these limitations), trust and scepticism (Hispanics reveal less trust in the doctor, not so much in their skill as in their professional integrity. Afro-Americans were more sceptical as to technological progress), paying for surgery (Afro-Americans mention this topic more frequently, and are more concerned with obtaining money lent to be able to pay for the operation, while Hispanics mention the possibility of first undergoing the operation and then paying later on). Ibrahim et al. (2004), in a sample of Afro-American men, found that in relation to the category "cultural aspects of the care of arthrosis", the emerging topics referred to religious beliefs of the doctor and patient, in addition to the doctor's sex and race. For the latter aspect, the majority of the sample said they felt indifferent towards the doctor's race as the important thing is their professional skill; however, approximately 10% of the sample preferred a doctor of their same race, arguing that in this way they could better understand their problems. Regarding the sex of the doctor, one fifth of people who mentioned this topic preferred a doctor of the same sex as they were uncomfortable discussing private issues with someone of the opposite sex.

Other studies have offered information on various clinical factors or related to the health system which also has an influence on patient preferences and taking decisions. The study by Ballantyne et al. (2007) reveals how the assessment of the severity of OA is performed in general in a framework of comorbidity; although OA is considered as debilitating, it is not usually the primary health concern. The impact of the symptoms of OA (pain, lack of functionality), and their possible relief following the operation are essential topics for consideration of arthroplasty, in addition to the risks or side effects of the treatments, and they appear like this in most studies (Bower et al., 2006; Campbell et al., 2001; Chang et al., 2004; Karlsson et al., 1997; Kroll et al., 2007; Thorstensson et al., 2006). Waiting lists are debated in the study by O´Neill et al. (2007). Although participants confide in arthroplasty as a means to relieve symptoms, the uncertainty generated by waiting time once they have decided to operate has a negative effect on patient quality of life. Examples of other emerging topics regarding medical aspects of the disease and treatment were: anatomy of OA and duration of the prosthesis (Chang et al., 2004), body abnormality (Kroll et al., 2007), surgical techniques and indication for surgery (Chang et al., 2004; Karlsson et al., 1997), or improvements to general physical function (Thorstensson et al., 2006).

The social networks of patients are also a very important aspect in the decision to operate (Ballantyne et al., 2007; Bower et al., 2006; Kroll et al., 2007); family members or other people relevant for patients play a notable influence on their decisions to handle the disease, both by means of instrumental and emotional support, in addition to strengthening or contravening the beliefs of patients or providing them with new information. The role of the spouse is decisive in one sense or the other, to the extent that this is the person who will adopt the role of carer, and who in some way "shares" the psycho-emotional impact produced by OA; in many cases decisions are taken in part based on the capacity of the spouse to face up to the disease (Ballantyne et al., 2007; O´Neill et al., 2007). In the same way, the knowledge of other people who have undergone arthroplasty and the results obtained from this process are important when taking decisions on treatment (Chang et al., 2004). In some cases, however, the validity of friends as a source of information is questioned by patients themselves (Bower et al., 2006).

Prior experience with the health system is also a highly determinant factor, to the extent that negative experiences may affect patient beliefs or expectations (Ballantyne et al., 2007). Other factors which will be included in this section would be financial/work-related aspects such as the effect of OA and/or the operation on working life (e.g. early retirement; Kroll et al., 2007), the cost of the operation (Chang et al., 2004; Ibrahim et al., 2004; Kroll et al., 2007), technical and structural support (accessibility to the health system, or specific contexts related to treatment; Thorstensson et al, 2006), etc.

Psychological variables comprise most topics generated in different studies, including knowledge, beliefs, expectations or emotional reactions to living with OA and its treatment. Beliefs on the nature of OA seem important when considering surgery. In many cases patients consider that OA is a natural age-related process and this belief has a negative effect on the expected success of the treatment (Ballantyne et al., 2007; Campbell et al., 2001; O´Neill et al., 2007). However, one possible positive consequence of these kinds of beliefs could be the fact that OA is not a threat to the sense of own identity, to the extent that it is considered "suitable" at one's current age and therefore integrates easily into one's own identity (Ballantyne et al., 2007). In other cases, however, the alterations in roles and social relationships, or the lack of autonomy and independence produced by OA represent an invasive characteristic of own identity which affects self-identity and self-esteem.

Beliefs about who is eligible for the operation also play an important role in their selection (O´Neill et al., 2007). Some people believe that to consider surgery, the pain should be constant and the incapacity to move, total; obviously, this reduces the probabilities of considering arthroplasty, although the expectations on their results are positive. In the same sense, it may also occur that patients consider there should be people in worse physical conditions, for which reason they should be priority for surgery. The experience of pain and incapacity produced by the OA has a strong subjective component (O´Neill et al., 2007). In this sense, it has been seen that there are differences in the way these aspects are assessed; for example, Afro-Americans report the disease as more disabling than Caucasians (Kroll et al., 2007). However, as mentioned above, this greater disability perceived is not translated into a greater disposition to operate, quite on the contrary. Expectations on the results of treatments whether on their benefits or on their risks/side effects, also play a determining role when taking decisions on OA (Bower et al., 2006; Kroll et al., 2007; O´Neill et al., 2007). These expectations may come from external sources (doctors, friends, acquaintances) or the patient's own experience, for example over medication (Bower et al., 2006) or practicing exercise (Thorstensson et al., 2006).

Different kinds of reaction to OA symptoms have also been detected (Karlsson et al., 1997). Reacting by means of adaptation would refer to the psychological acceptance of the disease by means of regulating one's own emotions with a positive attitude and trying to adapt lifestyle to the new physical condition. A response by means of action would also refer to trying out new treatments.

6. Conclusions

In the last few decades there has been a gradual change in models of healthcare and the way to understand the doctor-patient relationship. From a medical model based on the disease and symptoms there has been a gradual progression towards what has been called patient-focused care whose main features would be respect for the patient's choices and values, emotional support, providing information and education, coordination of clinical care or the involvement of the patient's family and friends (Gerteis et al., 1993)

From this new point of view, the patient's psychological attitude, reflected in beliefs and expectations on the disease, healthcare or the doctor-patient relationship, as well as emotional response and the establishment of socio-affective links with health professionals, turns into a highly relevant aspect which is necessary to incorporate into the healthcare process. Patient attitudes, beliefs, preferences and expectations are considered factors which may have an important influence on the treatment process and its results whether by means of behavioural factors such as compliance with treatment procedures or putting into practice certain lifestyles which may favour or, on the contrary, hinder the onset or development of the disease, whether because of the direct effect that beliefs and expectations could have on the results of medical interventions by means of psychological mechanisms still not well understood.

Regarding taking medical decisions, this new way of understanding the role of the patient and their relationship with health professionals has led to the concept of shared decision-making, a joint process of deliberation between the doctor and patient where preferences are incorporated into taking decisions on diagnostic or therapeutic procedures within a process of mutual communication between both, where the professional provides information based on scientific evidence on the efficacy and safety of available treatment options, while the patient incorporates their psychological experiences, concerns, preferences and expectations over reaching a consensual decision on the procedure to follow.

In the case of OA, research performed to date has been delimiting a series of factors which determine patient choices as to different treatment options for their disease. Race was the most frequently studied variable because of the consistent results on less frequent use of TJR by ethnic minorities, especially Afro-Americans. Other studies report sex-based differences in living with the disease, patient concerns regarding their quality of life and on the results of treatments. These studies have revealed the importance of dealing with the beliefs and expectations of patients on the disease and available treatment options to the extent that these factors account for a substantial part of the behaviour of patients regarding their disease and quest for healthcare.

The studies commented in this article used different methodologies which hinder the integration of results, which on the other hand lead to discrepancies in some cases. For example, studies which use preference elicitation techniques found, in general, that patients' preferences are more influenced by the risk of adverse effects than potential benefits (while this effect is moderated by variables such as severity level, as patients with more serious symptoms tend to agree to run a greater risk in exchange for obtaining symptomatic relief). This data is clearly reflected in the investigation by Fraenkel et al. (2004, 2008) regarding NSAIDs, which because of a greater possibility of adverse effects are less preferred by patients given less effective but safer options. However, studies which have analysed by means of self-reporting techniques patients' use and preferences on the different treatments find that NSAIDs are not only among the most frequently used but they also reveal a high degree of acceptance by patients. Studies which use Conjoint Analysis propose explicit trade-offs to patients between risks and benefits of treatments while preferences are made on the characteristics of treatments and not on these by themselves; therefore, the possibility of bias because of recognition of the product or commercial brand and the experience of patients with these treatments is removed. For their part, studies such as those by Wolfe et al. (2000) and Juby et al. (2005) ask patients about the use they have made of different therapeutic options and their satisfaction with these and do not oblige participants to establish trade-offs between treatment characteristics. In this sense, preference elicitation techniques enable a more "pure" measure of these, in the sense of not being explicitly influenced by experience (and satisfaction) of patients with the treatment assessed. However, we can ask ourselves to what extent these procedures offer a somewhat "artefactual" image of patients' preferences derived from trade-offs between the consequences of treatments based on population-related probabilities, compared to assessments made by people who have experienced both adverse effects and the benefits of treatments. Prior investigations have reported that people from the general population assess certain states of health more negatively than those patients who suffer them. In this context it would be interesting to analyse the results of the CA separately for people who have experienced adverse effects of treatments compared to those who have not suffered from them. Studies on communication of risks both in the health and other fields have also revealed that people are more insensitive to major variations in the likelihood of very life-threatening emotional events, such as cancer or a nuclear accident (Slovic et al., 2005; Rottenstreich & Hsee, 2001).

Participation of the patient in taking decisions on their own health has turned into an object of debate and research in the last few decades. Calls to involve the patient in the process of taking decisions is based on practical arguments, in the sense of achieving more quality and efficiency in health services, and from an ethical point of view as a consequence of the emphasis on rights of autonomy and patient participation. In this sense, the preferences and values of patients have to occupy a relevant place in the process of healthcare and both investigators and health professionals should develop strategies to incorporate these preferences into taking medical decisions. Although currently there is no absolute unanimity on the meaning of "shared decision-making", it may be generally accepted that this refers to a process of communication between patients and health professionals regarding reaching a consensus on diagnostic or therapeutic procedures to follow—a dynamic process both from a non-historical and historical point of view where the information, concerns, values and preferences are shared and debated for which, in fact, they may be modified during this process. This does not mean the patient lays down their own preferences; in fact, these may be based on erroneous perceptions of medical procedures. Therefore, for example, it has been commented that racial differences over disposition to undergo TJR are in large part explained by the worse expectations of Afro-American patients over the results of this operation when scientific evidence reveals that this is a highly effective procedure with a low level of risk. These erroneous perceptions may be modified during the process of communication which suggests SDM, but this will not occur unless they are debated explicitly by the actors in the healthcare process. These difficulties may be overcome by means of implementing interventions promoted by SDM, such as training professionals on a consultatory style which promotes participation of the patient or the use of patient decision aids (PtDAs). These are instruments designed to set out the scientific evidence in a understandable way for patients in addition to helping them clarify their values and preferences regarding the features of the diagnosis or treatment procedures in terms of efficacy, safety or other relevant aspects, with the aim of facilitating taking decisions alongside their doctor. There are few studies which have analysed the effect of the application of these tools to patients with OA, but results are promising. Therefore,

Weng et al. (2007), in an uncontrolled study, found an improvement in the expectations of the results of TJR in Afro-American patients in addition to a reduction in decision-related conflict in the overall sample following the application of a PtDA consisting of a video and booklet on OA and its treatments. In a randomised controlled trial where patients from the intervention group received the results of their scores in a CA test, Fraenkel et al. (2007) observed a significant increase in self-efficacy in the handling of OA and in preparedness to participate in decision-making with their physicians. Therefore, these tools represent a resource of major interest to encourage a more active role for patients, thereby improving their knowledge on the medical procedures in which they are involved, in addition to communication with their health professional on their values and preferences.

Healthcare in the 21st century must respond to new challenges in an increasingly complex society where the increase in life expectancy also entails an increase in chronic diseases with a more educated population and where the sources of information on health have quickly multiplied with the onset of new technologies. The change from a paternalistic model of healthcare to another where the patient adopts a more autonomous and active role seems unstoppable. The assessment and understanding of patients' values and preferences regarding their states of health and available medical procedures represents only part of the process of involving the patient in taking decisions on their health, but this is fundamental in order for this process to be successful. In the case of OA, research has shown that patients' preferences are influenced by a wide number of factors. Experimental tasks such as CA have pointed out the importance of treatment risks in patients' choices, since participants in those tasks tend to prefer options with lower risks although they involve a lower probability of benefit. However, survey based studies show that when patients are asked based on their experience, they are quite satisfied with more effective options although they involve a higher risk. Furthermore, these results are moderated by demographic or clinical variables such as age or disease severity. Future research must clarify these questions. Psychological and psychosocial variables such as beliefs about the disease and treatments, expectations about outcomes, trust in health professionals, previous experience with the Health System, social networks and perceived social support, conform a complex interaction of factors that play an important role in patients' preferences and choices, and therefore they should not be neglected in the health care of patients with OA.

7. References

Ang, D., Ibrahim, S., Burant, C., Siminoff, L. & Kwoh, C. (2002). Ethnic differences in the perception of prayer and consideration of joint arthroplasty, *Medical Care* Vol. 40 (No. 6): 471-476.

Ballantyne, P., Gignac, M. & Hawker, G. (2007). A patient-centered perspective on surgery avoidance for hip or knee arthritis: lessons for the future, *Arthritis & Rheumatism* Vol. 57 (No. 1): 27-34.

Bitton, R. (2009). The Economic Burden of Osteoarthritis, *The American journal of managed care* Vol. 15 (Suppl 8):230-235.

Blake, V., Allegrante, J., Robbins, L., Mancuso, C., Peterson, M., Esdaile, J., Paget, S. & Charlson, M. (2002). Racial differences in social network experience and perceptions of benefit of arthritis treatments among New York City medicare beneficiaries with self-reported hip and knee pain, *Arthritis & Rheumatism* Vol. 47 (No. 4): 366–371.

Bower, K., Frail, D., Twohig, P. & Putnam W. (2006). What influences seniors´choice of medications for osteoarthritis? Qualitative inquiry, *Canadian Family Physician* Vol. 52: 342-343.

Busija, L., Bridgett, L., Williams, S., Osborne, R., Buchbinder, R., March, L. & Fransen, M. (2010). Osteoarthritis, *Best practice & research. Clinical rheumatology* Vol. 24 (No. 6): 757–768.

Byrne, M., Souchek, J., Richardson, M. & Suarez-Almazor M. (2006). Racial/ethnic differences in preferences for total knee replacement surgery, *Journal of clinical epidemiology* Vol. 59: 1078-1086.

Campbell, R., Evans, M., Tucker, M., Quilty, B., Dieppe, P. & Donovan, J. (2001). Why don´t patients do their exercises? Understanding non-compliance with physiotherapy in patients with osteoarthritis of the knee, *Journal of epidemiology and community health* Vol. 55 (No. 2): 132-138.

Chang, J., Kauf, T., Mahajan, S., Jordan, J., Kraus, V., Vail, T., Reed, S., Omar, M., Kahler, K. & Schulman, K. (2005). Impact of disease severity and gastrointestinal side effects on the health state preferences of patients with osteoarthritis, *Arthritis and rheumatism* Vol. 52 (No. 8): 2366–2375.

Chang, H., Mehta, P., Rosenberg, A. & Scrimsham, S. (2004). Concerns of patiens actively contemplating total knee replacement: diferences by race and gender, *Arthritis care & research* Vol. 51 (No. 1): 117-123.

Charles, C., Gafni, A. & Whelan, T. (1997). Shared decision-making in the medical encounter: What does it mean? (Or it takes at least two to tango), *Social science & medicine* Vol. 44 (No. 5): 681-692.

Denegar, C., Dougherty, D., Friedman, J., Schimizzi, M., Clark, J., Comstock, B. & Kraemer, W. (2010). Preferences for heat, cold, or contrast in patients with knee osteoarthritis affect treatment response, *Clinical interventions in aging* Vol. 5: 199–206

Edwards, A. & Elwyn, G. Decision-Making in health care. *Achieving evidence-based patient choice*. Second edition, New York: Oxford University press; 2009; 17-22.

Comas, M., Sala, M., Román, R., Hoffmeister, L. & Castells, X. (2010). Variaciones en la estimación de la prevalencia de artrosis de rodilla según los criterios diagnósticos utilizados en los estudios poblacionales, *Gaceta sanitaria* Vol. 24 (No. 1): 28–32.

Elliott, A., Kraus, V., Fang, F., Renner, J., Schwartz, T., Salazar, A., Huguenin, T., Hochberg, M., Helmick, C. & Jordan J. (2007). Joint-specific hand symptoms and self-reported and performance-based functional status in African Americans and Caucasians: the Johnston County Osteoarthritis Project. *Annals of the rheumatic diseases* Vol. 66 (No. 12): 1622-1626.

Escalante, A., Espinosa-Morales, R., del Rincon, I., Arroyo, R. & Older, S. (2000). Recipients of hip replacement for arthritis are less likely to be Hispanic, independent of access to health care and socioeconomic status, *Arthritis and rheumatism* Vol. 43 (No. 2): 390-399.

Foster, N., Thomas, E., Hill, J. & Hay, E. (2010). The relationship between patient and practitioner expectations and preferences and clinical outcomes in a trial of exercise and acupuncture for knee osteoarthritis, *European journal of pain* Vol. 14 (No. 4): 402–409.

Fraenkel, L., Bogardus, Jr., S., Concato, J. & Wittink, D. (2004). Treatment options in knee osteoarthritis: the patient's perspective, *Archives of internal medicine* Vol. 164 (No. 12): 1299-1304

Fraenkel, L., Rabidou, N., Wittink, D. & Fried, T. (2007). Improving informed decision-making for patients with knee pain, *The Journal of rheumatology* Vol. 34 (No. 9): 1894-1898.

Fraenkel, L. & Fried, T. (2008). If You Want Patients with Knee Osteoarthritis (OA) to Exercise: Tell them about NSAIDS, *Patient* Vol. 1 (No. 1): 21–26.

Gerteis, M., Edgman-Levitan, S., Daley, J., Delbanco, T. *Through the Patient's Eyes: Understanding and Promoting Patient-Centered Care.* San Francisco: Jossey-Bass; 1993.

Hawker, G., Wright, J., Coyte, P., Williams, J., Harvey, B., Glazier, R., Wilkins, A. & Badley, E., (2001). Determining the need for hip and knee arthroplasty: the role of clinical severity and patients' preferences, *Medical Care* Vol. 39 (No.3): 206-216.

Hawker, G., Wright, J., Badley, E. & Coyte, P. (2004). Perceptions of, and willingness to consider, total joint arthroplasty in a population-based cohort of individuals with disabling hip and knee arthritis, *Arthritis and rheumatism* Vol. 51 (No. 4): 635-641.

Hawker, G., Wright, J., Glazier, R., Coyte, P., Harvey, B., Williams, J. & Badley, E. (2002). The effect of education and income on need and willingness to undergo total joint arthroplasty, *Arthritis and rheumatism* Vol. 46 (No. 12): 3331-3339.

Hawker, G., Guan, J., Croxford, R., Coyte, P., Glazier, R., Harvey, B., Wright, J., Williams, J. & Badley, E. (2006). A prospective population-based study of the predictors of undergoing total joint arthroplasty, *Arthritis and rheumatism* Vol. 54 (No. 10): 3212–3220.

Hannan, M., Felson, D. & Pincus, T. (2000). Analysis of the discordance between radiographic changes and knee pain in osteoarthritis of the knee. *The Journal of rheumatology* Vol. 27 (No. 6): 1513-1517.

Hausmann, L., Mor, M., Hanusa, B., Zickmund, S., Cohen, P., Grant, R., Kresevic, D., Gordon, H., Ling, B., Kwoh, C. & Ibrahim, S. (2010). The effect of patient race on total joint replacement: recommendations and utilization in the orthopedic setting, *Journal of general internal medicine* Vol. 25 (No. 9): 982-989.

Ibrahim, S., Siminoff, L., Burant, C. & Kwoh, C. (2002a). Understanding ethnic differences in the utilization of joint replacement for osteoarthritis: the role of patient-level factors, *Medical care* Vol. 40 (Suppl 1): 144-151.

Ibrahim, S., Siminoff, L., Burant, C. & Kwoh, C. (2002b). Differences in expectations of outcome mediate African American/white patient differences in "willingness" to consider joint replacement, *Arthritis and rheumatism* Vol. 46 (No. 9): 2429-2435.

Ibrahim, S., Zhang, A., Mercer, M., Baughman, M. & Kwoh, C. (2004). Inner city African-american elderly patients´ perceptions and preferences for the care of chronic knee and hip pain: findings from focus groups, *Journal of gerontology* Vol. 59 (No. 12): 1318-1322.

Ibrahim, S., Siminoff, L., Burant, C. & Kwoh, C. (2001). Variation in perceptions of treatment and self-care practices in elderly with osteoarthritis: a comparison between African American and white patients, *Arthritis care & research* Vol. 45 (No. 4): 340–345.

Jordan, J., Helmick, C., Renner, J., Luta, G., Dragomir, A., Woodard, J., Fang, F., Schwartz, T., Abbate, L., Callahan, L., Kalsbeek, W. & Hochberg, M. (2007). Prevalence of knee symptoms and radiographic and symptomatic knee osteoarthritis in African Americans and Caucasians: the Johnston County Osteoarthritis Project, *The Journal of rheumatology* Vol. 34 (No. 1): 172-180.

Juby, A., Skeith, K. & Davis, P. (2005). Patients' awareness, utilization, and satisfaction with treatment modalities for the management of their osteoarthritis, *Clinical rheumatology* Vol. 24 (No. 5): 535–538.

Jones, A., Kwoh, C., Kelley, M. & Ibrahim, S. (2005). Racial disparity in knee arthroplasty utilization in the veterans health administration, *Arthritis and rheumatism* Vol. 53 (No. 6): 979-981.

Karlson, E., Daltroy, L., Liang, M., Eaton, H. & Katz, J. (1997). Gender differences in patient preferences may underlie differential utilization of elective surgery. *The American journal of medicine* Vol. 102 (No. 6): 524-530.

Kopec, J., Richardson, C., Llewellyn-Thomas, H., Klinkhoff, A., Carswell, A. & Chalmers, A. (2007). Probabilistic threshold technique showed that patients' preferences for specific trade-offs between pain relief and each side effect of treatment in osteoarthritis varied, *Journal of clinical epidemiology* Vol. 60 (No. 9): 929-938.

Kotlarz, H., Gunnarsson, C., Fang, H. & Rizzo, J. (2009). Insurer and out-of-pocket costs of osteoarthritis in the US: evidence from national survey data, *Arthritis and rheumatism* Vol. 60 (No. 12): 3546-3553.

Kroll, T., Richardson, M., Sharf, B. & Suarez-Almazor, M. (2007). "Keep on truckin'" or "it's got you in this little vacuum": race-based perceptions in decision-making for total knee arthroplasty, *The Journal of rheumatology* Vol. 34 (No. 5): 1069-1075.

Lawrence, R., Felson, D., Helmick, C., Arnold, L., Choi, H., Deyo, R., Gabriel, S., Hirsch, R., Hochberg, M., Hunder, G., Jordan, J., Katz, J., Kremers, H. & Wolfe, F. (2008). Estimates of the prevalence of arthritis and other rheumatic conditions in the United States. Part II, *Arthritis and rheumatism* Vol. 58 (No. 1): 26-35.

Losina, E., Walensky, R., Kessler, C., Emrani, P., Reichmann, W., Wright, E., Holt, H., Solomon, D., Yelin, E., Paltiel, A. & Katz, J. (2009). Cost-effectiveness of total knee arthroplasty in the United States: patient risk and hospital volume, *Archives of internal medicine* Vol. 169 (No. 12): 1113-1121.

Mitchell, H. & Hurley, M. (2008). Management of chronic knee pain: survey of patient preferences and treatment received, *BMC musculoskeletal disorders* Vol. 9: 123.

Oishi, C., Hoaglund, F., Gordon, L. & Ross, P. (1998). Total hip replacement rates are higher among Caucasians than Asians in Hawaii, *Clinical orthopaedics and related research* Vol. 353: 166-174.

O'Neill, T., Jinks, C. & Ong, B. (2007) Decision-making regarding total knee replacement surgery: a qualitative meta-synthesis, *BMC health services research* Vol. 7: 52.

Ratcliffe, J., Buxton, M., McGarry, T., Sheldon, R. & Chancellor, J. (2004). Patient´s preferences for characteristics associated with treatment for osteoarthritis, *Rheumatology* Vol. 43 (No. 3): 337-345.

Rottenstreich, Y., & Hsee, C. (2001). Money, kisses and electric shocks: On the affective psychology of probability weighting, *Psychological science* Vol. 12 (No. 3): 185–190.

Salaffi, F., Carotti, M., Stancati, A. & Grassi, W. (2005). Health-related quality of life in older adults with symptomatic hip and knee osteoarthritis: a comparison with matched healthy controls, *Aging clinical and experimental research* Vol. 17 (No. 4): 255-263.

Scott, D. & Kowalczyk, A. (2007). Osteoarthritis of the knee, *Clinical evidence* Vol. 12:1121

Skinner, J., Weinstein, J., Sporer, S. & Wennberg, J. (2003). Racial, ethnic, and geographic disparities in rates of knee arthroplasty among Medicare patients, *The New England journal of medicine* Vol. 349 (No. 14): 1350–1359.

Slovic, P., Peters, E., Finucane, M. & MacGregor-Bates, D. (2005). Affect, Risk, and Decision Making, *Health psychology* Vol. 24 (Suppl): 35-40

Srikanth, V., Fryer, J., Zhai, G., Winzenberg, T., Hosmer, D. & Jones G. (2005). A meta-analysis of sex differences prevalence, incidence and severity of osteoarthritis, *Osteoarthritis and cartilage* Vol. 13 (No. 9): 769-781.

Suarez-Almanzor, M., Souchek, J., Kelly, P., O´Malley, K., Byrne, M., Richardson, M. & Pak, C. (2005). Ethnic variations in knee replacement: patients preferences or uninformed disparity?, *Archives of internal medicine* Vol. 165 (No. 10): 1117-1124.

Tallon, D., Chard, J., & Dieppe, P. (2000). Exploring the priorities of patients with osteoarthritis of the knee, *Arthritis care & research.*Vol. 13 (No. 5): 312-319.

Thorstensson, C., Roos, E., Petersson, I. & Arvidsson, B. (2006). How do middle-aged patients conceive exercise as a form of treatment for knee osteoarthritis? *Disability and rehabilitation* Vol. 28 (No. 1): 51-59.

Underwood, M., Ashby, D., Cross, P., Hennesy, E., Letley, L., Martin, J., Mt-Isa, S., Parsons, S., Vickers, M. & Whyte, K. (2007). Advice to use topical or oral ibuprofen for chronic knee pain in older people: randomised controlled trial and patient preference study, *British Medical Association* Vol. 336 (No. 7636): 138-142.

van Dijk, G., Veenhof, C., Schellevis, F., Hulsmans, H., Bakker, J., Arwert, H., Dekker, J., Lankhorst, G. & Dekker, J. (2008). Comorbidity, limitations in activities and pain in patients with osteoarthritis of the hip or knee, *BMC musculoskeletal disorders* Vol. 9: 95.

Weng, H., Kaplan, R., Boscardin, W., Maclean, C., Lee, I., Chen, W. & Fitzgerald, J. (2007). Development of a decision aid to address racial disparities in utilization of knee replacement surgery, *Arthritis and rheumatism*. Vol. 57 (No. 4): 568-575.

Wolfe, F., Zhao, S. & Lane, N. (2000). Preference for nonsteroidal antiinflammatory drugs over acetaminophen by rheumatic disease patients, *Arthritis and rheumatism.* Vol. 43 (No. 2): 378–385.

13

The Plica: Is a New Aetiological Factor in the Knee Osteoarthritis?

Ahmet Guney* and Ibrahim Kafadar
From the Department of Orthopaedics, Erciyes University Medical Faculty, Kayseri, Turkey

1. Introduction

Osteoarthritis is one of the most important diseases in the field of orthopedics worldwide. The disease is characterized by progressive loss of articular cartilage and formation of osteophytes, which lead to chronic pain and functional restrictions in the affected joints.

Different factors can be involved in the development of osteoarthritis including traumatic events, genetic predisposition, defective position of joints, and ageing and malnutrition.

The plica is the generic name of the ruins or folds of the synovial membrane in the knee joint. The incidence of the plicas in the knee joint is between 18,5-87 %. These plicas are named and classified according to their settlements in the knee joint (1-6).

The plicas sometimes come to a pathologic state, which gains clinical importance and causes the plica syndrome (7). When plica is symptomatic, the condition is called plica syndrome. The plicas are considered to be one of the potential causes of the complaints around the knee joint (8).

It is known that medial plica causes to degeneration of cartilage around the medial femoral condyle of the knee joint and / or the medial pole of the patella (2,8-14). Owing to the anatomic location of the medial plica, a loss of normal elasticity can cause it to impinge on the femoral medial condyle or the medial facet of the patella during flexion–extension motion of the knee. This kind of repetitive contact may result in a chondral lesion of varying severity, sometimes referred to as an impingement lesion (2,7,8,14-18).

It has also been suggested that normal-looking medial plica, not impinging on the articular surfaces, could be symptomatic as well . This is supported by recent findings which have demonstrated an increase in the amount of nerve endings in the plica after trauma or overuse, indicating increased pain sensitivity and sensation of pain (19,20).

The anatomy of the plicas or synovial folds was first described by Mayeda in 1918. In 1939, Lino first described the appearance of arthroscopic synovial folds in the cadaveric knees. In 1950 and 1971, Pipkin reported that the plicas should be distinguished from adhesions in the knee joint and those might cause clinical symptoms (21,22).

---

*Corresponding author

2. Embryology

The knee embryologically develops from mesoderm in several developement stages. At the first weeks of the fetal development, the mesenchymal origined intra-articular knee joint membrane separates the knee joint into three compartments, the medial and lateral tibiofemoral compartment, and the suprapatellar bursa. This membrane is usually resorbed between the weeks of 9.5 and 12. Later on, these compartments coalesce to form a single large cavity. However, if this membrane is not completely resorbed, membranous structure forms in different locations in the knee joint. These membranous structures, when persist as normal folds of synovial membrane in the knee joint, are termed as plica (10,22,23).

3. Anatomy, classification and incidence

Generally plicas have been classified into three predominant types based on their anatomical location; the infrapatellar plica or ligamentum mucosum, the suprapatellar plica and the medial patellar plica or the medial shelf. Lateral plica have also been described but are considered a much more rare entity. These can vary in morphology and can exist in combinations. Arthroscope is a boon in visualizing intra-articular anatomy and pathology, and it also allows precise assessment and dynamic examination of the plica (24).

3.1 Suprapatellar plica

This type of plica takes origin from the inferior face of tendon of quadriceps and lies transversly in the suprapatellar pouch and attaches to the superomedial and lateral walls of the knee joint. Different anatomical variations of the suprapatellar plica have been described. According to Kim and collegues there are different types, such as; absence of plica, vestigial shaped, medially cited, laterally cited, arch shaped, hole shaped and total septum. The most seen type of this group is medial suprapatellar plica (1,2).

Most arthroscopic studies have reported an incidence of some form of plica between 70% and 91%. Dandy in a study of 500 knees attempted to classify the suprapatellar plica arthroscopically. He described 10 variations with an overall incidence of 91% (1,2,4).

3.2 Mediopatellar plica

The medial plica has been given many names as it may reflect many variations of size, configurations, and attachments: Plica synovialis mediopatellaris, mediopatellar plica, medial shelf, Lino's band, Aoki's ledge, plica alaris elongata, medial intra-articular band meniscus of patella (2,8,12).

It originates on the medial wall of the knee joint and may or may not cross the suprapatellar plica passing obliquely, from the medial side of patella through to the distal, downward in the coronal plane to insert into the synovium surrounding the infrapatellar fat pad (1,2,7).

Lino first described four types of plica in 1939. And then Sakibara arranged these four types such as; Type A is a cord like structure in the synovial wall that can be traced to the fat

pad. Type B has a shelf like appearance but does not cover the femoral condyle. Type C has a large shelf like structure and can be seen to cover the anterior surface of the medial femoral condyle. Type D is a variation in which two insertions into the medial wall can be seen. There is a defect of plica that covers the whole medial femoral condyle (16).

Dandy reported difficulty in creating a classification to describe the medial patella plica and settled for a classification based upon the maximum width and position along with the incidence of each.

Dandy classification: type A, absence of any medial plica; type B, a narrow ridge at the medial wall of the knee joint; type C, width of the plica < 1 cm; type D, width of the plica 1-2 cm; type E, width of the plica >2 cm; type F, presence of a defect within the plica; type G, plica is high type but not contacting the medial femoral condyle; and type H, the plica is re-duplicated (4).

There are large variations in the reported incidence of medial plica ranging from 17 to 75%.

The incidence of the medial patella plica is difficult to define as different interpretations of its presence have been used with some authors considering a small fold of synovium as a plica and others indicating this as absent. The more recent arthroscopic studies where a fold of tissue was considered a plica give an overall incidence of 92% and 72% (1,4,25).

The medial plica is considered the most problematic by many authors (Muse et al,1985; Patel, 1986; Kim and Choe, 1996; Dupont, 1997) due to its close proximity to the medial border of the patella and medial femoral condyle where it can be'impinged'(1,2,24,26).

3.3 Infrapatellar plica

The infrapatellar plica is more commonly known as the ligamentum mucosum. It originates from the intercondylar notch, spreads paralel to the anterior cruciat ligament and inserts into the synovium around the infrapatellar fat pad.

The infrapatellar plica is a common finding at knee arthroscopy with Kim and Choe reporting an overall incidence of 86%. Kim et al. have been the first to describe an arthroscopic classification of the infrapatellar plica and used its relation to the ACL and morphology to classify it(1,25,27).

According to this classification;

Absent: no synovial fold between the condyles of the femur.

Separated: A complete synovial fold that was separate from the anterior cruciate ligament (ACL).

Split : Synovial fold that is separate from the ACL but is also divided into two or more cords.

Vertical septum: A complete synovial fold tht is attached to the ACL and divided the joint into medial and lateral compartments.

Fenestra: A vertical septum pattern that contains a hole or defect.

3.4 Lateral plica

The lateral plica is considered to be rare. Overall incidence was found 1,3% by Kim and collegues. It originates from the lateral wall of the knee above the popliteal hiatus and inserts into the synovium around the infrapatellar fat pad (1,2).

4. Pathophysiology

Normally plica exists as thin flexible soft tissue structures, mainly composed of elastic and areolar tissue. Due to this property, it changes its shape and length with knee movements (7). Inflammation of the synovial tissue makes plica edematous and thickened, and in chronic cases, it looses its inherent elastic nature and becomes thick and fibrosed. And even it hyalinize and rarely becomes calcified. Then plica can cause secondary mechanical synovitis around the femoral condyles. Mediopatellar plica is trapped between the anteromedial portion of the medial femoral condyle and the medial pole of the patella with flexion of the knee. This pathologic thickness of plica causes articular cartilage degeneration the anteromedial portion of the medial femoral condyle and the medial pole of the patella by the continuity of knee movements (2,9,28-32).

Plica become pathological when thickening and fibrosis occurs giving rise to relative inelasticity that can lead to it snapping over the femoral condyle causing synovitis, chondral damage and pain. The plica syndrome was described by Hardaker and defined as a painful impairment of knee function inwhich the only findingwas the presence of a thickened, hypertrophic plica (7).

Generally, direct injury to the knee leading to synovial hematoma and post-traumatic transient synovitis is one of the commonest factors coupled with the development of pathological medial plica (24). In some cases, repetitive and overuse of knee as per task-specific demands or athletic activities associated with minor irregularities of knee mechanics cause progressive inflammation with recurrent synovitis, edema, thickening, and fibrosis of plica (33).

It can also get involved in any primary disorder of knee capable of producing synovitis such as torn meniscus, loose bodies, and osteochondritis dissecans. Many authors accept that wider plicas are more often symptomatic and more frequently demonstrate pathologic changes at histological analysis than thinner plica (34). Normally, medial plica slides smoothly over medial femoral condyle in flexion and extension, and it remains in contact with the condyleduring whole range of motion. Thus, pathological plica, with movement of knee may generate some shearing force acting on the condyle, has a role in the pathogenesis of degeneration of the cartilage on the medial femoral condyle (35).

Being in close proximity to medial femoral condyle, plica may provoke secondary mechanical synovitis about the margins of condyle. The fibrotic plica can bowstring across the trochlea and condyle or can get impinged between the patella and medial femoral condyle, altering the patello-femoral mechanics (32,36).

However, this aberrant mechanics is directly related to degeneration of articular cartilage of patello-femoral joint. And there are high incidences of chondromalacia reported in pathological medial plica involving medial femoral condyle and medial patellar facet (37,38).

The severity of the degeneration was positively correlated with the severity of the medial plica and patients'age (15).

In the arthroscopy study of Christoforakis and Strachan on 1,000 patients, a total of 319 mediopatellar plicas were identified, and cartilage degeneration was found at medial femoral condyle and/or medial pole of patella in 24.7% of these cases (13).

In that study, isolated patellofemoral cartilage degeneration was present in 15.5% of knees not having mediopatellar plica. Authors concluded that mediopatellar plica leads to patellofemoral joint degeneration.

In an another study, cartilage degeneration was found in higher degrees patients at medial femoral condyle and medial pole of patella. Significant clinical and functional improvements were observed early after plica excision in patients with mediopatellar plica and associated cartilage degeneration. Pain score, physical function score, total score and the mean score of WOMAC were all decreased at 6 weeks compared to baseline (39).

Excessive exercises, sports activities and the chronic hyperflexion of the knee due to life style can cause the plica syndrome.

Even if plica does not touch the bone structures, it may disrupt the function of quadriceps tendon due to its tension and may cause pain by applying traction to the synovium and fat pad.
The function of plica has not been fully understood. However, plicas have neural elements according to some studies.
Quadriceps atrophy can occur in up to 45% of patients with a pathological plica. This concurs with the current view that atrophy is caused by chondromalacia and develops soon after the plica irritation (6,7).
In the case of medial plica trauma, biomechanical factors may cause it to enlarge, resulting in impingement between the medial border of the trochlea's medial facet and the medial facet of the patella. Impingement occurs during flexion of the knee between 40° and 80° when the gap between the patella and femoral joint is at its closest. Continued impingement of the plica with repeated flexion may cause chondromalacia, groove formation within the articular cartilage and a thickening of the plica. This is associated with a clicking or loud snapping sound on flexion/extension of the knee (2,26,40).

5. Clinical signs and symptoms

The most frequent complaint is pain (8). Most common presentation of medial plica syndrome is anteromedial knee pain. The pain is usually in front of the knee but it may also be on the the antero-medial and anterior-lateral, medial and lateral joint space. The pain is usually intermittent, and occurs with activity. Pain is significant while climbing stairs like other patellofemoral problems (10).
The cinema sign is positive. The increase of the pain when the knee is flexed for a long time, and then a relief by extension of the knee is decribed as positive cinema sign.
A pathological plica produces popping or catching in knee by snapping across patella or medial femoral condyle. Other symptoms associated with anteromedial pain include swelling of knee, feeling of tightness, and stiffness (7,24,36,37).
Sometimes pain and clicking of previously asymptomatic medial plica starts as a result of tear, due to rubbing of torned portion of plica over medial femoral condyle. Thus, one cause of anterior knee pain can be tear of plica along with thickening and fibrotic changes. A very rare presentation, hemearthrosis, caused by large medial plica has also been reported (41,42).
In physical examination when the knee is in extension posture, pain with the palpation of the medial lower pole of patella is specific. Sensitivity can be found in the medial joint space when the knee is in flexion.
Examination remains unreliable in most patients but common findings are quadriceps wasting, effusion, medial condyle tenderness, crepitus and decreased range of motion (26,37).
Provocative tests for meniscal tears are often positive but have poor specificity. Signs forpatellofemoral pathology are also often positive but again offer poor specificity (8). It is occasionally possible to palpate the thickened plica as a tight band mostly superomedially which will be tender to palpate and can be felt to click or catch with movement (43).
A number of provocative tests for pathological plica have been described.
Plica can be rolled over medial femoral condyle as it is thickened and fibrosed. A palpable or sometimes audible snap is present when knee passes from 30° to 60° of flexion(7,24).
Pipkin has described the pop that occurs, as the knee is extended from 90° of flexion with foot internally rotated and the patella pressed medially, between 60° and 45° of flexion of knee (22).

Two provocative tests described by Koshino and Okamato are helpful in diagnosing pathological medial plica. Rotation valgus test is elicited by flexing the knee and applying a valgus force on internally and externally rotating the tibia while simultaneously attempting to displace the patella medially. The other one is holding test, done by attempting to flex the knee against active resistance. If either test elicits pain, with or without a click, it is considered positive (32,44).
Kim et al. named his the medial patella plica test or MPP test (45). It is performed by applying a manual force to the infero-medial portion of the patellofemoral joint. Whilst maintaining the force the knee is flexed to 90 degrees. A positive test occurs when the patient experiences pain in extension but this is eliminated at 90 degrees of flexion.
Other provocative tests have previously been described by Pipkin, but this test relied upon no effusion being present and was often found to be negative later in the day, it therefore became dubbed the 'morning test'(22).
Shetty et al. in their prospective study over 66 knees, devised a system to diagnose symptomatic medial plica based on history and clinical examination. It includes five essential and four desirable criteria. Essential criteria are as follows: [1]. history of anteromedial knee pain, [2]. Pain primarily over medial femoral condyle, [3]. visible or palpable plica, [4]. tenderness over palpable plica, [5]. Exclusion of other causes of anteromedial knee pain. Desirable criteria are as follows: [1] onset blunt or trivial trauma, [2] Duvet test (use of a duvet placed between knees to prevent pain while sleeping, [3] audible snap during active range of motion, and [4] palpable snap during flexion. This systemHas diagnostic accuracy of 91.7%, sensitivity of 100%, and positive predictive value of 91.7% (32,38).
Diagnosis with routine blood tests may often be unhelpful as inflammatory markers almost invariably are normal. Radiographs of the knee do not demonstrate a plica but help to exclude other pathology. Double contrast arthrograms have historically been used and are able to demonstrate plica reliably but are unable to distinguish between pathological and non-pathological plica. It had been hoped that the advent of MRI would be useful in aiding the diagnosis of a pathological plica. Although it has been able to demonstrate plica reliably, it has not been able to predict the necessity of excision of that plica at arthroscopy, which limits its use as a screening tool (46-51).
Arthroscopy is still the gold standard modality to diagnose pathological medial plica.
Definitive diagnosis can only be made by arthroscopy, and it allows precise assessment of plica including dynamic examination. The normal plica is thin, pink, and pliable, whereaspathological plica is white, thickened, and fibrotic (7,32).

6. Treatment

6.1 Conservative treatment

In all cases, conservative treatment should be tried first (2,7-9). Rest and nonsteroidal anti-inflammatory drugs are used to resolve the pain and, after the removal of acute painful period rehabilitation program starts. Physical therapy is given in the form of local heat, ultrasound, short-wave diathermy, along with quadriceps and hamstring stretching exercises.
The basis of rehabilitation program includes quadriceps and hamstring strengthening and stretching exercises (3,28).
Objective of physiotherapy is to increase the structural flexibility of tissues and decrease compressive forces on the knee.

The response taken from the case determines the duration of the conservative treatment. Even if the improvement is visible partially with the treatment for two or three months, conservative treatment should be continued. If there is no reduction in pain, surgical treatment should be started. With the increase of pain in patients, early surgical treatment could be planned (3).

In addition injection of local anesthetic and corticosteroid can be given into the plica and surrounding synovial tissues. Rovere et al. reported overall success rate of 73% and poor results were obtained in chronic fibrotic plica (52).

Patients who do not respond to conservative therapy or have recurrence of symptoms are essentially the candidates for arthroscopic examination of knee joint.

6.2 Surgical treatment

The medial patella plica is most commonly associated with symptoms and is frequently considered to be pathological. There are very few reports in the literature of the infrapatellar plica being pathological. On the other hand, the suprapatellar plica has been implicated more commonly in pathology. Kyung Bae reported a series of 30 complete type suprapatellar plicae with 90% of the patients reporting good or excellent results following arthroscopic excision (53).

Patients who do not respond to conservative treatment, surgical treatment is applied. If a plica causes friction on medial femoral condyle or pinches between the patella and medial femoral condyle, it should be excised. But arthrotomy should not be done for excision.

According to Patel's surgical indications are as follows;

1. Palpation of clinically painful and sensitive band
2. Determination of thickened and subluxated mediopatellar plica existance with or without cartilage lesions at patella or femur
3. If arthroscopy is performed under local anesthesy, streching plica with a hook causes complaints of patient
4. Without the determination of other pathologies clinically and arthroscopically (2,3).

For arthroscopic surgery, usually standard portals like antero-medial, antero-lateral are used. Brief et al. described superolateral approach as a better arthroscopic portal for medial plica, and it offers a sweeping, unobstructed view of entire plica, and also good visualization of patello-femoral joint (7,54).

Visualisation of all the compartments of the knee and probing of the menisci should also be performed to ensure no other pathological cause of pain is present within the knee.

Accessory portals can be created to allow better visualisation of the patellofemoral and suprapatellar compartments. If any other pathology isfound, it needs to be treated appropriately (32).

Arthroscopic excision of medial plica is carried out as a day procedure. Complete resection of pathological plica to the capsular attachment is advisable. Many studies reported good to excellent results with this procedure(8,24,36-38). However, extensive excision of medial plica can lead to patellar subluxation (55,56).

During the medial plica surgery, knee should be in full extension. Mild flexion of the knee complicates the surgery.

The amount of excision is controversial. The main operations in the literature are; the division of the plica just as band, total excision and segmental resection. The division of the plica may cause recurrances. The radical resection may lead to formation of tense fibrotic tissue through the capsule and subcutaneous fat tissue. A thin peripheric edge is left in the procedure of subtotal resection. In this way capsule and synovium is not traumatised and because of this formation of fibrous tissue is not seen. As described by Dandy, segmental resection may be insufficent for large and hard plicas (4,9,28,29,36,37).

The normal or asymptomatic plicas should not be excised which are detected incidentally. Some researchers suggest the excision of plicas to prevent the complaints in the future except thin and distant plicas from bony structures.

Plicas have copious blood supply around the synovial attachments, and thus it is necessary to achieve hemostasis to prevent complications of intra-articular bleed post-operatively (10,54).

Post-operatively, compression bandage is applied over the joint. Mobilization is started on same day with the help of physical therapist, and early knee physiotherapy is encouraged to prevent stiffness and scarring of plica (7,10,55).

Plicas around the knee are common findings at arthroscopy but are rarely pathological. The plica syndrome is a cause of anterior knee pain and can be debilitating for patients. Inflammation and synovitis causes fibrosis and thickening of the plica. And then plica starts to behave like a bowstring causing to impingement and cartilage damage.

If a thickened and hypertrophic pathological plica is found at arthroscopy and completely excised good results from the artroscopical excision can be expected in the majority of the patients.

Surgical excision of mediopatellar plica associated with cartilage degeneration appears to result in substantial clinical improvement, thus representing an effective treatment modality for this group of patients.

7. References

[1] Kim SJ, Choe WS. Arthroscopic findings of the synovial plicae of the knee. Arthroscopy 1997;13:33-41.

[2] Patel D.Plica as a cause of anterior knee pain. Orthop Clin North Am. 1986;17 :273-7

[3] Pınar H. Plica Syndrome a case of anterior knee pain. Acta Orthop Traumatol Turc 1988;22:268

[4] Dandy DJ. Anatomy of the medial suprapatellar plica and medial synovial shelf.Arthroscopy. 1990;6:79-85.

[5] Alturfan A, Pınar H, Taşer Ö. Mediopatellar plika sendromunun tanı ve tedavisinde artroskopinin önemi. Acta Orthop Traumatol Turc 1991;25: 294

[6] Ammatuzzi MM, Fazzi A, Varella MH. Pathologic synovial plica of the knee. Results of conservative treatment. Am J Sports Med 1990; 18:466-9

[7] Hardaker WT, Whipple TL, Bassett FH III. Diagnosis and treatment of the plica syndrome of the knee. J Bone Joint Surg 1980; 62:221-5

[8] Tindel NL, Nisonson B. The plica syndrome. Orthop Clin North Am 1992;23:613

[9] Munzinger U, Ruckstuhl J, Scherrer H, Gschwend N. Internal derangement of the knee joint due to pathologic synovial folds: the mediopatellar plica syndrome. Clin Orthop Relat Res 1981;155:59-64

[10] Schindler OS. Synovial plicae of the knee. Current Orthopaedics 2004; 18: 210-9

[11] Sung-Jae K, Jae-Hoon J, Young-Min C, Sang-Wook R. MPP test in the diagnosis of the medial patellar plica syndrome. The Journal of the Arthroscopic and Related Surg 2004;20 :10101-3

[12] Vaughan-Lane T, Dandy DJ. The synovial shelf syndrome. J Bone Joint Surg 1982; 64: 475

[13] Christoforakis JJ, Strachan RK. Internal derangements of the knee associated with patellofemoral joint degeneration. Knee Surg Sports Traumatol Arthrosc. 2005 ;13:581-4
[14] Christoforakis JJ, Ballester J, Hunt N, Thomas R, Strachan RK. Synovial shelves of the knee: association with chondral lesions. Knee Surg Sports Traumatol Arthrosc. 2006 ;14:1292-8
[15] Lyu SR, Hsu CC. Medial plicae and degeneration of the medial femoral condyle. Arthroscopy 2006;22:17–26.
[16] Sakibara J. Arthroscopic study on Iinos's band (plica synovialis mediopatellaris) [In Japanese]. Nippon Seikeigekai Gakkai zasshi. 1976;513–22.
[17] Dorchak JD, Barrack RL, Kneisl JS, Alexander AH. Arthroscopic treatment of symptomatic synovial plica of the knee. Long-term followup. Am J Sports Med 1991;19:503–7.
[18] Hansen H, Boe S. The pathological plica in the knee. Results after arthroscopic resection. Arch Orthop Trauma Surg 1989;108:282–4.
[19] Irha E, Vrdoljak J. Medial synovial plica syndrome of the knee: a diagnostic pitfall in adolescent athletes. J Pediatr Orthop B 2003;12:44–8
[20] Farkas C, Hargitai Z, Gaspar L, Kuki A, Csernatony Z, Szepesi K. Histological changes in the symptomatic mediopatellar plica. Knee 2004;11:103–8.
[21] Aglietti P, Buzzi R, Insall JN. Disorders of the patellofemoral joint. In: Insall JN, Scott WN. (eds), Surgery of the knee (3rd ed) Curchill Livingstone, Pennsylvania 2001, 913-1043
[22] Pipkin G. Knee injuries: the role of the suprapatellar plica and suprapatellar bursa insimulating internal derangements.Clin Orthop Relat Res. 1971;74:161-76.
[23] Ogata S, Uhthoff HK. The development of synovial plicae in human knee joints: an embryologic study.Arthroscopy. 1990;6:315-21.
[24] Dupont JY Synovial plicae of the knee. Controversies and review. Clin Sports Med 1997;16(1):87-122
[25] Kent M, Khanduja V. Synovial plicae around the knee. Knee. 2010; 17(2):97-102.
[26] Muse, G, Grana, W and Hollingsworth, S. Arthroscopic treatment of medial shelf syndrome. Journal of Arthroscopy. 1985;1,63-7.
[27] Kim SJ, Min BH, Kim HK. Arthroscopic anatomy of the infrapatellar plica. Arthroscopy 1996; 12(5):561–4.
[28] Pınar H: Dizde sinovyal patolojiler ve plika sendromları. In: Tandoğan RN, Alpaslan M (ed), Diz cerrahisi, Haberal Eğitim Vakfı, Ankara 1999, 283-98.
[29] Kinnard P, Levesque RY. The plica syndrome. A syndrome of controversy. Clin Orthop Relat Res. 1984 ;183:141-3.
[30] Barry BP. Arthroscopy of lower extremity. In: Canale ST (ed), Campbell's Operative Orthopaedics (10th ed) Mosby, Pennsylvania 2003, 2515-2612
[31] Dorchak JD, Barrack RL, Kneisl JS, Alexander AH. Arthroscopic treatment of symptomatic synovial plicae of the knee . Long -term follow up. Am J Sports Med. 1991;19(5):503-7.
[32] Nigam A, Shetty VD. The medial plica: a clinical perspective. Eur J Orthop Surg Traumatol. 2011
[33] Blok A, Weiss W, Dolata T, Szczepaniec M Medial synovial plica. Ortop Traumatol Rehabil. 2005;7(4):397-40
[34] Zidorn T Classification of the suprapatellar septum considering ontogenetic development. Artroscopy.1992;8:459-64

[35] Lyu SR Relationship of medial plica and medial femoral condyle during flexion. Clin Biomech (Bristol,Avon).2007;22(9):1013-16
[36] Broom MJ, Fulkerson JP The plica syndrome: a new perspective. Orthop Clin North Am.1986;17(2):279-81
[37] Richmond JC, McGinty JB Segmental arthroscopic resection of the hypertrophic mediopatellar plica. Clin Orthop Relat Res.1983;178:185-89
[38] Shetty VD, Vowler SL, Krishnamurthy S, Halliday AE Clinical diagnosis of medial plica syndrome of the knee: a prospective study. J Knee Surg.2007;20(4):277-80
[39] Guney A,Bilal O, Oner M, Halici M, Turk Y, Tuncel M. Short- and mid-term results of plica excision in patients with mediopatellar plica and associated cartilage degeneration.Knee Surg Sports Traumatol Arthrosc. 2010; 18(11):1526-31.
[40] Aprin, H, Shapiro, J and Gerschwind, M. Arthrography (plica views). Clinical Orthopaedics and Related Research. 1983; 68,1,90-5.
[41] Kerimoglu S, Citlak A, Cavusoglu S, Turhan AU Bucket handle tear of medial plica. Knee. 2005;12(3):239-41
[42] Yamamoto Z, Fujita A, Minami G, Ishida R, Abe M Atraumatic hemarthrosis caused by a large mediopatellar plica. Arthroscopy.2001;17(4):415-17
[43] Kim SJ, Lee DH, Kim TE. The relationship between the MPP test and arthroscopicallyfound medial patellar plica pathology. Arthroscopy 2007;23(12):1303–8.
[44] Koshino T, Okamoto R Resection of painful shelf (plica synovialis mediopatellaris) under arthroscopy. Arthroscopy. 1995;11(6):738
[45] Kim SJ, Jeong JH, Cheon YM, Ryu SW. MPP test in the diagnosis of medial patellar plica syndrome. Arthroscopy 2004; 20(10):1101–3.
[46] Laissy JP, Schouman-Claeys E, Lacombe P, Dupont JY, Halimi P, Frija G. Value and limits of arthrography in the study of pathological mediopatellar plicae of the knee; a comparison with arthroscopy. Eur J Radiol 1990;11(2):93–7
[47] Lupi L, Bighi S, Cervi PM, Limone GL, Massari L. Arthrography of the plica syndrome and its significance. Eur J Radiol 1990;11(1):15–8.
[48] Boles CA, Butler J, Lee JA, Reedy ML, Martin DF. Magnetic resonance characteristics of medial plica of the knee: correlation with arthroscopic resection. J Comput Assist Tomogr 2004;28(3):397–401
[49] Kobayashi Y, Murakami R, Tajima H, Yamamoto K, Ichikawa T, Mase Y, et al. Direct MR arthrography of plica synovialis mediopatellaris. Acta Radiol 2001; 42 (3):286–90.
[50] Nakanishi K, Inoue M, Ishida T, Murakami T, Tsuda K, Ikezoe J, et al. MR evaluation of mediopatellar plica. Acta Radiol 1996;37(4):567–71
[51] Jee WH, Choe BY, Kim JM, Song HH, Choi KH. The plica syndrome: diagnostic value of MRI with arthroscopic correlation. J Comput Assist Tomogr 1998;22(5):814–8
[52] Rovere GD, Adair DM. Medial synovial shelf plica syndrome. Treatment by intraplical steroid injection.Am J Sports Med. 1985;13:382-6
[53] Bae DK, Nam GU, Sun SD, Kim YH. The clinical significance of the complete type of suprapatellar membrane. Arthroscopy 1998;14(8):830–5
[54] Brief LP, Laico JP The superolateral approach: a beter view of the medial patellar plica. Arthroscopy.1987;3(3):170-72
[55] Johnson DP, Eastwood DM, Witherow PJ Symptomatic synovial plicae of the knee. J Bone Joint Surg Am.1993; 75(10):1485-96
[56] Limbird TJ. Patellar subluxation following plica resection. Orthop Rev. 1988;17:282-85

14

Knee Osteoarthritis and Associated Periarticular Conditions: Iliotibial Band Friction and Baker Cyst

Violeta Vasilevska[1], Ulrike Szeimies[2], Milan Samardziski[1] and Axel Stäbler[2]
[1]*University Surgical Clinic "St Naum Ohrldski" Skopje,*
[2]*Radiologie in München Harlaching, Munich,*
[1]*Rep. Macedonia*
[2]*Germany*

1. Introduction

Osteoarthritis (OA) is a highly prevalent disease with markedly increasing impact worldwide because of the aging of populations (Center for disease control and prevention (CDC); Murphy L.et al., 2008). It affects more than 21 milion people in the U.S. (Handout on Health: Osteoarthritis), with 36% of elderly aged 70 or older having some degree of radiographic knee OA (D'Ambrosia et al., 2005; Felson et al., 1987). It is a major public health problem, with prevalence in the knee of approximately 30% in those over 65 years old (Felson et al., 1987).

The cause of knee pain in patients with OA remains unclear. Because hyaline cartilage has no innervations (Dye et al., 1998), the primary pathologic abnormality in OA (hyaline cartilage loss) could occur without pain. In MRI studies is reported an increase the prevalence of subchondral bone marrow edema, knee joint effusion, and synovial thickening in patients with symptomatic knee OA compared with patients with no symptoms (Hill et al., 2001; Felson et al., 2001). Knee with OA are biomechanically altered, and these changes may put stress on ligament and tendon insertion sites in and around the knee joint, creating pain (Hill et al., 2003). Some of the pain does not emanate from the joint itself but rather from the structures near the joint that contain pain fibers. Wide ranges of periarticular lesions occur around the knee joint, including popliteal Baker cyst (BC) (Vasilevska et.al., 2008, Janzen et al., 1994) and friction of the iliotibial band (ITBF) (Vasilevska et al., 2009).

Iliotibial band friction syndrome (ITBFS) is an inflammatory overuse disorder affecting soft tissue, interposed between the iliotibial band and the lateral femoral condyle, caused by chronic friction (Muhle et al., 1999). Recently, an anatomic study disclosed a fibrous anchorage of the iliotibial band to the femur preventing rolling over the epicondyle; therefore ITBFS is mainly caused by increased pressure to the richly innervated and vascularized fat and loose connective tissue beneath the tract (Fairclough et al., 2006, 2007). Either ITBFS has been shown to cause lateral knee pain in athletes, it may be a consequence of gait changes induced by knee OA and may occur together with symptomatic knee OA (presented only 3 cases with low grade ITBF, only one with symptom) (Hill et al., 2003).

Recent reports have suggested a 60% reduction in cartilage volume in severe knee osteoarthritis (Vahlensieck et al., 2001; Fritschy et al., 2006). Medial compartment cartilage loss leads to varus deformity, which can affect knee biomechanics by altering the relationship of the iliotibial band and the lateral epicondyle with the possibility of an increased friction and pressure between these structures.

In contrary it is well known that popliteal (Baker) cyst is the most frequent encountered lesion around the knee. Among older individual with asymptomatic OA, popliteal cyst have a high prevalence (20,8%) (Hill et al., 2001). Cystic lesions around the knee may present as a painless palpable mass (Kornaat et al., 2006; Hill et al., 2003), with pain, with symptoms of tenderness in the posterior fossa (Hill et al., 2003) or to be detected during the routine MR imaging of the knee with suspected internal joint derangement (Mc Carthy et al., 2004), eventually when is large can be painful.

Multiple studies confirmed that intraarticular derangement play an important role in pathogenesis of popliteal cyst. MR studies of popliteal cyst demonstrated connection to one or more intraarticular lesions in 87-98% of the cases, like osteoarthritis or inflammatory arthritis; often joint effusion, meniscus tear and degenerative disease of the joint are found (Miller et al., 1996).

During the routine practice in cases with advanced isolated medial osteoarthritis (with subsequent genu varum) presence of MR signs of friction of ITB have been noted. The purpose of the study was to describe the frequency of fibrovascular tissue between the iliotibial tract and the lateral epicondyle in patients with severe isolated medial compartment osteoarthritis of the knee (Vasilevska et al., 2009). From this cases were selected those with Baker cyst, and the correlation between sizes of Baker cyst in patients suffering from medial compartment osteoarthritis of the knee was recognized and evaluated. The purpose was to describe the significance of the associated medial compartment knee osteoarthritis: cartilage degeneration, different degree of medial meniscus degeneration, bone edema and knee effusion.

In a study which was done 2009, in a 128 patients retrospectively selected from 700 MR examinations of patients with advanced medial compartment osteoarthritis of the knee, with > 80% loss of articular cartilage at the femur and the tibia, a relationship with MR signs of ITBF was presented. In this study MR signs for ITBF were present in 95 patients (74.2%). Out of them 91 patient had moderate signs for ITBF and 4 had severe MR signs for presence of fibrovascular tissue (Table 1) (Vasilevska et al., 2009).

	ITBF 0 - absent	ITBF 1 - present	ITBF 2 - severe	total
Study group	33 (25.8%)	91 (71.1%)	4 (3.1%)	128
Control group	68 (72.3%)	26 (27.7%)	0	94

Table 1. Presence of MR signs of ITBF in the study group with severe medial compartment osteoarthritis and in the control group (consensus reading).

Patients with complete cartilage loss as well as patients with subtotal cartilage loss showed tendency to further increase the incidence of MR signs of ITBF, when advanced degeneration of the medial meniscus was present (Table 2).

Cartilage degneration	Meniscus degeneration	ITBF 0 - absent	ITBF 1 - present	ITBF 2 - severe	Total
complete loss	1st degree	0	2	0	2
complete loss	2nd degree	2	7	0	9
complete loss	3rd degree	14	42	2	58
	total	16 (12.5%)	51 (39.8%)	2 (1.6%)	*69 (53.9%)*
subtotal loss	1st degree	3	9	0	12
subtotal loss	2nd degree	3	12	1	16
subtotal loss	3rd degree	11	19	1	31
	total	17 (13.3%)	40 (31.3%)	2 (1.6%)	*59 (46.1%)*
	Column Total	33 (25.8%)	**91 (71.1%)**	**4 (3.1%)**	***128***

Table 2. Presence of MRI signs of ITBF in the group with severe medial compartment osteoarthritis correlated with cartilage degeneration and meniscal lesions.

Clinically, patients with medial sided osteoarthritis of the knee, occasionally also complain of laterally located pain. ITBF is unrecognized cause for lateral knee pain in patients with medial compartment knee osteoarthritis (Vasilevska et al., 2009).
When severe cartilage damage is associated with advanced degeneration of the medial meniscus, altered biomechanics probably with varus deformity, may contribute to the development of fibrovascular tissue between the iliotibial band and the lateral epicondyle on MR images as a recognized sign of ITBF (Fig.1) (Vasilevska et al., 2009).

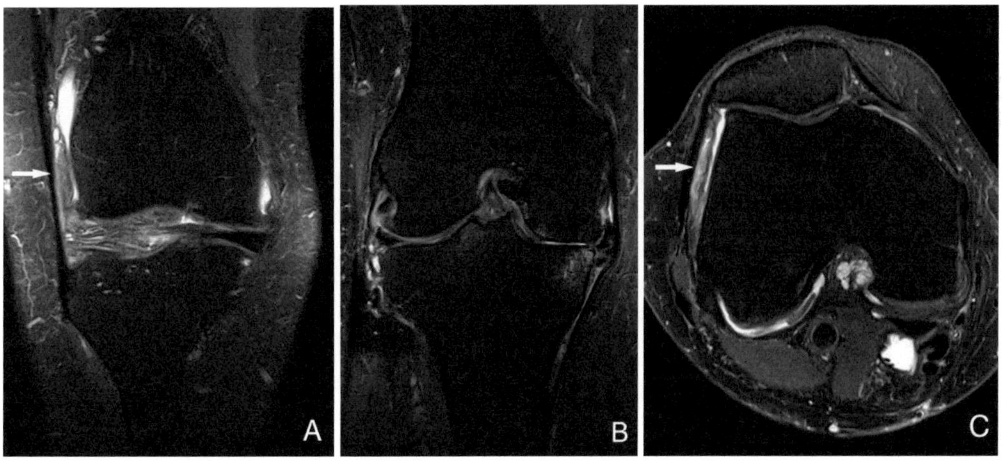

Fig. 1. A 72 y.o. woman with MR imaging signs of iliotibial band friction (ITBF) and medial osteoarthritis of the knee. Fibrovascular tissue (arrow) is seen between the lateral epicondyle and the ITB on PDw fatsat image (A). Some slices posterior the complete loss of hyaline cartilage at the medial femoral condyle and the tibia plateau with advanced degeneration of the medial meniscus is obvious. The lateral compartment is normal (B). On axial PDw fatsat image minor effusion and extensive firbovascular tissue between the lateral epicondyle and the ITB is present (arrow, C) (Vasilevska et al., 2009).

In another study 66 cases were retrospectively evaluated its MR study of the knee with medial compartment knee osteoarthritis and MR signs of Baker cyst. The median age was 56,42 years, (age range 34-84 years). We selected two groups according to the size of the Baker cyst on MRI. The first group was with palpable soft tissue mass on medial aspect of popliteal fosa with a large Baker cyst, and in the other group the Baker cyst was small and detected only on MRI (Table 3).

	Number of cases	Male/Female	Age (age range)
Large Baker Cyst	31	11/20	54 (37-78)
Small Baker Cyst	35	12/23	59 (34-84)
total:	66	23/43	56 (34-84)

Table 3. Sex and age distribution in cases with large and small Baker cysts

2. Imaging features

Magnetic resonance imaging (MRI) has enhanced our ability to examine patients non-invasively. This allows us to assess structural changes of osteoarthritis (OA) without risk to the patient. MRI enables to visualize and quantitate the changes in articular cartilage, the menisci, and other periarticular structures non-invasively (Wluka et al., 2001; Baranyay et al., 2007). MRI use in healthy populations and those with OA will detect a significant number of incidental lesions, some which are clinically significant and will require further imaging and clinical management (Grainger et al., 2008).

MRI may eventually eclipse plain radiography as the modality of choice for documenting structural progression of OA. Plain radiography remains the standard method for assessing progression. The measurement of radiographic joint space width is the most accepted and widely-used method of OA progression (Ravaud et al., 2008).

On MR images, cartilage thickness of the medial and lateral compartment should be measured centrally in the weight bearing zone. Degeneration of the medial meniscus had to be assessed, as well as subchondral bone marrow edema and effusion (Vasilevska et al., 2009).

The thickness of residual cartilage is measuring separately at the femur and at the tibia. The degree of degeneration of the meniscus is graded: 0- normal meniscus, 1- moderate degeneration with focal signal increase, 2- severe degeneration with some residual normal tissue and shape, 3-advanced degeneration of the meniscus with destroyed shape and no functional meniscal tissue.

Presence of MR signs for ITBF to be evaluated as well. For evaluation of MR signs of ITBF to be evaluated as well.

For evaluation of MR signs of ITBF (0-not present, 1-present, 2 severe changes) the following criteria can be used (Ekman et al., 1994; Muhle et al., 1999; Murphy et al., 1992; Nishimura et al., 1997; Vasilevska et al., 2009):

- poorly defined signal intensity abnormalities lateral, distal or proximal to the lateral epicondyle;

- signal intensity abnormalities superficial or deep to the ITT;
- localized fluid collection lateral, distal or proximal to the lateral epicondyle; (Fig.2).

To conclude that the reason of the lateral knee pain is ITBF in patients with osteoarthritis of the knee, which showed advanced medial compartment osteoarthritis with complete or subtotal (>80%) loss of articular cartilage at the femur and the tibia, lateral compartment should be normal including the articular cartilage and the lateral meniscus, without meniscal lesion or cartilage abnormalities (Vasilevska et al., 2009).

MR imaging allows confirmation of diagnosis of ITBFS and exclusion of other causes of lateral knee pain - such as meniscal tears or ligament injuries. Axial images are necessary to differentiate intraarticular fluid from ITBFS (Murphy et al., 1992).

Popliteal cysts on MR imaging are usually well defined, extending between the tendon of semimembranosus and the medial head of gastrocnemius into the gastrocnemius-semimembranosus bursa, situated superficial to the medial gastrocnemius muscle, along the medial side of the popliteal fosa (Torreggiani et al., 2002; Steiner et al., 1996). As cyst enlarge, the cystic fluid may extend in any direction. Inferomedial expansion is relatively common with a superficial location, which results in cysts becoming palpable (Torreggiani et al., 2002; Steiner et al., 1996). Baker cyst can be presented as a palpable soft tissue masses on the medial aspect of the popliteal fossa when it is distended and large (Fig.3) (Vasilevska et al., 2008).

On MRI, Baker cyst is presenting as a circumscribed mass with low signal on T1-weigted image, intermedal signal intensity on proton density (PD) image and high signal intensity comparing with skeletal muscle on PD-weithed fatsat image. The size of Baker cyst can be assessed by measuring the distension of the cyst, and when is thickened more than 1cm is a large cyst (Fig.4) (Vasilevska et al., 2008).

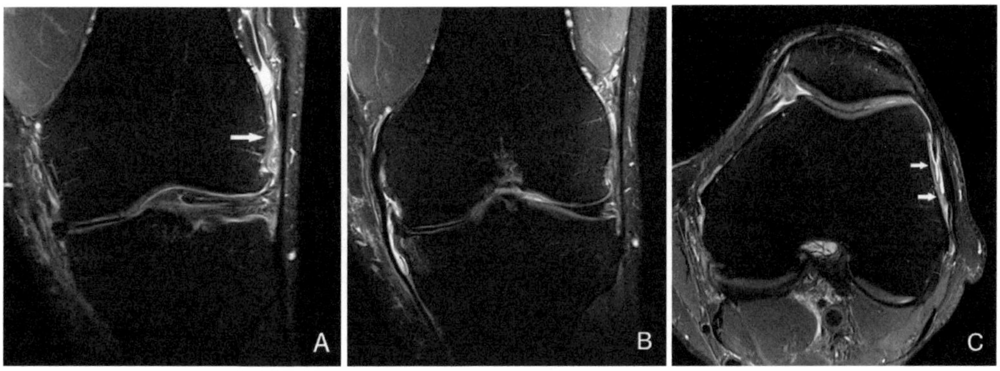

Fig. 2. A 61 y.o. man, medial sided osteoarthritis of the knee, associated with ITBF. Fibrovascular tissue and fluid collections (arrow) are located between the lateral epicondyle and the ITB at the lateral aspect of the left knee on PDw fatsat coronal image (A). Better seen on a section more posterior, osteoarthritis of the medial compartment is advanced with cartilage loss, vacuum phenomenon in the medial compartment and advanced degenerative desintegration of the medial meniscus (B). Axial PDw fatsat image again shows extraarticular fibrovascular tissues between the lateral epicondyle and the ITB (arrow, C) (Vasilevska et al., 2009).

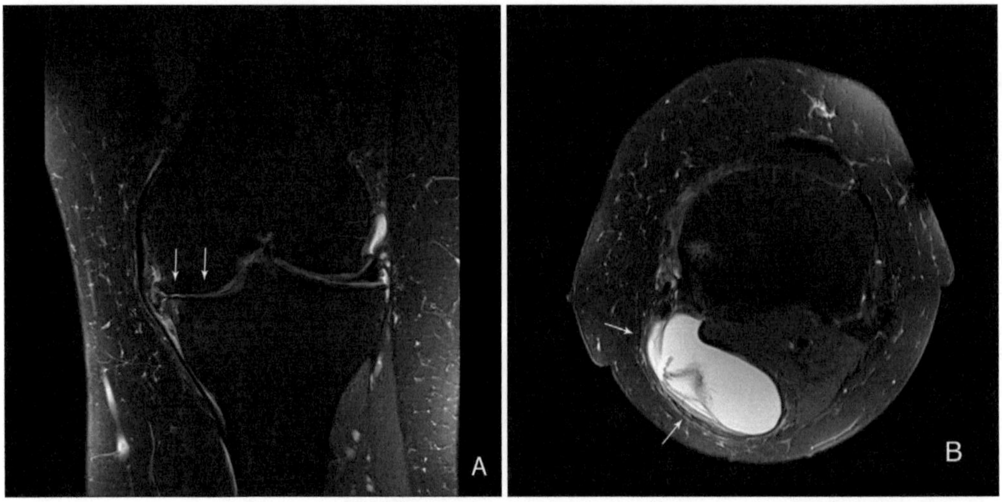

Fig. 3. Large Baker's cyst in a 59-year old woman; A) Coronal PDw fatsat image shows complete cartilage lose on the medial knee compartment with 3th degree medial meniscus degeneration with degenerative disintegration (arrows), the lateral compartment is normal including the hyaline cartilage and the lateral meniscus. B) Axial PDw fatsat image demonstrates a large Baker's cyst, with septum within the cyst (arrows) *(Vasilevska et al., 2008).*

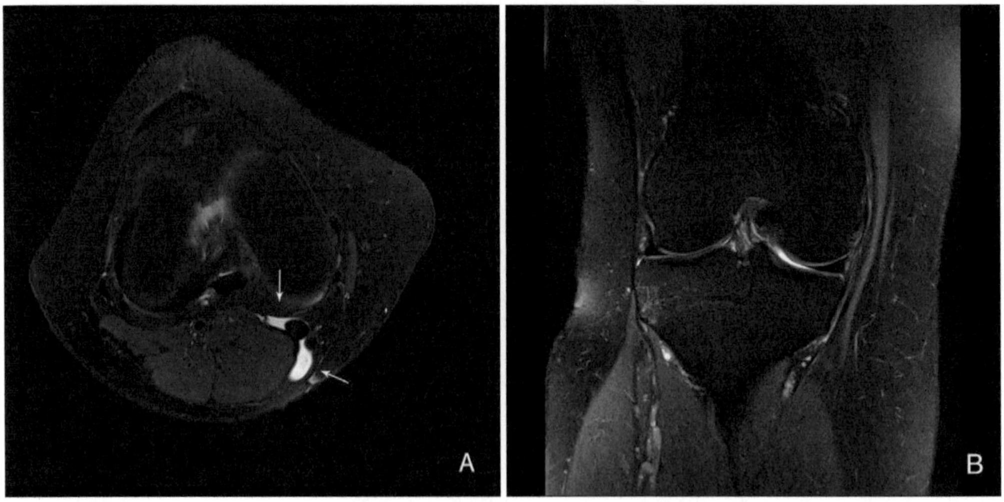

Fig. 4. Small Baker's cyst in a 35-year-old women; A) Axial fatsat PDw images. Small Baker cyst is shown with its subgastrocnemius bursa and gastrocnemius-semimembranosus bursa connected by a tin neck (arrow); B) Coronal PD fatsat image of the same patient exhibits normal hyaline cartilage thickness without defects. Minor mucoid degeneration is shown of posterior horn of the medial meniscus at its base without tear *(Vasilevska et al., 2008).*

3. Discussion

Some studies report an incidence of Baker cysts on MR images done for internal derangement of the knee of 5-58% with an increase in the prevalence with age, presence of arthritis, internal derangement and/or effusion (Miller et al., 1996; Ward et al., 2001). Sansone at al. noted that Baker's cyst were associated with one or more disorders detected by MRI in 94% of cases (Sansone et al., 1995). The results confirmed a strong association between popliteal cysts and intra-articular pathology (Sansone et al., 1995, 1999).

The popliteal cyst is almost never an isolated pathology in an adult knee (Fritschy et al., 2006). The probability of popliteal cysts increase with increasing number of associated knee conditions (Miller et al., 1996). Of 77 MRI-observed cysts, a statistical correlation existed with effusion, meniscus tears or "degenerative" arthropathy, or combination of these 3 maladies (Miller et al., 1996).

For fluid filled bursa have two etiological factors, knee joint effusion and persistence of one way valvular mechanism (Takahashi et al., 2005). Vahlensieck et al. mention that there is a communication with the joint in half of all cases, according to the anatomy literature. Therefore, a joint effusion may increase the size of the gastrocnemius bursae (Vahlensieck et al., 2001). Sowers MF et al. detected presence of joint effusion in 70% (507) in cases with the knee OA. They observed large baker cyst in 6,1% of the knee (Sowers et al., 2011). Marti-Bonmati L.et al. (2000) reported that the volume of Baker cyst was statistically related with presence of joint effusion in 70%. The presence and volume of the cyst is directly related with the quantity of the joint effusion, and the presence and type of meniscal lesion but not to the cartilage lesion (Marti-Bonmati et al., 2000). In isolated medial compartment knee osteoarthritis, there is no statistically significant difference between the size of the Baker cyst and degree of joint effusion (Vasilevska et al. 2008).

Other studies, in contrary, reported that there is a statistically significant correlation between Baker cyst and internal derangement of the joint without joint effusion. Internal derangement results from disturbed biomechanics with increased pressure to shift normal joint fluid into the bursa (Miller et al. 1996). The intraarticular pressure of the knee is increased with abnormal meniscus compared to healthy knees (Miller et al. 1996).

Almost all popliteal cyst are secondary cyst and degenerative cartilage lesions are responsible in 30-60% of the cases (Miller et al. 1996; Sansone et al. 1999). Articular cartilage lesion was the most frequent accompanying lesion with popliteal cysts and suggested an influence in pathogenesis of popliteal cyst (Rupp et al. 2002). An isolated degenerative alteration of the cartilage was present in 43% of the cases with Baker cyst (Sansone et al. 1995, 1999). Cartilage lesion, inflamatory and degenerative arthropaty are associated pathology with Baker cyst (Miller et al., 1996; Torreggiani et al., 2002; Ward et al., 2001; Handy et al., 2001; Vasilevska et al. 2008). In contrary, Marti-Bonmati et al. (2000) reported that they have not observed any statistically significant relation with presence and degree of the cartilage lesions.

In referred study of 30 patients with popliteal cyst in 90% had lesion of the posterior horn of medial meniscus (Sansone et al., 1999). Meniscal lesion was also directly related to the presence and quantity of fluid inside Baker cyst (Sansone et al. 1995; Marti-Bonmati et al., 2000). Although Baker cyst are more frequent with meniscus tear, their presence is also associated with menisci degeneration, especially of the posterior horn (Miller et al., 1996; Marti-Bonmati et al., 2000). Majority of cases with a Baker cyst usually were involved the medial meniscus (90%) and less frequently both menisci (17%) (Sansone et al., 1999).

Authors in study of 66 Baker cyst in cases with isolated medial compartment knee osteoarthritis concluded that in the cases with large Baker cyst, there is statistically significant difference between different degree of medial meniscus degeneration and distension of the cyst. The degree of medial meniscal degeneration has no influence on the distension of Baker cyst generally but an influence was found, when there is significant cartilage degeneration (Vasilevska et al., 2008). The same authors reported that the combination of medial compartment cartilage degeneration and medial meniscus degeneration are associated with large Baker cyst in 84%, but only 48% with small Baker cyst. In the group with large Baker cyst, isolated medial meniscus degeneration is present in 16%, comparing with association of medial meniscus degeneration in 52% from the cases with small cyst (Vasilevska et al., 2008).
Bone edema on medial compartment in isolated medial compartment osteoarthritis, can be present in 65% of the cases with large Baker cyst, only when cartilage degeneration is present. In cases with small Baker cyst, bone edema is present in 37% of the cases (Fig.5) (Vasilevska et al., 2008). In cases with both compartments knee OA, Sowers MF et al. reported the prevalence of bone marrow lesion in the medial compartment in 21,3% and in lateral 13,4 % (Sowers et al., 2011).

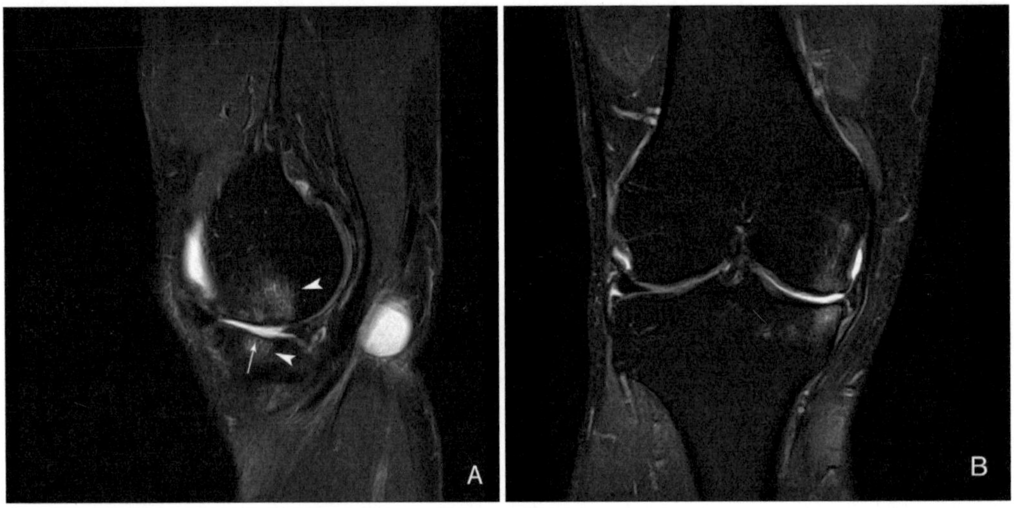

Fig. 5. Large Baker's cyst in a 67-year -old man; A) On a sagittal and B) coronal PDw fatsat image; complete cartilage lose on the femoral condyle and the tibial plateau of the medial compartment (arrows), with 3th degree of medial meniscus degeneration. Bone marrow edema (arrow heads) and effusion is present *(Vasilevska et al., 2008).*

There is a strong association between popliteal cysts and the severity of isolated medial compartment osteoarthritis, emphasizing the importance of cartilage degeneration for the distension of Baker cysts (Vasilevska et al., 2008).
It is well known that ITBFS is associated with overuse in long distance runners, cyclists, military personnel, football players, and weight lifters (Barber et al., 2007; Kirk et al., 2000; Fredericson et al., 2006,2007;). In runners the reported incidence is as high as 22,2% of all lower extremity injuries (Linenger et al., 1992), and it is 15% of all overuse injuries of the knee from cycling (Holmes et al., 1993). Excessive running in the same direction on a track,

downhill running, a lack of running experience, long distance running are the most often mentioned etiologic factors for ITBFS (Linenger et al., 1992; Messier et al., 1995). Weakness of the hip abductor muscles is also believed to play a role in the development of ITBFS (Fredericson et al., 2006; MacMahon et al., 2000). Football players and weight lifters can also suffer from chronic inflammation and fibrovascular tissue at the ITB proximal to its insertion into the anterolateral tibia. The causes of the ITBFS can be extrinsic (related to training technique) or intrinsic (related to the patient's anatomic alignment) (Farell et al., 2003; Fredericson et al., 2006; Nishimura et al., 2003).

Farell et al. (2003) emphasized that ITBFS usually occurs as a result of overuse. If, however, the patient has certain anatomical conditions (leg length discrepancies, varus knee alignment or excessive pronation and external tibial rotation of more than 20%), he/she will be more inclined to experience ITBFS. They concluded that knee-flexion repetition was more likely to result in the onset of the overuse injury ITBFS during cycling (Farell et al., 2003).

ITBFS is predominantly a clinical diagnosis.

Several other anatomical abnormalities, including leg length discrepancy and functional overpronation of the food have been postulated as predisposing factors (Nishimura et al., 2003). Nishimura et al. (2003) described also two no athletic patients with ITBFS.

As a possible factor contributing to the development of ITBFS, genus varus has been described, in runners and in athlete that may increase the tension and thus a frictional force over the lateral femoral condyle (Jones et al., 1987; Sutker et al., 1981).

The finding of predominant cartilage degeneration on the medial rather than the lateral tibia plateau side suggests a close relation to the varus- knee osteoarthritis present in most of the cases (Kleemann et al., 2005). Recent reports have suggested a 60% reduction in cartilage volume in severe knee osteoarthritis (Burgkart et al., 2001; Cicuttini et al., 2001).

Significant correlation between joint space narrowing and cartilage volume was reported (Cicuttini et al., 2001). Medial compartment cartilage loss leads to varus deformity, which can affect knee biomechanics by altering the relationship of the iliotibial band and the lateral epicondyle with the possibility of an increased friction and pressure between these structures. An association of ITBFS with genu varum in runners has been previously established (Farell et al., 2001).

There is only one study in literature of 128 MR of the knee, we published a 2009, that describe the correlation of advanced isolated medial compartment knee osteoarthritis (with subsequent genu varum) and MR signs of friction of ITB (Vasilevska et al., 2009). Cartilage volume was not measured but the cartilage thickness in the weight bearing zone, to assess if there was a significant difference on cartilage thickness between the medial and the lateral compartment. There was a significant difference in cartilage thickness between medial and lateral compartment which led to joint space narrowing when standing and varus deformity of the knee. Varus knee alignment may be one of the causes for permanent stretching of the ITB and even during walking, to cause friction of the ITB on the femoral lateral condyle which leads to inflammation of the fibrovascular tissue, thus presenting signs of ITBF on MRI (Vasilevska et al., 2009).

4. Conclusion

Advanced reduction of cartilage thickness combined with severe degeneration of the meniscus at the medial compartment probably leads to biomechanical changes, and varus knee alignment. It may be the cause for stretching of the ITB, and may be one of the reasons for ITBF. A latest statement for the so frequent presence of MR signs of ITBF in patients with isolated medial compartment knee osteoarthritis, give us a rights to put this entity in the list of an important associated entities with knee osteoarthritis. We should always think about it as the reason for lateral knee pain in those cases. This can be an explanation for the presence of lateral knee pain, when lateral knee compartment is unaffected.

Baker cyst is not a single joint lesion, but it is associated with cartilage and meniscus degeneration on the medial compartment of the knee joint. Its size is strongly correlated with degenerative changes of the cartilage on the medial compartment and medial meniscus degeneration. It is not connected with a joint effusion. The size of Baker cyst had a strong correlation with degenerative changes of the cartilage and with the degree of meniscus degeneration on the medial compartment of the knee joint. Presence of distended Baker cyst can be one of the reasons of the pain and discomfort in the posterior aspect of the knee.

5. References

Baranyay FJ, Wang Y, Wluka AE, English DR, Giles GG, Sullivan RO, Cicuttini FM. (2007) Association of bone marrow lesions with knee structures and risk factors of bone marrow lesions in the knee of clinically healthy, community-based adults. *Semin Arthritis Reum* 37:112-118.

Barber FA, Boothby MH, Troop RL. (2007) Z-plasty lengthening for iliotibial band friction syndrome. *J Knee Surg* 20:281-284

Burgkart R, Glaser C, Hyhlik-Drr A, Englmeier K, Reiser M, Eckstein F. (2001) Magnetic resonance imaging based assessment of cartilage loss in severe osteoarthritis: accuracy, precision and diagnostic value. 44:2072-2077

Center for disease control and prevention (CDC). (2003) Public health and aging: projected prevalence of self reported arthritis or chronic joint symptoms among persons aged >65-United States,2005-2030.*MMWR Morb Mortal Wkly Rep.*52:489-91.

Cicuttini FM, Wluka AE, Stuckey SL. (2001) Tibial and femoral cartilage changes in knee osteoarthritis. *ANN Rheum Dis* 60:977-980

D'Ambrosia RD. (2005) Epidemiology of osteoarthritis. *Orthopedics* 28(suppl.):s201-205

Dye SF, Vaupel GL, Dye CC. (1998) Conscious neurosurgery mapping of the internal structures of the human knee without intraarticular anesthesia. *Am J Sports Med* 26:773-7

Ekman EF, Pope T, Martin DF, Curl WW. (1994) Magnetic resonance imaging of iliotibial band syndrome. *Am J Sports Med* 22:851-854

Fairclough J, Hayashi K, Toumi H, Lyons K, Bydder G, Phillips N, Best TM, Benjamin M. (2006) The functional anatomy of the iliotibial band during flexion and extension of the knee: implications for understanding iliotibial band syndrome. *J Anat* 208:309-316

Fairclough J, Hayashi K, Toumi H, Lyons K, Bydder G, Phillips N, Best TM, Benjamin M. (2007) Is iliotibial band syndrome really a friction syndrome? *J Sci Med Sport* 10:74-76

Farell KC, Reisinger KD, Tillman MD. (2003) Force and repetition in cycling: possible implications for iliotibial band friction syndrome. *The Knee* 10:103-109

Felson DT, Naimark A, Anderson J, Kazis L, Castelli W, Meenan RF. (1987) The prevalence of knee osteoarthritis in elderly. The Framingham Osteoarthritis Study. *Arthritis Rheum* 30(8):914-918

Felson DT, Chaisson CE, Hill CL, Totterman SM, Gale ME, Skinner KM, et al. (2001) The association of bone marrow lesion with pain in knee osteoarthritis. *Ann Intern Med* 134:541-9.

Fredericson M, Weir A. (2006) Practical management of iliotibial band friction syndrome in runners. *Clin J Sport Med* 16:261-268

Fredericson M, Misra AK. (2007) Epidemiology and aetiology of marathon running injuries. *Sports Med* 37:437-439

Fritschy D, Fasel J, Umbert JC, Bianchi S, Verdonk R, Wirth CJ. (2006) The popliteal cyst. *Knee Surg Sport Traumatol Arthrosc* 14:623-628.

Grainger R, Stuckey S, O'Sullivan R, Davis SR, Ebeling PR, Wluka AE. (2008) What is the clinical and ethical importance of incidental abnormalities found by knee MRI? *Arthritis Research & Therapy* 10:R18

Handout on Health: Osteoarthritis. www.niams.nih.gov

Handy JR. (2001) Popliteal cysts in adults: a review. *Semin Arthritis Rheum* 31:108-118.

Hill CL, Gale DG, Chaisson CE, Skinner K, Kazis L, Gale ME, et al. (2001) Knee effusion, popliteal cyst, and synovial thickening : association with knee pain in osteoarthritis. *J Reumatol*28:1330-7.

Hill CL, Gale DG, Chaisson CE, Skinner K, Kazis L, Gale ME, Felson DT. (2003) Periarticular lesions detected on magnetic resonance imaging. prevalence in knees with and without symptoms. *Arthritis & Reumatism* 48:2836-2844.

Holmes JC, Pruitt AL, Whalen NJ. (1993)Iliotibial band syndrome inIliotibial band friction syndrome in cyclists. *Am Orthop Soc Sports Med* 21:419-424

Janzen DL, Peterfy CG, Forbes JR, Tirman PF, Genant HK. (1994) Cystic lesions around the knee joint: MR imaging findings. *AJR Am J Roendgenol*163:155-61

Jones DC, James SL. (1987) Overuse injuries of the lower extremity: shin splints, iliotibial band friction syndrome and exertional compartment syndromes. *Clin Sports Med* 6:273-290

Kirk LK, Kuklo T, Klemme W. (2000) Iliotibial band friction syndrome. *Orthopedics* 23:1209-1214

Kleemann RU, Krocker D, Cedraro A, Tuischer J, Duda GN. (2005) Altered cartilage mechanics and histology in the knee osteoarthritis: relation to clinical assessment (ICRS Grade). *OsteoArthritis and Cartilage* 13:958-963

Kornaat PR, Bloem JL, Ceulemans RY, Riyazi N, Rosendaal FR, Nelissen RG, Carter WO, Le Graverand MPH, Kloppenburg M. (2006) Osteoarthritis of the knee: Association between Clinical Features and MR Imaging Findings. *Radiology* vol.239: No 3-June.

Linenger IMCC. (1992) Is iliotibial band syndrome overlooked? *Phys Sport Med* 20:98-108

MacMahon JM, Chaudhari AM, Andriacchi TP. (2000) Biomechanical injury predictors for marathon runners; striding towards iliotibial band syndrome injury prevention. Conference of the International Society of Biomechanics in Sports, Hong Kong.

Marti-Bonmati L, Molla E, Dosda R, Casillas C, Ferrer P. (2000) MR imaging of Baker cyst-prevalence and relation to internal derangement of the knee. *Magnetic Resonance Materials in Physics, Biology and Medicine* 10:205-210.

Mc Carthy C.L., Mc Nally E.G. (2004) The MRI appearance of cystic lesions around the knee. *Skeletal Radiol* 33: 187-209.

Messier SP, Edwards DG, Martin DF, et al. (1995) Etiology of iliotibial band friction syndrome in distance runners. *Med Sci Sports Exerc* 27:951-960

Miller TT, Staron RB, Koenigsberg T, Levin TL, Feldman F. (1996) MR imaging of Baker cysts:association withinternal derangement, effusion and degenerative arthropathy. *Radiology* 201:247-450.

Murphy L, Schwartz TA, Helmick CG, Renner JB, Tudor G, Koch G, Dragomir A, Kalsbeek WD, Luta G, Jordan JM. (2008) Lifetime risk of symptomatic knee osteoarthritis. *Arthritis Rheum.* 59:1207-13.

Muhle C, Ahn JM, Yeh L, Bergman GA, Boutin RD, Schweitzer M, Jacobson JA, Haghighi P, Trudell DJ, Resnick D. (1999) Iliotibial band friction syndrome: MR imaging findings in 16 patients and MR arthrographic study of six cadaveric knees. *Radiology* 212:103-110

Murphy BJ, Hechtman KS, Uribe JW, Selesnick H, Smith RL, Zlatkin MB. (1992) Iliotibial band friction syndrome: MR imaging findings. *Radiology* 185:569-571

Nishimura G, Yamato M, Tamai K, Takahashi J, Uetani M. (1997) MR findings in iliotibial band syndrome. *Skeletal Radiol* 26:533-537

Ravaud P, Giraudeau B, Aulely GR, Chastang C, Poiraudeau S, Ayral X, et al. (1996) Radiographic assessment of the knee osteoarthritis: reproducibility and sensitivity to change. *J Reumatol* 23(10):1756-1764.

Rupp S, Seil R, Jochum P, Kohn D. (2002) Popliteal cyst in adults. Prevalence, associated intraarticular lesions and results after arthroscopic treatment. *Am J Sport Med* 30:112-115.

Sansone V, de Ponti GM, del Maschio A. (1995) Popliteal cyst and associated disorder of the knee: critical review with MR imaging. *Int Orthop* 19:275-279

Sansone V, De Ponti A. (1999) Arthroscopic treatment of popliteal cyst and associated intra-articular knee disorders in adults. *Arthroscopy*15:368-372.

Steiner E, Steinbach LS, Schnarkowski P, Tirman PFJ, Ganant HK. (1996) Ganglia and cysts around joints. *Radiol Clin North Am* 34:400-410.

Sowers MF, Karvonen-Gutierrez CA, Jacobson JA, Jiang Y, Yosef M. (2011) Associations of anatomical measures from MRI with radiographically defined knee osteoarthritis, score, pain and physical function. *J Bone Joint Surg Am*93:241-51.

Sutker AN, Jackson DW, Pagliano JW. (1981) Iliotibial band syndrome in long distance runners. *Phys Sportsmed* 9:69-73

Takahashi M, Nagano A. (2005) Arthroscopic treatment of popliteal cyst and visualization of its cavity through the posterior portal of the knee. *The Journal of Arthroscopic and Related Surgery* vol 21, No 5: 638e1-638e4.

Torreggiani WC, Al-Ismail K, Munk PL, et al. (2002) The imaging spectrum of Baker's (popliteal) cysts. *Clin Radiol* 57:681-691.

Vahlensieck M, Linneborn G, Schild HH, Schmidt HM. (2001) Magnetic resonance imaging(MRI) of the bursa around the knee joint[in German]. *Rofo Fortschr Geb - Rontgenstr Neuen Bildgeb Verfahr*173:195-199.

Vasilevska V, Szeimies U, Staebler A. (2008) MRI diagnosis of Baker cyst and significance of associated medial compartment knee osteoarthritis. *Radiol Oncol* 42(2);51-8.

Vasilevska V, Szeimies U, Staebler A. (2009) Magnetic resonance imaging signs of ilitibial band friction in patients with isolated medial compartment osteoarthritis of the knee. *Skeletal Radiol* 38:871-875.

Ward EE, Jacobson JA, Fessel DP, Hayes CW, Van Holsbeeck M. (2001) Sonographic detection of Baker's cysts: comparison with MR imaging. *AJR Am J Roentgenol* 176:373-380.

Wluka AE, Stuckey S, Snaddon J, Cicuttini FM. (2002) The determinants of change in tibial cartilage volume in osteoarthritic knees. *Arthritis Rheum* 46:2065-2072.

15

Evaluation of *In Vivo* Proteolytic Activity

Wataru Yoshida, Akihisa Kamataki, Miwa Uzuki and Takashi Sawai
Iwate Medical University,
Japan

1. Introduction

Osteoarthritis (OA) is a degenerative articular disease primarily observed in older adults, and is the leading cause of physical disability and impaired quality of life. OA is characterized by softening, fibrillation, erosion, defect of the articular cartilage, bone hypertrophy at the margins with osteophyte formation, subchondral sclerosis, and chronic inflammation of the synovial membrane and joint capsule (Zhang et al., 2010).

These alterations are thought to be caused by biochemical and biomechanical factors leading to a failure in the balance of synthesis and degradation (Martel-Pelletier et al., 2010). Pathogenesis of OA is based on an imbalance of the functional requirements and morphologic alterations, and these statuses progressively and chronically evoke subsequent alterations (Lorenz et al., 2005).

Although the etiology of OA is not completely understood, the accompanying biochemical, structural, and metabolic alterations of the articular cartilage have been well described (de Seny et al., 2011; Kraus 2010; Reeves et al., 2011; Sobczak et al., 2010). Recently, it has been revealed that proteolytic enzymes, cytokines, biomechanical stress, and altered genetics are involved in its pathogenesis, and proteolytic activity is particularly important in regards to the morphologic alterations of the articular structures, and is considered as an internal-factor of the disease (Takei et al., 1999; Kevorkian et al., 2004). It has been suggested that proteolytic activity in the constituent of the joint, such as synovium, joint fluid, cartilage, is continuously involved in the articular alterations of the disease, as its progression is gradual.

Although it is extremely difficult to accurately predict future articular OA alterations, it is possible to evaluate the present phenomenon, which may lead to speculation of possible further alterations by evaluating proteolytic activity in the joint.

2. Evaluation of *in vivo* proteolytic activiy

2.1 *In situ* zymography

There have been many studies of proteolytic activity, using gelatin zymography. This method is a valuable and effective tool for examining and analyzing proteolytic activity, as gelatin degrades over the course of the disease (Hattori et al., 2003; Cha et al., 2004; Sun et al., 2003). However, most current zymography methods are used to qualitatively examine this activity, and are thus not adequate for histological evaluation or quantification.

In situ zymography was developed to determine the *in vivo* proteolytic activity and determine its histological location. However, this method has only been used to demonstrate a qualitative analysis as the gelatin does not sufficiently coat the film with a uniform thickness of substrate to allow precise quantification of the *in vivo* proteolytic activity (Senzaki et al., 2000; Yi et al., 2001; Galis et al., 1995; Viemard-Barone et al., 2000; Goodall et al., 2001).

A newly method, "film *in situ* zymography (FIZ)", has been developed specially to evaluate the histological distribution the *in vivo* proteolytic activity (Ikeda et al., 2000; Takano et al., 2001; Zheng et al., 2002; Kaji et al., 2003) .

This new method works by applying unfixed frozen tissues (or fluid) to the recently developed FIZ film (Fuji Film. Co., Tokyo, Japan) which is uniformly coated with cross-bridge gelatin at a thickness of 7 µm. In our study, the synovial tissue specimens were embedded in Tissue-Tek OCT Compound (Lab-Tek Products, Elkhart, IN, USA) and frozen in the cryostat's refrigerated chamber. Then, frozen sections were cut at 4 µm, and applied to the FIZ film, followed by flushing with water for a few seconds. After incubation for 6 hours at 37°C, the film was stained with 0.2% Ponceau solution (which is commonly used for protein staining), (Sigma-Aldrich, St. Louis, MO, USA) for 3 minutes and fixed with 1% acetate for 5 minutes. After flushing with water for 15 minutes, the film was stained with hematoxylin for nuclear staining. Gelatinolyzed areas caused by the proteolytic activity in the synovium were detected as pale in color, and non-gelatinolyzed areas were stained red (Figure 1). In several studies, this method was successful in achieving reproducible quantification of gelatinolyed areas (Iwata et al., 2001; Furuya et al., 2001; Yamanaka et al., 2000).

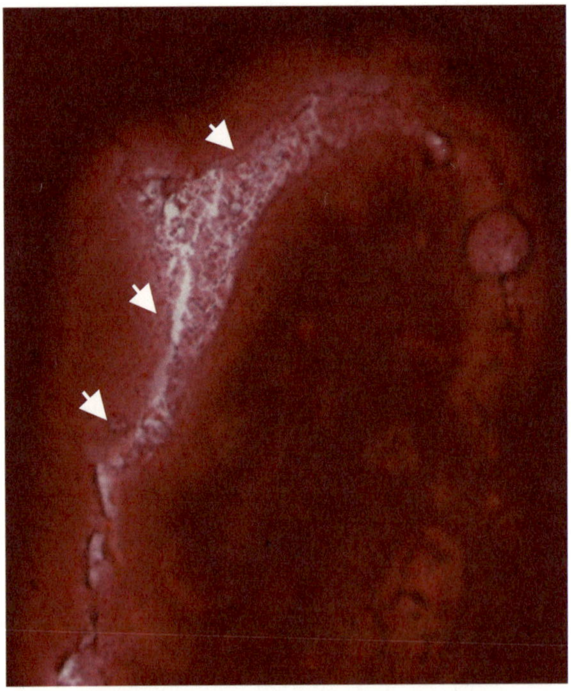

Fig. 1. Film *in situ* zymography of OA synovium. Arrows indicate the proteolytic lesions as pale in color in the Ponceau-stained FIZ film.

2.2 Quantification by image analyzer

Furthermore, it is possible to quantify the degree of this activity using a digital image analyzer (Image Processor for Analytical Pathology, IPAP, Sumitomo Tech, Osaka, Japan). The IPAP system is comprised of a conventional microscope, a CCD color video camera, an IBM-compatible microcomputer and a specialized image analysis board, Matrox Image-1280 (Dorval, Quevec, Canada) to convert microscopic photographic images into digital images, and allows us to analyze many samples, fields and parameters (Figure 2). For each Ponceau-stained FIZ film image, the analyzer can measure the approximate optical density of gelatinolyzed area as optical density of gelatinolyzed area (ODG) and ratio of gelatinolyzed area (RGA). The ODG is the mean optical density of the red-stained component at 50 random points in the gelatinolyzed area. The RGA is the ratio of the gelatinolyzed area to the entire synovium stained on the FIZ films as background reference (ODG and RGA were measured blindly at a magnification of ×4). As such, implementing both FIZ and IPAP enable the histological evaluation and quantification of the *in vivo* proteolytic activity to analyze the gelatinolyzed area (Uzuki et al., 1999; Yoshida et al., 2009).

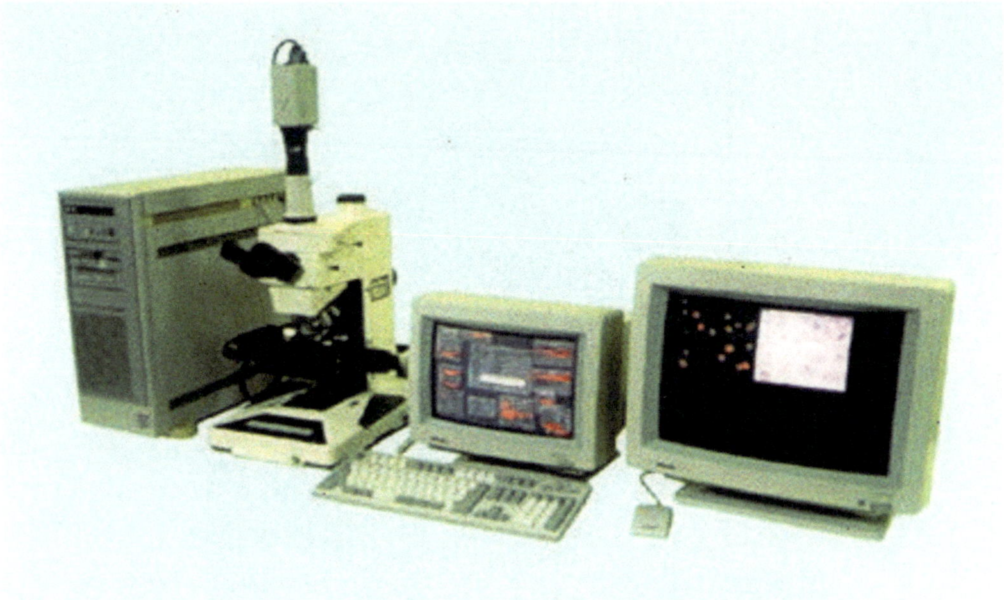

Fig. 2. IPAP system. This system is comprised of a microscope, a CCD color video camera and an analyzing computer for converting microscopic photographic images into digital images.

3. *In vivo* proteolytic activity on OA synovium

It was revealed through FIZ the *in vivo* proteolytic activity on OA synovium was mainly distributed in the layer of the lining rather than in the stroma, although this histological feature is predominant and consisted of uniform fibrous proliferation with chronic inflammation. Furthermore, distribution of the proteolytic area in rheumatoid arthritis (RA) synovium, which showed obvious inflammatory changes, also detected in layer of the lining (Yoshida et al., 2009).

Comparing the *in vivo* proteolytic activity using FIZ and IPAP, there was a significant difference between OA and RA synovium in regards to the ODG (Figure 3) and RGA (Figure 4)(Yoshida et al., 2009). These findings suggest that there is also a difference on the proteolytic potential per one active-cell and the proteolytic-cell number between OA and RA synovium, and this might reflect that the articular alteration in OA is less progressive than in RA.

Furthermore, the proteolytic area is mostly localized in the layer of the lining and similar to both OA and RA articular disease, although they have different degrees of activity. The proteolytic area is constantly exposed to the articular space, and this finding suggests that the *in vivo* proteolytic activity in synovium might be affected in the interaction with the constituents of articular space as an internal-factor of the articular alterations.

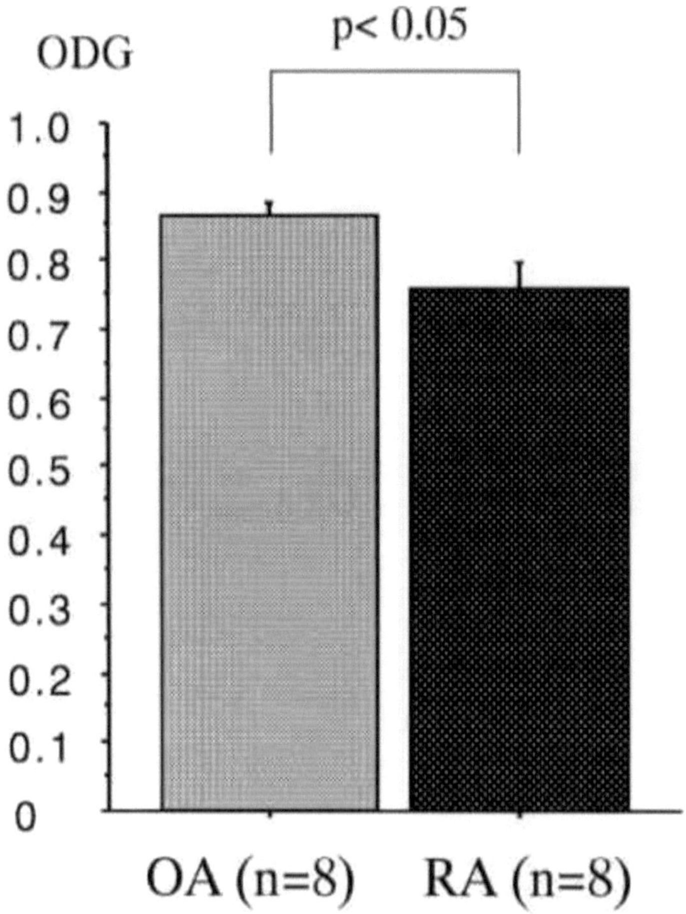

Fig. 3. Optical density of the gelatinolyzed area (ODG) as produced by FIZ and IPAP the synovium of OA and RA. OA synovium had a significantly higher ODG (0.864±0.037) than RA synovium (0.758±0.019). All OA cases were classified as grade 4 using Kellgren and Lawrence classification and all RA cases were classified as stage IV using the Steinbrocker classification.

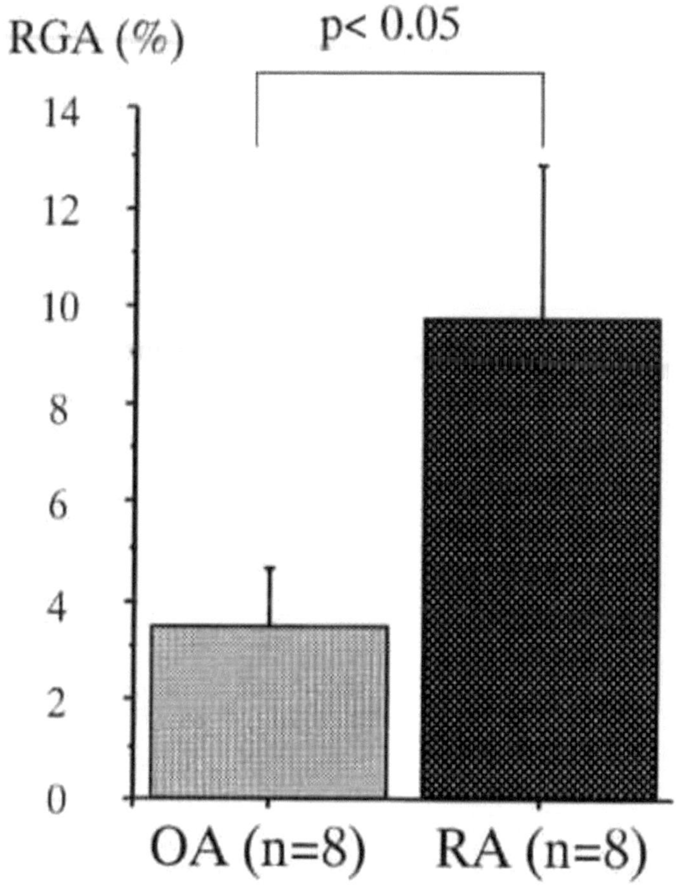

Fig. 4. Ratio of gelatinolyzed areas (RGA) as produced by FIZ and IPAP the synovium of OA and RA. The synovium of OA had a significantly lower RGA (3.5±1.1%) than RA synovium (9.7±3.1%). All OA cases were classified as grade 4 using Kellgren and Lawrence classification and all RA cases were classified as stage IV using the Steinbrocker classification.

In examination of enzyme expression by immunohistochemistry using serial sections, matrix metalloproteinase (MMP)-2, MMP-9, also known as gelatinase-A and -B, were mainly expressed by fibroblast- or macrophage-like cells of the synovial-lining layer (Figures 5a and 5b). Interestingly, these same cells also expressed tissue inhibitor of metalloproteinase (TIMP) -1 and TIMP-2 (Figures 5c and 5d). In addition, the distribution of cells expressing MMPs and TIMPs corresponded to the proteolytic areas detected by FIZ investigation (Figure 5a, 5b, 5c, and 5d as serial sections showed the expression of the enzymes by immunohistochemisty in lining layer of RA synovium). These findings indicate that synovial cells simultaneously produce proteolytic enzymes and their inhibitors, and suggest that the *in vivo* proteolytic activity might be dependent on "imbalances" in enzymes-inhibitors production of the individual cells.

Utilizing FIZ and IPAP may further help to understand biological enzymatic activity on articular manifestations of OA.

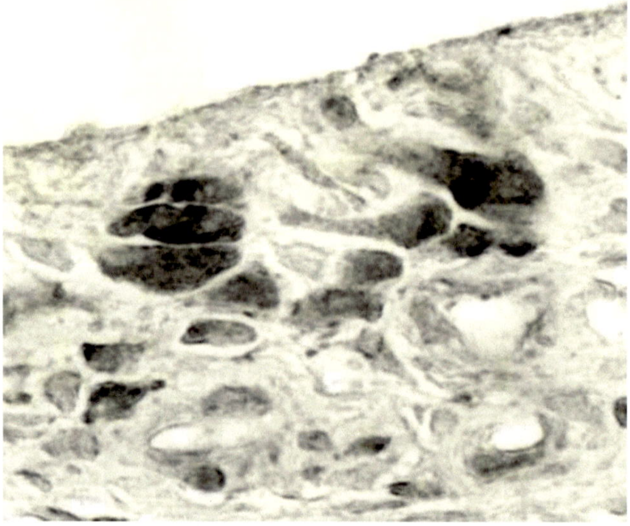

Fig. 5a. Expression of MMP-2 by immunohistochemistry.

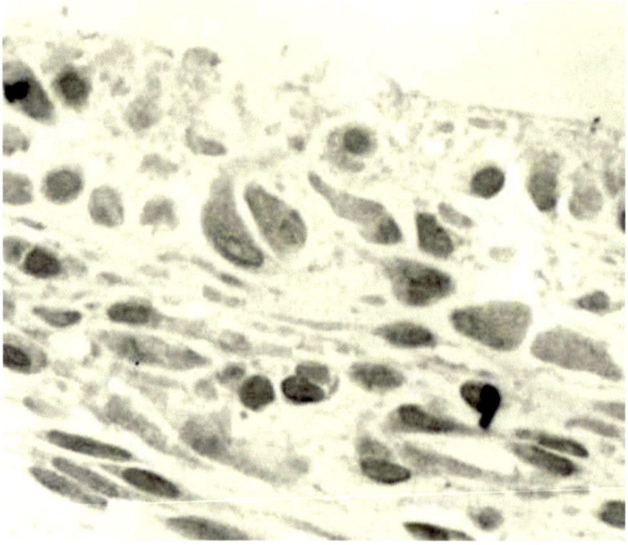

Fig. 5b. Expression of MMP-9 by immunohistochemistry.

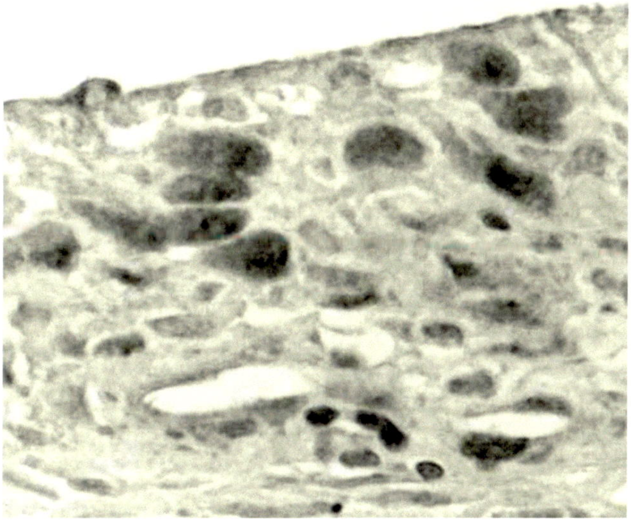

Fig. 5c. Expression of TIMP-1 by immunohistochemisry.

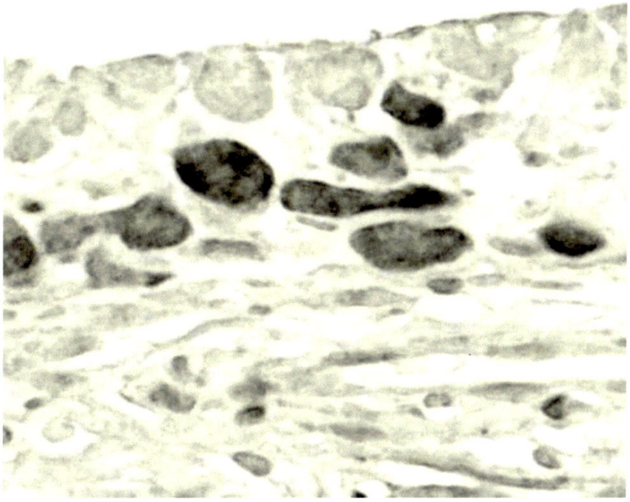

Fig. 5d. Expression of TIMP-2 by immunohistochemisry.

4. References

Cha H.S., Ahn K.S., Jeon C.H., Kim J., Koh E.M. (2003). Inhibitory effect of cyclo-oxygenase-2 inhibitor on the production of matrix metalloproteinases in rheumatoid fibroblast-like synoviocytes. *Rheumatol Int*, Vol. 24, No. 4, (Jul 2004) pp. 207-211, ISSN 0172-8172

de Seny D., Sharif M., Fillet M., Cobraiville G., Meuwis M.A., Marée R., Hauzeur J.P., Wehenkel L., Louis E., Merville M.P., Kirwan J., Ribbens C., Malaise M. (2011). Discovery and biochemical characterisation of four novel biomarkers for osteoarthritis. *Ann Rheum Dis*, Vol., 70, No. 6, (Jun 2011) pp. 1144-1152, ISSN 0003-4967

Furuya M., Ishikura H., Nemori R., Shibata M., Fujimoto S., Yoshiki T. (2001). Clarification of the active gelatinolytic sites in human ovarian neoplasms using in situ zymography. *Hum Pathol*, Vol. 32, No. 2, (Feb 2001) pp. 163-168, ISSN 0046-8177

Galis Z.S., Sukhova G.K., Libby P. (1995). Microscopic localization of active proteases by in situ zymography: detection of matrix metalloproteinase activity in vascular tissue. *FASEB J*, Vol. 9, No. 10 (Jul 1995) pp. 974-980, ISSN 0892-6638

Goodall S., Crowther M., Hemingway D.M., Bell P.R., Thompson M.M. (2001). Ubiquitous elevation of matrix metalloproteinase-2 expression in the vasculature of patients with abdominal aneurysms. *Circulation*, Vol. 104, No. 3, (Jul 2001) pp.304-309, ISSN 0009-7322

Hattori T., Kawaki H., Kubota S., Yutani Y., de Crombrugghe B., von der Mark K., Takigawa M. (2003). Downregulation of a rheumatoid arthritis-related antigen (RA-A47) by ra-a47 antisense oligonucleotides induces inflammatory factors in chondrocytes. *J Cell Physiol*, Vol. 197, No. 1, (Oct 2003) pp. 94-102, ISSN 0021-9541

Ikeda M., Maekawa R., Tanaka H., Matsumoto M., Takeda Y., Tamura Y., Nemori R., Yoshioka T. (2000). Inhibition of gelatinolytic activity in tumor tissues by synthetic matrix metalloproteinase inhibitor: application of film in situ zymography. *Clin Cancer Res*, Vol. 6, No. 8, (Aug 2000) pp. 3290-3296, ISSN 1078-0432

Iwata H., Yamamoto M., Nemori R., Mizutani M., Iwase T., Miura S., Obata Y., Hara Y., Omoto Y., Toyama T., Yamashita H., Iwase H., Kobayashi S. (2001). Localization of gelatinolytic activity can be detected in breast cancer tissues by film in situ zymography. *Breast Cancer*, Vol. 8, No. 2, (2001) pp. 111-115, ISSN 1340-6868

Kaji M., Moriyama S, Sasaki H., Saitoh Y., Kiriyama M., Fukai I., Yamakawa Y., Mitsui A., Toyama T., Nemori R., Fujii Y. (2003). Gelatinolytic activity of matrix metalloproteinase in lung cancer studied using film in situ zymography stamp method. *Lung Cancer*, Vol. 39, No. 2, (Feb 2003) pp. 125-130, ISSN 0169-5002

Kevorkian L., Young D.A., Darrah C., Donell S.T., Shepstone L., Porter S., Brockbank S.M., Edwards D.R., Parker A.E., Clark I.M. (2004) Expression profiling of metalloproteinases and their inhibitors in cartilage. *Arthritis Rheum*, Vol. 50, No. 1, (Jan 2004) pp. 131-141, ISSN 0004-3591

Kraus V.B. (2010). Osteoarthritis year 2010 in review: biochemical markers. *Osteoarthritis Cartilage*, Vol 19, No. 4, (Apr 2011) pp. 346-353, ISSN 1063-4584

Lorenz H., Wenz W., Ivancic M., Steck E., Richter W. (2005). Early and stable upregulation of collagen type II, collagen type I and YKL40 expression levels in cartilage during early experimental osteoarthritis occurs independent of joint location and histological grading. *Arthritis Res Ther*, Vol. 7, No. 1, (2005) pp. 156-165, ISSN 1478-6354

Martel-Pelletier J., Pelletier J.P. (2010). Is osteoarthritis a disease involving only cartilage or other articular tissues? *Eklem Hastalik Cerrahisi*, Vol. 21, No. 1, (Apr 2010) pp. 2-14, ISSN 1305-8282

Reeves N.D., Bowling F. L. (2011). Conservative biomechanical strategies for knee osteoarthritis. *Nat Rev Rheumatol*, Vol. 7, No. 2, (Feb 2011) pp. 113-122, ISSN 1759-4790

Senzaki H., Paolocci N., Gluzband Y.A., Lindsey M.L., Janicki J.S., Crow M.T., Kass D.A. (2000). Beta-blockade prevents sustained metalloproteinase activation and diastolic stiffening induced by angiotensin II combined with evolving cardiac dysfunction. *Circ Res*, Vol. 86, No. 7, (Apr 2000) pp. 807-815, ISSN 0009-7330

Sobczak S., Baillon B., Feipel V., Van Sint Jan S., Salvia P., Rooze M. (2010). In vitro biomechanical study of femoral torsion disorders: effect on tibial proximal epiphyseal cancellous bone deformation. *Surg Radiol Anat*, Vol. 33, No. 5, (Jul 2010) pp. 439-449, ISSN 0930-1038

Sun H.B., Nalim R., Yokota H. (2003). Expression and activities of matrix metalloproteinases under oscillatory shear in IL-1-stimulated synovial cells. *Connect Tissue Res*, Vol. 44, No. 1, (2003) pp. 42-49, ISSN 0300-8207

Takano S., Tsuboi K., Matsumura A., Sato H., Nose T. (2001). Localization of gelatinase activities in glioma tissues by film in situ zymography. *Brain Tumor Pathol*, Vol. 18, No. 2, (2001) pp. 145-150, ISSN 1433-7398

Takei I., Takagi M., Santavirta S., Ida H., Hamasaki M., Ishii M., Fukushima S., Ogino T., Konttinen Y.T. (1999). Matrix metalloproteinases and tissue inhibitors of metalloproteinases in joint fluid of the patients with loose artificial hip joints. *J Biomed Mater Res*, Vol. 45, No. 3, (Jun 1999) pp. 175-183, ISSN 0021-9304

Uzuki M., Watanabe T., Katsura Y., Sawai T. (1999). Quantitative histochemical study of hyaluronic acid binding protein and the activity of uridine diphosphoglucose dehydrogenase in the synovium of patients with rheumatoid arthritis. *Anal Quant Cytol Histol*, Vol. 21, No. 1, (Feb 1999) pp. 75-80, ISSN 0884-6812

Vieillard-Baron A., Frisdal E., Eddahibi S., Deprez I., Baker A.H., Newby A.C., Berger P., Levame M., Raffestin B., Adnot S., d'Ortho M.P. (2000). Inhibition of matrix metalloproteinases by lung TIMP-1 gene transfer or doxycycline aggravates pulmonary hypertension in rats. *Circ Res* 2000, Vol. 87, No, 5, (Sep 2000) pp. 418-425. ISSN 0009-7330

Yamanaka H., Makino K., Takizawa M., Nakamura H., Fujimoto N., Moriya H., Nemori R., Sato H., Seiki M., Okada Y. (2000). Expression and tissue localization of membrane-type 1, 2, and 3 matrix metalloproteinases in rheumatoid synovium. *Lab Invest*, Vol. 80, No. 5, (2000) pp. 677-687, ISSN 0023-6837

Yi C.F., Gosiewska A., Burtis D., Geesin J. (2001). Incorporation of fluorescent enzyme substrates in agarose gel for in situ zymography. *Anal Biochem*, Vol. 291, No.1, (Apr 2001) pp. 27-33, ISSN 0003-2697

Yoshida W., Uzuki M., Nishida J., Shimamura T., Sawai T. (2009). Examination of in vivo gelatinolytic activity in rheumatoid arthritis synovial tissue using newly developed in situ zymography and image analyzer. *Clin Exp Rheumatol*, Vol. 27, No. 4, (Jul-Aug 2009) pp. 587-593, ISSN 0392-856X

Zhang W., Doherty M., Peat G., Bierma-Zeinstra M.A., Arden N.K., Bresnihan B., Herrero-Beaumont G., Kirschner S., Leeb B.F., Lohmander L.S., Mazières B., Pavelka K., Punzi L., So A.K., Tuncer T., Watt I., Bijlsma J.W. (2010). EULAR evidence-based recommendations for the diagnosis of knee osteoarthritis. *Ann Rheum Dis*, Vol. 69, No. 3, (Mar 2010) pp. 483-489, ISSN 0003-4967

Zheng K., Nagai Y., Kishimoto T., Yamazawa K., Tate S., Nemori R., Hirai Y., Sekiya S., Ishikura H. A quantitative evaluation of active gelatinolytic sites in uterine endometrioid adenocarcinoma using film in situ zymography: association of stronger gelatinolysis with myometrial invasion. *Jpn J Cancer Res*, Vol. 93, No. 5, (May 2002) pp. 516-522, ISSN 0910-5050

16

Phonoarthrography: A New Technique for Recording Joint Sounds

Hassan M. Bassiouni
Al-Azhar University
Egypt

1. Introduction

In Medicine there are a lot of sounds emerging from the human body. Many of them are used either for diagnosing the condition such as heart murmurs or following up cases of ileus by hearing nascent intestinal borboregmi or even hearing bruits traversing the skull in cases with brain angiomatous malformation and many more. There is one sound of interest to both rheumatologists and orthopedic surgeons which is the one heard and felt when osteoarthritic knees are moved. As knee sounds were regarded as an accompaniment to OA, the idea of recording knee sounds seemed interesting and plausible to many investigators.

The historical background was handsomely written before (Mollan et al, 1982). An early report dates back to 1882, when Heuter reported the first study involving the evaluation of sounds from the locomotory system, as he described hearing and localizing loose bodies within the knee, using a stethoscope. Blodgett reported in 1902 his experiences on auscultation of the knee using a stethoscope fitted with a rubber diaphragm to prevent slipping and skin friction noises. He could classify different joint sounds, graphically linking each to joint position .In 1906, Ludloff claimed a possible diagnosis on spinal arthritis on auscultatory basis .Bircher in 1913 investigated meniscal lesions of the knee and concluded that each type of injury had a specific sound emission .Walters in 1929, reported the auscultation of 1600 joints and suggested that these sounds might be a sign of early arthritis and promoted the use of joint auscultation in early phases of arthritis . Later, microphones have been used to reduce subjectivity; that step was taken by Erb (1933), when he used a contact microphone obtaining the clearest sound, with the exception of cases of meniscal tears, when he placed the sensor over the patella.

Most of the joints recorded were the knees (M H Bassiouni & El-Feki, 1986;M H Bassiouni et al., 1995; Krishnan et al., 2000; Nagata, 1988) and temporomandibular joints (Ciancaglini et al., 1987; Guler et al., 2003). The first reason, they are superficial thus perfect for auscultation and recording and the second reason is that they produce sounds when diseased.

In 1986, a detailed report was published on phonoarthrography, performed using a special sensor, amplifier, special recorder tape, and a memory oscilloscope (M H Bassiouni & El-Feki, 1986). This device, however, had many disadvantages, such as tape noise imposed on the knee signal; the limited memory storage of the oscilloscope, which did not allow storage of the full motion of the knee; and finally, the incapacity of auto-analysis of the obtained signals.

In 1995 a full report was published on a computerized program used to record knee sounds with a sensor; the results were reproducible and were expressed as average amplitude (units/recording) or frequency/second (M H Bassiouni et al., 1995). The average amplitude was calculated per 2 seconds of recording, while the frequency was measured per 1 second.

When sound engineers deal with this specific area of research, they prefer to name it, externally detected vibroarthrographic signals (VAG) .They concentrate basically on the study of sound definitions rather on the medical point of view. In a paper of that kind, the authors concluded that VAG could provide quantitative indices for non-invasive diagnosis of knee osteoarthritis. They also proposed the use of statistical parameters of VAG signals including the form factor involving the variance of the signal and its derivatives, skewness, kurtosis and entropy to classify the VAG signals into normal or abnormal (Krishnan et al.,2000). Unfortunately, this may not serve rheumatologists as it is not clearly related to the pathophysiology of the disease, or to other investigative tools and treatment impacts.

2. Nomenclature

All sounds are vibrations, but not all vibrations are sounds, that is why the nomenclatures given to the technique included the word vibration such as joint vibrational analysis (JVA) and vibroarthrographic signals (VAG) (Krishnan et al.,2000). Phonoarthrography is the most widely accepted term to describe the medical process as it refers to sounds (phono), originating from joints (arthro) and appearing on a graph.

3. Briefing on sounds

3.1 Definition

Sound is a mechanical wave that is an oscillation of pressure transmitted through a solid, liquid, or gas, composed of frequencies within the range of hearing and of a level sufficiently strong to be heard, or the sensation stimulated in organs of hearing by such vibrations (The American Heritage Dictionary, 2008).

3.2 Propagation of sound inside a joint

Sound is a sequence of waves of pressure that propagates through compressible media such as air or water. Inside the joint the tissues will allow propagation of sounds easily even through the thin patella. During propagation, waves can be reflected, refracted, or attenuated by the medium (The propagation of sound).

Sound propagation during phonoarthrography may be affected by the relationship between density and pressure. This relationship, affected by temperature, determines the speed of sound within the medium. For joint recording, the density of structures do not seem to vary between individuals, nevertheless the intra-articular pressure is increased in cases of OA due to effusion (H M Bassiouni et al., 1992). That is why it is recommended to aspirate excess synovial fluid before recording. The propagation of sound may be affected by the motion of the medium which is not applicable to recording of joint sounds since there is no medium to be moving during recording.

3.3 Sound wave properties and characteristics

Sound waves are often simplified to a description in terms of sinusoidal waves, with some characteristics such as:

- Frequency
- Wavelength
- Wave number
- Amplitude

The important ones used by investigators were the frequency/second, and the amplitude. The wavelength and individual wave number carry no importance to researchers recording joint sounds.

3.4 Speed of sound

The speed of sound depends on the medium traversed by the waves . In general, the speed of sound is proportional to the square root of the ratio of the elastic modulus (stiffness) of the medium to its density. And since the velocity of sound in water is approximately 1,482 m/s then it is assumed that the sound originating from the cartilage surface would take a negligible time to reach the sensor (http://library.thinkquest.org/19537/Physics4.html).

3.5 Noise

Noise is a term often used to refer to an unwanted sound. In science and engineering, noise is an undesirable component that obscures a wanted signal. The problem of noise recording during the process of recording the joint sounds has been dealt with properly. The solution to avoiding the noise background level is either to record in an anechoic chamber or recording first the noise then subtracting it from the joint recording.

3.6 Equipment for dealing with sound

Equipment for generating or recording sound includes transducers such as microphones and loudspeakers. The latter may help to listen to the joint recording afterwards.

4. Joint tissues producing sounds

4.1 Cartilage

Cartilage friction is the mostly accused of producing sounds. If it wears out it produces a complex sound known as crepitus (figure 4) but if there is a torn meniscus it produces one sharp sound during flexion and same on extension (figure 5). The cartilage covering the patella and the femur is also incriminated in sound production together with the femoro-tibial articulations in the knee joint. In the temporomandibular joint, the articulating disc is usually the source of sound production in disorders of mastication, while pain and tenderness come from the synovial lining of the joint.

4.2 Muscles

Muscles acting on knee for flexion and extension as well as those for mastication in the temporomandibular joint may produce sounds during contraction. That is why during recording of the knee sounds flexion and extension are done passively by the examiner to annul the muscle noise. Recording the sounds originating from the temporomandibular joint necessitate active opening and closure of the mouth, while the microphone is put directly on the superficial part of the joint far from the 4 muscles causing jaw movements.

4.3 Ligaments

Ligaments do not move hence they are not major sound contributors.

5. Different recording techniques

The use of a special sensor together with a recording tape and a memory oscilloscope was done in 1986 with many disadvantages such as the inability to get rid of the background noise; also the oscilloscope had a small memory insufficient to complete the full recording of knee flexion- extension at one time. The Inability to analyze the waves was also a disappointment (M H Bassiouni & El-Feki, 1986). A couple of years later another work was able to analyze the joint sounds using a narrow-band spectrum analyzer and a computer. The authors could subtract the spectrum of background noise from the linear averaged spectrum to obtain the phopnoarthrograph (Nagata, 1988). Nevertheless; this work carried some disadvantages. First the authors had to divide the sounds into two levels, the (L type) representing the low level less than 2.5 kHz and the high frequency sound (H type) lower than 3.5 kHz. This did not permit enough flexibility for diagnosing the cartilage condition regarding degeneration, and furthermore it did not help to classify the degree of degeneration. The authors concluded that the sounds emerging were due to thickness and hardness of the cartilage surface.

In 1987, a study was conducted to evaluate the dysfunctional temporomandibular joint (TMJ) by recording the joint sounds heard by a microphone during full mouth opening then closure done repeatedly. The main objective of the authors being dentists was to evaluate masticatory disorders attributed to TMJ disorders. They also correlated the phonoarthrographic values with pain in the TMJ area and also the radiological arthropathic index finding a high degree of correlation between the phonoarthrographic values and the arthropathic index (Ciancaglini et al., 1987).

The first report on phonoarthrography using a sensitive microphone and a computer with a special program came in 1995 with me as a co-author (M H Bassiouni et al., 1995). We proposed the following steps for recording the knee joint:

1. The selected and fixed time for the recording was two seconds. One second for flexion and the other for extension. It was done to be similar to what we do in clinical examination of the knee to feel the crepitus.
2. The patient was seated on a chair with the knee bent in order to fix a constant load (that of the lower limb) and to avoid noises coming from the hip joint Figure 1.
3. A recording of the background noise in the room was done. After its analysis, a standard value for the noise is now obtained. If the device is placed in a sound-proof room (anechoic), there will be no need for standardization of the noise.
4. Ultrasound gel was applied over the shaved patellar skin to avoid friction noises.
5. The sensor was put over the center of the patella in a fixed point.
6. The signals now appear on the monitor after flexing and extending the knee in two seconds.
7. Signals are analyzed and printed.

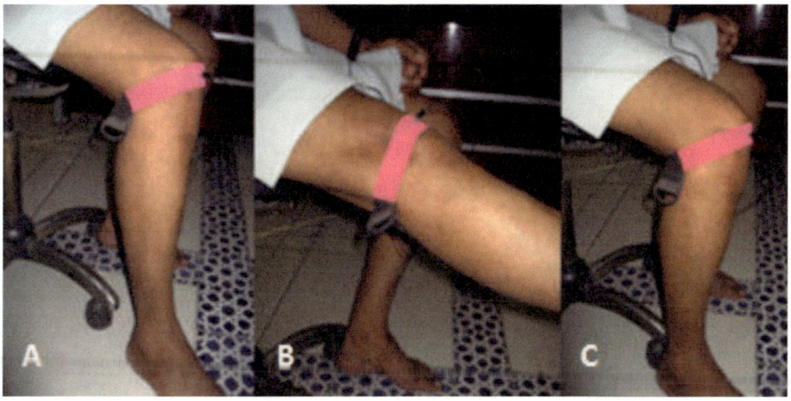

Fig. 1. Showing the microphone attached to a rubber band fixed around the knee so as to be centered on the patella. A –The knee is resting at 90°flexion. B- The knee is fully extended passively. C- Return to resting 90° flexion.

In another work done by some researchers from a department of electronics engineering (Kim et al., 2010), the authors recorded the knee sounds in 2 sec as stated above but they repeated the motion of knee flexion extension during a 20 seconds period. Unfortunately, this method did not add to the outcome of the recording, not to mention muscle fatigue and change in the velocity of movement which renders the test not precisely reproducible. The authors also did the recording using 2 postures the first while the patient is sitting and the second while the patient was standing. The values obtained while on standing were larger than those obtained while sitting; the authors attributed this result to the effect of the patient's weight or stress or both on the knee joint. During knee flexion and extension in standing mode, the different agonist muscles contributed to these movements, such as the hamstrings, biceps femoris, quadriceps femoris, muscles needed a more forceful contraction than in sitting position which increased the sounds recorded. Additionally, during these movements, the exposed area within the patella (which generates the knee sounds due to friction), could become relatively larger producing more waves.

For all researchers working in this field, reproducibility of phonoarthrographic values was a major concern. For that purpose ten knees were selected randomly and recorded 5 consecutive times. The mean values for every single reading were obtained and then readings were compared. The P values were insignificant between the readings assuring reproducibility (M H Bassiouni, 1995).

In an attempt to link modern therapies with phonoarthrography, recording the knee sounds was done before and after hyaluronic acid intraarticular injections (Matsuura & Masatoshi, 2000) two microphones were used in this piece of work, the authors placed them over the patella, 10 mm apart. The work was done on cases with end stage OA of the knees patellofemoral disorders and bucket-handle meniscal tears. The patients were divided into two groups, the first was given hyaluronic acid injections and the second was given steroid injections, both intraarticular. It was found that the sound frequency was significantly reduced (p=0.001) immediately and 24 hours after the hyaluronic acid administration while it did not differ after steroid injections. The frequency returned to pre-administrative levels when the recording was done 48h and 1 week after the administration of hyaluronic acid. The authors attributed the frequency lowering to a better joint lubrication.

In an attempt to explain the previous results, it must be remembered that the molecular structure of glycosaminoglycans allows them to attract and hold countless water molecules through electrostatic forces and weak chemical interactions as hydrogen bonds, which are easily formed and broken. The water-holding capacity of these glycosaminoglycans is so great that, when they are incorporated into the molecular complex, they can hold up to 50 times its own weight in water. This enables the complex to cushion the effects of physical impacts, which when occur, water is squeezed out of the glycosaminoglycans, and when the compressive force dissipates, the water rebinds to these thirsty molecules (Kawano et al., 2003). An important finding also is the fast return of frequency to pre-administrative levels which may suggest a short action of the injected hyaluronic acid.

6. Calibration of signals

The waves obtained in phonoarthrography like others have a frequency/recording and amplitude. Figure 2 shows a control case while figure 3 and 4 show moderate and severe case of osteoarthritis respectively. The frequency will be the number of waves crossing the midline every second and will be measured as number of waves/second. When the number gets higher it means directly more degenerated areas in cartilage. As for the amplitude, it is simply the difference between the highest and lowest points of the wave. The specially designed software has the capability to analyze the waves in average and extreme amplitude. Analogue scale divided into units was used to compare the different amplitudes. When using the amplitude, it is best to use the average values for the all waves in the same recording and this is known as the average amplitude (M H Bassiouni et al. 1995). In some cases where the click of a torn meniscus is recorded, the sound will appear once during flexion and repeated again during extension. The rest of the recording time will not record any other sounds if the knee was healthy until the meniscal problem happened (Figure 5).

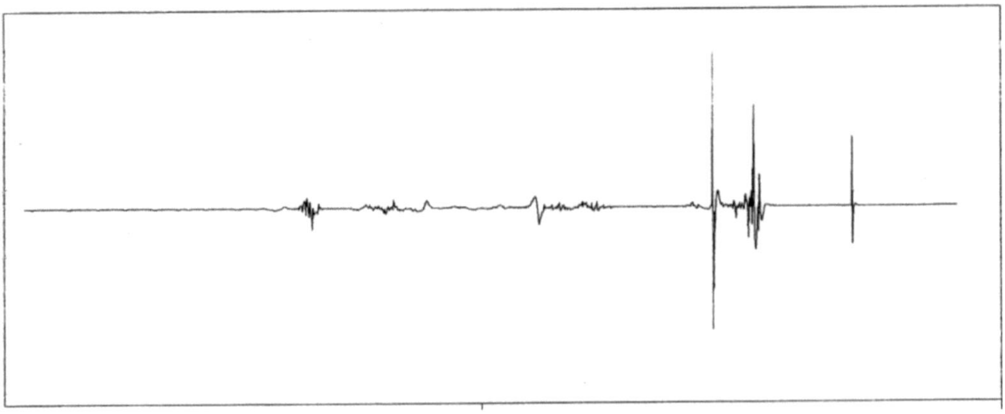

Fig. 2. Phonoarthrography of a control knee with average amplitude of 27.55 units/recording.

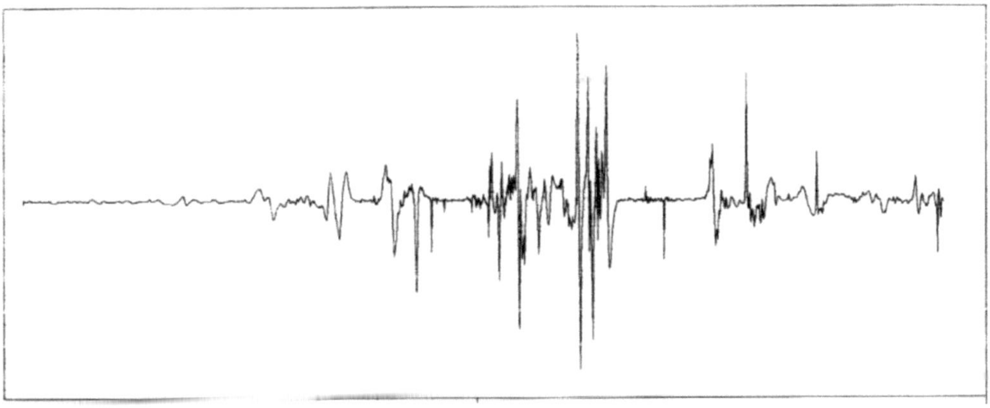

Fig. 3. Phonoarthrography of a moderate case of osteoarthritis (OA), with average amplitude of 47.53 units/recording.

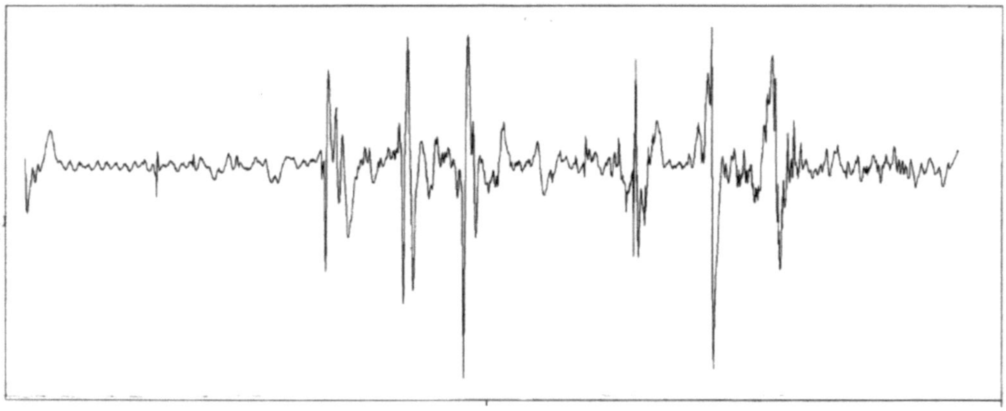

Fig. 4. Phonoarthrography of a severe case of OA, with average amplitude of 64.65 units/recording

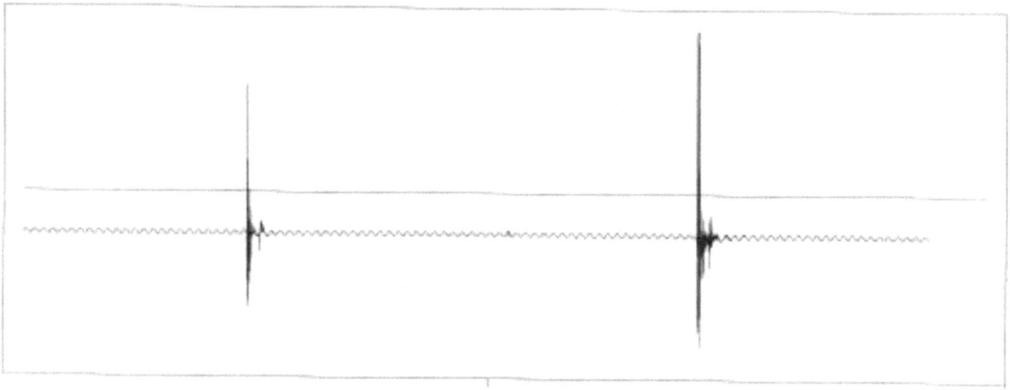

Fig. 5. Phonoarthrograph of a case of torn meniscus showing the sharp sound wave appearing twice during the recording of flexion and extension.

7. Cracking knee sounds

These sounds may be confusing with others. Actually what we call "normal joint sounds" may be produced through a mechanism different from a degenerated cartilage. When the two articulating surfaces, of a synovial joint are forcefully separated from each other, the volume within the joint capsule increases suddenly, creating a negative pressure within. Synovial fluid normally present cannot fill the created extra space and the gases dissolved in the synovial fluid- such as carbon dioxide) are liberated swiftly to fill the space leading to the formation of a bubble (Unsworth et al, 1971). This process is known as cavitation. Cavitation in synovial joints results in a high frequency 'cracking' sound (Watson et al., 1989).

8. Phonoarthrography, a simple parameter for cartilage degeneration

Aging must impose its print on cartilage as it does to many other organs in the human body. In a previous work that performed phonoarthrography on normal controls, rising values went side by side with advancement of age (Figure 6). Logically thinking, this could be expected, however, it still was statistically less than those who had clinically symptomatic osteoarthritis. Another important observation in the same work was that phonoarthrography was found to show abnormally high values in all cases with radiological OA, proving to be 100% sensitive for radiology. Positive values were also present in 32.5% of cases with normal radiology, giving more credit to phonoarthrography as being more sensitive than radiology for detecting cartilage degeneration. All Cases with clinically felt crepitus had abnormal phonoarthrographic values while in those with no felt crepitus, 13% had high phonoarthrographic values (M H Bassiouni et al., 1995).

9. Relating phonoarthrography to other standard investigative tools

9.1 Phonoarthrography versus standard knee radiology

Being relatively a new parameter, phonoarthrography had to be tested against standard used parameters such as radiology in order to discover its potentials properly. The work done by M H Bassiouni et al in 1995, dealt with this point; as the patients had their knees phonoarthrographied and classified using the radiological Kellgren-Lawrence classification grades (K-L) (Kellgren & Lawrence, 1957). The K-L classification as previously known is presented into 4 grades according to radiological severity of the knee joints. The average amplitude and frequency were defined for each K-L grade. A marked statistical difference was found between the phonoarthrography values in each grade and the following grade (P =0.0001) denoting a positive correlation between both parameters (M H Bassiouni et al., 1995).

In a recent work (H M Bassiouni et al., 2011), comparing phonoarthrographic values obtained from patients with bilateral OA of the knees with K-L classification, the authors plotted the average amplitude against each grade and found that it rose steadily with higher radiological grades (35.04 in grade 1, 39.55 in grade 2, 44.27 in grade 3, 50.53 in grade 4) (table 1).

TMJ has a clinico-radiologicalarthropathic index (CRAI) that includes the duration of the occurrence of noise, pain in the TMJ area, the tenderness on lateral palpation of the TMJ, and linear and computer tomography of the craniomandibular complex. The CRAI ranged from

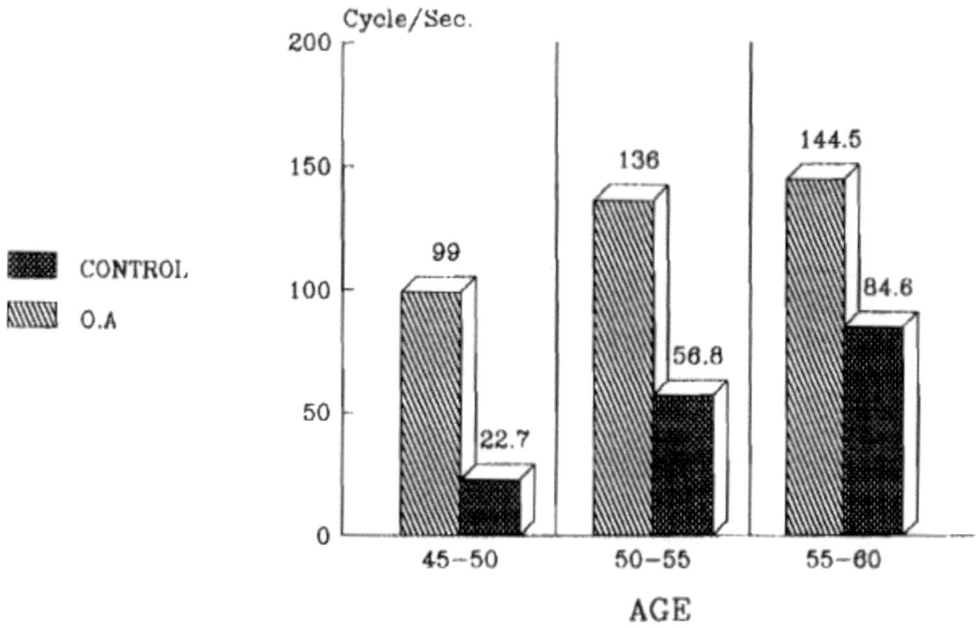

Fig. 6. Showing the frequency/sec from normal controls and from OA patients in different age groups.

O (no arthropathy) to 13 (severe arthropathy). A previous paper where the authors used clinical exam, tomograms and JVA to diagnose TMJ internal derangement versus an artificial neural network (ANN) program trained to recognize vibration patterns. The results of this work showed that ANN correctly identified 98.2% of the diagnosis made previously (Knutson & Radke, 1995).

9.2 Phonoarthrography versus musculoskeletal ultrasonography and MRI

Musculoskeletal ultrasonography (MSUS) has been proposed previously for assessing periarticular and intra- articular abnormalities involved in the pathophysiology of knee OA (Naredo et al., 2005).Before linking parameters to each other, one must know what the capabilities of each are. Musculoskeletal ultrasonography (MSUS) has the capability of studying many structures around the knee joint; it can also measure the thickness of the cartilage peripherally but cannot give information about the surface of the cartilage. On the other hand Phonoarthrography provides an evaluation about the smoothness or roughness of the articular cartilage.

The cartilage thickness from the 4 condyles was measured by MSUS in cases of OA of the knees and Phonoarthrography was performed to same patients (H M Bassiouni et al., 2011). The study provides important information about the thickness of cartilage in both OA patients and control groups and it shows clearly that there was a high statistical difference between the thickness in both groups (P=0.0001). This difference was present in all 4 condyles. Table 1 shows the cartilage thickness from the patients group measured from the 4 condyles in each grade of OA. There was also an inverse correlation between thickness of cartilage and radiological grading.

Phonoarthrography inversely correlated with the thickness of cartilage i.e. the lesser thickness (denoting more degeneration), the higher the average amplitude. An example correlating the medial femoral cartilage thickness to the average amplitude shows r =-0.77, p=0.01.

In a single work in literature that was done to correlate magnetic resonance imaging (MRI) findings of effusion, disc displacement, condylar bony changes and disc form with clinical findings of pain and sounds in patients with bruxing and non-bruxing behavior, the authors found that a higher prevalence of condylar bony changes occurred in reducing joints in patients with bruxing behavior and also they highlighted the importance of phonoarthrography in diagnosing unilaterally affected joints. In non-reducing joints, 30% of painful joints in the patient group and 59% of controls showed a strong signal in the joint space on T_2 weighted imaging (Guler et al., 2003).

9.3 Phonoarthrography versus cartilage biomarkers

In the same work where the authors correlated the cartilage thickness with the average amplitudes (H M Bassiouni net al., 2011); they also measured the MMP-3 and TIMP-1 as to detect if changes in these markers would influence the outcome of phonoarthrography (table 1). MMp-3 was selected because many proteolytic enzymes, secreted by chondrocytes and synovial cells, cause degeneration and destruction of the cartilage matrix of the joints. Matrix metalloproteinase-3 (MMP-3) (stromelysin) is a major player in cartilage destruction; it degrades proteoglycan and collagen types II, IX, and XI (Wu et al., 1991), and also activates other MMPs (Okada et al., 1989).

Parameters Percentage of cases in each grade	OA grade 1 10%	OA grade 2 36%	OA grade 3 30%	OA grade 4 24%
TIMP1 Mean ±SD Median	7570±1678.76 7350	6719.44±2682.1 6300	8356.67±2447.1 8250	9808.33±4135.4 9975
P		F = 2.68, p=0.0662	MW= 6.56, p=0.0871	
MMP3 Mean ± SD Median	36.06±4.98 36.44	109.18±54.61 100.31	121.73±56.43 130.56	93.93±59.78 73.45
P		F=3.33, p=0.0274	MW=12.77, p=0.0051	
Phono-A Rt Mean ± SD Median	35.04±1.85 35.53	39.55±1.55 39.38	44.27±1.5 43.5	50.53±4.57 49.39
P		F=59.87, p=0.0000	MW=44.68, p=0.0000	
Phono-A Lt Mean ± SD Median	35.71± 0.85 35.25	40.54±1.23 40.77	45.04±1.41 44.78	49.62±1.59 49.99
		F=171.55, p=0.0000	MW=44.55, p=0.0000	
MFC Rt Mean ± SD Median	2.73±0.17 2.71	2.37±0.25 2.36	1.97±0.26 1.86	1.38±0.31 1.33
		F=46.86, p=0.0000	MW=36.28, p=0.0000	
MFC Lt Mean ± SD Median	2.93±0.27 3	2.48±0.2 2.49	2.04±0.42 2.01	1.38±0.32 1.22
		F=41.18, p=0.0000	MW=35.17, p=0.0000	
LFC Rt Mean ± SD Median	2.88±0.44 3.1	2.72±0.24 2.76	2.58±0.24 2.65	1.86±0.33 1.79
		F=26.48, p=0.0000	MW=29.05, p=0.0000	
LFC Lt Mean ± SD Median	3.17±0.26 3.04	2.77±0.31 2.69	2.48±0.33 2.6	1.86±0.34 1.98
		F=27.54, p=0.0000	MW=31.21, p=0.0000	
MTC Rt Mean ± SD Median	2.9±0.43 2.94	3.43±0.29 2.37	2.05±0.17 2.12	1.45±0.33 1.41
		F=41.16, p=0.0000	MW=34.93, p=0.0000	
MTC Lt Mean ± SD Median	2.88±0.35 3	2.57±0.24 2.54	2.19±0.24 2.31	1.74±0.42 1.56
		F=25.49, p=0.0000	MW=28.66, p=0.0000	
LTC Rt Mean ± SD Median	3.19±0.29 3.37	2.9±0.31 2.86	2.63±0.32 2.71	2.0±0.34 1.95
		F=25.2, p=0.0000	MW=32.82, p=0.0000	
LTC Lt Mean ± SD Median	3.44±0.19 3.55	2.77±0.25 2.84	2.49±.32 2.59	1.91±0.68 2.02
		F=19.62, p=0.0000	MW=29.46, p=0.0000	

Table 1. This table shows the 4 OA grades in relation to biomarkers (MMp-3 and TIMP-1), phonoarthrography, and cartilage thickness from the 4 condyles.

Interestingly, MMP-3 did not correlate with the real-time status of cartilage elaborated by phonoarthrography, and the reason for that is that this marker denotes only episodes of joint destruction, while Phonoarthrography describe the present cartilage condition.

10. Conclusion

Phonoarthrography is a simple, non-invasive tool that should be present in any rheumatology clinic. A trained doctor or nurse can perform the test easily. A point of strength for Phonoarthrography is that it provides early and sensitive information about cartilage that other imaging machines cannot do, except when the disease is prominent. This information is related to motion, which involves two articulating surfaces gliding over each other at the same time. Magnetic resonance imaging (MRI), a known strong tool for the diagnosis and follow-up of OA, remains handicapped in the domain of detecting any changes related to cartilage surfaces' functioning together, which is provided by Phonoarthrography.

So far only 2 joints have been studied which are the knees and temporomandibular joints. Other joints such as the elbow, metacarpophalangeal, shoulder and other articulations should be candidates for phonoarthrography.

More works are needed to prove that we can use phonoarthrography in diagnosis and follow ups of patients in diseases where the etiologies are different from OA such as in rheumatoid arthritis.

11. Acknowledgement

The idea of recording knee sounds is fully credited to the late Prof. Mohamed Bassiouni who strived to make the idea possible and clinically achievable. The devices and programming were attributed to Prof Fahmy E Fahmy and Prof Mohamed B El-Feki. Delta Software Company also provided the latest version of the program used currently for the recording.

12. References

Bassiouni H, El-Dahan M and El-Gioushy M(1992). Intra-articular pressure in osteoarthritis and its effect on synovial membrane demonstrated by histopathology . *Egypt Rheum & Rehab*;19:317.

Bassiouni H M , El-Deeb M, Kenawy N, Abdul-Azim E, Khairy M(2011). Phonoarthrography, musculoskeletal ultrasonography, and biochemical biomarkers for the evaluation of knee cartilage in osteoarthritis. *Mod Rheumatol* DOI 10.1007/s10165-011-0441-8.

Bassiouni M, Bassiouni H, El-Feki M. (. 1995). Sensitivity versus specificity in phonoarthrography as an indicator for cartilage degen eration. *Clin Rheumatol;* 14:135–42.

Bassiouni MH, El-Feki MB. (1986). Phonoarthrography of the knee in health and diseases. MSc thesis. Department of Rheumatology and Rehabilitation, Al-Azhar University. pp. 97–102.

Bircher, E(, 1929).: Zur Diagnose der Menisculuxationen und des Meniscusabrusses. *Zentrablatt Chir.* 40:1852- 1913.

Blodgett, W.E (1902): Auscultation of the knee joint. *Boston Med. Surg.* J 46-63.

Ciancaglini R, Sorini M, De Cicco L, and Brodolini F. (1987) Digital phonoarthrography of temporomandibular joint sounds: a preliminary report. *J Oral Rehab;* 14:385-392.

Erb, K.H. (1933) Auscultation and recording of knee joint noises (English translation) *Deutsche Ztschr Chir,* 241,237-245.

Guler,N, Yatmaz P,I,, Ataoglu, H, Emlik D and Uckan S. (2003) Temporomandibular internal derangement: correlation of MRI findings with clinical symptoms of pain and joint sounds in patients with bruxing behavior. *Dentomaxillofacial Radiology)* 32, 304–310.

Heuter C. (1882). Grundriss der chirurgic, 3rd ed. Leipzig, FCW Vogel.

Ippe Matsuura and Masatoshi Naito(2000). An analysis of knee sound in cases of OA, PF disorders and meniscal lesions. *Med Bull Fukuoka Univ.* 27(2);78-92.

Kawano T, Miura H, Mawatari T, Moro-Oka T, Nakanishi Y, Higaki H, Iwamoto Y.(2003). Mechanical effects of the intraarticular administration of high molecular weight hyaluronic acid plus phospholipid on synovial joint lubrication and prevention of articular cartilage degeneration in experimental osteoarthritis. *Arthritis Rheum* ;48(7):1923-9.

Kellgren JH, Lawrence JS. (1957). Radiological assessment of osteoar throsis. *Ann Rheum Dis.;* 16:494–502.

Keo Sik Kim & Jeong Hwan Seo & Chul Gyu Song(2010). An Acoustical Evaluation of Knee Sound for Non-invasive Screening and Early Detection of Articular Pathology. *J Med Syst.*17.

Knutson, M., Radke, J (1995). Artificial Neural Network Classification of TMJ Internal Derangement. Abstract. *J Dent Res* 74 (AADR Abstracts) March.

Krishnan S, Rangayyan RM, Bell GD and Frank CB. (2000) Adaptive time-frequency analysis of knee joint vibroarthrographic signals for noninvasive screening of articular cartilage pathology. *IEEE TRANS BIOMED ENG;* 47:773-783.

Ludloff, K (1906): Die auscultation der wirbelsacule des kruezbeines und des Beckheus. *Munchner Med. Wockenschrift.* 53:1197.

Mollan R, McCullough B and Wlison R. (1982) A critical appraisal of auscultation of human joints. *Clin Orthop & related Res.*170; 231-237.

Nagata Y. (1988) joint sounds in gonarthrosis. Clinical application of phonoarthrography for the knees. *J UOEH;* 10(1):47-58.

Naredo E, Cabero F, Palop MJ, Collado P, Cruz A, Crespo M. (2005).Ultrasonographic findings in knee osteoarthritis: a comparative study with clinical and radiographic assessment. *Osteoarthritis Cartilage;*13:568–74.

Okada Y, Konomi H, Yada T, Kimata K, Nagase H.(1989) Degradation of type IX collagen by matrix metalloproteinase 3 (stromelysin) from human rheumatoid synovial cells. *FEBS Lett* ;244:473–77.

Unsworth A, Dowson D, Wright V. (1971). "'Cracking joints'. A bioengineering study of cavitation in the metacarpophalangeal joint.". *Ann Rheum Dis* 30 (4): 348–58.

Walters, C.F(1929). : The value of joint auscultation. *Lancet* 1:920.

Watson P, Kernoham WG, Mollan RAB.(1989) A study of the cracking sounds from the metacarpophalangeal joint. *Proceedings of the Institute of Mechanical Engineering [H]*;203:109-118.

Wu J-J, Lark MW, Chun LE, Eyre DR(1991). Sites of stromelysin cleavage in collagen types II, IX, X, and XI of cartilage. *J Biol Chem.* ;266:5625–8.

The American Heritage Dictionary of the English Language, *Fourth Edition*, Houghton Mifflin Company, 2000, archived from the original on June 25, 2008, http://web.archive.org/web/20080625012016/http://www.bartleby.com/61/65/S0576500.html, retrieved May 20, 2010.

http://www.jhu.edu/virtlab/ray/acoustic.htm

The Soundry: The Physics of Sound The propagation of sound. http://library.thinkquest.org/19537/Physics4.html

Part 5

Sugery of OA in Lower Extremity (Hip, Knee, and Ankle)

17

Surgery for Osteoarthritis of the Knee

J.R. Lewis[1] and R.L. Carey Smith[2]
[1]*Allograft Fellow, Perth Orthopaedic Institute, Perth*
[2]*Trauma and Orthopaedic Surgery, Sir Charles Gairdner Hospital, The University of Western Australia, Perth*
Australia

1. Introduction

Osteoarthritis (OA) of the knee is a common joint disorder affecting nearly a third of the elderly population.

[Felson 1987] The chance of suffering from knee OA increases with advancing age. In a world with an aging population, the prevalence is set to increase further. Conservative management for Osteoarthritis of the knee is often successful and should always be considered initially. However, it is not uncommon for the situation to arise where conservative management has failed or indeed is futile. This chapter will outline, categorize and detail the surgical options available for knee OA. Key results from the literature will be used to demonstrate the current reasoning behind evidence-based practice in surgery for knee Osteoarthritis. In particular we shall focus on evidence comparing surgical options for knee OA.

2. Definition, aetiology and diagnosis

Osteoarthritis (OA), also known as osteoarthrosis and degenerative joint disease is a progressive disorder of the articular cartilage. The aetiology of knee OA is multifactorial. Contributory factors include age, sex, obesity and previous trauma. There is a genetic component to the aetiology of knee OA. It is thought that genetic variations lead to chondrocyte abnormalities resulting in osteoarthritis. [Valdes 2010] Twin studies have demonstrated an increase in prevalence independent of other confounding factors. [Spector 1996]

Diagnosis of knee OA is generally made from a combination of history, examination and radiographic findings. Plain radiographs are usually diagnostic, particularly if they are weight-bearing views. The four classic features are joint space narrowing, osteophyte formation, subchondral sclerosis and the presence of subchondral cysts. Not all of these are required for the diagnosis to be made. In some situations, additional imaging in the form of Computer Tomography (CT), Magnetic Resonance Imaging (MRI) and isotope bone scans can be helpful in providing further diagnostic information.

3. Basic science of articular cartilage

Osteoarthritis is principally a disorder of articular cartilage. The proteoglycan structure of articular cartilage can be damaged by trauma, or by enzymatic degradation secondary to inflammation or infection. If this occurs, the water holding ability of articular cartilage is disturbed. This in turn leads to progressive breakdown of the collagen meshwork exposing the subchondral bone beneath the articular cartilage. It is this exposure of bone, which is responsible for the symptoms of pain in OA.

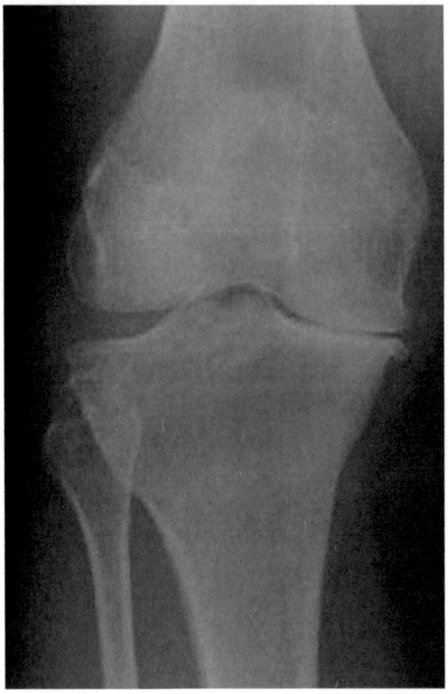

Fig. 1. Knee Osteoarthritis. Medial joint space narrowing, subchondral sclerosis and osteophyte formation.

Articular cartilage is avascular, aneural and alymphatic. Nutrition is derived by diffusion from the synovial fluid or via the blood vessels in the subchondral bone. Articular cartilage unfortunately cannot significantly repair once damaged. Partial thickness injuries do not heal as they stimulate only a minimal reaction in adjacent chondrocytes. Full thickness injuries penetrating the subchondral bone cause bleeding and heal with fibrocartilage as opposed to hyaline cartilage. Unfortunately, the mechanical properties of fibrocartilage are inferior to the specialized hyaline cartilage. The above-described mechanism of fibrocartilage production is the surgical goal of the marrow stimulation techniques, which will be described later.

4. When is surgical intervention warranted in knee OA?

Initial treatment of knee OA is with non-operative measures. When these measures fail, surgical options can be considered. The choice of procedure is based on the symptoms, the severity of OA and patient factors such comorbidities and physical demands on the knee.

The radiological findings are helpful in making an overall assessment of the patient, but do not dictate the treatment option alone. Many patients have severe radiological OA changes but with minimal symptoms. Similarly, some patients can be severely disabled by their knee OA symptoms with minimal changes on plain radiographs.

Pain that is not responding to conservative measures along with decreasing function and mobility are the predominant features in the history that help guide when surgical treatment is required. Inability to sleep due to pain is used by many surgeons as a guide, but occasionally progressive deformity or instability symptoms dictate when the time is chosen for surgery.
There is no globally accepted timing point for surgery to be performed. Patient and surgeon factors along with availability of local resources all play their part.
This chapter will identify and discuss the surgical treatment options in knee OA.

5. Surgical options

5.1 Arthroscopy

Arthroscopy or "key hole" surgery involves the examination and treatment of intra-articular conditions of the knee. Small incisions or portals are made to allow the insertion of an arthroscope. A camera within the arthroscope, a fibre optic light source and irrigation allow visualization of the articular surfaces of the knee. Small instruments that are capable of probing, cutting, shaving and ablating can be passed through the portals to allow assessment and treatment of the osteoarthritic knee.

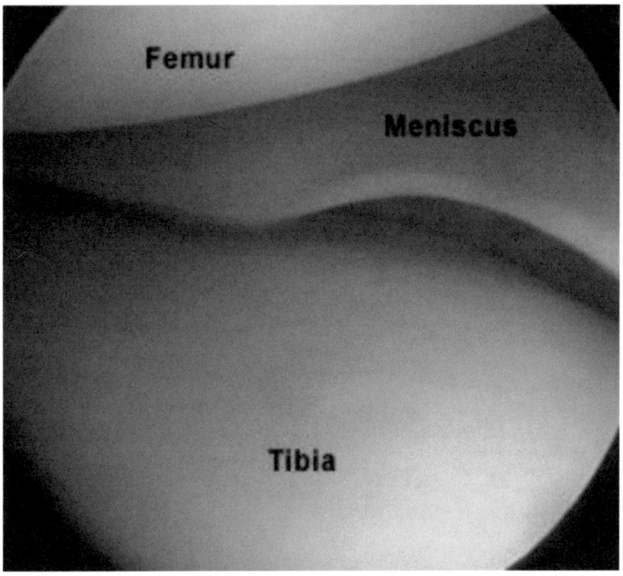

Fig. 2. Normal knee arthroscopic appearances

5.1.1 Classification of cartilaginous lesions

In 1961, Outerbridge [Outerbridge 1961] detailed a grading for patellar chondral lesions. Since then it has become accepted for lesions in other areas of the knee and remains a useful classification in the assessment of cartilaginous lesions of the knee.
Grade 1: Softening and swelling
Grade 2: Fragmentation and fissuring of 0.5 inch or less
Grade 3: Fragmentation and fissuring of 0.5 inch or more
Grade 4: Erosion of cartilage to bone

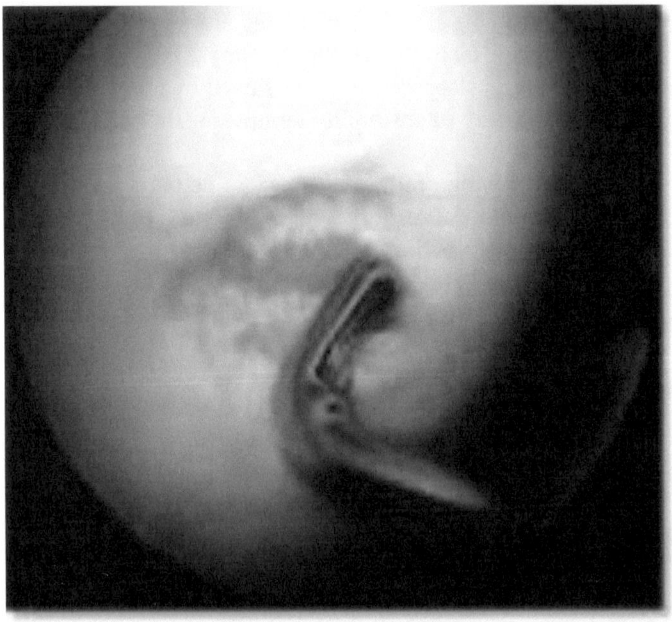

Fig. 3. Erosion of cartilage to bone. Medial femoral condyle.

5.1.2 Arthroscopic lavage and debridement

Arthroscopic lavage involves simply irrigating and washing out the knee joint. The lavage effect was first noted by Burman in 1934. [Burman 1934] Theoretically, it has been proposed that lavage is effective by removing debris and inflammatory cytokines that can cause synovitis. [Chang 1993] [OgilvieHarris 1991]

Arthroscopic debridement can remove loose chondral flaps. The removal of mechanical irritants by debridement of any roughened surface was pioneered by Magnuson in 1941. [Magnuson 1941]

In well-selected middle-aged patients with grade 3 or 4 changes in the medial femoral condyle, a better outcome can be expected with arthroscopic debridement as opposed to arthroscopic lavage. [Hubbard 1996]

It remains controversial as to whether arthroscopic lavage or debridement has a significant role to play in the treatment of knee OA. [Zhang 2007] [Zhang 2008] [Zhang 2010]

Moseley demonstrated no significant benefit to arthroscopic lavage or debridement compared to placebo surgery. [Moseley 2002] The placebo effect was also shown to be significant in the treatment of OA in a systematic literature review. [Zhang 2008a]

A recent Cochrane review of arthroscopic debridement and lavage concluded from these that the procedure has no benefit for OA arising from mechanical or inflammatory changes. [Laupattarakasem 2008]

Despite the lack of evidence in favour for this procedure, it is easy to see why it continues to part of the surgical armamentarium for knee OA for many patients and surgeons. It is evident that it cannot prevent the progression of OA, but it may offer some temporary symptomatic relief. It is a low risk procedure with a short postoperative recovery and doesn't "burn any bridges" in terms of further procedures.

5.1.3 Arthroscopic bone marrow stimulating techniques

The following procedures are not curative. They all aim to create bleeding which in turn will produce a fibrin clot on the exposed bony surface. Undifferentiated cells from the bone marrow proliferate with an end result a fibrocartilage (scar tissue). The procedures do not address the issue of why a weight bearing area of articular cartilage has been denuded. If there is an underlying element of instability or malalignment, the fibrocartilage layer filling the defect is likely to fail.

5.1.4 Drilling

Pridie first described this technique using an arthrotomy incision. [Pridie 1959] He used a 0.25 inch drill bit to penetrate the vascular cancellous bone beneath the sclerotic subchondral lamina. This technique has been adapted to the use of a kirschner wire via arthroscopic portals. Two studies using this technique in rabbits have failed to demonstrate long-term coverage of the denuded bone. [Meachim 1971] [Mitchell 1976]

5.1.5 Abrasion arthroplasty

In this technique a motorized burr is used to create an intracortical abrasion in areas where the chondral surface is deficient. Similar in nature to the drilling technique, the process causes localized bleeding and consequent healing with fibrocartilaginous tissue. During the immediate postoperative phase, the healing fibrocartiaginous tissue is protected from shearing forces by a period of non-weight bearing for the patient.

One study found abrasion arthroplasty was beneficial in the short term in 60% of 110 patients who had full thickness cartilage defects in the knee. Better results were noticed in patients less than 40 years of age. [Friedman 1984]

A comparative 5 year retrospective review of 126 patients with unicompartmental osteoarthritis, undergoing arthroscopic treatment, demonstrated a satisfactory result in only 67% of 59 patients who had been managed with abrasion arthroplasty with debridement as opposed to a satisfactory result in 79% of 67 patients who had been managed with arthroscopic debridement alone. [Bert 1989]

5.1.6 Microfracture

This technique is currently the most widely accepted of the bone marrow stimulating techniques.

Microfracture is the process of making multiple small holes in an area of denuded articular surface with small picks by hand rather than using drills or pins under power. In this low energy technique the awl theoretically causes microfracture of the trabeculae rather than destruction of the bone. Steadman et al [Steadman 1997] describe the technique where the exposed bone is debrided of loose articular cartilage to a stable articular margin. The base of the defect should also be debrided to remove the calcified layer of cartilage. Three to four perforations per square centimeter are made at a depth of approximately 4 mm and spaced 3-4 mm apart. Post operatively range of movement exercises are encouraged, but weight bearing is restricted to protect the healing cartilaginous zone. Histological evaluation of the healed tissue following second look arthroscopy has demonstrated a hybrid of fibrocartilaginous and hyaline-like cartilage. [Bae 2006]

This is a relatively simple, low cost arthroscopic technique. Steadman [Steadman 2002] [Steadman 2003] reported 80% of 75 knees were improved by microfracture with respect to

function and pain at a minimum of 7 years follow up. Other studies suggest a shorter duration of improvement. Kreuz et al found that in their 85 patients, a deterioration in results began at 18 months post surgery. They also reported that the clinical results appear age dependent with better results in patients less than 40 years of age. [Kreuz 2006]
With the development of chondrocyte implantation techniques, inevitably the question arises as to which technique is superior in terms of clinical results. Numerous studies have attempted to address this. A recent systematic review [Harris 2010] evaluated 7 studies [Basad 2010] [Basad 2004] [Knutsen 2007] [Knutsen 2004] [Saris 2009] [Saris 2008] [Kon 2009] comparing autologous chondrocyte implantation with microfracture. Intermediate term (with follow up times ranging from 1 to 5 years) clinical outcome analysis demonstrated a trend towards autologous chondrocyte implantation having improved outcomes as compared with microfracture.

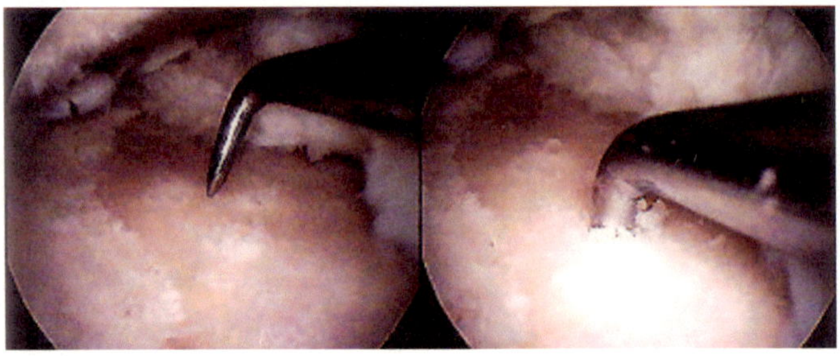

Fig. 4. Microfracture technique.

5.1.7 Arthroscopic Osteochondral Autograft Transplantation System (OATS or Mosaicplasty)

Transplantation of hyaline cartilage from one area of the knee to another will not heal to the underlying bone. An osteochondral graft provides a bony surface to anchor the attached cartilage to the recipient area. The bony area can then be replaced by creeping substitution.
This technique was first described in 1993 by Matsusue et al. [Matsusue 1993] Single or multiple cylindrical plugs from a relatively non weight-bearing region of the knee are harvested. These plugs are then inserted into the chondral surface defect. It is possible to perform the procedure either as an open procedure or arthroscopically.
The main disadvantages are donor site morbidity and the limited options for donor site. The donor site is usually the edge of the patellar groove or the area just proximal to the intercondylar notch. Although larger grafts have been performed, [Karataglis 2005] the limited possible donor sites available, generally restrict the use of this technique to small focal areas of articular cartilage loss.
Outerbridge [Outerbridge 1995] demonstrated an improvement in knee function and symptoms at an average of 6.5 years following osteochondral grafts for defects of the femoral condyle. The procedure does not seem to disturb the main nutritional pattern of articular cartilage. The donor sites fill in with fibrocartilage.
Hangody [Hangody 2003] reported the results of a large series of mosaicplasty. 597 femoral condyles, 76 tibial plateau and 118 patellofemoral joints at up to 10 years postoperatively were assessed. Good or excellent results were reported in 92%, 87%, and 79% of patients who underwent mosaicplasty of the femoral condyle, tibial plateau and patellofemoral joint respectively.

When compared to other cartilage repair techniques, a randomized study by Gudas et al [Gudas 2005] demonstrated a more reliable improvement in clinical outcome with OATS compared to microfracture. In a recent systematic review [Harris 2010] autologous chondrocyte implantation and mosaicplasty were compared in 2 studies. [Dozin 2005] [Horas 2003] Analysis demonstrated equivalent clinical outcomes, but a more rapid treatment response was seen with the mosaicplasty patients.

5.1.8 Autologous chondrocyte implantation

In 1994 Brittberg [Brittberg 1994] described the technique whereby cultivated and proliferated autologous chondrocytes are re-implanted underneath a periosteal flap. An initial arthroscopy following visualization of the chondral defect provides the opportunity to harvest chondrocytes with a small probe. The harvested cells are then grown in a monolayer culture enriched with growth factors over a 3-4 week period. The cells can be suspended in a liquid medium or cultured directly into a three-dimensional collagen scaffold which itself can be implanted. A collagen membrane now replaces the periosteal flap that was initially described. The second stage of the procedure is performed through an open arthrotomy. The main advantage of the procedure is the potential for the restoration of normal hyaline cartilage. The disadvantages are the need for 2 procedures and the cost of the cell culture.

Similar to other cartilage repair techniques, success depends on patient selection. The ideal candidate is a young patient, with a short duration of symptoms and an isolated small chondral defect. [Krishnan 2006]

Instability, malalignment and patellofemoral maltracking will almost certainly jeopardize the final result. An improvement over recent years in Magnetic Resonance Imaging techniques is helpful in patient selection and assessment. [Potter 2009]

Histological analysis studies [Roberts 2003] have demonstrated tissue which is hyaline-like, but the tissue is not morphologically or histochemically identical to normal hyaline cartilage and may include some fibrocartilage.

In a clinical review of 244 patients [Brittberg 2003] with 2-10 years' follow up, subjective and objective improvements were seen in high numbers of patients with femoral condyle lesions. There was a high percentage of good to excellent results (84-90%) in patients with different types of single femoral condyle lesions while other types of lesions had a lower degree of success. Other reports have shown similar levels if success in terms of symptomatic improvement [Erggelet 2003] [Gillogly 2006]. However it has been suggested [Lohmander 2003] that results should be compared with other cartilage repair techniques in randomized trials.

In a randomized trial of 100 patients comparing autologous chondrocyte implantation (58 patients) with mosaicplasty (42 patients), Bentley [Bentley 2003] demonstrated a significant difference between the 2 groups with 88% excellent or good results in the autologous chondrocyte implantation group and 69% excellent or good in the mosaicplasty group. A recent systematic review [Harris 2010] comparing these two techniques, looked at two other studies [Horas 2003] [Dozin 2005] concluding that clinical outcomes were similar.

The same systematic review [Harris 2010] evaluated 7 studies [Basad 2010] [Basad 2004] [Knutsen 2007] [Knutsen 2004] [Saris 2009] [Saris 2008] [Kon 2009] comparing autologous chondrocyte implantation with microfracture. Intermediate term (with follow up times ranging from 1 to 5 years) clinical outcome analysis demonstrated a trend towards autologous chondrocyte implantation having improved outcomes as compared with microfracture.

Despite the increasingly widespread use of autologous chondrocyte implantation, it remains unclear as to whether there is a significant difference between this and other cartilage repair techniques. A Cochrane Database Systematic Review [Vasiliadis 2010] concluded that there was insufficient evidence to draw conclusions on the use of autologous chondrocyte implantation in the knee.

5.2 Osteotomy

Osteotomies around the knee alter the weight-bearing axis of the lower extremity. The surgical goal is to unload the damaged compartment and to transfer the weight load from the affected areas by slightly overcorrecting into a valgus or varus alignment. The aims of the procedure are to reduce pain, slow the degenerative process and delay joint replacement.

The concept gained acceptance in the 1960s after studies by Jackson and Waugh [Jackson 1961]. They demonstrated that a correction in the knee deformity relieved the pain. Many surgeons believe that the mechanism for symptomatic improvement is entirely mechanical [Harris 1970]. Others believe that this biomechanical concept is spurious. Shaw and Moulton demonstrated in their biomechanical cadaveric study, that to unload the medial compartment, a valgus correction of 25 degrees would be required. [Shaw 1996]

During the 1960s and 1970s, the use of osteotomy was the recommended surgical treatment for osteoarthritis of the knee. As the mid term and long-term excellent results of knee replacements became apparent, the use of osteotomy became less widespread.

The advantages of osteotomy over total joint arthroplasty are the preservation of bone stock and intra-articular structures. The classic indication is an osteoarthritic knee with single compartment disease (most commonly the medial compartment) accompanied by a varus or valgus alignment. Patient selection is fundamental to achieving a satisfactory result. The knee should have a good range of movement. The patellofemoral joint should not be significantly involved. Ligamentous stability is ideal, but cruciate ligament instability is not an absolute contraindication. Combining an osteotomy with a cruciate ligament reconstruction is possible. Changing the slope of the proximal tibia at the time of the osteotomy can also improve cruciate ligament laxity. [Aqueskirchner 2002] [Paley 2000]

Osteotomies around the knee have generally been suited to young active patients in place of joint replacement. An osteotomy once united allows unlimited activity. The polyethylene is a cause for concern in highly active patients with knee joint replacements. High loads from running and jumping may exceed the tolerance of polyethylene. Repetitive loading may loosen or damage a total knee replacement.

In unicompartmental osteoarthritis, it is possible to correct the mechanical axis with different techniques. These include proximal tibia and supracondylar distal femoral osteotomies. Both can be performed with an additive (opening wedge) or subtractive (closing wedge) technique. Most commonly, the osteotomy is performed on the proximal tibia for varus medial compartment osteoarthritis. This can be a lateral closing wedge or a medial opening wedge osteotomy.

Traditionally, a closing wedge, valgising osteotomy was performed for medial compartment osteoarthritis. Described by Coventry [Coventry 1965], the osteotomy is made proximal to the tibial tuberosity and incorporates a fibula osteotomy also.

One disadvantage of a lateral closing proximal tibial osteotomy is the associated risk of peroneal nerve injury at the time of fibula osteotomy. This is reported to be as high as 11%. [Staubli 2003] Other concerns are the propensity for loss of bone stock, patella baja and leaving the joint line in an oblique position, making subsequent joint replacement more challenging.

For these reasons, the medial opening wedge osteotomy has gained in popularity.

5.2.1 Outcome following high tibial osteotomy

There are numerous studies available on the outcome following high tibial osteotomy. Differing techniques and evaluation methods make pooling and comparison of this data challenging. A Cochrane review [Brouwer 2007] concluded that there is "silver" level evidence that a valgising high tibial osteotomy improves knee function and reduced pain, but there is no evidence whether an osteotomy is more effective than conservative treatment.

Coventry describes good results in several studies. [Coventry 1979] [Coventry 1982] [Coventry 1993] Coventry also states that high tibial osteotomy not only improves the knee function, but also allows healing of the articular cartilage. [Coventry 1984]

Multiple studies have demonstrated that the early good results of high tibial osteotomy gradually deteriorate with time. A meta-analysis [Virolainen 2004] demonstrated good or excellent results in 75% of patients after 60 months and 60% of patients after 100 months. Unchanged and mild pain were defined as unsatisfactory results.

It is generally accepted that age is an important factor in predicting outcome. Patients greater than 50 years old are less likely to have a satisfactory result. [Naudie 1999] [Flecher 2006]

The degree of correction has repeatedly been shown to correlate with survivorship. Overcorrecting the femorotibial angle to more than 15 degrees has been shown to give a better clinical outcome, but the cosmetic appearance is generally not acceptable to patients. [Rudan 1990] Under correction is associated with a poorer outcome. [Naudie 1999] [Ivarsson 1990] [Matthews 1988] [Sprenger 2003]. Consequently, most surgeons aim for a correction of between 5 and 12 degrees.

5.2.2 Closing versus opening wedge high tibial osteotomy

For many years, the closing wedge osteotomy was considered the gold standard. Over recent years the medial open wedge osteotomy technique has been developed. This procedure is considered technically less demanding and more precise. The use of modern angular stable locking plates for fixation of the osteotomy makes the need for bone grafting potentially dispensable. [Lobenhoffer 2003] [Staubli 2003]. Long-term results for open wedge techniques, with modern implants using locking screws are not yet available. One randomized controlled trial [Brouwer 2006] comparing the two techniques reports at one year follow up, an improvement in knee function and pain in both groups but no significant differences. Until further studies become available, it is not possible to state which technique should be preferred.

5.2.3 Total knee replacement after high tibial osteotomy

Understandably, the outcome of Total Knee Replacement following High Tibial Osteotomy raises concerns amongst surgeons and patients. The two concerns generally raised, relate to the technical difficulty of total knee replacement following high tibial osteotomy and the whether there is a negative effect on functional outcome of total knee replacement if there has been a previous high tibial osteotomy.

It is generally accepted that Total Knee Replacement can be more challenging following lateral closing wedge High Tibial Osteotomy. [Mont 1994] [Karabatsos 2002] The difficulties relate to loss of bone stock, surgical exposure, obliquity of the joint line, soft tissue balancing and patella baja.

Amendola [Amendola 2010] reviewed all published data relating to this and concluded that there is no statistically significant difference between patients treated with a primary total knee replacement or with a total knee replacement following a high tibial osteotomy. A systematic review by Van Raaij [VanRaaij 2009] also concluded that previous osteotomy does not compromise subsequent total knee replacement.

There have been no studies reporting Total Knee Replacement results following opening wedge high tibial osteotomy.

5.2.4 Unicompartmental knee arthroplasty versus high tibial osteotomy

Although there is a large difference in the philosophy between these two procedures, the indications can overlap. Consequently, a number of comparative studies have been performed. Most of these studies compare Unicompartmental Knee Arthroplasty to lateral closing wedge high tibial osteotomy.

A retrospective review of 49 lateral closing wedge high tibial osteotomies and 42 unicompartmental knee arthroplasties reported 76% good results with Unicompartmental Knee arthroplasty and 43% with high tibial osteotomy at 5-10 years. [Broughton 1986]

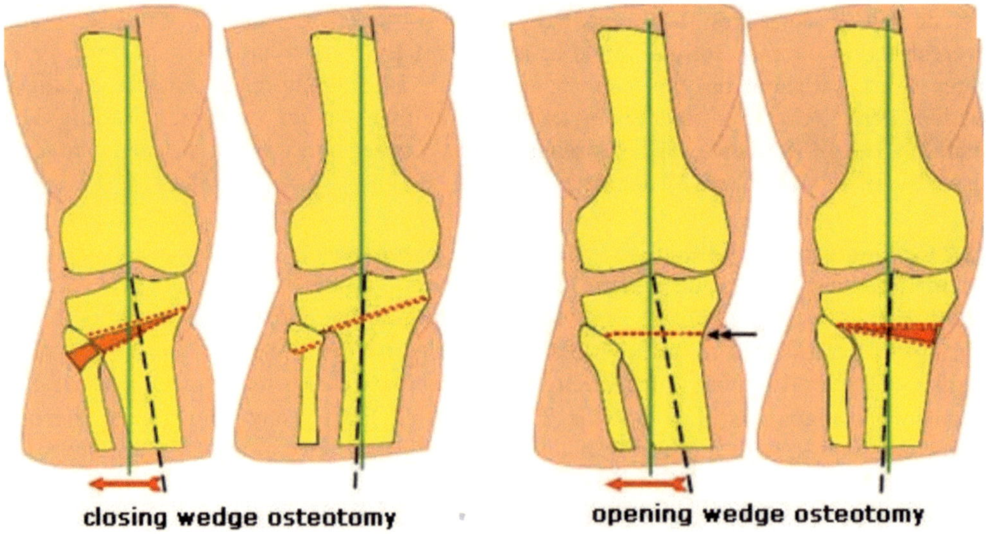

Fig. 5. Closing and opening wedge osteotomies of the proximal tibia

A prospective randomised comparison between 32 high tibial osteotomies and 28 unicompartmental knee arthroplasties reported improved long term success with unicompartmental knee arthroplasty with 77% 10 year survival compared with 60% in the osteotomy group. [StukenborgColsman 2001]

A comparison of 54 consecutive opening wedge high tibial osteotomies and 56 unicompartmental knee arthroplasties found no difference in the midterm clinical or radiological results. [Dettoni 2010]
The latest Cochrane review [Brouwer 2007] states that there is no significant difference in pain, function and gait analysis between HTO and UKA.

5.3 Arthroplasty

Arthroplasty or joint replacement is a well-accepted and effective treatment modality for advanced knee osteoarthritis. The number of knee arthroplasties performed has increased exponentially over the last few decades.

5.3.1 History of knee arthroplasty

Themistocles Gluck implanted a primitive hinge joint made of ivory in 1860. The next significant step was the acrylic Walldius hinge joint in 1951, followed by a cobalt and chrome implant in 1958. [Walldius 1953]
Gunston in the 1960s designed an unhinged knee that that incorporated separate medial and lateral condylar components. [Gunston 1971] Gunston recognized that the knee does not rotate on a single axis and has more complex kinematics than a simple hinge. By preserving the cruciate ligaments, the polycentric knee design allowed the femoral condyles to roll and glide on the tibia with multiple instant centres of rotation. The failure mechanism related to inadequate fixation of prosthesis to bone.
The so-called "kinematic conflict" arose as further designs became available. Some designers opting to follow Gunston's principle of attempting to recreate normal knee kinematics. Others opting for a conforming articulation and constraint. A highly conforming design acts like a simple hinge, which increases the torsional stress across the joint leading to loosening of the prosthesis.
Insall designed and introduced the Total Condylar Prosthesis at the Hospital for Special Surgery in 1973. This initial design did not attempt to recreate normal knee kinematics. Subsequently, the design was altered to improve knee range of movement. Improvements in component geometry, instrumentation, bearing materials and fixation techniques continue to be made.

5.3.2 Indications and assessment for knee arthroplasty

The functional impact of the knee osteoarthritis is the key factor in determining the timing of knee replacement surgery. Severity of symptoms are classically assessed by how disabling the pain is, noting a decreased walking distance, increased analgesic use and disturbance of sleep.
Examination should assess gait, limb alignment, range of movement and the neurovascular status of the limb. Other sources of knee pain such as the hip and lumbar spine should routinely be assessed to exclude dual pathology.
Up to date radiographs should be available including weight bearing anteroposterior views as well as a true lateral and skyline view. Radiographs of the ipsilateral hip are necessary if clinical examination raises the suspicion of hip pathology.

5.3.3 Total knee arthroplasty – Current designs

Most current primary knee replacement designs fall into the category of unconstrained knee replacements. There are two design types in this category: the posterior cruciate retaining and the posterior cruciate substituting (or posterior stabilized) implants. Both types include a metal femoral component, a metal tibial component with a polyethylene insert (or an all polyethylene tibial component) and if used a polyethylene patella component. The implants can be cemented or uncemented.

The posterior cruciate retaining design is controversially thought to replicate knee kinematics more closely because the native posterior cruciate ligament causes femoral rollback. They have low conformity with a round femoral surface and a relatively flat tibial polyethylene surface.

The posterior cruciate substituting designs have increased conformity. They employ a tibial polyethylene post in the middle of the knee together with a cam situated between the femoral condyles. During flexion the femoral cam engages against the tibial post. With further flexion controlled mechanical rollback is achieved.

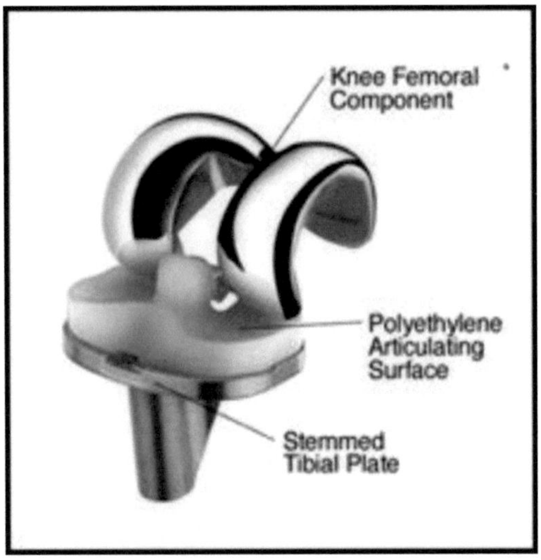

Fig. 6. Cruciate substituting Total Knee Replacement prosthesis

5.3.4 Total knee arthroplasty – Surgical goals

A pain free, mobile, stable joint replacement with a long life span is the overall aim of knee replacement surgery. The achievement of several biomechanical goals can contribute towards this overall aim. Implant design and surgical technique are crucial in how these goals are achieved.

5.3.4.1 Restoration of mechanical axis

The proximal tibia and distal femur are cut in such a way that at the end of the operation the mechanical axis of the limb should pass from the centre of the hip through the centre of the knee to the centre of the ankle. This allows the equal passage of forces through the joint replacement optimizing its longevity. [Fang 2009]

5.3.4.2 Preserve the level of the joint line

The femur and tibia are cut at a depth that is equal to the thickness of the prosthesis that is inserted. Optimal function of ligaments, muscles and tendons can be expected if the joint line level is preserved.

5.3.4.3 Soft tissue balancing in the coronal plane

An osteoarthritic knee with a varus or valgus deformity has soft tissues that are contracted on one side of the joint and stretched on the other side. If the deformity is not corrected by the bony cuts, a soft tissue release is performed on the concave side of the deformity. If the knee is well balanced at the end of the procedure, load transmission should be approximately equal through both sides of the joint.

5.3.4.4 Balancing the flexion and extension gaps in the sagittal plane

At the end of the procedure, the gap between the tibia and femur should be the same in extension and in flexion. A gap that is too tight in extension or flexion will prevent full extension or flexion respectively. A gap too loose in extension will allow hyperextension of the knee; too loose in flexion will allow instability in flexion.

5.3.4.5 Maintenance of Q angle

The most common complication in Total Knee replacement involves the patellofemoral articulation.
The Q angle is the angle formed by a line drawn from the Anterior Superior Iliac Spine to the central patella and a second line drawn from the central patella to the tibial tubercle. An increased Q angle is a risk factor for patellar subluxation.
Positioning of the femoral, tibial and patella component (if used) all can influence the stability of the patellofemoral articulation.

5.3.5 Total knee arthroplasty – Results

Total knee arthroplasty is an effective treatment for advanced knee osteoarthritis, resulting in substantial improvement in patient function and health related quality of life. [Buly 1995]
The success of the procedure can be judged by patient satisfaction and by the lifespan of the implant before a revision procedure is required. (Survivorship)
Patient satisfaction can be assessed by questionnaires. A study using data from the British National Joint Registry demonstrated 81.8% of 8095 patients were satisfied, 11.2% (906 of 8095) were unsure and 7% (566 of 8095) were not satisfied with their new knee. [Baker 2007]
The total condylar knee design continues to be successful. At 15 years follow up, survivorship can be expected to be as high as 95%. [Ranawat 1993] [Ritter 2001].

5.3.6 Total knee arthroplasty – Controversial topics and recent developments

5.3.6.1 Cemented versus uncemented fixation

Cemented fixation of total knee replacement is a standard procedure with good long-term durability. Despite the predominance of cemented fixation, there is increasing interest in using cementless fixation. The principal advantage to using uncemented implants is the shorter operating times.
A meta-analysis compared the two techniques by outcome. [Gandhi 2009] For implant survival without aseptic loosening, cemented prostheses lasted longer. Both designs shared similar complications and produced similar results.
The advantages of cemented fixation are that it is less costly and gives immediate stable fixation, preventing early migration. [Nilsson 1999] Cemented fixation has the added advantage of filling in small voids, whereas uncemented fixation requires perfect bony cuts to allow a perfect fit between prosthesis and bone.

5.3.6.2 Cruciate retaining versus cruciate sacrificing design

Good long-term results are reported in both posterior cruciate retaining (CR) and posterior cruciate substituting (PS) Total Knee Replacement designs. [Ritter 2007] [Bourne 2007]
The role of the posterior cruciate ligament (PCL) in total knee replacement remains controversial. Those in favour of retaining the PCL propose maintenance of normal knee kinematics, particularly with reference to femoral rollback. Others believe that the PCL's proprioceptive properties should encourage its retention. [Scott 1986] [Conditt 2004] [Insall 1988] [Swanik 2004] Those in favour of sacrificing the PCL argue that the ligament is degenerative in arthritic knees and that removing it makes soft tissue balancing more straight forward. If the PCL is excised, most surgeons will use a posterior cruciate substituting design, although this is not essential as long as a reasonably conforming insert is used. [Straw 2003] Proponents of the PS design argue that the central polyethylene post engages on the femoral cam during flexion providing mechanical femoral rollback. [Dennis 1996]The central post may also provide some additional stability in the anteroposterior plane and act as a secondary stabiliser to varus or valgus stress. [Matsuda 1996]
Multiple comparative studies have shown no demonstrable difference in knee scores, patient satisfaction or radiographic parameters. [Dorr 1988] [Clark 2001] [Tanzer 2002] A systematic literature review within the Cochrane framework [Jacobs 2005] identified an increased average range of motion in the posterior stabilised group (113 degrees) compared with the PCL retention group (105 degrees). No other differences were found. The review does not conclude superiority of one technique over the other.

5.3.6.3 Patella resurfacing versus non-resurfacing

Management of the patella in Total Knee Replacement for osteoarthritis remains controversial. Currently, there are three options available: Routine resurfacing, non-resurfacing and selective resurfacing. Proponents of patellar resurfacing propose that this procedure will decrease the incidence of anterior knee pain postoperatively and lower the risk of reoperation following Total Knee Replacement.
Some surgeons avoid routine resurfacing on the basis of a variety of complications that have been attributed to the procedure. These include instability of the patellofemoral joint, avascular necrosis, patellar fracture, patella tendon injury, aseptic loosening and polyethylene wear of the patella component. These complications although relatively uncommon have been associated with difficult revision procedures. [Barrack 1998] [Rand 2005]
Some surgeons opt to selectively resurface the patella, but it has been shown that the appearance of the articular cartilage is an unreliable predictor for a successful outcome. [Waters 2003]
There have been a substantial number of comparative studies on this subject. Indeed, several meta-analyses have collated this evidence, demonstrating a lower risk of reoperation for resurfaced implants, but not demonstrating firm evidence of superiority of one technique over the other. [Nizard 2005] [Forster 2004] [Pakos 2005] [Parvizi 2005] A critical appraisal of the available evidence suggests that patellar resurfacing reduces the risk of anterior knee pain and patella related reoperation, but found methodological limitations in all the studies examined. It concludes that no single option for patella treatment in total knee replacement is clearly superior. [Calvisi 2009]

5.3.6.4 Computer assisted surgery

Over recent years, there has been considerable development in computer-assisted navigation systems for total knee replacement.

Current navigation systems are comprised of several components. An optical tracking system measures the position and orientation of optical reference frames that are attached to the femur and tibia, typically with bicortical threaded pins. The camera also tracks a stylus that the surgeon uses to digitize bony landmarks and an instrumented plate that records the position and orientation of the cutting blocks and bone surfaces. The navigation system is controlled by a computer and accompanying software. Anatomical reference frames are created that relate the position mad orientation of the optical reference frames to the underlying bony anatomy.

Although navigation in total knee replacement has increased in popularity over recent years, it remains controversial as to whether it is superior to traditional mechanical instrumentation techniques.

Most would accept that demonstrating improvements in results for a successful procedure such as total knee replacement is not easy.

The main arguments against the routine use of computer-assisted navigation relate to cost and time. The cost is variable, but has been shown to be in the region of an additional 200 to 1400 Euros per case, compared with the manual technique [Cerha 2009]. Cost effectiveness is difficult to judge until long-term outcome studies are available. It has been estimated that an annual reduction in revision rates of 2 % would be required over 20 years in a centre performing 250 navigated total knee replacements per year, in order to be cost effective [Slover 2008]. Additional operating time is required. This has been demonstrated as being between 8 to 14 minutes per case. [Bäthis 2004] [Jenny 2005] [Haaker 2005]

A fundamental premise of computer-assisted navigation relates to one of the surgical goals of total knee replacement surgery. It has been proposed that more accurately restoring the mechanical axis of the limb will promote greater implant durability. Previous studies have suggested that restoring overall limb alignment to a mechanical axis of less than 3° varus/valgus will improve the longevity of the implant [Jeffery 1991] [Ritter 1994]. Consequently, several studies have focused on this and demonstrated that the use of computer navigation can lead to a significant reduction in the number of outliers outside of this range. [Jenny 2005] [Bäthis 2004] A systematic review incorporating twenty nine studies comparing alignment outcomes in computer assisted knee replacements with conventional techniques demonstrated a 3° varus/valgus malalignment occurred in 9% of computer assisted cases and 32% in conventional knee replacements.

More recently, this concept this has been contested with evidence to suggest that fifteen year survival of knee replacements is unaffected by variations in the postoperative limb mechanical axis. [Parratte 2010]

Some surgeons favour physiological reasons rather than alignment reasons in their reasoning to navigate a total knee replacement. Computer navigation techniques can avoid the need to instrument the femoral or tibial canals as with intramedullary jigs. Studies have demonstrated decreases in blood loss, systemic emboli and generalized systemic inflammatory response with the use of navigation techniques. [Kalairajah 2005] [Kalairajah 2006] [Church 2007] [Shen 2009].

Definitive conclusions regarding differences in clinical outcome between navigated and conventional techniques can only be made with long-term results of well-conducted randomised controlled trials. These are not yet available, but there is some evidence suggesting that rehabilitation is quicker and short-term function within the first postoperative year is improved with a greater accuracy in implant alignment. [Choong 2009] [Longstaff 2009]

5.3.6.5 Mobile versus fixed bearing inserts

Surgeons make a choice between monoblock all polyethylene tibial components and metallic tibial components with a modular polyethylene insert. The insert as described earlier can either be posterior stabilizing (with a post, to articulate with a cam on the femoral component) or cruciate retaining (no post). Either way, the insert can be of fixed bearing or mobile bearing design.

Mobile-bearing inserts can be further subdivided into rotating platform types or meniscal bearing types. A rotating platform rotates by utilizing a peg on its undersurface that fits into a socket on the base plate. In contrast to this, meniscal bearing inserts also allow anterior – posterior translation of the insert over the base plate.

Theoretically, mobile bearing designs have greater total congruency of the femur/tibial articulation. This leads to less contact stress and potentially less polyethylene wear. Knee simulation studies have demonstrated less wear with rotating platform designs. [Mcewen 2001] The other proposed advantage is that the freedom of movement at the polyethylene/tibial tray interface should decrease the stresses at the tibial tray/bone interface.

There have been a large number of publications attempting to determine whether the theoretical advantages of a mobile bearing insert are transformed into clinical advantages. These studies consistently fail to demonstrate any significant advantage for either design. [Evans 2006] [Biau 2006] [Kim 2007] [Kim 2007a]

5.3.6.6 Patient specific cutting blocks

This new technique relies on patient specific cutting blocks. These are engineered by using a computer template of the patient's own anatomy. Preoperative imaging with a Magnetic Resonance Imaging scan and mechanical axis radiographs are used. These individualized cutting blocks allow precise bone resections to be made, allowing implantation of standard knee replacement implants. Advantages are a shortened operation time and a smaller surgical inventory requirement (sizes of implants determined preoperatively). Disadvantages are the additional costs for the preoperative imaging and the production of the custom made cutting blocks. Long-term results using this technique are awaited.

5.3.7 Unicompartmental Knee Arthroplasty (UKA)

UKA is the partial surface replacement of the knee joint. Osteoarthritic changes can be predominantly confined to one of the three compartments of the knee. In this scenario, a UKA can be performed in the medial tibiofemoral joint, the lateral tibiofemoral joint or the patellofemoral joint. By far the most common site for osteoarthritis in the knee is the medial tibiofemoral joint. The biggest experience to date with UKA has been with the medial tibiofemoral joint. Here, a metallic femoral component and a metallic tibial component replace the medial side of the knee joint. The components can be cemented or uncemented. In between the two metal components, a polyethylene insert is positioned. This can be a mobile bearing or a fixed bearing design. In the mobile bearing design, the polyethylene insert has a flat undersurface to allow it to slide over the flat tibial component. The top surface is concave allowing a congruent articulation with the spherical femoral component above. The proposed benefits of this articulation are larger contact areas; resulting in lower contact pressures and decreased polyethylene wear rates. The disadvantages of the mobile bearing design are that it is technically more challenging to implant and the potential risk for bearing dislocation. The fixed bearing design has a polyethylene insert which locks into the tibial tray. A meta-analysis pooling data from five studies concluded that there was no significant difference in outcome or complication rates between mobile and fixed bearing UKAs. [Smith 2009]

The ideal indications for UKA include unicompartmental osteoarthritis; age over 60 years; low demand patient; no obesity; range of motion arc over 90 degrees with less than 5 degrees fixed flexion contracture; less than 10 degrees of axial malalignment in the coronal plane which is passively correctable. [Borus 2008]

One perceived advantage of UKA over Total Knee Replacement is a less extensive surgical dissection. Generally, there is no need for eversion of the patella and the soft tissue disruption is less. Preservation of bone stock, decreased blood loss and an end result with more normal knee kinematics are also quoted as advantages. [Robinson 2003]

Unicompartmental knee arthroplasty (UKA), total knee arthroplasty (TKA) and high tibial osteotomy (HTO) may all be used to treat unicompartmental osteoarthritis, but they are often used for different patient groups. However, there is considerable overlap in indications for all three options.

A systematic review [Griffin 2007] focused on the safety and efficacy of UKA compared with TKA and HTO in unicompartmental osteoarthritis. Studies that compared UKA with either TKA or HTO were identified and included for review. They conclude that UKA is considered at least as safe as TKA and HTO. For function, UKA appears to be at least as efficacious as TKA and HTO. The survival of UKA compared with TKA and HTO could not be determined based on the available evidence.

The first published series of UKA documented a 70% 10-year survival rate. [Marmor 1988] [Marmor 1988a]

Improvements in implant design; materials and instrumentation combined with clearer patient selection criteria may have been partially responsible for some of the better-reported results. Up to 98% survivorship has been reported at 10 years in both fixed and mobile bearing designs. [Berger 1999] [Murray 1998]

On the other hand a prospective study of 1819 patients from the Finnish Arthroplasty Register demonstrated an overall 10-year survival of 73% between four different implants. This supports the view of many, that the long-term survival of UKAs remains significantly poorer than that of TKA. [Koskinen 2007]

Isolated lateral compartment osteoarthritis of the knee is less common. Consequently, outcome studies reporting results of lateral UKA are less abundant. Results appear to be less predictable with a higher complication rate than the medial UKA. [Gunther 1996]

Isolated patellofemoral osteoarthritis occurs in approximately 10% of patients with knee osteoarthritis. There is often a previous diagnosis of trauma, patellar maltracking or trochlear dysplasia. Arthroplasty options include TKA with patellar resurfacing, TKA without patella resurfacing [Thompson 2001] and isolated patellofemoral replacement. The number of isolated patellofemoral replacements is increasing. The commonest complication identified is radiological progression of arthritis. [Ackroyd 2007] [Odumenya 2010]

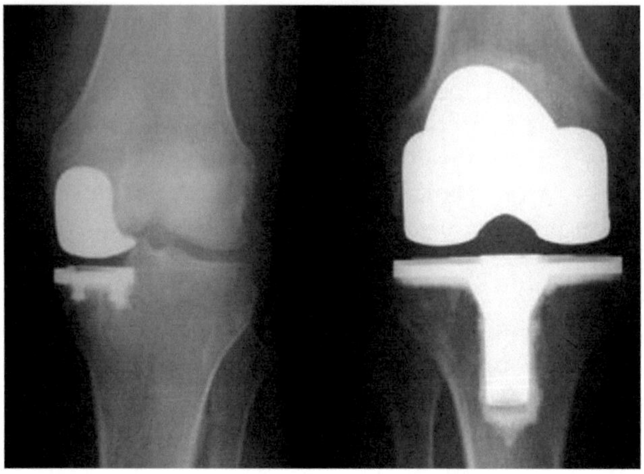

Fig. 7. Unicompartmental Knee Arthroplasty (UKA) and Total Knee Replacement (TKR)

6. Conclusion

Osteoarthritis of the knee is a common condition. The chances of developing symptoms increase with age. Initially treatment is with non-operative measures. Surgical options are considered when conservative measures have failed. We have discussed the options of arthroscopy, bone marrow stimulating techniques, chondrocyte transplantation, osteotomy and arthroplasty. Determining which of these procedures is most appropriate depends on a number of different variables. Age, comorbidities, patient activity levels and expectations, severity of symptoms and surgeon expertise and preference all contribute to the decision process.

Arthroscopic lavage and debridement is a procedure that is often carried out, but it does not alter the disease progression. Single compartment disease may be amenable to offloading osteotomy or unicompartmental knee arthroplasty. Total knee arthroplasty is a reliable treatment option for end stage osteoarthritis of the knee.

7. References

Ackroyd, C.E., Newman, J.H., Evans, R., Eldridge, J.D. & Joslin, C.C., 2007, The Avon patellofemoral arthroplasty: five-year survivorship and functional results, *The Journal of bone and joint surgery. British volume*, 89(3), pp. 310-5.

Amendola, A. & Bonasia, D.E., 2010, Results of high tibial osteotomy: review of the literature, *International orthopaedics*, 34(2), pp. 155-60.

Aqueskirchner, J.D., Bernau, A., Burkart, A.C. & Imhoff, A.B., 2002, [Knee instability and varus malangulation - Simultaneous cruciate ligament reconstruction and osteotomy (Indication, planning and operative technique, results)], *Zeitschrift für Orthopädie und ihre Grenzgebiete*, 140(2), pp. 185-93.

Bae, D.K., Yoon, K.H. & Song, S.J., 2006, Cartilage healing after microfracture in osteoarthritic knees, *Arthroscopy: The Journal of Arthroscopic & Related Surgery*, 22(4), pp. 367-74.

Baker, P.N., van der Meulen, J.H., Lewsey, J., Gregg, P.J. & National Joint Registry for England and Wales, 2007, The role of pain and function in determining patient satisfaction after total knee replacement. Data from the National Joint Registry for England and Wales, *The Journal of bone and joint surgery. British volume*, 89(7), pp. 893-900.

Barrack, R.L., Matzkin, E., Ingraham, R., Engh, G. & Rorabeck, C., 1998, Revision knee arthroplasty with patella replacement versus bony shell, *Clinical orthopaedics and related research*(356), pp. 139-43.

Basad, E., Ishaque, B., Bachmann, G., Stürz, H. & Steinmeyer, J., 2010, Matrix-induced autologous chondrocyte implantation versus microfracture in the treatment of cartilage defects of the knee: a 2-year randomised study, *Knee surgery, sports traumatology, arthroscopy : official journal of the ESSKA*, 18(4), pp. 519-27.

Basad, E., Stürz, H. & Steinmeyer, J., 2004, Die Behandlung chondraler Defekte mit MACI oder Microfracture--erste Ergebnisse einer vergleichenden klinischen Studie, *Orthopädische Praxis*, 40, pp. 6-10.

BÄTHIS, H., Perlick, L., Tingart, M., LÜRING, C. & Grifka, J., 2004, CT-free computer-assisted total knee arthroplasty versus the conventional technique: radiographic results of 100 cases, *Orthopedics*, 27(5), pp. 476-80.

Bentley, G., Biant, L.C., Carrington, R.W., Akmal, M., Goldberg, A., Williams, A.M., Skinner, J.A. & Pringle, J., 2003, A prospective, randomised comparison of autologous chondrocyte implantation versus mosaicplasty for osteochondral defects in the knee, *The Journal of bone and joint surgery. British volume*, 85(2), pp. 223-30.

Berger, R.A., Nedeff, D.D., Barden, R.M., Sheinkop, M.M., Jacobs, J.J., Rosenberg, A.G. & Galante, J.O., 1999, Unicompartmental knee arthroplasty. Clinical experience at 6- to 10-year followup, *Clinical orthopaedics and related research*(367), pp. 50-60.

Bert, J.M. & Maschka, K., 1989, The arthroscopic treatment of unicompartmental gonarthrosis: a five-year follow-up study of abrasion arthroplasty plus arthroscopic debridement and arthroscopic debridement alone, *Arthroscopy : the journal of arthroscopic & related surgery : official publication of the Arthroscopy Association of North America and the International Arthroscopy Association*, 5(1), pp. 25-32.

Biau, D., Mullins, M.M., Judet, T. & Piriou, P., 2006, Mobile versus fixed-bearing total knee arthroplasty: mid-term comparative clinical results of 216 prostheses, *Knee surgery, sports traumatology, arthroscopy : official journal of the ESSKA*, 14(10), pp. 927-33.

Borus, T. & Thornhill, T., 2008, Unicompartmental knee arthroplasty, *The Journal of the American Academy of Orthopaedic Surgeons*, 16(1), pp. 9-18.

Bourne, R.B., Laskin, R.S. & Guerin, J.S., 2007, Ten-year results of the first 100 Genesis II total knee replacement procedures, *Orthopedics*, 30(8 Suppl), pp. 83-5.

Brittberg, M. & Peterson, L., 2003, Articular cartilage engineering with autologous chondrocyte transplantation: a review of recent developments, *The Journal of Bone and Joint Surgery*, 85(Supplement 3), p. 109.

Brittberg, M., Lindahl, A., Nilsson, A., Ohlsson, C., Isaksson, O. & Peterson, L., 1994, Treatment of deep cartilage defects in the knee with autologous chondrocyte transplantation, *The New England journal of medicine*, 331(14), pp. 889-95.

Broughton, N.S., Newman, J.H. & Baily, R.A., 1986, Unicompartmental replacement and high tibial osteotomy for osteoarthritis of the knee. A comparative study after 5-10 years' follow-up, *The Journal of bone and joint surgery. British volume*, 68(3), pp. 447-52.

Brouwer, R.W., Bierma-Zeinstra, S.M.A., Van Raaij, T.M. & Verhaar, J.A.N., 2006, Osteotomy for medial compartment arthritis of the knee using a closing wedge or an opening wedge controlled by a Puddu plate: a one-year randomised, controlled study, *Journal of Bone and Joint Surgery-British Volume*, 88(11), p. 1454.

Brouwer, R.W., Raaij van, T.M., Bierma-Zeinstra, S.M., Verhagen, A.P., Jakma, T.S. & Verhaar, J.A., 2007, Osteotomy for treating knee osteoarthritis, *Cochrane database of systematic reviews (Online)*(3), p. CD004019.

Buly, R.L. & Sculco, T.P., 1995, Recent advances in total knee replacement surgery, *Current opinion in rheumatology*, 7(2), pp. 107-13.

Burman, M.S., FINKELSTEIN, H. & MAYER, L.E.O., 1934, Arthroscopy of the knee joint, *The Journal of Bone and Joint Surgery*, 16(2), p. 255.

Calvisi, V., Camillieri, G. & Lupparelli, S., 2009, Resurfacing versus nonresurfacing the patella in total knee arthroplasty: a critical appraisal of the available evidence, *Archives of orthopaedic and trauma surgery*, 129(9), pp. 1261-70.

Cerha, O., Kirschner, S., Günther, K.P. & Lützner, J., 2009, [Cost analysis for navigation in knee endoprosthetics], *Der Orthopäde*, 38(12), pp. 1235-40.

Chang, R.W., Falconer, J., Stulberg, S.D., Arnold, W.J., Manheim, L.M. & Dyer, A.R., 1993, A randomized, controlled trial of arthroscopic surgery versus closed-needle joint lavage for patients with osteoarthritis of the knee, *Arthritis and rheumatism*, 36(3), pp. 289-96.

Choong, P.F., Dowsey, M.M. & Stoney, J.D., 2009, Does accurate anatomical alignment result in better function and quality of life? Comparing conventional and computer-assisted total knee arthroplasty, *The Journal of arthroplasty*, 24(4), pp. 560-9.

Church, J.S., Scadden, J.E., Gupta, R.R., Cokis, C., Williams, K.A. & Janes, G.C., 2007, Embolic phenomena during computer-assisted and conventional total knee replacement, *The Journal of bone and joint surgery. British volume*, 89(4), pp. 481-5.

Clark, C.R., Rorabeck, C.H., MacDonald, S., MacDonald, D., Swafford, J. & Cleland, D., 2001, Posterior-stabilized and cruciate-retaining total knee replacement: a randomized study, *Clinical orthopaedics and related research*(392), pp. 208-12.

Conditt, M.A., Noble, P.C., Bertolusso, R., Woody, J. & Parsley, B.S., 2004, The PCL significantly affects the functional outcome of total knee arthroplasty, *The Journal of arthroplasty*, 19(7 Suppl 2), pp. 107-12.

Coventry, M.B., 1965, Osteotomy of the upper portion of the tibia for degenerative arthritis of the knee. a preliminary report, *The Journal of bone and joint surgery. American volume*, 47, pp. 984-90.

Coventry, M.B., 1979, Upper tibial osteotomy for gonarthrosis. The evolution of the operation in the last 18 years and long term results, *The Orthopedic clinics of North America*, 10(1), pp. 191-210.

Coventry, M.B., 1984, Upper tibial osteotomy, *Clinical orthopaedics and related research*, 182, p. 46.

Coventry, M.B. & Bowman, P.W., 1982, Long-term results of upper tibial osteotomy for degenerative arthritis of the knee, *Acta orthopaedica Belgica*, 48(1), p. 139.

Coventry, M.B., Ilstrup, D.M. & Wallrichs, S.L. 1993, Proximal tibial osteotomy. A critical long-term study of eighty-seven cases, in *The Journal of Bone and Joint Surgery*, JBJS, p. 196.

Dennis, D.A., Komistek, R.D., Hoff, W.A. & Gabriel, S.M., 1996, In vivo knee kinematics derived using an inverse perspective technique, *Clinical orthopaedics and related research*(331), pp. 107-17.
Dettoni, F., Bonasia, D.E., Castoldi, F., Bruzzone, M., Blonna, D. & Rossi, R., 2010, High tibial osteotomy versus unicompartmental knee arthroplasty for medial compartment arthrosis of the knee: a review of the literature, *The Iowa orthopaedic journal*, 30, pp. 131-40.
Dorr, L.D., Ochsner, J.L., Gronley, J. & Perry, J., 1988, Functional comparison of posterior cruciate-retained versus cruciate-sacrificed total knee arthroplasty, *Clinical orthopaedics and related research*(236), pp. 36-43.
Dozin, B., Malpeli, M., Cancedda, R., Bruzzi, P., Calcagno, S., Molfetta, L., Priano, F., Kon, E. & Marcacci, M., 2005, Comparative evaluation of autologous chondrocyte implantation and mosaicplasty: a multicentered randomized clinical trial, *Clinical journal of sport medicine : official journal of the Canadian Academy of Sport Medicine*, 15(4), pp. 220-6.
Erggelet, C., Sittinger, M. & Lahm, A., 2003, The arthroscopic implantation of autologous chondrocytes for the treatment of full-thickness cartilage defects of the knee joint, *Arthroscopy : the journal of arthroscopic & related surgery : official publication of the Arthroscopy Association of North America and the International Arthroscopy Association*, 19(1), pp. 108-10.
Evans, M.C., Parsons, E.M., Scott, R.D., Thornhill, T.S. & Zurakowski, D., 2006, Comparative flexion after rotating-platform vs fixed-bearing total knee arthroplasty, *The Journal of arthroplasty*, 21(7), pp. 985-91.
Fang, D.M., Ritter, M.A. & Davis, K.E., 2009, Coronal alignment in total knee arthroplasty: just how important is it? *The Journal of arthroplasty*, 24(6 Suppl), pp. 39-43.
Felson, D.T., Naimark, A., Anderson, J., Kazis, L., Castelli, W. & Meenan, R.F., 1987, The prevalence of knee osteoarthritis in the elderly. The Framingham Osteoarthritis Study, *Arthritis and rheumatism*, 30(8), pp. 914-8.
Flecher, X., Parratte, S., Aubaniac, J.M. & Argenson, J.N.A., 2006, A 12-28-year followup study of closing wedge high tibial osteotomy, *Clinical orthopaedics and related research*, 452, p. 91.
Forster, M.C., 2004, Patellar resurfacing in total knee arthroplasty for osteoarthritis: a systematic review, *The Knee*, 11(6), pp. 427-30.
Friedman, M.J., Berasi, C.C., Fox, J.M., Del Pizzo, W., Snyder, S.J. & Ferkel, R.D., 1984, Preliminary results with abrasion arthroplasty in the osteoarthritic knee, *Clinical orthopaedics and related research*(182), pp. 200-5.
Gandhi, R., Tsvetkov, D., Davey, J.R. & Mahomed, N.N., 2009, Survival and clinical function of cemented and uncemented prostheses in total knee replacement: a meta-analysis, *The Journal of bone and joint surgery. British volume*, 91(7), pp. 889-95.
Gillogly, S.D., Myers, T.H. & Reinold, M.M., 2006, Treatment of full-thickness chondral defects in the knee with autologous chondrocyte implantation, *The Journal of orthopaedic and sports physical therapy*, 36(10), pp. 751-64.
Griffin, T., Rowden, N., Morgan, D., Atkinson, R., Woodruff, P. & Maddern, G., 2007, Unicompartmental knee arthroplasty for the treatment of unicompartmental osteoarthritis: a systematic study, *ANZ journal of surgery*, 77(4), pp. 214-21.

Gudas, R., Kalesinskas, R.J., Kimtys, V., Stankevicius, E., Toliusis, V., Bernotavicius, G. & Smailys, A., 2005, A prospective randomized clinical study of mosaic osteochondral autologous transplantation versus microfracture for the treatment of osteochondral defects in the knee joint in young athletes, *Arthroscopy : the journal of arthroscopic & related surgery : official publication of the Arthroscopy Association of North America and the International Arthroscopy Association*, 21(9), pp. 1066-75.

Gunston, F.H., 1971, Polycentric knee arthroplasty. Prosthetic simulation of normal knee movement, *The Journal of bone and joint surgery. British volume*, 53(2), pp. 272-7.

Gunther, T.V., Murray, D.W., Miller, R., Wallace, D.A., Carr, A.J., O'Connor, J.J., McLardy-Smith, P. & Goodfellow, J.W., 1996, Lateral unicompartmental arthroplasty with the Oxford meniscal knee, *The Knee*, 3(1-2), pp. 33-9.

Haaker, R.G., Stockheim, M., Kamp, M., Proff, G., Breitenfelder, J. & Ottersbach, A., 2005, Computer-assisted navigation increases precision of component placement in total knee arthroplasty, *Clinical orthopaedics and related research*(433), pp. 152-9.

Hangody, L. & Füles, P., 2003, Autologous osteochondral mosaicplasty for the treatment of full-thickness defects of weight-bearing joints: ten years of experimental and clinical experience, *The Journal of bone and joint surgery. American volume*, 85-A Suppl 2, pp. 25-32.

Harris, J.D., Siston, R.A., Pan, X. & Flanigan, D.C., 2010, Autologous chondrocyte implantation: a systematic review, *The Journal of bone and joint surgery. American volume*, 92(12), pp. 2220-33.

Harris, W.R. & Kostuik, J.P., 1970, High tibial osteotomy for osteo-arthritis of the knee, *The Journal of bone and joint surgery. American volume*, 52(2), pp. 330-6.

Horas, U., Pelinkovic, D., Herr, G., Aigner, T. & Schnettler, R., 2003, Autologous chondrocyte implantation and osteochondral cylinder transplantation in cartilage repair of the knee joint. A prospective, comparative trial, *The Journal of bone and joint surgery. American volume*, 85-A(2), pp. 185-92.

Hubbard, M.J.S., 1996, Articular debridement versus washout for degeneration of the medial femoral condyle: a five-year study, *Journal of Bone and Joint Surgery-British Volume*, 78(2), p. 217.

Insall, J.N., 1988, Presidential address to The Knee Society. Choices and compromises in total knee arthroplasty, *Clinical orthopaedics and related research*(226), pp. 43-8.

Ivarsson, I., Myrnerts, R. & Gillquist, J., 1990, High tibial osteotomy for medial osteoarthritis of the knee. A 5 to 7 and 11 year follow-up, *The Journal of bone and joint surgery. British volume*, 72(2), pp. 238-44.

Jackson, J.P. & Waugh, W., 1961, Tibial osteotomy for osteoarthritis of the knee, *Journal of Bone and Joint Surgery-British Volume*, 43(4), p. 746.

Jacobs, W.C., Clement, D.J. & Wymenga, A.B., 2005, Retention versus removal of the posterior cruciate ligament in total knee replacement: a systematic literature review within the Cochrane framework, *Acta orthopaedica*, 76(6), pp. 757-68.

Jeffery, R.S., Morris, R.W. & Denham, R.A., 1991, Coronal alignment after total knee replacement, *The Journal of bone and joint surgery. British volume*, 73(5), pp. 709-14.

Jenny, J.Y., Clemens, U., Kohler, S., Kiefer, H., Konermann, W. & Miehlke, R.K., 2005, Consistency of implantation of a total knee arthroplasty with a non-image-based navigation system: a case-control study of 235 cases compared with 235 conventionally implanted prostheses, *The Journal of arthroplasty*, 20(7), pp. 832-9.

Kalairajah, Y., Cossey, A.J., Verrall, G.M., Ludbrook, G. & Spriggins, A.J., 2006, Are systemic emboli reduced in computer assisted knee surgery?: a prospective, randomised, clinical trial, *Journal of Bone and Joint Surgery-British Volume*, 88(2), p. 198.

Kalairajah, Y., Simpson, D., Cossey, A.J., Verrall, G.M. & Spriggins, A.J., 2005, Blood loss after total knee replacement: effects of computer-assisted surgery, *Journal of Bone and Joint Surgery-British Volume*, 87(11), p. 1480.

Karabatsos, B., Mahomed, N.N. & Maistrelli, G.L., 2002, Functional outcome of total knee arthroplasty after high tibial osteotomy, *Canadian journal of surgery. Journal canadien de chirurgie*, 45(2), pp. 116-9.

Karataglis, D. & Learmonth, D.J., 2005, Management of big osteochondral defects of the knee using osteochondral allografts with the MEGA-OATS technique, *The Knee*, 12(5), pp. 389-93.

Karolin, R., 2011, Current Surgical Treatment of Knee Osteoarthritis, *Arthritis*, 2011.

Kazakos, K.J., Chatzipapas, C., Verettas, D., Galanis, V., Xarchas, K.C. & Psillakis, I., 2008, Mid-term results of total knee arthroplasty after high tibial osteotomy, *Archives of orthopaedic and trauma surgery*, 128(2), pp. 167-73.

Kim, Y.H., Kim, D.Y. & Kim, J.S., 2007a, Simultaneous mobile- and fixed-bearing total knee replacement in the same patients. A prospective comparison of mid-term outcomes using a similar design of prosthesis, *The Journal of bone and joint surgery. British volume*, 89(7), pp. 904-10.

Kim, Y.H., Yoon, S.H. & Kim, J.S., 2007b, The long-term results of simultaneous fixed-bearing and mobile-bearing total knee replacements performed in the same patient, *The Journal of bone and joint surgery. British volume*, 89(10), pp. 1317-23.

Knutsen, G., Drogset, J.O., Engebretsen, L., Grøntvedt, T., Isaksen, V., Ludvigsen, T.C., Roberts, S., Solheim, E., Strand, T. & Johansen, O., 2007, A randomized trial comparing autologous chondrocyte implantation with microfracture. Findings at five years, *The Journal of bone and joint surgery. American volume*, 89(10), pp. 2105-12.

Knutsen, G., Engebretsen, L., Ludvigsen, T.C., Drogset, J.O., Grøntvedt, T., Solheim, E., Strand, T., Roberts, S., Isaksen, V. & Johansen, O., 2004, Autologous chondrocyte implantation compared with microfracture in the knee. A randomized trial, *The Journal of bone and joint surgery. American volume*, 86-A(3), pp. 455-64.

Kon, E., Gobbi, A., Filardo, G., Delcogliano, M., Zaffagnini, S. & Marcacci, M., 2009, Arthroscopic second-generation autologous chondrocyte implantation compared with microfracture for chondral lesions of the knee: prospective nonrandomized study at 5 years, *The American journal of sports medicine*, 37(1), pp. 33-41.

Koskinen, E., Paavolainen, P., Eskelinen, A., Pulkkinen, P. & Remes, V., 2007, Unicondylar knee replacement for primary osteoarthritis: a prospective follow-up study of 1,819 patients from the Finnish Arthroplasty Register, *Acta orthopaedica*, 78(1), pp. 128-35.

Kreuz, P.C., Erggelet, C., Steinwachs, M.R., Krause, S.J., Lahm, A., Niemeyer, P., Ghanem, N., Uhl, M. & Südkamp, N., 2006, Is microfracture of chondral defects in the knee associated with different results in patients aged 40 years or younger? *Arthroscopy: The Journal of Arthroscopic & Related Surgery*, 22(11), pp. 1180-6.

Krishnan, S.P., Skinner, J.A., Bartlett, W., Carrington, R.W., Flanagan, A.M., Briggs, T.W. & Bentley, G., 2006, Who is the ideal candidate for autologous chondrocyte implantation? *The Journal of bone and joint surgery. British volume*, 88(1), pp. 61-4.

Laupattarakasem, W., Laopaiboon, M., Laupattarakasem, P. & Sumananont, C., 2008, Arthroscopic debridement for knee osteoarthritis, *Cochrane database of systematic reviews (Online)*(1), p. CD005118.

Lobenhoffer, P. & Agneskirchner, J.D., 2003, Improvements in surgical technique of valgus high tibial osteotomy, *Knee surgery, sports traumatology, arthroscopy : official journal of the ESSKA*, 11(3), pp. 132-8.

Lohmander, L.S., 2003, Tissue engineering of cartilage: do we need it, can we do it, is it good and can we prove it? *Novartis Foundation symposium*, 249, pp. 2-10; discussion 10-6, 170-4, 239-41.

Longstaff, L.M., Sloan, K., Stamp, N., Scaddan, M. & Beaver, R., 2009, Good alignment after total knee arthroplasty leads to faster rehabilitation and better function, *The Journal of arthroplasty*, 24(4), pp. 570-8.

Magnuson, P.B., 1941, Joint debridement. Surgical treatment of degenerative arthritis, *Surg Gynecol Obstet*, 73(1).

Marmor, L., 1988a, Unicompartmental arthroplasty of the knee with a minimum ten-year follow-up period, *Clinical orthopaedics and related research*(228), pp. 171-7.

Marmor, L., 1988b, Unicompartmental knee arthroplasty. Ten- to 13-year follow-up study, *Clinical orthopaedics and related research*(226), pp. 14-20.

Matsuda, S., Whiteside, L.A., White, S.E. & McCarthy, D.S., 1996, TRANSACTIONS OF THE ANNUAL MEETING-ORTHOPAEDIC RESEARCH SOCIETY, *Knee kinematics of posterior cruciate ligament sacrificed total knee arthroplasty*. pp. 722-.

Matsusue, Y., Yamamuro, T. & Hama, H., 1993, Arthroscopic multiple osteochondral transplantation to the chondral defect in the knee associated with anterior cruciate ligament disruption, *Arthroscopy: The Journal of Arthroscopic & Related Surgery*, 9(3), pp. 318-21.

Matthews, L.S., Goldstein, S.A., Malvitz, T.A., Katz, B.P. & Kaufer, H., 1988, Proximal tibial osteotomy. Factors that influence the duration of satisfactory function, *Clinical orthopaedics and related research*(229), pp. 193-200.

McEwen, H.M., Fisher, J., Goldsmith, A.A., Auger, D.D., Hardaker, C. & Stone, M.H., 2001, Wear of fixed bearing and rotating platform mobile bearing knees subjected to high levels of internal and external tibial rotation, *Journal of materials science. Materials in medicine*, 12(10-12), pp. 1049-52.

Meachim, G. & Roberts, C., 1971, Repair of the joint surface from subarticular tissue in the rabbit knee, *Journal of anatomy*, 109(Pt 2), pp. 317-27.

Microfracture technique for full thickness chondral defects: technique and clinical results, .

Mitchell, N. & Shepard, N., 1976, The resurfacing of adult rabbit articular cartilage by multiple perforations through the subchondral bone, *The Journal of Bone and Joint Surgery*, 58(2), p. 230.

Mont, M.A., Alexander, N., Krackow, K.A. & Hungerford, D.S., 1994, Total knee arthroplasty after failed high tibial osteotomy, *The Orthopedic clinics of North America*, 25(3), pp. 515-25.

Moseley, J.B., O'Malley, K., Petersen, N.J., Menke, T.J., Brody, B.A., Kuykendall, D.H., Hollingsworth, J.C., Ashton, C.M. & Wray, N.P., 2002, A controlled trial of arthroscopic surgery for osteoarthritis of the knee, *The New England journal of medicine*, 347(2), pp. 81-8.

Murray, D.W., Goodfellow, J.W. & O'Connor, J.J., 1998, The Oxford medial unicompartmental arthroplasty: a ten-year survival study, *The Journal of bone and joint surgery. British volume*, 80(6), pp. 983-9.

Naudie, D., Bourne, R.B., Rorabeck, C.H. & Bourne, T.J., 1999, The Install Award. Survivorship of the high tibial valgus osteotomy. A 10- to -22-year followup study, *Clinical orthopaedics and related research*(367), pp. 18-27.

Nilsson, K.G., Kärrholm, J., Carlsson, L. & Dalén, T., 1999, Hydroxyapatite coating versus cemented fixation of the tibial component in total knee arthroplasty: prospective randomized comparison of hydroxyapatite-coated and cemented tibial components with 5-year follow-up using radiostereometry, *The Journal of arthroplasty*, 14(1), pp. 9-20.

Nizard, R.S., Biau, D., Porcher, R., Ravaud, P., Bizot, P., Hannouche, D. & Sedel, L., 2005, A meta-analysis of patellar replacement in total knee arthroplasty, *Clinical orthopaedics and related research*(432), pp. 196-203.

Odumenya, M., Costa, M.L., Parsons, N., Achten, J., Dhillon, M. & Krikler, S.J., 2010, The Avon patellofemoral joint replacement: Five-year results from an independent centre, *The Journal of bone and joint surgery. British volume*, 92(1), pp. 56-60.

Ogilvie-Harris, D.J. & Fitsialos, D.P., 1991, Arthroscopic management of the degenerative knee, *Arthroscopy : the journal of arthroscopic & related surgery : official publication of the Arthroscopy Association of North America and the International Arthroscopy Association*, 7(2), pp. 151-7.

Outerbridge, H.K., Outerbridge, A.R. & Outerbridge, R.E., 1995, The use of a lateral patellar autologous graft for the repair of a large osteochondral defect in the knee, *The Journal of bone and joint surgery. American volume*, 77(1), pp. 65-72.

Outerbridge, R.E., 1961, The etiology of chondromalacia patellae, *Journal of Bone and Joint Surgery-British Volume*, 43(4), p. 752.

Pakos, E.E., Ntzani, E.E. & Trikalinos, T.A., 2005, Patellar resurfacing in total knee arthroplasty. A meta-analysis, *The Journal of bone and joint surgery. American volume*, 87(7), pp. 1438-45.

Paley, D. & Pfeil, J., 2000, [Principles of deformity correction around the knee], *Der Orthopäde*, 29(1), pp. 18-38.

Parratte, S., Pagnano, M.W., Trousdale, R.T. & Berry, D.J., 2010, Effect of postoperative mechanical axis alignment on the fifteen-year survival of modern, cemented total knee replacements, *The Journal of bone and joint surgery. American volume*, 92(12), pp. 2143-9.

Parvizi, J., Rapuri, V.R., Saleh, K.J., Kuskowski, M.A., Sharkey, P.F. & Mont, M.A., 2005, Failure to resurface the patella during total knee arthroplasty may result in more knee pain and secondary surgery, *Clinical orthopaedics and related research*, 438, pp. 191-6.

Potter, H.G. & Chong, l.e. .R., 2009, Magnetic resonance imaging assessment of chondral lesions and repair, *The Journal of bone and joint surgery. American volume*, 91 Suppl 1, pp. 126-31.

Pridie, K.H., 1959, A method of resurfacing osteoarthritic knee joints, *The Journal of bone and joint surgery. British volume*, 41(3), pp. 618-9.

Ranawat, C.S., Flynn, W.F., Saddler, S., Hansraj, K.K. & Maynard, M.J., 1993, Long-term results of the total condylar knee arthroplasty. A 15-year survivorship study, *Clinical orthopaedics and related research*(286), pp. 94-102.

Rand, J.A., 2005, Extensor mechanism complications after total knee arthroplasty, *Instructional course lectures*, 54, pp. 241-50.

Ritter, M.A., Berend, M.E., Meding, J.B., Keating, E.M., Faris, P.M. & Crites, B.M., 2001, Long-term followup of anatomic graduated components posterior cruciate-retaining total knee replacement, *Clinical orthopaedics and related research*(388), pp. 51-7.

Ritter, M.A., Faris, P.M., Keating, E.M. & Meding, J.B., 1994, Postoperative alignment of total knee replacement its effect on survival, *Clinical orthopaedics and related research*, 299, p. 153.

Ritter, M.A., Lutgring, J.D., Davis, K.E., Faris, P.M. & Berend, M.E., 2007, Total knee arthroplasty effectiveness in patients 55 years old and younger: osteoarthritis vs. rheumatoid arthritis, *The Knee*, 14(1), pp. 9-11.

Roberts, S., McCall, I.W., Darby, A.J., Menage, J., Evans, H., Harrison, P.E. & Richardson, J.B., 2003, Autologous chondrocyte implantation for cartilage repair: monitoring its success by magnetic resonance imaging and histology, *Arthritis research & therapy*, 5(1), pp. R60-73.

Robinson, B.J., Price, A.J., Murray, D.M. & McLardy-Smith, P., 2003, Indications and results of unicompartmental arthroplasty, *Current Opinion in Orthopaedics*, 14(1), p. 41.

Rudan, J.F. & Simurda, M.A., 1990, High tibial osteotomy. A prospective clinical and roentgenographic review, *Clinical orthopaedics and related research*(255), pp. 251-6.

Saris, D.B., Vanlauwe, J., Victor, J., Almqvist, K.F., Verdonk, R., Bellemans, J., Luyten, F.P. & TIG/ACT/01/2000&EXT Study Group, 2009, Treatment of symptomatic cartilage defects of the knee: characterized chondrocyte implantation results in better clinical outcome at 36 months in a randomized trial compared to microfracture, *The American journal of sports medicine*, 37 Suppl 1, pp. 10S-9S.

Saris, D.B., Vanlauwe, J., Victor, J., Haspl, M., Bohnsack, M., Fortems, Y., Vandekerckhove, B., Almqvist, K.F., Claes, T., Handelberg, F., Lagae, K., van der Bauwhede, J., Vandenneucker, H., Yang, K.G., Jelic, M., Verdonk, R., Veulemans, N., Bellemans, J. & Luyten, F.P., 2008, Characterized chondrocyte implantation results in better structural repair when treating symptomatic cartilage defects of the knee in a randomized controlled trial versus microfracture, *The American journal of sports medicine*, 36(2), pp. 235-46.

Scott, R.D. & Volatile, T.B., 1986, Twelve years' experience with posterior cruciate-retaining total knee arthroplasty, *Clinical orthopaedics and related research*(205), pp. 100-7.

Shaw, J.A. & Moulton, M.J., 1996, High tibial osteotomy: an operation based on a spurious mechanical concept. A theoretic treatise, *American journal of orthopedics (Belle Mead, NJ)*, 25(6), p. 429.

Shen, H., Zhang, N., Zhang, X. & Ji, W., 2009, C-reactive protein levels after 4 types of arthroplasty, *Acta orthopaedica*, 80(3), pp. 330-3.

Slover, J.D., Tosteson, A.N., Bozic, K.J., Rubash, H.E. & Malchau, H., 2008, Impact of hospital volume on the economic value of computer navigation for total knee replacement, *The Journal of bone and joint surgery. American volume*, 90(7), pp. 1492-500.

Smith, T.O., Hing, C.B., Davies, L. & Donell, S.T., 2009, Fixed versus mobile bearing unicompartmental knee replacement: a meta-analysis, *Orthopaedics & traumatology, surgery & research : OTSR*, 95(8), pp. 599-605.

Spector, T.D., Cicuttini, F., Baker, J.R., Loughlin, J.A. & Hart, D.J., 1996, Genetic influences on osteoarthritis in females: a study of twins, *Br. Med. J*, 312, pp. 940-4.

Sprenger, T.R. & Doerzbacher, J.F., 2003, Tibial osteotomy for the treatment of varus gonarthrosis. Survival and failure analysis to twenty-two years, *The Journal of bone and joint surgery. American volume*, 85-A(3), pp. 469-74.

Staubli, A.E., De Simoni, C., Babst, R. & Lobenhoffer, P., 2003, TomoFix: a new LCP-concept for open wedge osteotomy of the medial proximal tibia--early results in 92 cases, *Injury*, 34 Suppl 2, pp. B55-62.

Steadman, J.R., Briggs, K.K., Rodrigo, J.J., Kocher, M.S., Gill, T.J. & Rodkey, W.G., 2003a, Outcomes of microfracture for traumatic chondral defects of the knee: average 11-year follow-up, *Arthroscopy : the journal of arthroscopic & related surgery : official publication of the Arthroscopy Association of North America and the International Arthroscopy Association*, 19(5), pp. 477-84.

Steadman, J.R., Miller, B.S., Karas, S.G., Schlegel, T.F., Briggs, K.K. & Hawkins, R.J., 2003b, The microfracture technique in the treatment of full-thickness chondral lesions of the knee in National Football League players, *The journal of knee surgery*, 16(2), pp. 83-6.

Steadman, J.R., Rodkey, W.G. & Briggs, K.K., 2002, Microfracture to treat full-thickness chondral defects: surgical technique, rehabilitation, and outcomes, *The journal of knee surgery*, 15(3), p. 170.

Steadman, J.R., Rodkey, W.G., Singleton, S.B. & Briggs, K.K., 1997, Microfracture technique forfull-thickness chondral defects: Technique and clinical results, *Operative techniques in orthopaedics*, 7(4), pp. 300-4.

Straw, R., Kulkarni, S., Attfield, S. & Wilton, T.J., 2003, Posterior cruciate ligament at total knee replacement. Essential, beneficial or a hindrance? *The Journal of bone and joint surgery. British volume*, 85(5), pp. 671-4.

Stukenborg-Colsman, C., Wirth, C.J., Lazovic, D. & Wefer, A., 2001, High tibial osteotomy versus unicompartmental joint replacement in unicompartmental knee joint osteoarthritis: 7-10-year follow-up prospective randomised study, *The Knee*, 8(3), pp. 187-94.

Swanik, C.B., Lephart, S.M. & Rubash, H.E., 2004, Proprioception, kinesthesia, and balance after total knee arthroplasty with cruciate-retaining and posterior stabilized prostheses, *The Journal of bone and joint surgery. American volume*, 86-A(2), pp. 328-34.

Tanzer, M., Smith, K. & Burnett, S., 2002, Posterior-stabilized versus cruciate-retaining total knee arthroplasty: balancing the gap, *The Journal of arthroplasty*, 17(7), pp. 813-9.

Thompson, N.W., Ruiz, A.L., Breslin, E. & Beverland, D.E., 2001, Total knee arthroplasty without patellar resurfacing in isolated patellofemoral osteoarthritis, *The Journal of arthroplasty*, 16(5), pp. 607-12.

Valdes, A.M., Spector, T.D., Tamm, A., Kisand, K., Doherty, S.A., Dennison, E.M., Mangino, M., Tamm, A., Kerna, I., Hart, D.J., Wheeler, M., Cooper, C., Lories, R.J., Arden, N.K. & Doherty, M., 2010, Genetic variation in the SMAD3 gene is associated with hip and knee osteoarthritis, *Arthritis and rheumatism*, 62(8), pp. 2347-52.

van Raaij, T., Reijman, M., Furlan, A. & Verhaar, J.A.N., 2009, Total knee arthroplasty after high tibial osteotomy. A systematic review, *BMC musculoskeletal disorders*, 10(1), p. 88.

Vasiliadis, H.S. & Wasiak, J., 2010, Autologous chondrocyte implantation for full thickness articular cartilage defects of the knee, *Cochrane database of systematic reviews (Online)*(10), p. CD003323.

Virolainen, P. & Aro, H.T., 2004, High tibial osteotomy for the treatment of osteoarthritis of the knee: a review of the literature and a meta-analysis of follow-up studies, *Archives of orthopaedic and trauma surgery*, 124(4), pp. 258-61.

Walldius, B., 1953, Arthroplasty of the knee joint using an acrylic prosthesis, *Acta orthop. scand*, 23, p. 121.

Waters, T.S. & Bentley, G., 2003, Patellar resurfacing in total knee arthroplasty. A prospective, randomized study, *The Journal of bone and joint surgery. American volume*, 85-A(2), pp. 212-7.

Zhang, W., Moskowitz, R.W., Nuki, G., Abramson, S., Altman, R.D., Arden, N., Bierma-Zeinstra, S., Brandt, K.D., Croft, P., Doherty, M., Dougados, M., Hochberg, M., Hunter, D.J., Kwoh, K., Lohmander, L.S. & Tugwell, P., 2007, OARSI recommendations for the management of hip and knee osteoarthritis, part I: critical appraisal of existing treatment guidelines and systematic review of current research evidence, *Osteoarthritis and cartilage / OARS, Osteoarthritis Research Society*, 15(9), pp. 981-1000.

Zhang, W., Moskowitz, R.W., Nuki, G., Abramson, S., Altman, R.D., Arden, N., Bierma-Zeinstra, S., Brandt, K.D., Croft, P., Doherty, M., Dougados, M., Hochberg, M., Hunter, D.J., Kwoh, K., Lohmander, L.S. & Tugwell, P., 2008, OARSI recommendations for the management of hip and knee osteoarthritis, Part II: OARSI evidence-based, expert consensus guidelines, *Osteoarthritis and cartilage / OARS, Osteoarthritis Research Society*, 16(2), pp. 137-62.

Zhang, W., Nuki, G., Moskowitz, R.W., Abramson, S., Altman, R.D., Arden, N.K., Bierma-Zeinstra, S., Brandt, K.D., Croft, P., Doherty, M., Dougados, M., Hochberg, M., Hunter, D.J., Kwoh, K., Lohmander, L.S. & Tugwell, P., 2010, OARSI recommendations for the management of hip and knee osteoarthritis: part III: Changes in evidence following systematic cumulative update of research published through January 2009, *Osteoarthritis and cartilage / OARS, Osteoarthritis Research Society*, 18(4), pp. 476-99.

Zhang, W., Robertson, J., Jones, A.C., Dieppe, P.A. & Doherty, M., 2008, The placebo effect and its determinants in osteoarthritis: meta-analysis of randomised controlled trials, *Annals of the rheumatic diseases*, 67(12), p. 1716.

18

High Tibial Open-Wedge Osteotomy – New Techniques and Early Results

Werner Kolb[1], Hanno Guhlmann[2], Christoph Windisch[2] and Klaus Kolb[3]
[1]*Department of Trauma and Orthopaedic Surgery, Bethesda Hospital, Stuttgart*
[2]*Department of Trauma Surgery, Friedrich-Schiller-University, Jena*
[3]*Department of Trauma Surgery, Klinikum am Steinenberg, Reutlingen, Germany*

1. Introduction

High tibial osteotomy was first described by Langenbeck in 1854 (Langenbeck 1854). It is an efficient method to treat unicondylar osteoarthrosis. High tibial osteotomy allows one to interrupt the circular reasoning of unicondylar osteoarthrosis (Fig. 1) (Jakob & Jacobi, 2004).

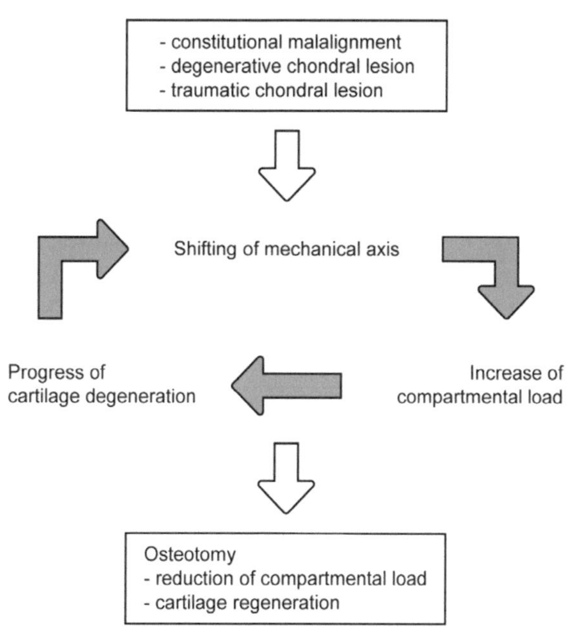

Fig. 1. The circular reasoning of unicondylar arthrosis (from Jakob & Jacobi, 2004).

Following high tibial osteotomy, osteosclerosis in the medial compartment of the arthritic knee is significantly reduced, and the degenerated portions of the articular surface are completely covered by a fibrocartilagenous layer (Akamatsu et al., 1997; Fujisawa et al., 1979; Koshino, & Tsuchiya, 1979; Koshino, 2010; Odenbring et al. 1992; Takahashi et al. 2002-2003).

An open-wedge high tibial osteotomy proximal to the tibial tuberosity was first described by Debeyre and Patte in 1951 (Debeyre & Patte, 1962). A disadvantage of this method is the need for bone grafts and the resulting risk of donor-site morbidity (Becker et al., 2011). Thus, because of its inherent stability, closed-wedge osteotomy has become the treatment of choice for unicompartmental osteoarthritis (Coventry, 1965).

Unicompartmental (or total knee) arthroplasty has been the treatment of choice because osteotomy is considered a demanding procedure with an unpredictable outcome and is associated with significant complications. The biological internal fixation of fractures using the indirect reduction technique could improve the outcome in treating fractures (Mast et al., 1989). The "minimally invasive plate osteosynthesis (MIPO) technique" further improves the results of plate osteosynthesis . Locked-plate fixators significantly improve the stability of plate osteosynthesis. The combination of locked-plate fixators and the MIPO technique makes it possible to perform plateosteosynthesis without the need for bone grafts. Menisceal and chondral lesions both as ligament instabilities have an increased risk for osteoarthritis (Hofmann et al., 2009). In young patients with a varus malalignment, the treatment of menisceal or chondral lesions both as ligament instabilites can be combined with a high tibial osteotomy (Noyes et al., 1993; Imhoff et al., 2004). The combination of varus malalignment with chronic posterolateral instability was defined as triple varus by Noyes and Simon (Noyes & Simon, 1994).

The keys to a successful osteotomy are basic biomechanics, careful patient selection, and precise planning combined with a skilful surgical technique and stable osteosynthesis for early mobilisation (Hanssen, 2001; Hofmann et al., 2009). Remarkably, the patient selection process and the specific indications for osteotomy are more standardised than the various preoperative planning methods and operative techniques currently being used (Hanssen, 2001). Given the positive long-term outcome of osteotomy when strict selection criteria are implemented and the compliance with a rigorous technique, it appears that these procedures have their place in the treatment of the early stages of gonarthrosis that arise from axial deviation (Poilvache, 2001). Careful planning of the axis of correction and the osteotomy, the degree of correction and the implant allow one to avoid complications such as nerve injury, instability and pseudoarthrosis (Lichte et al. 2010).

Periarticular corrective osteotomies have grown in importance since the advent of locking compression plates (Köck et al., 2011)

New planning methods as well as new techniques for open-wedge high tibial osteotomies and custom-designed internal fixators have improved upon the early results and have led to a trend towards high tibial open-wedge osteotomy. Medial open-wedge high tibial osteotomy secured by a TomoFix plate (Synthes, West Chester, Pennsylvania) provides stability that is equal to the lateral closing-wedge technique (Luites et al., 2009). The TomoFix plate is an anatomically pre-contoured locked plate for the medial aspect of the tibia and is inserted into a subcutaneous tunnel with minimal bone exposure (Kolb et al., 2009).

The aim of this report is to (1) describe new planning methods and (2) describe new techniques for open-wedge high tibial osteotomy.

2. Indication

The typical indication for deformity correction is a combination of morphological, functional and radiographic results in terms of both the personal situation of the patient (e.g., expectation, compliance, general factors such as smoking, peripheral vascular status, nutritional status, comorbidities such as diabetes, occupational situation and sports activities) and the length of rehabilitation (Hofmann et al., 2009; Tunggal et al., 2010). The primary indications are active patients who are between 40 and 60 years of age with varus malalignment of the limb with no radiographic evidence of subluxation, no patellofemoral symptoms, isolated medial activity-related joint line pain, full extension, and a knee arc of motion that is >100°. In reality, however, there are many other patients who would benefit from osteotomy but fall short of these idealised criteria (Hanssen & Chao, 1994) (Table 1).

Absolute Indications	Relative Indications	Absolute Contraindications
Patients 40-60 years of age	Patients >60 or <40 years of age	Open growth plates
Varus malalignment of the limb <15°	Varus malalignment >15° (sometimes double osteotomy)	Rheumatoid arthritis
No patellofemoral symptoms	Moderate patellofemoral symptoms	Severe patellofemoral symptoms
Isolated medial activity-related joint line pain		Lateral joint line pain
Full extension	Flexion contracture >15°	Flexion contracture >25°
Range of motion >100°	Range of motion >90°	Range of motion <75°
Medial soft tissue coverage	Previous infection	Inflammatory disease
Stable knee	ACL, PCL or PLC insufficiency	Mediolateral insufficiency
No patellofemoral arthrosis	Patellofemoral arthrosis grade II – III*	Patellofemoral arthrosis grade IV-V*
Non-smoker	Smoker (<15 cigarettes/day)	Smoker (>15 cigarettes/day)
BMI<30	BMI 30-40	BMI >40
High-demand activity but no running or jumping	Wish to continue all sports	Severe osteoporosis
Metaphyseal tibial varus (TBVA+ >5°)	Metaphyseal femoral varus and tibial valgus	Extraarticular deformity
Normal lateral component, arthrosis grade I-III* medial component	Arthrosis grade IV* medial	Lateral gonarthrosis, Arthrosis grade V* medial
No meniscectomy	Partial medial meniscectomy	Lateral meniscectomy
No cupula	Osteochondritis dissecans	Bad peripheral vascular status (no foot pulse)
	Condylar osteonecrosis	Bone healing disorders

*Ahlbäck Grading System for Degenerative Arthritis
+ tibial bone varus angle

Table 1. Ideal and possible patients for high tibial osteotomy and patients not suited for the procedure, modified from the International Society of Arthroscopy, Knee Surgery and Orthopaedic Sports Medicine (Brinkman et al., 2008; Frey et al., 2008; Hofmann et al., 2009; Kolb et al., 2009; Rand & Neyret, 2005; Song et al., 2010)

3. Preoperative evaluation

A preoperative clinical evaluation of the knee and adjacent joints is mandatory. The gait pattern of the patient, including additional varus, must be assessed (Müller, 2001). Limited mobility of the hip-, especially its rotation, -may influence both the gait pattern and dynamic load (Müller, 2001). A varus knee with internal rotation requires more valgus correction than in cases in which the foot is in its normal position (Müller, 2001). A preoperative gait analysis should become part of the routine preoperative patient assessment (Lind et al., 2011). High tibial osteotomy can reduce significantly the external adduction moment (Bhatnagar & Jenkyn, 2010). According to the magnitude of the knee-adduction moment, (Prodomos et al., 1985) classified patients into low and high adduction moment groups, and patients with a low preoperative adduction moment had substantially better clinical results than did patients with high adduction moments. The dynamic situation may therefore be an important consideration in helping to explain certain failures or recurrences despite a good initial correction, as the static alignment of the knee cannot account for dynamic loading (Tunggal et al., 2010).
Radiographic assessment includes standard knee radiographs, full-length A-P view standing radiographs with the patella facing directly anterior with the patient standing on both legs, a lateral view, a flexed weightbearing tunnel view (Rosenberg's view) and skyline views of the patella with both knees in 30° flexion (Merchant's view, Table 2). Patients with a positive varus stress test, increased varus during thrust, increased tibial external rotation at 30° of flexion, or varus recurvatum during standing or walking should receive stress radiographs (Dugdale et al., 1992). If the radiographs are positive, the patient should receive supine full-length A-P radiographs of both legs to evaluate their true alignment (Noyes et al., 2000). The routine use of magnetic resonance imaging (MRI) to evaluate and manage meniscal tears, cartilage lesions or ligament injuries in patients with osteoarthritis of the knee is recommended (Bhattacharyya et al., 2003; Jakob & Jacob, 2004; Englund et al., 2008). Bone marrow oedema in MRI is a potent risk factor for structural deterioration in knee osteoarthritis, and its relation to progression is explained in part by its association with limb alignment (Felson et al., 2003). Preoperative planning of the osteotomy using the MRI data is not recommended, as full-length views of the leg are not possible.

Standard radiograph	**Purpose**
Full-length double stance A-P-radiograph (Moreland et al., 1987)	To evaluate the femorotibial alignment
Full-length double supine A-P-radiograph (Moreland et al., 1987)	To eliminate the added varus due to deficiency of the lateral and PL structures
Real lateral view radiograph (Dejour & Bonnin, 1994)	To evaluate the posterior tibial slope
Merchant's view radiograph (Merchant et al., 1974)	To evaluate the patellofemoral joint
Rosenberg's view (Rosenberg et al., 1988)	To evaluate the lateral compartment of the knee
Stress radiograph	**Purpose**
Lateral stress view according to the Telos method (Jacobsen, 1976; Strobel et al., 2002)	To evaluate the anterior and posterior tibial translation with respect to the femur
Lateral stress view according to the kneeling method (Louisia et al., 2005)	To evaluate the anterior and posterior tibial translation with respect to the femur
Lateral stress view with hamstring contraction method (Chassaing et al., 1995)	To evaluate the anterior and posterior tibial translation with respect to femur
Lateral stress view according to the gravity method (Stäubli & Jakob, 1990)	To evaluate the anterior and posterior tibial translation with respect to the femur
Axial stress view (Puddu et al., 2000)	To evaluate the anterior and posterior tibial translation with respect to the femur

Table 2. Imaging views and their purpose for standard and stress radiographs (Savarese et al., 2011).

4. Preoperative planning

Preoperative planning of the osteotomy is mandatory (Freiling et al., 2010; Pape et al., 2007). The outcome will depend strongly on achieving an optimal and exact degree of correction (Pape et al., 2004). An analysis of knee malalignment includes 5 criteria as listed in Table 3 (Hofmann & Pietsch, 2007).

1.	Frontal mechanical axis
2.	Joint line
3.	Sagittal mechanical axis
4.	Patellofemoral joint
5.	Malrotation

Table 3. The 5 criteria for analysing knee deformities (Hofmann & Pietsch, 2007).

The malalignment test is used for cases in which there is a frontal mechanical axis deviation (Paley et al., 1994). The normal axis passes 10 mm medial of the centre of the knee joint in the region of the tibial spine (ranging from 3 to 17 mm) (Paley et al., 1992) (Table 4). Frontal malalignment may result from a femoral deformity, a tibial deformity, knee joint laxity and luxation, an intra-articular condylar deficiency of the knee joint, reduced joint space due to meniscus or cartilage lesions, or any combination of the above (Dugdale et al., 1992; Paley et al., 1994). The intersection point of the proximal and distal mechanical axes is called the centre of rotation of angulation (CORA) (Paley et al., 1994). The axis of correction of angulation and the osteotomy should pass through the same CORA to avoid displacement of the bone ends. The osteotomy should maintain neutral joint-line obliquity and thus not increase the shear stresses at the joint surface (Babis et al., 2002). Excessive obliquity prevents the shift of weight bearing to the lateral compartment and may cause a recurrence of the varus deformity following high tibial osteotomy (Terauchi et al., 2002). (Levigne and Bonnin, 1991) differentiated congenital tibial bone varus (TBVA) from acquired tibial varus malalignment, which results from bone wear in medial gonarthrosis. A high tibial osteotomy can cure tibial bone varus, whereas in acquired tibial varus malalignment it is only a palliative procedure (Bonnin & Chambat, 2004). Patients with varus malalignment and normal TBVA (<5°) and medial proximal tibial angle (MPTA, 85-90°) have a bone varus of the distal femur (lateral distal femoral angle, LDFA >90°) (Hofmann et al., 2009).

1.	Mechanical tibiofemoral angle
2.	Mechanical axis (Mikulicz-line)
3.	The total transverse line through the knee (joint line is given as 100%)
4.	Lateral distal femoral angle (LDFA) 88° (85-90°)
5.	Medial proximal tibial angle (MPTA) 87° (85-90°)
6.	Joint line convergence angle (JLCA) 2° (1-3°)
7.	Joint line (JL) 87° (84-90°)
8.	Mechanical axis deviation (MAD) 10 mm medial (3-17 mm)
9.	Centre of rotation of angulation (CORA)
10.	Tibial bone varus angle (TBVA) 0° (<0-5°)

Table 4. Biomechanical parameters in the frontal plane (Bonnin & Chambat, 2004; Brown & Amendola, 2000; Fick, 1911; Hofmann & Pietsch, 2007; Paley et al., 1994)

The posterior distal femoral angle (PDFA) helps one to differentiate between bone- and soft tissue-dependant hyperextension or a flexion contracture (Bonin et al., 2004). Changes in the posterior proximal tibial angle (PPTA) or the posterior tibial slope have a strong effect on cartilage pressure and kinematics of the knee (Agneskirchner et al., 2004). With the exception of rare circumstances, the normal tibial slope should not be changed (Hofmann et al., 2009) (Table 5).

Posterior distal femoral angle (PDFA) 83° (79-87°)
Posterior proximal tibial angle (PPTA, posterior tibial slope) 81° (77-84°)

Table 5. Biomechanical parameters in the sagittal plane (Paley et al., 1994)

A closing-wedge high tibial osteotomy decreases the posterior slope, translates the tibia in the posterior direction and stabilises a knee that has anterior instability, whereas a medial opening wedge high tibial osteotomy increases the posterior tibial slope, translates the tibia in the anterior direction, and stabilises a knee that has posterior instability (Giffin et al., 2007; Hohmann et al., 2006; Lerat et al., 1993; Savarese et al., 2011). The slope must be raised only slightly, as an elevation in the slope of more than 10° can cause a chronic insufficiency in the anterior cruciate ligament (Dejour et al., 2000).
Changes in the mechanics of the patellofemoral joint can also result in changes in the tibiofemoral compartments (Feller et al., 2007) (Table 6). A medial open-wedge high tibial osteotomy improves the symptoms of patellofemoral osteoarthritis because the anterior translation of the tibia reduces the tension on the patellar tendon, the patella becomes less horizontal, and pressure decreases in the lateral facet (Kumagai et al., 2002; Li et al., 2002; Savarese et al., 2011). When faced with a patellofemoral malfunction, it is important to check all of the soft tissues and the articular geometry factors that relate to the patella locally and to not neglect the overall alignment and function of the lower limb (Feller et al., 2007). Weight bearing skyline views of the patella with both knees at 30° flexion, both as the tibial tuberosity-trochlear groove (TT-TG) distance that measured with the CT-scan is an important factor for analysing patellofemoral malfunction (Dejour et al., 1994).

No trochlear dysplasia (no crossing sign with trochlea bump >3 mm and trochlea depth <4 mm)
No quadriceps dysplasia with no patellar tilt >20% in extension
Caton-Deschamps Index 1.0 (0.8-1.2) (Caton, 1989)
Insall-Salvati Index 1.0 (0.8-1.2) (Insall & Salvati, 1971)
Blackburne-Peel Index 0.8 (0.5-1.0) (Blackburne & Peel, 1977)
Tibial tuberosity-trochlea groove (TT-TG) distance <15 mm
Congruence angle -6° + 11° (Merchant et al., 1974)
Axial linear patellar displacement (Urch et al., 2009)
Patellar tilt angle 2° + 5° (Grelsamer et al., 1993)
Sulcus angle (Brattstroem, 1964)

Table 6. Biomechanical parameters in the patellofemoral joint

A CT scan or MRI of the leg is recommended in malrotations during the preoperative clinical evaluation.

5. Planning of post-operative correction

The post-operative correction is typically planned with the use of full-length A-P view standing radiographs with the patella facing directly anterior with the patient standing on both legs according to the method of Miniaci et al. (M Galla & Lobenhoffer, 2004; Miniaci et al., 1989). Alternatively, the post-operative correction can be planned according to the methods of (Dugdale et al., 1992 or Coventry, 1985). (Coventry, 1985) recommended a postoperative anatomical valgus of at least 8°. The correction that is achieved can also be verified by measuring the mechanical tibiofemoral angle (Hernigou et al., 1987; Ivarsson et al., 1990). The point where the mechanical axis crosses the transverse diameter of the tibial plateau is the recommended planning method (Pape et al., 2007) Table 6 (Noyes et al., 1993). The mechanical axis is shifted to a point that is 62% of the transverse diameter of the tibial plateau (Fujisawa et al., 1979) (Table 7). In a biomechanical study under reproducible dynamic loading conditions using pressure-sensitive films with the corrected axis running through the "Fujisawa point", the load changed only after the complete release of the MCL from medial to lateral (64%) (Agneskirchner et al., 2007). An individual correction of varus deformities between 0° and 6° of the mechanical valgus or shifting the mechanical axis to a point between 55% and 67.5% on the transverse diameter of the tibial plateau according to the intra-articular disease is also recommended (Fig. 2 and Table 8). Post-operative correction can also be planned with an arthroscopy before the osteotomy based on the Outerbridge classification (Fig. 3) (Müller & Strecker, 2008; Outerbridge, 1961). Digital radiographs require calibration before planning (Freiling et al., 2010). A large flexion deformity in varus knees precludes the precise planning of deformity correction, as the degree of the varus malalignment will be overestimated (Pape et al., 2004). To support planning deformities with TomoFix (Synthes, West Chester, Pennsylvania), the tool PreOp-Plan was developed by Siemens.

Authors (Reference)	Preoperative planning	Recommended postoperative correction angle (°)	Point where the mechanical axis crosses the tibial plateau (%)
Coventry (Coventry, 1985)	Anatomical tibiofemoral angle	8-10	-
Koshino et al. (Koshino et al., 1989)	Anatomical tibiofemoral angle	6-15	-
Engel & Lippert (Engel & Lippert, 1981)	Anatomical tibiofemoral angle	5-10	-
Kettelkamp (Kettelkamp et al., 1976)	Anatomical tibiofemoral angle	>5	-
Aglietti et al. (Aglietti et al., 2003)	Anatomical tibiofemoral angle	8-15	
Hernigou et al. (Hernigou et al., 1987)	Mechanical tibiofemoral angle	3-6	-
Ivarson et al. (Ivarson et al., 1990)	Mechanical tibiofemoral angle	3-7	-
Myrnerts (Myrnerts, 1980)	Mechanical tibiofemoral angle	3-7	-
Miniaci et al. (Miniaci et al., 1989)	Mechanical axis	-	60-70
Dugdale (Dugdale et al., 1992)	Mechanical axis	-	50-75
Noyes (Noyes et al. 1993)	Mechanical axis	-	62

Table 7. Recommended correction angles and lines (Pape et al., 2004; Pape et al., 2007)

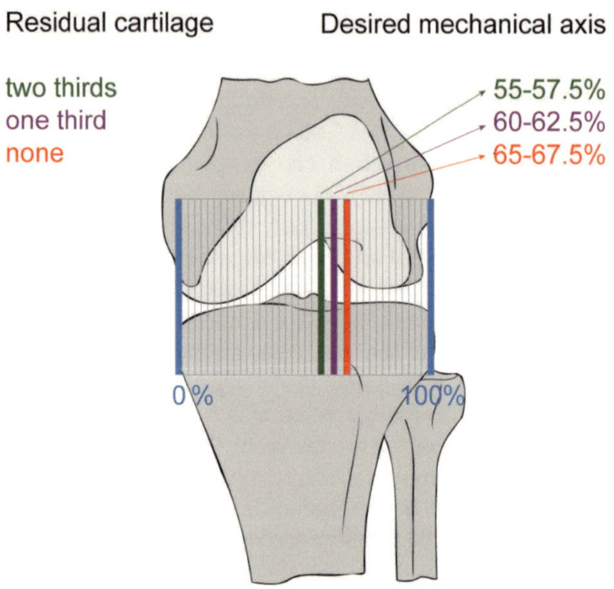

Fig. 2. Correction of varus deformities (Marti et al., 2004; Jakob &Jacobi, 2004)

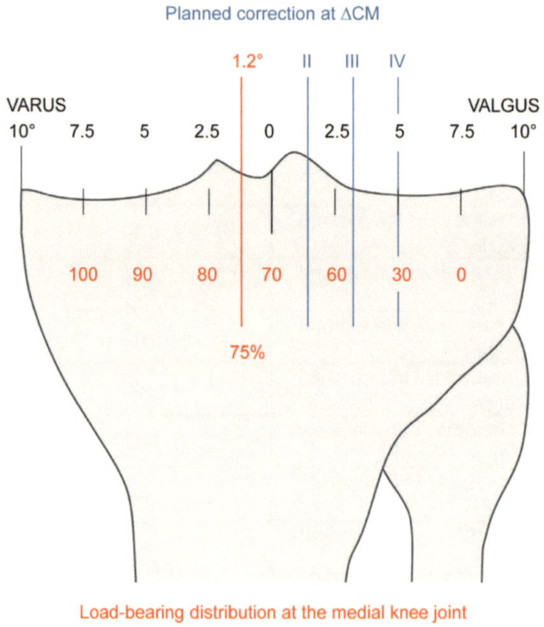

Fig. 3. Planned correction in high tibial valgus osteotomies. The load bearing distribution at the medial knee depending on the frontal axis of the leg (normal 75% according to Hsu et al., 1990) is in red, and the correction angle depending on ΔCM (Cartilage lesion) according to the Outerbridge classification (Outerbridge, 1961) is in blue. The planned correction angles were as follow: at ΔCM=IV° 5° of valgus, at ΔCM=III° the Fujisawa point (3.3° of valgus) and at ΔCM =II° 1.7° of valgus (Müller & Strecker, 2008; Strecker et al. 2009).

Posttraumatic malalignment without osteoarthritis	0-2°
ACL insufficiency	0-2°
PCL insufficiency	2-4 (5)°
Surgery of chondral lesions	3-5°

Table 8. Correction angles of varus deformities for the different types of disorders (Müller, 2001; Hofmann et al., 2009)

The first step is to draw the z-line from the centre of the femoral head to the centre of the talus (Fig. 4). In varus malalignment, the mechanical axis passes the tibial plateau more medially than the physiological mechanical axis deviation (MAD) of 10 mm (ranging from 3 to 17 mm). Next, a line that is parallel to the tibial plateau is drawn. A third line is drawn with the desired mechanical axis from the centre of the femoral head to a point 62% lateral on the transverse diameter of the tibial plateau (Fujisawa et al., 1979). The desired mechanical axis is continued to the centre of the ankle in its postoperative position. The centre of rotation of angulation (CORA) lies in the lateral cortex at the tip of the fibula. Line 1 connects CORA with the middle of the ankle joint. Line 2 is drawn from CORA to the centre of the ankle in its postoperative position and crosses the desired mechanical axis at the centre of the ankle. The angle between lines 1 and 2 forms the correction angle. The degree of lateral separation (the joint line convergence angle, or JLCA) from the apparent deformity in the preoperative planning of the correction angle is subtracted (Kolb et al., 2010).

Alternatively the JLCA can be determined preoperatively from the full-length A-P view standing radiographs of both knees. The difference Δa between both JLCAs is measured (Pape et al., 2004). By taking the width of the tibial plateaus (WTP) and a constant K (76.4) into consideration, the varus malalignment that is caused by the ligamentous instability (β) can be determined using the following equation: $\beta = K \times (\Delta a)/WTP$ (Galla & Lobenhoffer, 2004). The angle β is then subtracted from the measured angle of correction (Pape et al., 2004; Galla & Lobenhoffer, 2004).

Ideal correction of the leg of the leg is difficult to achieve, and postoperative malalignment is often observed following high tibial osteotomy (Dahl, 2000; Noyes et al., 2000). The challenge for achieving a permanent surgical solution is to achieve the planned axis intraoperatively (Gebhard et al., 2011). Computer-assisted navigation systems may improve the precision and accuracy of the leg axis correction while offering simulation tools that can predict the postoperative alignment (Gebhard et al., 2011) (Fig. 5). The integration of "computer-aided design/computer-aided manufacturing (CAD/CAM)" planning into computer-assisted surgery allows one to plan complex orthopaedic surgical procedures (Wong et al., 2010).

6. Surgical technique

An arthroscopy is first performed to check the indication for an osteotomy, to modify the planned correction according to the intra-articular findings and to rule out and treat the intra-articular pathologies (Fig. 3) (Strecker et al., 2009). Meniscal tears, loose bodies, osteophytic spurs, and chondral flaps can cause mechanical symptoms that can be treated successfully with arthroscopy (Iorio & Healy, 2003). In 51 out of 300 cases (17%), the procedure was changed to a total knee arthroplasty due to finding of advanced osteoarthritis in the intended compartment during the preoperative arthroscopy (Strecker et al., 2009).

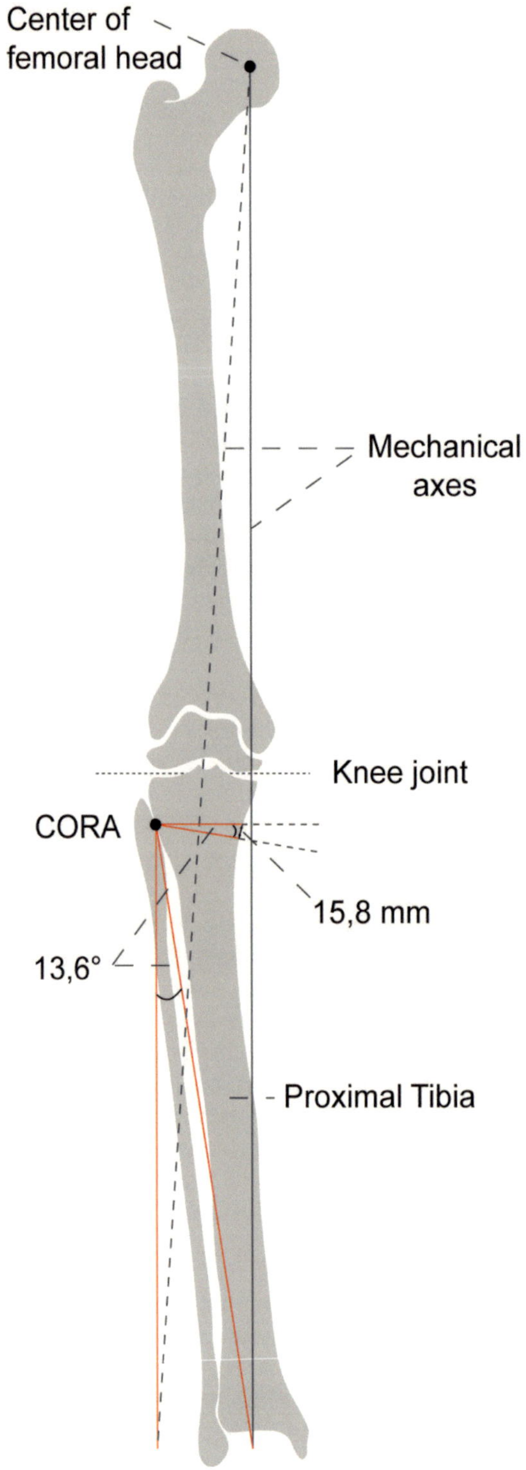

Fig. 4. Planning of post-operative correction for an open wedge high tibial osteotomy.

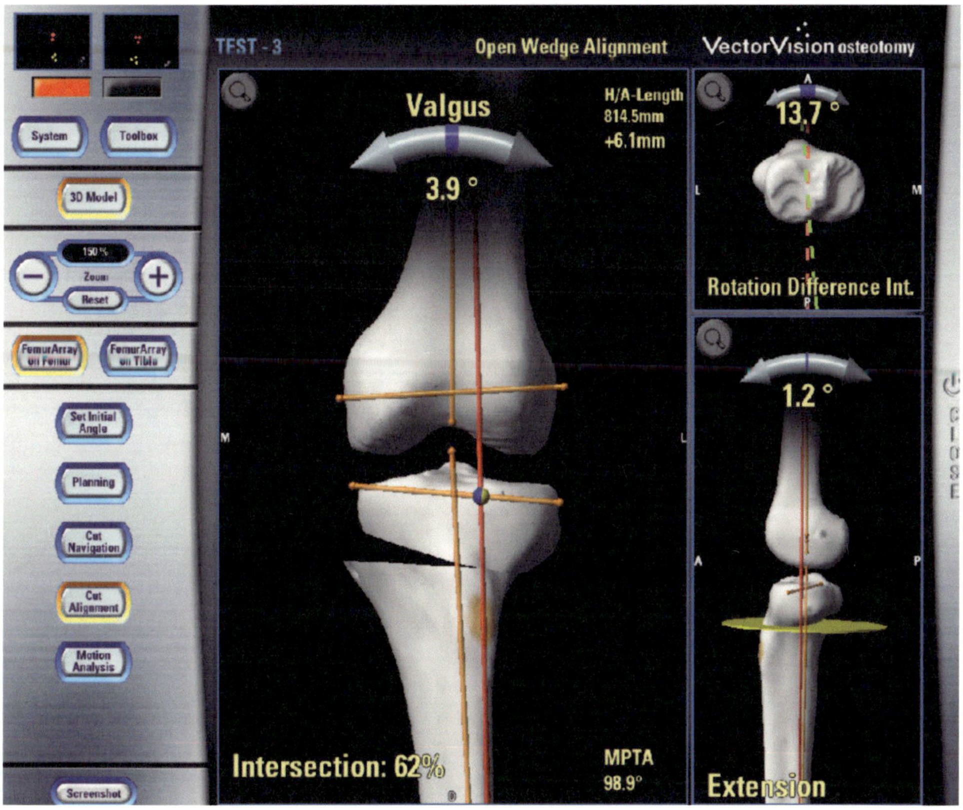

Fig. 5. High tibial osteotomy with a computer-assisted navigation system (From BRAINLAB with permission)

Lateral open-wedge high tibial osteotomies are rarely performed. There is a paucity reports regarding the use of a reconstructive osteotomy to treat depression and valgus malunions of the proximal tibia (Kerkhoffs et al., 2008).

Barrel-vault (dome) osteotomies, lateral-closed-wedge, medial open-wedge high tibial osteotomies or a procedure that combines these techniques are used to treat varus deformities of the knee (Coventry, 1965; M Galla & Lobenhoffer, 2004; Hernigou et al. 1987; Maquet, 1976; Nagi et al., 2007; Watanabe et al., 2008; Weber & Wörsdörfer, 1980). Patellofemoral pain due to patella baja, large deformities or high tibial slope is an indication for performing a closed-wedge osteotomy (Marti et al., 2004). Small deformities and medial instability are indications for open-wedge osteotomies.

Lateral closed-wedge high tibial osteotomies have been the treatment of choice since 1965 (Coventry, 1965). The closed wedge is the most stable high tibial osteotomy technique when compared with the open-wedge osteotomy and the barrel-vault (dome) osteotomy, as the periosteum and cortex adjacent to the apex of the removed wedge act as a tether when the osteotomy is closed (Hansen & Chao, 1994, Kolb et al., 2009). Several lateral tensioning systems such as 1/3 tubular plates with cortical bone screws, a 4.5-mm L-plate, bone staples, external fixation devices, Giebel plates and locked plates are used (Billings et al., 2000; Coventry, 1969; Giebel et al., 1985; Jackson & Waugh, 1961; Kessler et al. 2002; Luites et al., 2009; Perusi et al., 1994; Weber & Wörsdörfer, 1980).

We have used the modified Weber-technique (Weber & Wörsdörfer, 1980), which provides several advantages, including high stability of the osteotomy through the tension band principle with large bone contact areas and the possibility of bone impaction, intraoperative correction of the osteotomy, no large implant (in particular, no removal of the implant is necessary), no increase in pressure in the medial compartment through tensioning of the MCL, no increase of pressure in the patellofemoral joint and no bone graft (Frey et al., 2008).
The most common problems associated with this procedure are difficulty in achieving an accurate correction of the osseous malalignment, the need for fibular osteotomy or separation of the proximal tibiofibular joint, contracture of the patellar tendon leading to patellar baja, leg shortening, and a high rate of other complications (Aydogdu et al., 2000; Kirgis & Albrecht, 1992; Tunggal et al., 2010) (Tables 9 and 10). Large corrections may cause marked shortening of the leg and a large offset of the tibia, which may compromise the later placement of the tibial component during a total knee replacement (Brinkman et al., 2008).
(Shaw et al., 2004) conducted an anatomical study and found that an osteotomy angle greater than 10° rendered the lateral collateral ligament non-functional and allowed the knee to swing back to its native alignment with varus loading, thus negating much of the bony correction.

Infection	0.8-10.4%
Thromboembolic disease	2-5%
Compartment syndrome	Rare
Fracture of the medial cortex	82%
Intra-articular fractures	0-20%
Non-union	1-5%
Delayed union	4-8.5%
Peroneal nerve palsy	0-27%

Table 9. Complications (and their incidence) of closed-wedge high tibial osteotomy (Staubli & Jacob, 2010, Tunggal et al., 2010)

-	No difference in the incidence of infection, deep vein thrombosis, peroneal nerve palsy, non-union or revision to knee arthroplasty ($p>0.05$)
-	Significantly greater posterior tibial slope and mean angle of correction, reduced patellar height and hip-knee-ankle angle following opening-wedge HTO ($p<0.05$)
-	No significant difference was found for any clinical outcome including pain, functional score or complications ($p>0.05$)

Table 10. Differences in complications between Open- or closed-wedge high tibial osteotomies (Smith et al. 2010).

The open-wedge high tibial osteotomy gained recognition after the encouraging reports of (Hernigou et al., 1987). A medial open-wedge osteotomy proximal to the tibial tubercle was performed, and appropriate-size wedges of bone that were obtained from the iliac crest were inserted into the defect (Hernigou et al., 1987; Poignard et al., 2010). No internal fixation or plaster was used. A crack in the lateral cortex during or after the osteotomy may cause a displacement and a subsequent loss of correction (Hernigou et al., 1987). Therefore, we now perform internal fixation using a plate and screws for all osteotomies (Poignard et al., 2010). Modern techniques involve sawing and chiselling through the bone and the application of an internal (or external) splint to fix the fragments in the required juxtaposition until bone healing is complete (Staubli & Jacob, 2010; Merian et al., 2005; Weale et al., 2001). Because of the well-known morbidity of the relevant donor site, bone substitutes such as DUOWEDGE (from Intrauma, Rivoli, Italy) can be employed (Poignard et al., 2010). However, the outcome often falls short of the expected result, and much effort is currently being expended to improve this outcome. The surgical technique was improved by applying a combination of the MIPO-technique with a V-shaped osteotomy and an internal fixator. The V-shaped osteotomy provides additional room for the adequate fixation of any device to the proximal fragment (i.e., 5 cm distal to the joint line rather than only 3.5 cm) (Hernigou et al., 1987; Lobenhoffer et al., 2002). The V-shaped osteotomy further improves the rotational and sagittal stability (Lobenhoffer et al., 2002). The anterior bone contact supports healing of the osteotomy and prevents intraoperative malrotation, forward slipping and tilting (Freiling et al., 2010; Van Heerwarden et al., 2007). Lastly, the force transmission of the patellar tendon is not compromised (Staubli & Jacob, 2010).

The TomoFix internal fixator is anatomically pre-contoured for the proximal-medial aspect of the tibia, which allows healing of the osteotomy without compression between the plate and bone and promotes osteogenesis through angular stable fixation with the precise amount of elasticity (Brinkman et al., 2008; Kolb et al., 2009; Nelissen et al., 2010). The angle of correction is maintained, thereby avoiding a later loss of correction (Kolb et al., 2009; Staubli et al., 2003; Stoffel et al., 2004).

The following surgical technique was developed by Lobenhoffer et al., 2002 and Staubli et al., 2003 (Kolb et al., 2009, 2010)

The procedure is performed with the patient placed in a supine position on a radiolucent table with a lateral support. With the knee held at 90° of flexion, the medial side of the proximal tibia is exposed by a 6 to 8 cm oblique incision 4 cm distal to the joint line extending from the medial aspect of the tibial tuberosity to the posterior border of the tibial plateau.

The superficial fibres of the medial collateral ligament are mobilised and released (Fig. 6). The knee is then extended, and two 2.5-mm Kirschner wires mark the oblique osteotomy starting proximal to the pes anserinus 5 cm distal to the joint line (Figs. 6 and 7).

The wires then extend to the tip of the fibula. A V-shaped osteotomy is then performed with the knee flexed again. The oblique osteotomy is performed in the posterior two-thirds of the tibia while leaving a 10-mm lateral bone bridge intact. To prevent an unintentded increase in the posterior tibial slope, special attention should be paid in locating the intact cortical hinge on the lateral - not posterolateral - side of the tibia (Wang et al., 2009)

The second osteotomy begins in the anterior one-third of the tibia at an angle of 135° while leaving the tibial tuberosity intact (a proximal-tuberosity osteotomy, or PTO, Fig. 8). When jigs are not available, a significant improvement in cutting accuracy can be achieved using a navigating system or an industrial robot that is integrated into the freehand bone-cutting (Cartiaux et al., 2010).

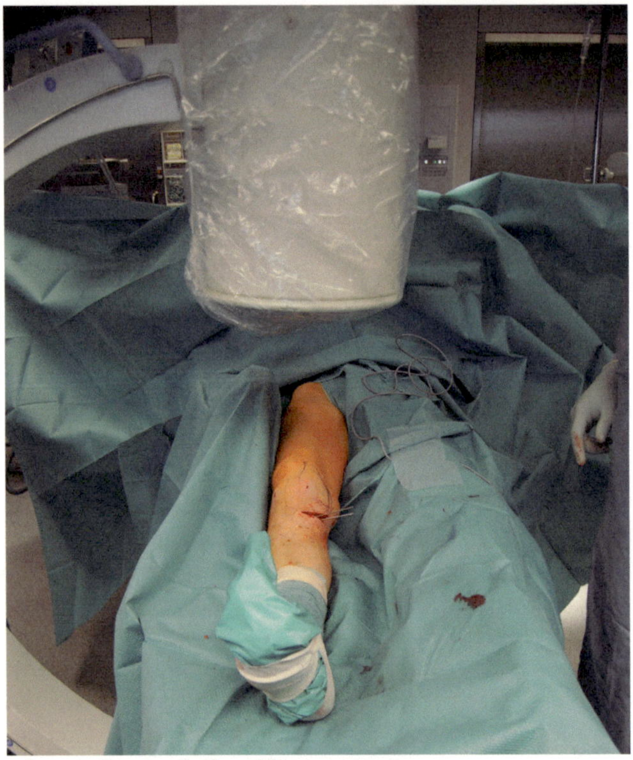

Fig. 6. 2.5 mm Kirschner wire mark the oblique osteotomy

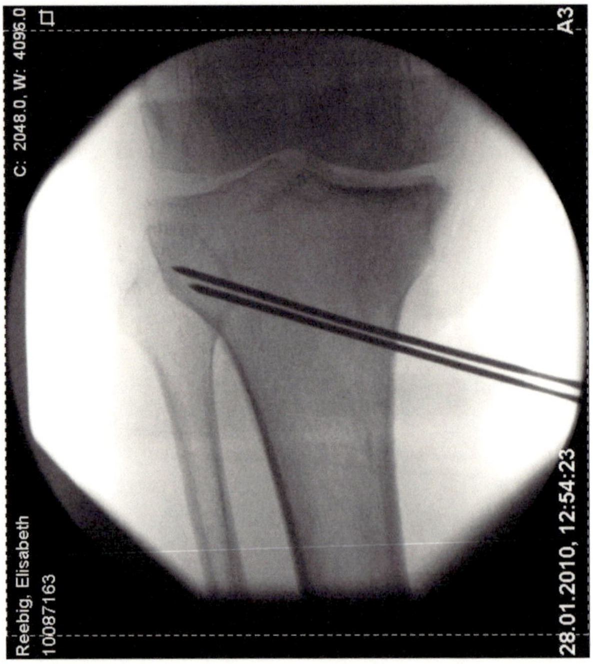

Fig. 7. 2.5 mm Kirschner wire mark the oblique osteotomy

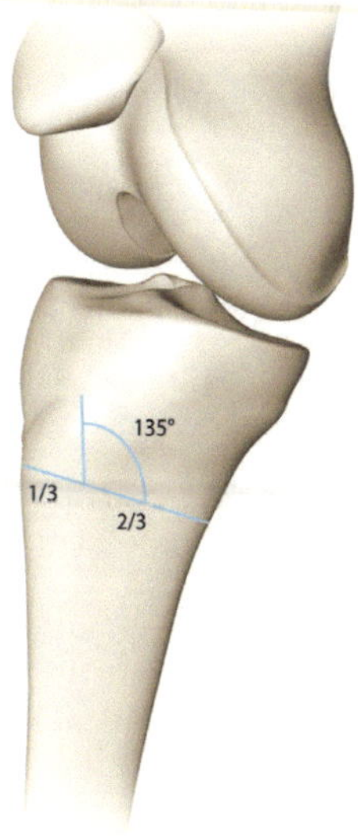

Fig. 8. V-shaped open-wedge high tibial osteotomy

We open the oblique osteotomy stepwise using three stacked osteotomes and a calibrated wedge spreader. The alignment is verified using the cable method (Krettek et al., 1997) or, alternatively, a rigid bar (Brinkman et al., 2008) or an axis-board (Liodakis et al., 2010). The axis-board is a simple and convenient option for intraoperative evaluation of the mechanical axis (Liodakis et al., 2010); however, for complex corrections, the use of navigation systems is still recommended (Liodakis et al. 2010). In recent studies, computer-assisted surgery has proven to be a helpful tool for the intraoperative control of the leg axis (Bae et al., 2009; Lützner et al., 2010; Gebhard et al., 2011), as it provides additional information regarding the lateral plane, ligaments and extension (Heijens et al., 2009). Moreover, 3D navigation can provide surgeons with reliable information both to determine the appropriate coronal alignment and to maintain the anatomical tibial slope during the open-wedge high tibial osteotomy procedure (Yamamoto et al., 2008). With the addition of arthroscopy, the anatomy and landmarks of the proximal tibia can be fully utilised to determine the frontal alignment and tibial slope (Lo et al., 2009). In a first prospective case series, approximately 85%, of patients achieved perfect result in terms of deviaton of the planned mechanical axis using computer assistance as an intraoperative guiding tool (Gebhard et al., 2011).

The alignment is checked with the knee fully extended. The TomoFix internal fixator is inserted into a subcutaneous tunnel on the anteromedial aspect of the tibia (Fig. 9).

The posterior tibial slope depends on the position of the plate that is used to stabilise the osteotomy (Rodner et al., 2006, Saverese et al., 2011). An anterior plate position results in an increase in the posterior tibial slope by an average of 6.6° (Rodner et al., 2006). In a large open-wedge correction (i.e., >8° to 10°) or in the cases of a preoperative patella infera, the tibial tuberosity is cut distally with a modified distal-tuberosity osteotomy (DTO) (Gaasbeek et al., 2004; Brinkman et al., 2008). (Poignard et al., 2010) recommend open medially and posteriorly to avoid increasing the posterior slope and unducing patella baja. We use cancellous bone grafts for open-wedge osteotomies that exceed 15 mm, whereas (Brinkman et al. 2008) uses these bone grafts when the open-wedge osteotomy exceeds 20 mm. (Poignard et al., 2010) recently reported the use of the porous beta-tricalcium phosphate (Beta-TCP) DOUWEDGE.

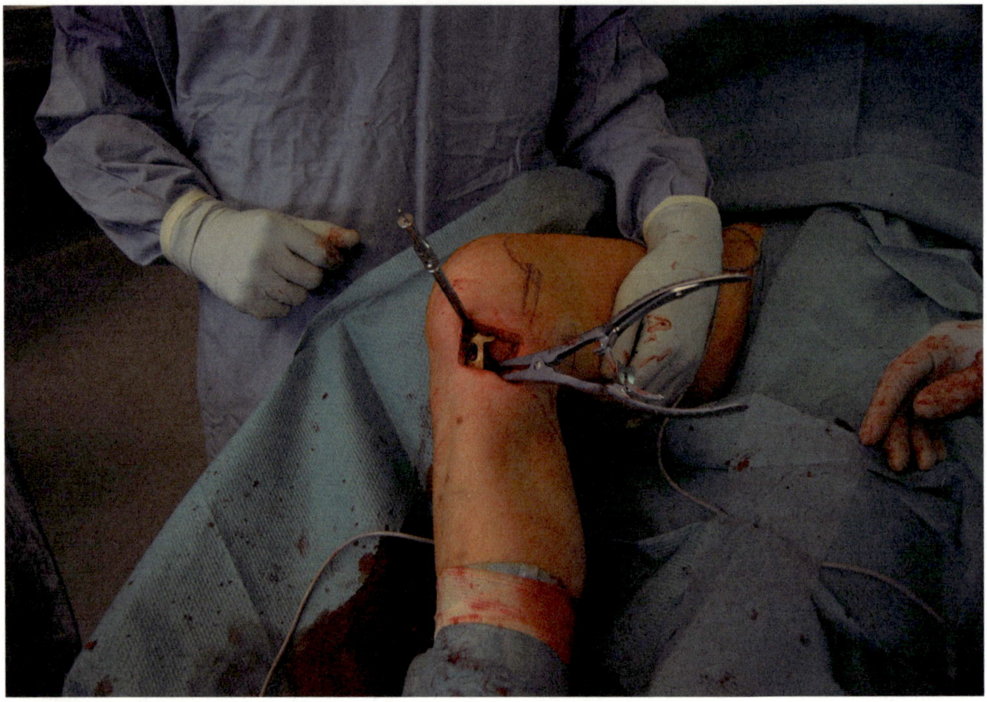

Fig. 9. The TomoFix is inserted into a subcutaneous tunnel

6.1 Postoperative care

Beginning on their first postoperative day, the patient is limited to partial weight bearing (15 kg to 20 kg) for six weeks, after which the patient can begin full weightbearing. According to (Brinkman et al., 2010) patients can typically begin full weight bearing-depending on pain-after two to three weeks (Brinkman et al., 2010).

7. Results

The open-wedge high tibial osteotomy with the MIPO technique using the TomoFix internal fixator obtained significant improved clinical results after a short to medium term follow-up (Table 10). Postoperatively, the infection rate, the rate of delayed and non-unions, the intra-articular fracture rate and the rate of implant failures were low (Table 11). Smokers had a higher rate of non-unions (Meidinger et al., 2009) (Table 12). The reason for the low complication rate of the MIPO technique with the TomoFix internal fixator was its high stability that allows a larger distance between the two screws that are adjacent to the osteotomy, thereby resulting in less elastic deformation of the plate and interfragmantary tissue. A high percentage of patients (41%) complained of local irritation that was associated with the implant in the clinical course after high tibial osteotomy (Table 13, Meidinger et al., 2011). In all cases, irritation disappeared after implant removal upon consolidation of the osteotomy gap (Meidinger et al., 2011). In the meantime, the design of the TomoFix has been modified.

Author	Patients (n) for Follow-up (n, %), age (years)	Mean Follow-up	Mean results pre-op (range)	Mean result at Follow-up (range)	Scoring system
Staubli et al., 2003	90/90 (100%), 50 (18-75) Years	9 (2-24) months	4 (3.5-5)	2 (1.5-3) significant	Visual Analogue Scale
Galla & Lobenhoffer, 2004, Lobenhoffer et al., 2004	262/262 (100%), mean 40 years	Osteotomy healing	ND	ND	ND
Takeuchi et al., 2009	52/52 (100%), 69 (54-82) years, 57 knees	40 (24-62) months	50.9 ± 12.3	91.7 ± 6.9 significant	American Knee Society Score and Function Score
Valkering et al., 2009	40/40 (100%)	Mean 10.4 months	ND	ND	ND
Zaki & Rae, 2009	46(46 (100%), 50 knees	60 (36-72) months	48 (38-54) 38 (30-55) 35 (25-55)	22 (17-31) ($p < 0.05$) 82 (45-92) ($p < 0.05$) 75 (50-95) ($p < .0\%$)	Oxford knee score, Knee Society score, functional score
Kolb et al., 2009	51/49 (96%)	52 (28-66) months	65.8 (50-98) 60.2 (43-86)	92.9 (73-100) 90.6 (71-100)	HSS score, Lysholm score
Niemeyer et al., 2010	73/69 (95%), 46.73± 9.99 years	Minimum 36 months	47.25 ± 18.71 54.26 + 20.76	72.72 ± 17.15 ($p < .001$) 79.14 + 16.63 ($p < .001$)	IKDC score, Lysholm score
Gebhard et al., 2011	51/50 (98%), 45.4 ± 8.6 (22-59)	6 weeks	ND	ND	ND
Meidinger et al., 2011	182, 142 men, 40.3 ± 10.6 years, 40 women, 43.7 ± 8.9 years	3 months	ND	ND	ND

ND means not determined

Table 11. The results of open-wedge high tibial osteotomy with the TomoFix internal fixator from various studies.

Author	Alignment/Correction losses	Osteotomy healing (weeks)	Infection (n, %)	Implant failure (n, %)	Secondary surgical procedure
Staubli et al., 2003	>slope p.o. mean 0.99, one loss of correction in both knees	10	1 (1%)	0	Implant removal due to infection
Galla & Lobenhoffer, 2004, Lobenhoffer et al., 2004	No loss of correction	2 delayed union (0.8%)	1 (0.4%) deep infection 4 months postoperative	Breakage 1 screw (3%)	2 secondary bone grafts (0.8%), 4 (2%) hematomas, one (0.4%) implant removal due to infection, one revision (0.4%) due to malalignment
Takeuchi et al., 2009	Mean femorotibial angle pre-op 181.3 ± 2.4°, p.o. 169.6 ± 2.3°	No non-union	ND	0	ND
Valkering et al., 2009	Mean loss of correction 0.3°, no loss of correction after implant removal	10.4 months	4 (10%) superficial infection	ND	ND
Zaki & Rae, 2009	Tibio-femoral 7 (5-8)° varus pre-op, 6 (5-8)° valgus p.o.		2 superficial infections (4%)	ND	ND
Kolb et al., 2009	9.5 (15-0)° varus pre-op, 1.3 (-1-5)° valgus, no loss of correction	12.9 (8-16) weeks, one non-union (2%)	0	No implant failure	One revision osteosynthesis with bone graft (2%)
Niemeyer et al., 2010	3 (4%) overcorrection mechanical axis >70% transverse diameter of proximal tibia,	2 (3%) delayed union	1 (1%) superficial wound infection	28 (41%) local irritation due to the implant	1 (1%) additional osteosynthesis due to intra-articular fracture, 2 (3%) bone graft, 3 (4%) revision osteosyntheses due to overcorrection
Gebhard et al., 2011	p.o. mean leg axis deviation 1.5° (22 (48%) patients <2.5°, 39 (85%) patients <3.5°	1 (2%) severe bone complication	2 (4%) superficial infections	ND	ND
Meidinger et al. 2011	Correction degree 7.5 (3-15)°	10 (5%) non-union, fracture lateral hinge 49 (26%)	ND	ND	10 (5%) revision surgery with debridement and bone graft including 4 (2%) plate exchanged

ND means not determined

Table 12. Complications from open-wedge high tibial osteotomy with the TomoFix internal fixator I from various studies.

Author	Nerve lesion (n, %)	Total knee arthroplasty (n, %)	Implant removal (n, %)
Staubli et al., 2003	10 hyposensitivity of the saphenous nerve (11%)	3 TKA (3%)	37 (41%) after 12 (2.5-17) months
Galla & Lobenhoffer, 2004, Lobenhoffer et al., 2004	ND	ND	10 (38%)
Takeuchi et al., 2009	ND	ND	ND
Valkering et al., 2009	ND	ND	ND
Zaki & Rae, 2009	ND	1 (2%)	ND
Kolb et al., 2009	ND	4 (8%)	2 (4%)
Niemeyer et al., 2010	ND	ND	68 (93%)
Gebhard et al., 2011	ND	ND	ND
Meidinger et al. 2011	ND	ND	ND

Table 13. Complications from open-wedge high tibial osteotomy with the TomoFix internal fixator II from various studies.

8. References

Aglietti, P.; Buzzi, R.; Vena, L.M.; Baldini, A.; & Mondaini, A. (2003). High tibial valgus osteotomy for medial gonarthrosis: a 10- to 21-Year study, J Knee Surg, Vo.16, No.1, pp.21-26.

Agneskirchner, J.D.; Hurschler, C.; Stukenborg-Colsman, C.; Imhoff, A.B.; Lobenhoffer, P. (2004). Effect of high tibial flexion osteotomy on cartilage pressure and joint kinematics: a biomechanical study in human cadaveric knees. Winner of the AGA-DonJoy Award 2004, Arch Orthop Trauma Surg, Vol.124, No.9, pp.575-584.

Agneskirchner, J.D.; Hurschler, C.; Wrann, C.D.; Lobenhoffer, P. (2007). The effects of valgus medial opening wedge high tibial osteotomy on articular cartilage pressure of the knee: a biomechanical study, Arthroscopy, Vol.23, No.8, pp.852-861.

Ahlbäck, S. (1968). Osteoarthrosis of the knee. A radiographic investigation, Acta Radiol Diagn (Stockh), Suppl 277, pp.7-72.

Akamatsu, Y.; Koshino, T.; Saito, T.; & Wada, J. (1997). Changes in osteosclerosis of the osteoarthritic knee after high tibial osteotomy, Clin Orthop Relat Res, Vol.334, No.1, pp.207-214.

Aydogdu, S.; Cullu, E.; Arac, N.; Varolgunes, N.; & Sur, H. (2000). Prolonged peroneal nerve dysfunction after high tibial osteotomy: pre- and postoperative electrophysiological study, Knee Surg Sports Traumatol Arthrosc, Vol.8, No.5, pp.305-308.

Babis, G.C.; An, K.N.; Chao, E.Y.; Rand, J.A.; & Sim, F.H. (2002). Double level osteotomy of the knee: a method to retain joint-line obliquity. Clinical results,. J Bone Joint Surg Am, Vol.84, No.8, pp.1380-1388.

Bae, D.K.; Song, S.J.; & Yoon, K.H. (2009). Closed-wedge high tibial osteotomy using computer-assisted surgery compared to the conventional technique, J Bone Joint Surg Br, Vol.91, No.9, pp.1164-1171.

Becker S.T., Warnke P.H., Behrens E., & Wiltfang, J. (2011). Morbidity after iliac crest bone graft harvesting over an anterior versus posterior approach, J Oral Maxillofac Surg, Vol.69, pp.48-53.

Bhatnagar, T.; & Jenkyn, T.R. (2010). Internal kinetic changes in the knee due to high tibial osteotomy are well-correlated with change in external adduction moment: an osteoarchritic knee model, J Biomech, Vol.43, No.12, (August 2010), pp. 2261-2266.

Bhattacharyya, T.; Gale, D.; Dewire, P.; Totterman, S.; Gale, M.E.; McLaughlin, S.; Einhorn, T.A.; & Felson, D.T. (2003). The clinical importance of meniscal tears demonstrated by magnetic imaging in osteoarthritis of the knee, J Bone Joint Surg Am, Vol.85, No.1 pp.4-9.

Billings, A.; Scott, D.F.; Camargo, M.P.; & Hofmann, A.A. (2000). High tibial osteotomy with a calibrated osteotomy guide, rigid internal fixation, and early motion. Long-term follow-up, J Bone Joint Surg Am, Vol.82, No.1, pp.70-79.

Blackburne, J.S.; & Peel, T.E. (1977). A new method of measuring patellar height, J Bone Joint Surg Br, Vol.59, No.2, (May 1977), pp.241-242.

Bonin, N.; Ait Si Selmi, T.; Dejour, D.; & Neyret, P. (2004). [Knee para-articular flexion and extension osteotomies in adults], Orthopäde, Vol.33, No.2, pp.193-200. German.

Bonnin, M.; & Chambat, P. (2004). [Current status of valgus angle, tibial head closing wedge osteotomy in media gonarthrosis]. Orthopäde, Vol.33, No.2, (February 2004), pp. 135-142.

Brattstroem, H. (1964). Shape of the intercondylar groove normally and in recurrent dislocation of patella. A clinical and x-ray anatomical investigation, Acta Orthop Scand, Vol.68, Suppl, pp.1-148.

Brinkman, J.M., Lobenhoffer, P.; Agneskirchner, J.D.; Staubli, A.E.; Wymenga, A.B.; & van Heerwarden. R.J. (2008). Osteotomies around the knee: patient selection, stability of fixation and bone healing in high tibial osteotomies, J Bone Joint Surg Br, Vol.90, No.12, (December 2008), pp.1548-1557.

Brinkman, J.M.; Luites, J.W; Wymenga, A.B.; & van Heerwarden, R.J. (2010) Early full weight bearing is safe in open-wedge high tibial osteotomy, Acta Orthop, Vol.81, No.2, (April 2010), pp.193-198.

Brown, G.A.; & Amendola, A. (2000). Radiographic evaluation and preoperative planning for high tibial osteotomies, Oper Techn Sports Med, Vol.8, No.1, pp.2-19.

Cartiaux, O.; Paul, L.; Docquier, P.L.; Raucent, B.; Dombre, E.; & Banse, X. (2010). Computer-assisted and robot-assisted technologies to improve bone-cutting accuracy when integrated with a freehand process using an oscillating saw, J Bone Joint Surg Am, Vol.92, No.11, pp.2076-2082.

Chassaing, V.D.F.; Touzard, R.; Ceccaldi, J.P.; & Miremad, C. (1995). Étude radiologique du L.C.P. à 90 de flexion, Rev Chir Orthop, Vol.81, pp.35-38.

Caton, J. (1989) [Method of measuring the height of the patella], Acta Orthop Belg, Vol.55, No.3, pp.385-386. French.

Coventry, M.B. (1965) Osteotomy of the upper portion of the tibia for degenerative arthritis of the knee: a preliminary report. J Bone Joint Surg Am, Vol.47, No.5, pp.984-990.

Coventry, M.B. (1969). Stepped staple for upper tibial osteotomy, J Bone Joint Surg Am, Vol.51, No.5, pp.1011.

Coventry, M.B. (1985). Upper tibial osteotomy for osteoarthritis, J Bone Joint Surg Am, Vol.67, No.7, pp.1136-1140.

Dahl, M.T. (2000). Preoperative planning in deformity correction and limb lengthening surgery, Instr Course Lect, Vol.49, pp.503-509.

Debeyre, J, & Patte, D. (1962). Intérêt des ostéotomies de correction dans le traitement de certaines gonarthroses avec deviation axiale. Rev Rhum Mal Osteoartic, Vol.29, pp.722-729.

Dejour, H.; Walch, G.; Nove-Josserand, L.; & Guier, C. (1994). Factors of patellar instability: an anatomic radiographic study, Knee Surg Sports Traumatol Arthosc, Vol.2, No.1, pp.19-26.

Dejour, H.; & Bonnin, M. (1994). Tibial translation after anterior cruciate ligament rupture. Two radiological tests compared, J Bone Joint Surg Br, Vol.76, No.5, pp.745-749.

Dejour, D.; Bonin, N.; & Locatelli, E. (2000). Tibial antirecurvatum osteotomies, Oper Techn Sports Med, Vol.8, No.1, pp.67-70.

Dugdale, T.W.; Noyes, F.R.; & Styer, D. (1992). Preoperative planning for high tibial osteotomy. The effect of lateral tibiofemoral separation and tibiofemoral length, Clin Orthop Relat Res, Vol.274, No.1, pp.248-264.

Engel, G.M.; & Lippert, F.G. (1981). Valgus tibial osteotomy: avoiding the pitfalls, Clin Orthop Relat Res, Vol.160, pp.137-143.

Englund, M.; Guermazi, A.; Gale, D.; Hunter, D.J.; Aliabadi, P.; Clancy, M.; & Felson, D.T. (2008). Incidental meniscal findings on knee MRI in middle-aged and elderly persons, N Engl J Med, Vol.359, No.11, (September 2008), pp.1108-1115.

Feller, J.A.; Amis, A.A.; Andrish, J.T.; Arendt, E.A.; Erasmus, P.J.; & Powers, C.M. (2007). Surgical biomechanics of the patellofemoral joint, Arthroscopy, Vol. 23, No.5, pp.542-553.

Felson, D.T.; McLaughlin, S.; Goggins, J.; LaValley, M.P.; Gale, M.E.; Totterman, S.; Li, W.; Hill, C.; & Gale, D. (2003). Bone marrow edema and its relation to progression of knee osteoarthritis, Ann Intern Med, Vol.139, No.5 Pt 1, pp.330-336.

Fick, R. (1911). Handbuch der Anatomie und Mechanik der Gelenke, Vol.3, Gustav Fischer, Jena.

Freiling, D.; van Heerwarden, R.; Staubli, A.; & Lobenhoffer, P. (2010). [The medial closed-wedge osteotomy of the distal femur for the treatment of unicompartmental lateral osteoarthritis of the knee], Oper Orthop Traumatol, Vol.22, pp.317-334. German.

Frey, P.; Müller, M.; & Munzinger, U. (2008). [Closing-wedge high tibial osteotomy with a modified Weber technique], Oper Orthop Traumatol, Vol.20, No.1, pp.75-88. German.

Fujisawa, Y.; Masuhara, K.; & Shiomi, S. (1979). The effect of high tibial osteotomy on osteoarthritis of the knee, Orthop Clin North Am, Vol.10, pp.585-608.

Gaasbeek, R.D.; Sonneveld, H.; van Heerwaarden, R.J.; Jacobs, W.C.; & Wymenga, A.B. (2004). Distal tuberosity osteotomy in open wedge high tibial osteotomy can prevent patella infera: a new technique, Knee, Vol.11, pp.457-461.

Galla, M.; & Lobenhoffer, P. (2004). High tibial open wedge valgus osteotomy stabilized with the TomoFix plate fixator, Operat Orthop Traumatol, Vol.16, No.4, pp.397-416. English, German.

Gebhard, F.; Krettek, C.; Hüfner, T.; Grützner, P.A.; Stöckle, U.; Imhoff, A.B.; Lorenz, S.; Liungqvist, J.; & Keppler, P. (2011). The AO CSEG. Reliability of computer-assisted surgery as an intraoperative ruler in navigated high tibial osteotomy, Arch Orthop Trauma Surg, Vol.131, pp.297-302.

Giebel, G.; Tscherne, H.; & Daiber, M. (1985). [Tibial head osteotomy in the treatment of gonarthrosis, Orthopäde, Vol.14, No.3, pp.144-153. German.

Giffin, J.R.; Stabile, K.J.; Zantop, T.; Vodrin, T.M.; Woo, S.L.; & Harner, C.D. (2007). Importance of tibial slope for stability of the posterior cruciate ligament deficient knee, Am J Sports Med, Vol.35, No.9, pp.1443-1449.

Grelsamer, R.P.; Bazos, A.N.; & Proctor, C.S. (1993). Radiographic analysis of patellar tilt, J Bone Joint Surg Br, Vol.75, No.5, (September 1993), pp.822-824.

Hankemeier, S.; Mommsen, P.; Krettek, C.; Jagodzinski, M.; Brand, J.; Meyer, C.; & Meller, C. (2010). Accuracy of high tibial osteotomy: comparison between open- and closed-wedge technique, Knee Surg Sports Traumatol Arthrosc, Vol.18, No.10, pp.1328-1333.

Hanssen, A.D.; & Chao, E.Y.S. (1994). High Tibial Osteotomy, In Knee Surgery, Vol. 2, F.H. Fu, C.D. Harner & K.G. Vince, (Eds.), pp.1121-1134, Williams & Wilkins, ISBN 0-683-03389-1, Baltimore, USA.

Hanssen, A.D. (2001). Osteotomy About the Knee: American Perspective. In Surgery of the knee, J.N. Insall, W.N. Scott, (Eds.), Vol 2, pp. 1447-1464, Churchill Livingstone, ISBN, New York, USA.

Van Heerwarden, R.J.; Wymenga, A.; Freiling, D.; & Lobenhoffer, P. (2007). Distal medial closed wedge varus femur osteotomy stabilized with the TomoFix plate fixator, Oper Tech Orthop, Vol.17, No.1, pp.12-21.

Heijens, E.; Kornherr, P.; & Meister, C. (2009). The role of navigation in high tibial osteotomy: a study of 50 patients, Orthopedics, Vol.32, No.10 Suppl, pp.40-43.

Hernigou, P.; Medevielle, D.; Debeyre, J.; & Goutallier, D. (1987). Proximal tibial osteotomy for osteoarthritis with varus deformity. A ten to thirteen-year follow-up study, J Bone Joint Surg Am, Vol.69, No.3, pp.332-354.

Hofmann, S.; & Pietsch, M. (2007). [Principles and indications of osteotomies around the knee], Arthroskopie Vol.20, No.4, (November 2007), pp. 270-276.

Hofmann, S.; Lobenhoffer, P.; Staubli, A.; & Van Heerwarden, P. (2009). [Osteotomies of the knee joint in patients with monocompartimental arthritis, Orthopäde, Vol.38, No.8, pp.755-769; quiz 770. German.

Hohmann, E.; Bryant, A.; & Imhoff, A.B. (2006). The effect of closed wedge high tibial osteotomy on tibial slope: a radiographic study, Knee Surg Sports Traumatol Arthrosc, Vol.14, No.5, pp.454-459.

Hsu, R.W.; Himeno, S.; Coventry, M.B.; & Chao, E.Y. (1990). Normal axial alignment of the lower extremity and load-bearing distribution at the knee, Clin Orthop Relat Res, Vol.225, pp.215-227.

Imhoff, A.B.; Linke, R.D.; & Agneskirchner, J. (2004). [Corrective osteotomy in primary varus, double varus and triple varus knee instability with cruciate ligament replacement], Orthopäde, Vol.33, No.2, pp. 201-207. German.

Insall, J., & Salvati, E. (1971). Patella position in the normal knee joint, Radiology, Vo.101, No.1, (October 1971), pp.101-104.

Iorio, R.; & Healy, W.L. (2003). Unicompartmental arthritis of the knee, J Bone Joint Surg Am, Vol.85, No.7, pp.1351-1364. Review.

Ivarsson, I.; Myrnerts, R.; & Gillquist, J. (1990). High tibial osteotomy for medial osteoarthritis of the knee. A 5 to 7 and 11 year follow-up, J Bone Joint Surg Br, Vol.72, No.2, pp.238-244.

Jakob, R.P.; & Jacobi, M. (2004). [Closing wedge osteotomy of the tibial head in the treatment of single compartment arthrosis], Orthopäde, Vol.33, No.2, pp. 143-152. German.

Jacobsen, K. (1976). Stress radiographical measurement of the anteroposterior, medial and alteral stability of the knee joint, Acta Orthop Scand, Vol.47, No.3, pp.334-335.

Jackson, J.P.; & Waugh, W. (1961). Tibial osteotomy for osteoarthritis of the knee, J Bone Joint Surg Br, Vol.43, No.4, pp.746-751.

Kerkhoffs, G.M.; Rademakers, M.V.; Altena, M.; & Marti, R.K. (2008). Combined intra-articular and varus opening wedge osteotomy for lateral depression and valgus malunion of the proximal part of the tibia, J Bone Joint Surg Am, Vol.90, No.6, pp.1252-1257.

Kessler, O.C.; Jacob, H.A.; & Romero, J. (2002). Avoidance of medial cortical fracture in high tibial osteotomy: improved technique, Clin Orthop Relat Res, Vol.395, No.2, pp.180-185.

Kettelkamp, D.B.; Wenger, D.R.; Chao, E.Y.; & Thompson, C. (1976). Results of proximal tibial osteotomy. The effects of tibiofemoral angle, stance-phase flexion-extension, and medial-plateau force, J Bone Joint Surg Am, Vol.58, No.10, pp.952-960.

Kirgis, A.; & Albrecht, S. (1992). Palsy of the deep peroneal nerve after proximal tibial osteotomy. An anatomical study, J Bone Joint Surg Am, Vol.74, No.8, pp.1180-1185.

Köck, F.X.; Weingärtner, D.; Beckmann, J.; Anders, S.; Schaumburger, J.; Grifka, J.; & Lüring, C. [Operative treatment of unicompartmental knee arthritis - Results of a Nationwide survey in 2008], Z Orthop Unfall, Vol.149, No.2, (February 2011), pp.153-159. [Article in German].

Kolb, W.; Guhlmann, H.; Windisch, C.; Marx, F.; Kolb, K.; & Koller, H. (2008). Fixation of distal femoral fractures with the Less Invasive Stabilization System: a minimally invasive treatment with locked fixed-angled screws, J Trauma, Vol.65, No.6, (December 2008), pp.1425-1434.

Kolb, W.; Guhlmann, H.; Windisch, C.; Kolb, K.; Koller, H.; & Grützner, P. (2009). Opening-wedge high tibial osteotomy with a locked low-profile plate, J Bone Joint Surg Am, Vol.91, pp.2581-2588.

Kolb, W.; Guhlmann, H.; Windisch, C.; Koller, H.; Grützner, P.; & Kolb, K. (2010). Opening-wedge high tibial osteotomy with a locked low-profile plate: surgical technique, J Bone Joint Surg Am, Vol.92, Suppl 1, pp.197-207.

Koshino, T.; & Tsuchiya, K. (1979). The effect of high tibial osteotomy on osteoarthritis of the knee. Clinical and histological observations, Int Orthop, Vol.3, No.1, pp.37-45.

Koshino, T.; Morii, T.; Wada, J.; Saito, H.; Ozawa, N.; & Noyori, K. (1989). High tibial osteotomy with fixation by a blade plate for medial compartment osteoarthritis of the knee, Orthop Clin North Am, Vol.20, No.2, pp.227-243.

Koshino, T. (2010). Osteotomy around young deformed knees: 38-year super-long-term follow-up to detect osteoarthritis, Int Orthop, Vol.34, No.2, pp.263-269.

Krettek, C.; Schandelmaier, P.; Miclau, T.; & Tscherne, H. (1997). Minimally invasive percutaneous plate osteosynthesis (MIPPO) using DCS in proximal and distal femoral fractures, Injury, Vol.28, (Suppl 1), pp.S-A20-30.

Lichte, P.; Kobbe, P.; Lörken, M.; & Pape, H.C. (2010). [Planning of corrective osteotomies of the lower limb], Unfallchirurg, Vol.113, No.7, pp. 573-583, quiz 584. German.

Lind, M.; McClelland, J.; Wittwer, J.E.; Withehead, T.S.; Feller, J.A.; & Webster, K.E. (2011). Gait analysis of walking before and after medial opening wedge high tibial osteotomy. Knee Surg Sports Traumatol Arthrosc, Apr 12, [Epub ahead of print].

Liodakis, E.; Kenawey, M.; Liodaki, E.; Mommsen, P.; Krettek, C.; & Hankemeier, S. (2010). The axis-board: an alternative to the cable technique for intraoperative assessment of lower limb alignment, Technol Health Care, Vol.18, pp.165-171.

Langenbeck, B. (1854). Die subkutane Osteotomie, Dtsch Klin, Vol.6, pp.327-330.

Lerat, J.L.; Moyen, B.; Garin, C.; Mandrino, A.; Besse, J.L.; & Brunet-Guedi, E. (1993). [Anterior laxitiy and internal arthritis of the knee. Results of the reconstruction of the anterior cruciate ligament associated with tibial osteotomy], Rev Chir Orthop App Mot, Vol.79, No.5, pp.365-374.

Levigne, C. ; & Bonnin, M. (1991). Ostéotomie tibiale de valgisation pour AFTI, Journées Lyonnaises de Chirurgie du Genou, Lyon.

Louisia, S.; Siebold, R.; Canty, J.; & Bartlett, R.J. (2005). Assessment of posterior stability in total knee replacement by stress radiographs: prospective comparison of two different types of mobile bearing implants, Knee Surg Sports Traumatol Arthrosc, Vol.13, No.6, pp.476-482.

Luites, J.W.; Brinkman, J.M.; Wymenga, A.B.; & van Heerwarden, R.J. (2009). Fixation stability of opening-versus closing-wedge high tibial osteotomy: a randomised clinical trial using radiostereometry, J Bone Joint Surg Br, Vol. 91, No.11, (November 2009), pp. 1459-1465.

Lo, W.N.; Cheung, K.W.; Yung, S.H.; & Chiu, K.H. (2009). Arthroscopy-assisted computer navigation in high tibial osteotomy for varus knee deformity, J Orthop Surg (Hong Kong), Vol.17, No.1, pp.51-55.

Lobenhoffer, P.; De Simoni, C.; & Staubli, A.E. (2002). Open-wedge high tibial osteotomy with rigid plate fixation, Tech Knee Surg, Vol.1, pp.93-105.

Lobenhoffer, P.; Agneskirchner, J.; & Zoch, W. (2004). [Open valgus alignment osteotomy of the proximal tibia with fixation by medial plate fixator], Orthopäde, Vol.33, No.2, pp.153-160.

Lützner, J.; Gross, A.F.; Günther, K.P.; & Kirschner, S. (2010). Precision of navigated and conventional open-wedge high tibial osteotomy in a cadaver study, Eur J Med Res, Vol.15, pp.117-120.

Maquet, P. (1976). Valgus osteotomy for osteoarthritis of the knee, Clin Orthop Relat Res, Vol.120, pp.143-148.

Marti, C.B.; Gautier, E.; Wachtl, S.W.; & Jakob, R.P. (2004). Accuracy of frontal and sagittal plane correction in open-wedge high tibial osteotomy, Arthroscopy, Vol.20, No.4, pp.366-372. Review.

Mast, J.W.; Jakob, R. & Ganz, R. (1989). Planning and Reduction Techniques in Fracture Surgery, Springer, Berlin, Germany.
http://www.medical.siemens.com/webapp/wcs/stores/servlet/ProductDisplay~q_catalogId~e_-3~a_catTree~e_100010,1007665,12760,1032265~a_langId~e_-3~a_productId~e_202741~a_storeId~e_10001.htm

Meidinger, G.; Imhoff, A.B.; Paul, J.; Kirchhoff, C.; Sauerschnig, M.; & Hinterwimmer, S. (2011). May smokers and overweight patients be treated with medial open-wedge HTO? Risk factors for non-union, Knee Surg Sports Traumatol, Vol.19, No.3, pp.333-339.

Merchant, A.C.; Mercer, R.L.; Jacobsen, R.H.; & Cool, C.R. (1974). Roentgenographic analysis of patellofemoral congruence, J Bone Joint Surg Am, Vol.56, No.7, pp.1391-1396.

Merian, M.; Schäfer, D.; & Hintermann, B. (2005) Proximal tibial valgus osteotomy with callus distraction. Oper Orthop Traumatol, Vol.17, No.3, pp.313-325.

Miniaci, A.; Ballmer, F.T.; Ballmer, P.M.; & Jakob, R.P. (1989). Proximal tibial osteotomy. A new fixation device, Clin Orthop Relat Res, Vol.246, pp.250-259.

Moreland, J.R.; Bassett, L.W.; & Hanker, G.J. (1987). Radiographic analysis of the axial alignment of the lower extremity, J Bone Joint Surg Am, Vol.69, No.5, pp.745-749.

Müller, M.; & Strecker, W. (2008). Arthroscopy prior to osteotomy around the knee? Arch Orthop Trauma Surg, Vol.128, No.11, pp.1217-1221.

Müller, W. (2001). Osteotomies around the knee. Instructional Courses, EFFORT, pp.34-39.

Myrnerts, R. (1980). Failure of the correction of varus deformity obtained by high tibial osteotomy, Acta Orthop Scand, Vol.51, No.3, pp.569-573.

Nagi, O.N.; Kumar, S.; Aggarwal, S. (2007). Combined lateral closing and medial opening-wedge high tibial osteotomy, J Bone Joint Surg Am, Vol.89, No.3, pp.542-549.

Nelissen, E.M.; van Langelaan, E.J.; & Nelissen, R.G. (2010) Stability of medial opening wedge high tibial osteotomy: a failure analysis, Int Orthop, Vol.34, No.2, pp.217-223.

Niemeyer, P.; Schmal, H.; Hauschild, O.; von Heyden, J.; Südkamp, N.P.; & Köstler, W. (2010). Open-wedge osteotomy using an internal plate fixator in patients with medial-compartment gonarthritis and varus malalignment: 3-year results with regard to preoperative arthroscopic and radiographic findings, Arthroscopy, Vol. 26, No.12 (December 2010), pp.1607-1616.

Noyes, F.R.; Barber, S.D. & Simon, R. (1993). High tibial osteotomy and ligament reconstruction in varus angulated, anterior cruciate ligament-deficient knees. A two- to seven-year follow-up study, Am J Sports Med, Vol.21, No.1, Jan-Feb, pp.2-12.

Noyes, F.R.; & Simon, R. (1994). The role of high tibial osteotomy in the anterior cruciate ligament-deficient knee with varus alignment. In Orthopaedic Sports Medicine, Principles and Practice, J.C. DeLee, D. Drez, (Eds.), pp.1401-1443, W.B. Saunders, ISBN 0721628346, Philadelphia, USA.

Noyes, F.R.; Barber-Westin, S.D.; & Hewett, T.E. (2000). High tibial osteotomy and ligament reconstruction for varus angulated anterior cruciate ligament-deficient knees, Am J Sports Med, Vol.28, No.3, pp.282-296.

Odenbring, S.; Egund, N.; Lindstrand, A.; Lohmander, L.S.; & Willén, H. (1992). Cartilage regeneration after proximal tibial osteotomy for medial gonarthrosis. An arthroscopic, roentgenographic, and histologic study, Clin Orthop Relat Res, Vol.277, No.4, pp.210-216.

Outerbridge, R.E. (1961). The etiology of chondromalacia patellae, J Bone Joint Surg Br, Vol.43, No.4, pp.752-757.

Paley, D.; & Tetsworth, K. (1992). Mechanical axis deviation of the lower limbs. Preoperative planning of multiapical frontal plane angular and bowing deformities of the femur and tibia, Clin Orthop Relat Res, Vol.280, No.7, pp.65-71.

Paley, D.; Herzenberg, J.E.; Tetsworth, K; McKie, J.; & Bhave, A. (1994). Deformity planning for frontal and sagittal plane corrective osteotomies, Orthop Clin North Am, Vol.25, pp.483-498.

Pape, D.; Seil, R.; Adam, F.; Rupp, S.; Kohn, D.; & Lobenhoffer, P. (2004). [Imaging and preoperative planning of osteotomy of tibial head osteotomy], Orthopäde, Vol.33, No.2, pp.122-134. German.

Pape, D.; Adam, F.; Rupp, S.; Seil, R.; & Kohn, D. (2004). [Stability, bone healing and loss of correction after valgus realignment of the tibial head. A roentgen stereometry analysis], Orthopäde, Vol.33, No.2, pp.208-217. German.

Pape, D.; Lorbach, O.; & Steimer, O. (2007). Analyse der Deformität und präoperative Planung einer knienahen Osteotomie, Arthroskopie, Vol.20, No.4, pp.277-290. [German].

Perusi, M.; Baietta, D.; & Pizzoli, A. (1994). [Surgical correction of osteoarthritic genu varum by the heimcallotasis technique], Rev Chir Orthop Raparatrice Appar Mot, Vol.80, No.8, pp.739-743. French.

Poignard, A.; Flouzat Lachaniette, C.H.; & Amzallag, J P. (2010) Revisiting high tibial osteotomy: fifty years of experience with the opening-wedge technique, J Bone Joint Surg Am, Vol.92, Suppl 2, pp.187-195.

Poilvache, P. (2001). Osteotomy for the Arthritic Knee: A European Perspective. In Surgery of the Knee, Vol. 2, J.N. Insall, W.N. Scott, (Eds.), pp.1465-1505, Churchill Livingstone, ISBN 0-443-06545-4, New York, USA.

Prodomos, C.C.; Andriacchi, T.P.; & Galante, J.O. (1985). A relationship between gait and clinical changes following high tibial osteotomy. J Bone Joint Surg Am, Vol.67, No.8, pp. 1188-1194.

Puddu, G.; Gianni, E.; Chambat, P.; & De Paulis, F. (2000). The axial view in evaluating tibial translation in cases of insuffiency of the posterior cruciate ligament, Arthroscopy, Vol.16, No.2, pp.217-220.

Rand, J.A.; & Neyret, P. (2005). ISAKOS meeting on management of osteoarthritis of the knee prior to total knee arthroplasty. ISAKOS, pp.1-8, Hollywood, Florida, USA.

Rodner, C.M.; Adams, D.J.; Diaz-Doran, V.; Tate, J.P.; Santangelo, S.A.; Mazzocco, A.D.; & Arcieno, R.A. (2006). Medial opening wedge osteotomy and the sagittal plane: the effect of increasing tibial slope on tibiofemoral pressure, Am J Sports Med, Vol.34, No.9, pp.1431-1441.

Rosenberg, T.D.; Paulos, L.E.; Parker, R.D.; Coward, D.B.; & Scott, S.M. (1988). The forty-five-degree posteroanterior flexion weight-bearing radiograph of the knee, J Bone Joint Surg Am, Vol.70, No.10, pp.1479-1483.

Savarese, E.; Bisicchia, S.; Romeo, R.; & Amendola, A. (2011). Role of high tibial osteotomy in chronic injuries of posterior cruciate ligament and posterolateral corner, J Orthop Traumatol, Vol.12, No.1, pp.1-17.

Seitlinger, G.; Scheurecker, G.; Högler, R.; Kramer, J.; & Hofmann, S. (2010). Bildgebende Diagnostik des Patellofemoralgelenks, Arthroskopie, Vol.23, pp.176-183.

Seitlinger, G.; Beitzel, K.; Scheurecker, G.; Imhoff, A.; & Hofmann, S. (2011). [The painful patellofemoral joint. Biomechanics, diagnosis and therapy], Orthopäde, Vol.40, No.4, pp.353-368; quiz 369-370. German.

Shaw, J.A.; Dungy, D.S.; & Arsht, S.S. (2004). Recurrent varus angulation after high tibial osteotomy: an anatomic analysis, Clin Orthop Relat Res, Vol.420, pp.205-212.

Smith, T.O.; Sexton, D.; Mitchell, P.; & Hing, C.B. (2010). Opening- or closing-wedge high tibial osteotomy: A meta-analysis of clinical and radiological outcomes. Knee, Oct 28, [Epub ahead of print].

Song, E.K.; Seon, J.K.; Park, S.J.; & Jeong, M.S. (2010). The complications of high tibial osteotomy: closing - versus opening-wedge methods, J Bone Joint Surg Br, Vol.92, No.9, pp. 1245-1252.

Stäubli, H.U.; & Jakob, R.P. (1990). Posterior instability of the knee near extension. A clinical and stress radiographic analysis of acute injuries of the posterior cruciate ligament, J Bone Joint Surg Br, Vol.72, No.2, pp.225-230.

Staubli, A.E.; De Simoni, C.; Babst, R.; & Lobenhoffer, P. (2003). TomoFix: a new LCP-concept for open wedge osteotomy of the medial proximal tibia-early results in 92 cases, Injury, Vol.34, Suppl 2, pp.B55-62.

Staubli, A.E.; & Jacob, H.A. (2010). Evolution of open-wedge high-tibial osteotomy: experience with a special angular stable device for internal fixation without interposition material, Int Orthop, Vol.34, No.2, pp.167-172.

Stoffel, K.; Stachowiak, G.; & Kuster, M. (2004). Open wedge high tibial osteotomy: a biomechanical investigation of the modified Arthrex Osteotomy Plate (Puddu Plate) and the TomoFix Plate, Clin Biomech, Vol.19, No.9, pp.944-950.

Strecker, W.; Dickschas, J.; Harrer, J.; & Müller, M. (2009). [Arthroscopy prior to osteotomy in cases of unicondylar osteoarthritis], Orthopäde, Vol.38, No.3, pp.263-268. German.

Strobel, M.J.; Weiler, A.; Schulz, M.S.; Russe, K.; & Eichhorn, H.J. (2002). Fixed posterior subluxation in posterior cruciate ligament-deficient knees: diagnosis and treatment of a new clinical sign, Am J Sports Med, Vol. 30, No.1, pp.32-38.

Takahashi, S.; Tomihisa, K.; & Saito, T. (2002-2003). Decrease of osteosclerosis in subcondral bone of medial compartmental osteoarthritic knee seven to nineteen years after high tibial valgus osteotomy, Bull Hosp Jt Dis, Vol.61, No.1-2, pp.58-62.

Takeuchi, R.; Ishikawa, H.; Aratake, M.; Bito, H.; Kumagai, K.; Akamatsu, Y.; & Saito, T. (2009). Medial opening wedge high tibial osteotomy with early full weight bearing, Arthroscopy, Vol.25, No.1, pp.46-53.

Terauchi, M.; Shirakura, K.; Katayama, M.; Higuchi, H.; Takagishi, K.; & Kimura, M. (2002). Varus inclination of the distal femur and high tibial osteotomy, J Bone Joint Surg Br, Vol.84, No.2, pp.223-226.

Tunggal, J.A.; Higgins, G.A.; & Waddell, J.P. (2010). Complications of closing wedge high tibial osteotomy, Int Orthop, Vol.34, No.2, pp.255-261.

Urch, S.E.; Tritle, B.A.; Shelbourne, K.D.; & Gray, T. (2009). Axial linear patellar displacement: a new measurement of patellofemoral congruence, Am J Sports Med, Vol.37, No.5, (May 2009), pp.970-973.

Valkering, K.P.; van den Bekerom, M.P.; Kappelhoff, F.M.; & Albers, G.H. (2009). Complications after medial opening wedge high tibial osteotomy, J Knee Surg, Vol.22, No.3, pp.218-225.

Weber, B.G., & Wörsdorfer, O. (1980). Zuggurtungsosteosynthese bei Tibiakopfosteotomie, Z Orthop, Vol.118, pp.637.

Wagner M.; & Frigg, R. (2006). AO Manual of Fracture Management. Internal Fixators. Concepts and Cases Using LCP and LISS, Thieme, ISBN-10; 3-13-1435551-8, New York, USA.

Wang, J.H.; Bae, J.H.; Lim, H.C.; Shon, W.Y.; Kim, C.W.; & Cho, J.W. (2009). Medial open wedge high tibial osteotomy: the effect of the cortical hinge on posterior tibial slope, Am J Sports Med, Vol.37, No.12, pp.2411-2418.

Watanabe, K.; Tsuchiya, H.; Sakurakichi, K.; Matsubara, H.; & Tomita, K. (2008). Acute correction using focal dome osteotomy for deformity about knee joint, Arch Orthop Trauma Surg, Vol.128, No.12, pp.1373-1378.

Weale, A.E.; Lee, A.S.; & MacEachern, A.G. (2001). High tibial osteotomy using a dynamic external fixator, Clin Orthop Relat Res, Vol.382, pp.154-167.

Windsor, R.E.; Insall, J.N.; & Vince, K.G. (1988). Technical considerations of total knee arthroplasty after proximal tibial osteotomy, J Bone Joint Surg Am, Vol.70, No.4, pp.547-555.

Wong, K.C.; Kumta, S.M.; Leung, K.S.; Ng, K.W.; Ng, E.W.; Lee, K.S. (2012). Integration of CAD/CAM planning into computer assisted orthopaedic surgery, Comput Aided Surg, Vol.15, No.4-6, pp.65-74.

Yamamoto, Y.; Ishibashi, Y.; Tsuda, E.; Tsukada, H.; Kimura, Y.; & Toh, S. (2008). Validation of computer-assisted open-wedge high tibial osteotomy using three-dimensional navigation, Orthopedics, Vol.31, No.10 Suppl 1, pp. pii: orthosupersite.com/view.asp?rID=35551.

Zaki, S.H.; & Rae, P.J. (2009). High tibial valgus osteotomy using the Tomofix plate – medium-term results in young patients, Acta Orthop Belg, Vol.75, No.3, pp.360-367.

Part 6

Treatment of OA in Lower Extremity (Hip, Knee, and Ankle)

19

Ultrasound Guided Hip Injection Techniques

Micu Mihaela Cosmina
Rehabilitation Clinical Hospital Cluj, Rehabilitation Department II, Rheumatology Division
Romania

1. Introduction

Current development of medical practice has shown that imaging-guided interventional invasive techniques are superior to blind manoeuvres. Moreover, a safe nonradiant and cheap imaging guidance method is always preferred (Aliabadi P et al., 1988; Ozonoff MB, 1973; Sofka CM et al., 2005; Picano & Matucci Cerinic, 2010). In addition to its primary use as a very useful diagnostic tool and natural extension of the clinical examination, musculoskeletal ultrasound is now frequently used in clinical rheumatological practice for guiding interventional manoeuvres.

Interventional musculoskeletal ultrasound guided manoeuvres refer to a variety of invasive procedures performed percutaneously covering diagnostic as well as therapeutic injection of joints, tendon sheats or other peri-articular structures up to more complex manoeuvres like biopsies, removal of foreign bodies and intratumoral therapeutic injections.

Ultrasonography has a very important advantage over other imaging methods because it allows the concomitant visualization of the target structure, the needle penetration and tip positioning as well as the drug deposition (Bradley MJ, 2001). Indeed, musculoskeletal ultrasound evaluation is an accurate and reliable method in depicting articular and periarticular lesions, has no radiation, is cheap and quick to perform and allows repeated examinations at baseline and during follow up (Bierma-Zeinstra et al., 2001; Koski JM et al., 1989; Iagnocco A et al., 2006; Qvistgaard E et al., 2001). Moreover, a modular flexible training strategy to achieve competence in diagnostic as well as in interventional musculoskeletal ultrasound showed a fast learning curve among rheumatologists, thus encouraging its employment in daily practice (Atchia I et al., 2007).

Hip joint pathology is very frequently encountered in clinical practice. Hip joint pain is the main symptom generated by several pathological conditions including primary osteoarthritis (OA), inflammatory diseases like rheumatoid arthritis, spondylarthropaties, crystal deposition diseases as well as congenital and traumatic disorders with potential evolution to secondary OA.

Recently, several studies have shown an increase in the general population of hip OA incidence in parallel with an increase of obesity incidence and higher life expectancy worldwide. Chronic hip pain on walking is the most important factor impacting on patient quality of life and is complicated by functional disability due to structural damage. The management of hip pain is therefore burdened by long term high treatment costs. In fact, the increasing number of total hip replacements with elevated surgery costs and prolonged rehabilitation procedures are challenging the health care systems all over the world (Birrell F et al., 2003; Brooks PM, 2006). For this reason, various diagnostic and treatment strategies are continuously tested in order to obtain maximum efficacy and minimize the total management costs .

In the outpatient rheumatological setting, diagnostic aspiration and therapeutic intra-articular hip joint injections are frequently required. In fact, the guided aspiration of the fluid from the coxofemoral joint is of paramount importance to obtain laboratory analyses (microscopy-culture and Gram stain) that may rapidly differentiate septic arthritis from other inflammatory joint conditions like rheumatoid arthritis, spondilarthropaties and crystal deposition diseases. Other imaging techniques do not differentiate a septic effusion from other kind of effusions because of the non-specific appearance. (Foldes K et al., 1995)

The current Osteoarthritis Research Society International (OARSI) and Assessment of SpondyloArthritis International Society (ASAS) / European League Against Rheumatism (EULAR) therapeutic guidelines include hip corticosteroid injection, which is still a rare therapeutic approach because standardized criteria for patients selection are still missing and because of the small number of performing physicians. These are clear limitation in using the method. (Zhang W et al., 2005, 2008) On the other hand, the use of intraarticular hip viscosupplementation is still under study because of the low number of existing trials, most of them with contradictory results and is still waiting for approval in some countries. (Migliore A et al., 2004; Qvistgaard E et al., 2006; Richette P et al., 2009)

It is well known that deep joints, like the hip, are difficult to reach and inject and therefore require imaging guided needle techniques that are currently preferred to the blind injections guided only by anatomical landmarks. In fact, musculoskeletal ultrasound guided technique allows a correct needle penetration (avoiding neurovascular structures injury), joint aspiration, and a more accurate drug deposition which assures a higher efficacy. (Leopold SS et al., 2001 ; Iagnocco A & Naredo E , 2010; Naredo E et al., 2005)

The first data about the use of musculoskeletal ultrasound guided hip aspiration of synovial fluid were reported by Komppa in 1985. (Komppa GH et al., 1985) Ultrasound guided injections were introduced much later in clinical trials and practice, when it became evident that joint ultrasound facilitates a quick, accurate diagnosis and operative safe local treatment showing extraordinary advantages over the other imaging techniques. Despite several efforts made in many countries to implement the invasive musculoskeletal ultrasound guided techniques as a part of the rheumatology curriculum, this procedure still remains insufficiently exploited among rheumatologists.

The aim of this chapter is to describe the basic techniques of the ultrasound guided hip joint injection and to update the therapeutic standards, indications and contraindications, efficacy and safety of the method.

2. Anatomy of the hip

The hip is a "ball and socket" synovium lined joint between the spherical femoral head covered by hyaline articular cartilage and the cup- shaped acetabulum. The capsule, superficially reinforced in the anterior aspect by the ilio- femoral ligament and covered by synovial tissue, extends around the joint attaching superiorly to the acetabulum and labrum and inferiorly to the intertrochanteric area. The deep synovial layer reflects back from the intertrochanteric area to the head neck junction delineating the anterior joint recess. The ilio-psoas muscle is superficial to the anterior aspect of the capsule.

3. Sonoanatomy, patient position and scanning technique

To perform an ultrasound guided procedure, the patient should be supine with the heels together and slightly (10-20 °degrees) externally rotated legs. The examination is performed with a low frequency 3.5- 7.5 MHz linear array probe or a convex one (2.5-5 MHz) for obese or muscular patients, following EULAR ultrasound evaluation guidelines with multiplanar structure scanning, in grey scale and Doppler mode. (Iagnocco A & Naredo E, 2010; Leopold SS et al., 2001; Naredo E et al., 2005; Qvistgaard E et al., 2006) The anterior longitudinal view as well as the transversal one are fundamental.

The anterior (superior collicular recess) and the supero- anterior recesses are the most important in musculoskeletal ultrasound assessment because of the sensitivity in depicting synovitis. (Backhaus M et al., 2001; Iagnocco A et al., 2006; Qvistgaard E et al., 2001) Femoral neuro- vascular structures are located medial to the joint and easily depicted in transversal view. (Figures 1, 2)

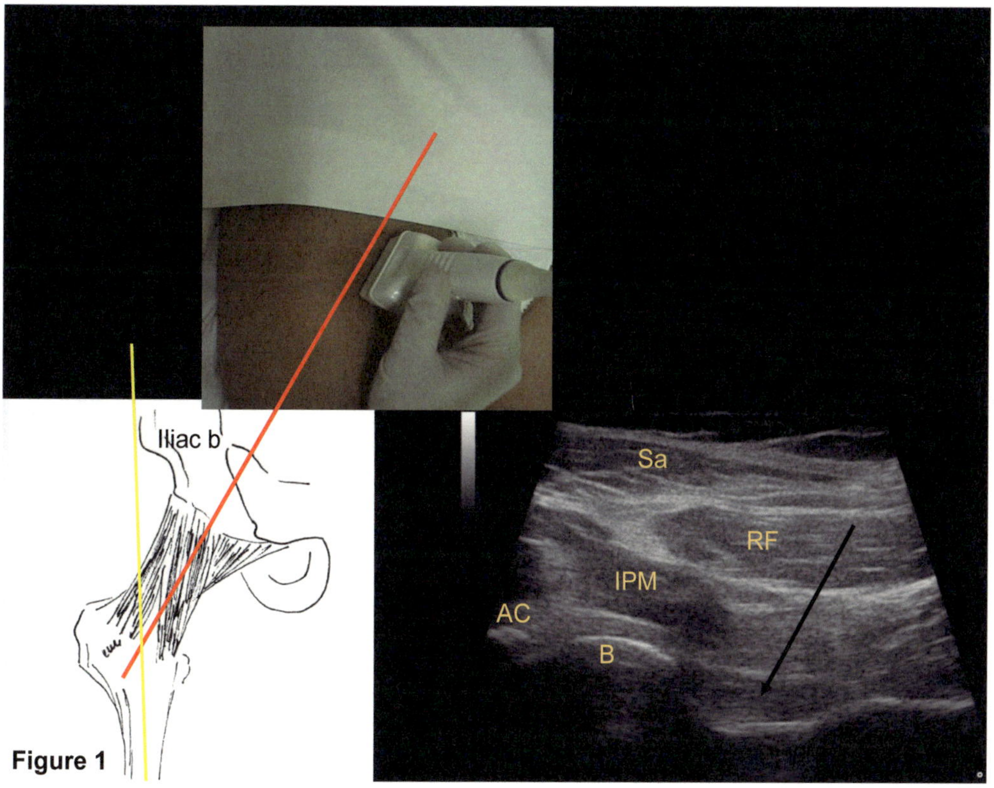

Fig. 1. Anterior longitudinal scanning and view of the hip. Patient photo in scanning position and correct position of the probe; drawing of the hip region showing the probe position parallel to the femoral neck (red line); sonoanatomy of the hip in trapezoidal view- anterior joint recess (black arrow). Legend: B- bone (femoral head), AC- acetabulum, RF- rectus femoris muscle, IPM- ilio-psoas muscle, Sa- sartorius muscle, iliac b- iliac bone.

4. Ultrasound guided hip injection

Generally, two types of US joint injection techniques may be performed: an indirect method (half blind) and a real time procedure which may be further divided in a "hand free" technique and a device guided one.

4.1 Indirect method

The indirect method uses ultrasound for establishing the puncture site, the depth of the target structure but without following the needle penetration. After performing two perpendicular scans, the site of the needle insertion is marked with a skin marking pen and the dept of the target is measured with the ultrasound machine callipers. After the probe removal and proper skin disinfection, the needle is perpendicularly inserted progressing blindly up to the depth previously measured, followed by aspiration and/or drug injection. The blind injection, despite previous imaging location of the target structure, may expose to inaccurate needle positioning. (Cantini F et al., 2005)

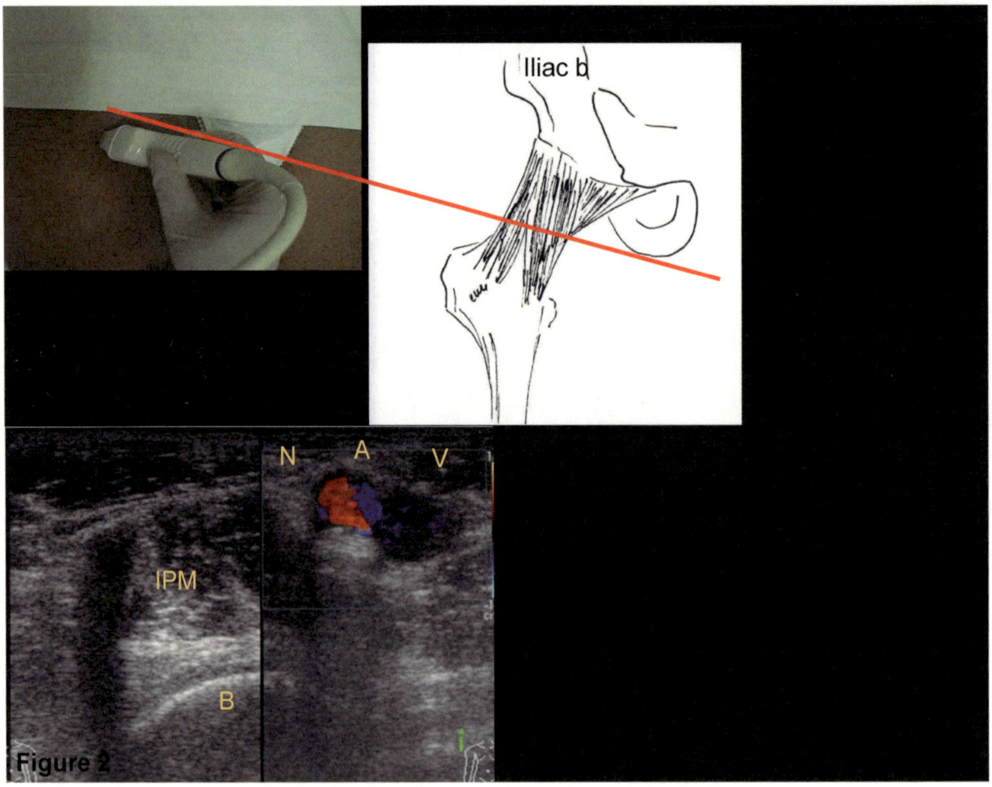

Fig. 2. Anterior transversal scanning and view of the hip. Patient photo and correct position of the probe perpendicular to the femoral neck (red line); drawing of the hip region and sonoanatomy of the hip. Medial to the joint (right side of the ultrasound image), the neurovascular structures can be recognized. Legend: B- bone, IPM- ilio-psoas muscle, N- femoral nerve, A- femoral artery, V- femoral vein, iliac b- iliac bone.

4.2 Real time method

With the real time injection methods, the probe is placed in close proximity of the puncture site and the progression of the needle is followed having direct ultrasound control of the position and depth.

4.2.1 Device guided technique

The device guided technique is used less frequently in clinical practice because of the supplementary cost of the biopsy device and further sterile preparation before each punction manoeuvre. Instead, the penetration of the needle is more precisely and easier to use even for beginners in the field of invasive guided manoeuvres, the insertion of the needle is made always from the lateral side of the probe, in older models. Attachable guiding kits are easier to use and became more popular in the last years. The procedure can be easily performed by a single person , but the method has a certain limitation due to the fixed angle relative to the transducer.

4.2.2 Hand free technique

The "hand free" technique requires more experienced practitioners but is more flexible, allows multiple angle repositioning of the probe and may allow, if necessary, to redirect the needle during the manoeuvre. The site of needle insertion can be placed in fact anywhere in relation with the probe and allows the choice of the most convenient position for the performing doctor. The method is performed usually by two or, more rarely, by a single physician but is burdened by higher learning costs.

5. Approach to the hip joint

Nowadays, two real time musculoskeletal ultrasound guided hip injection approaches are used (Migliore A et al., 2001, 2004). The *longitudinal antero- inferior* approach, suggested mostly for aspiration of synovial fluid and corticosteroid deposition and the *longitudinal antero- superior* approach having the femoral head as target, proposed for viscosupplementation drug deposition.

As a rule, before starting the interventional procedure, an ultrasound evaluation of the hip joint must be repeated in order to reconfirm the diagnostic selection criteria for the invasive manoeuvre and to choose the most appropriate approach. An adequate but also comfortable scanning position is required for the patient as well as for the doctor.

6. Written consent of the patient

The patient must be informed about the injection indication, about potential side effects or complications and must sign a written consent.

7. Antiseptic rules

All punction techniques must fulfil the antiseptic rules. After wearing of sterile gloves, the preparation of the skin above the hip with iodine or clorhexidine gluconate is made. In addition to these requests, a large variation in using supple-mentary antiseptic methods is present among doctors. Some use a sterile condom to isolate the transducer followed by application of sterile gel on the scanning area. The needle insertion is possible through it. Other practitioners prefer nonsterile gel commonly used for musculoskeletal ultrasound evaluations, with application strictly under the probe footprint and needle insertion at a distance of 1-2 cm from the transducer margin through previous disinfected skin surface.

8. Visualisation of the needle

The progression of the needle through different tissue layers (fat tissue, rectus femoris and ilio- psoas muscle, capsule) can be followed if it is kept inside the ultrasound beam, with maximum accuracy if the penetration direction is perpendicular to the ultrasound beam. When linear array probes are used in standard view, the horizontal position of the needle allows a better visualisation of the progression in the tissues but in deep structures, like the hip joint, it is impossible to position the needle horizontal. The use of very long needles has a breaking risk during tissue penetration. Today, new developed steering based imaging techniques obtained by activating consecutive elements in the linear array are now able to generate oblique lines of sights along the dept axis creating the trapezoid shaped image display. In this case, due to the characteristics of the ultrasound beam or by using curvilinear probes, the 45° up to 60° degree angulation of the needle obtains good visualisation of the needle position. In clinical practice, it is proven that the visualisation of the relationship between the needle tip and target structure is more important in comparison to the visualisation of the entire needle body.

For aspiration, spinal-needle gauge 18-20 are used, while for injection only, a 22 gauge needle is sufficient. For better visualisation due to increased reflectivity, some performing physicians scratch the needle surface with a sterile scalpel and keep the mandrin inside while inserting the needle. (Sofka CM et al., 2005)

9. Artifacts

Some artefacts, like anisotropy can occur, creating difficulties in needle visualisation. This artefact may appear when the needle is not strictly perpendicular to the ultrasound beam: in this case, the needle is not visualised as a shiny hyperechoic line but it appears as a hypo-anechoic line. Also the comet tail artefact characteristic for the needle insertion in a fluid collection can be very much attenuated while penetrating a solid structure. Some practitioners activate the Doppler mode while penetrating the skin and underlying layers to follow the needle tip up to the bony cortex. (Hamper UM et al., 1991)

10. Hip injection techniques

10.1 Antero- inferior longitudinal approach

The *antero- inferior longitudinal* approach is designed for hip aspiration of the anterior recess content in inflammatory or septic conditions as well as for corticosteroid injections in cases of synovitis refractory to traditional treatment. (Iagnocco A et al., 2006; Micu MC et al., 2010; Zhang W et al., 2005, 2008)

In our daily practice, the "free hand" technique is used with the following steps: the patient lays in supine position and legs slightly external rotated , the image of the hip is obtained in longitudinal view (probe placed parallel to the femoral neck and lateral to the femoral neuro- vascular structures) and transversal view for the last check. After proper disinfection of the area, the image is obtained in longitudinal view by placing nonsterile gel exactly under the probe footprint, the needle is inserted 2 cm from the distal part of the probe with an angle of 45° degrees to the horizontal skin plane having as target the head neck junction. The needle insertion can be traced from the moment it enters in the ultrasound beam, approximately 1 cm below the skin, through the fat tissue, rectus femoris and ilio-psoas muscle, capsule up to the bone. (Figure 3, 4)

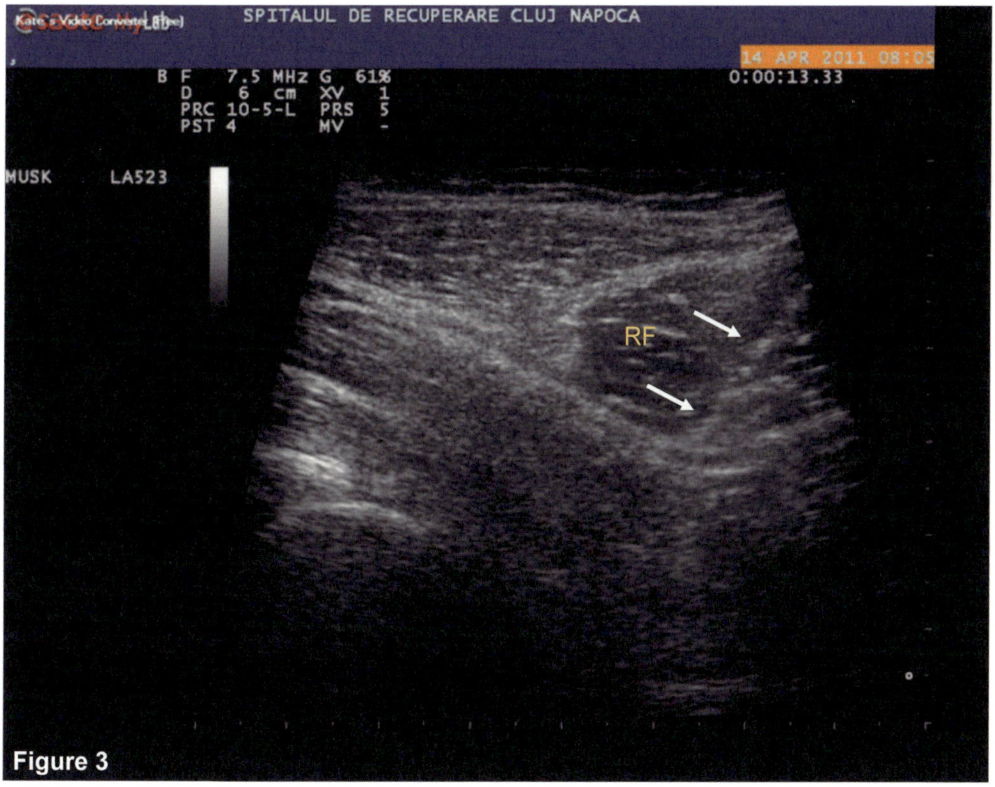

Fig. 3. Anterior longitudinal view of the hip; visualisation of the needle as a hyperechoic line penetrating the rectus femoris muscle (white arrows)

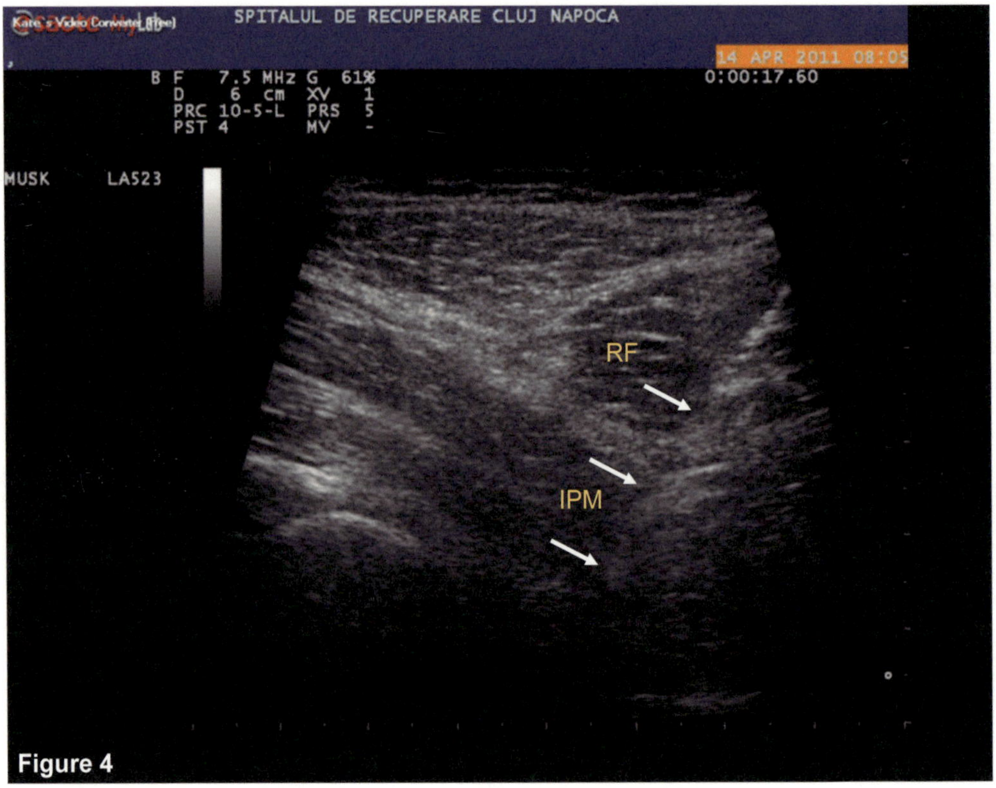

Fig. 4. Anterior longitudinal view of the hip; visualisation of the needle as a hyperechoic line penetrating the rectus femoris and ilio-psoas muscle (white arrows)

After bony cortex contact, the needle is retracted 3-4 mm in order to avoid engaging the tip in the posterior synovial layer and facilitate the tip placement inside the anterior joint recess. In this position, the effusion can be aspirated and/ or corticosteroids can be injected. (Micu MC et al., 2010) (Figures 5, 6, 7)

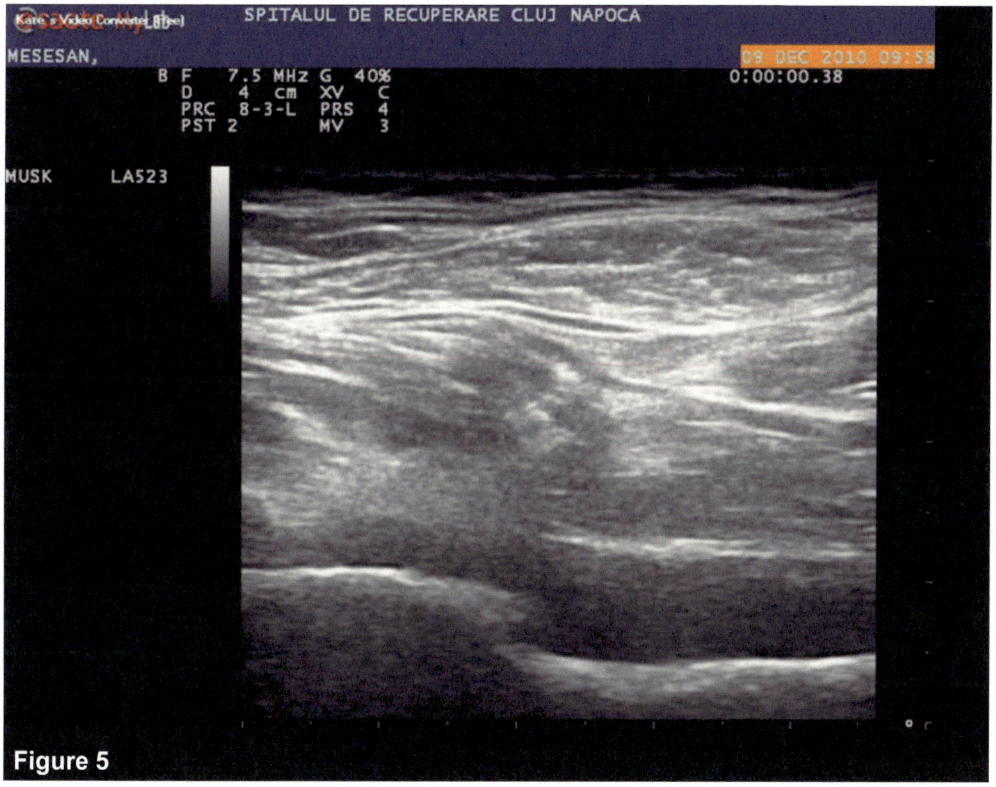

Fig. 5. Anterior longitudinal view of the hip; irregularities of the bony cortex and synovitis with capsule distension can be seen.

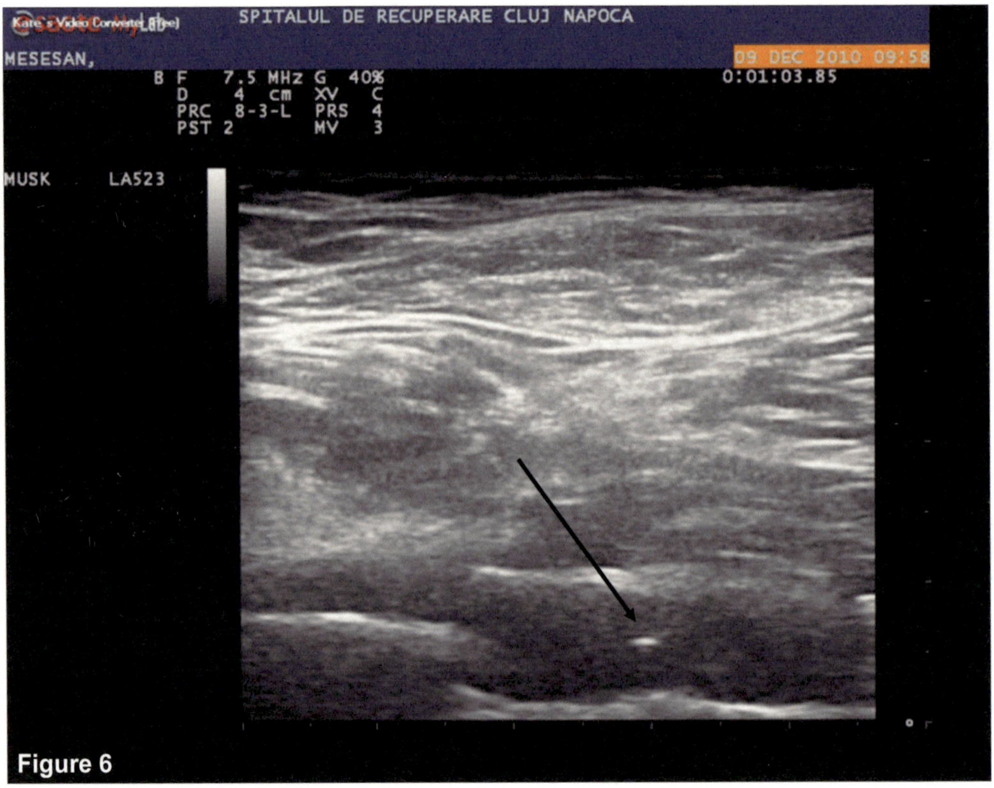

Fig. 6. Anterior longitudinal view of the hip; the needle tip can be identified as a hyperechoic dot inside the anterior recess (black arrow).

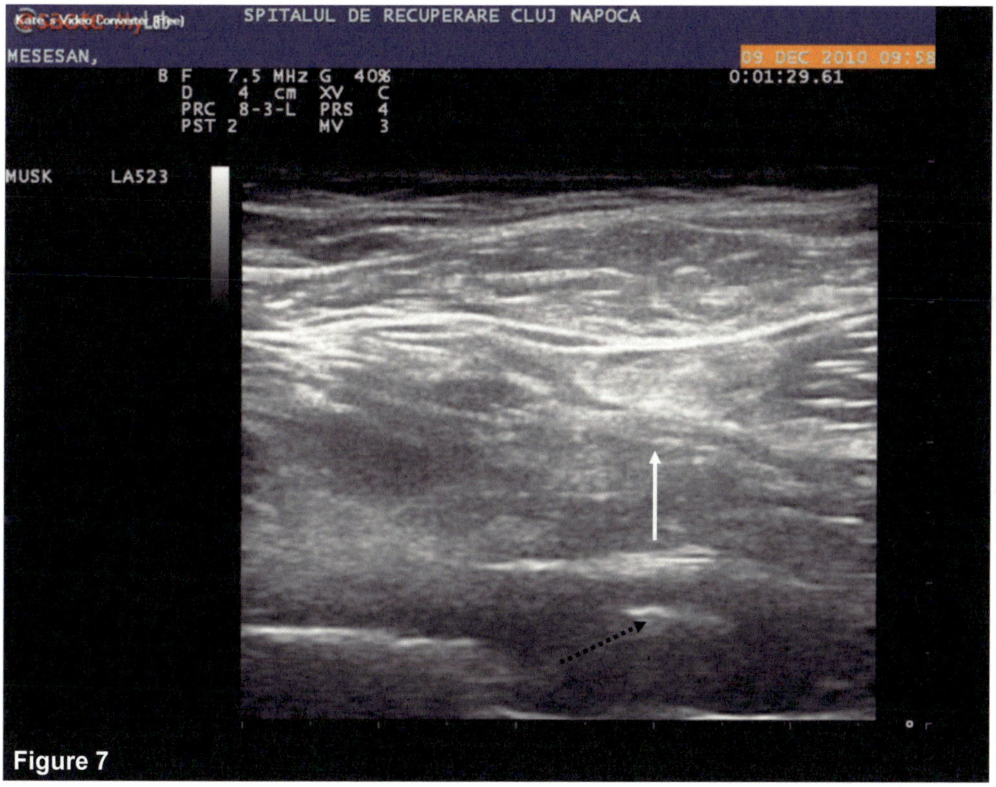

Fig. 7. Anterior longitudinal view of the hip; visualisation of the corticosteroid drug as a hyperechoic mass while being injected (black punctured arrow); distension of the capsule after corticosteroid deposition in direction of the white arrow.

It is extremely important to visualize the progression of the needle through the capsule because sometimes this structure can become very thick after repeated inflammatory episodes, giving the sensation of bony contact inducing subsequent extracapsular drug deposition. A potential advantage of the *antero- inferior longitudinal* approach is the anatomical position of the ilio- femoral ligament with and inverted "Y" shape so that the needle can be inserted between the two ligament branches, in a thinner part of the capsule. This allows a less traumatic perforation.

The aspiration of hip effusions is possible only in some cases, partly explicable due to its gravitational movement inside the recess while laying supine (Iagnocco A et al., 2006; Micu MC et al., 2010). The injection of different corticosteroid products alone or with Lidocaine, with or without a small amount of air, is visualized in real time as a growing hyperechoic mass generated by the injected drug crystals and air bubbles creating the reverberation and ring down artifacts. The detection of the antigravitational movement of the drugs in the supero- anterior recess is also possible. (Figures 8, 9)

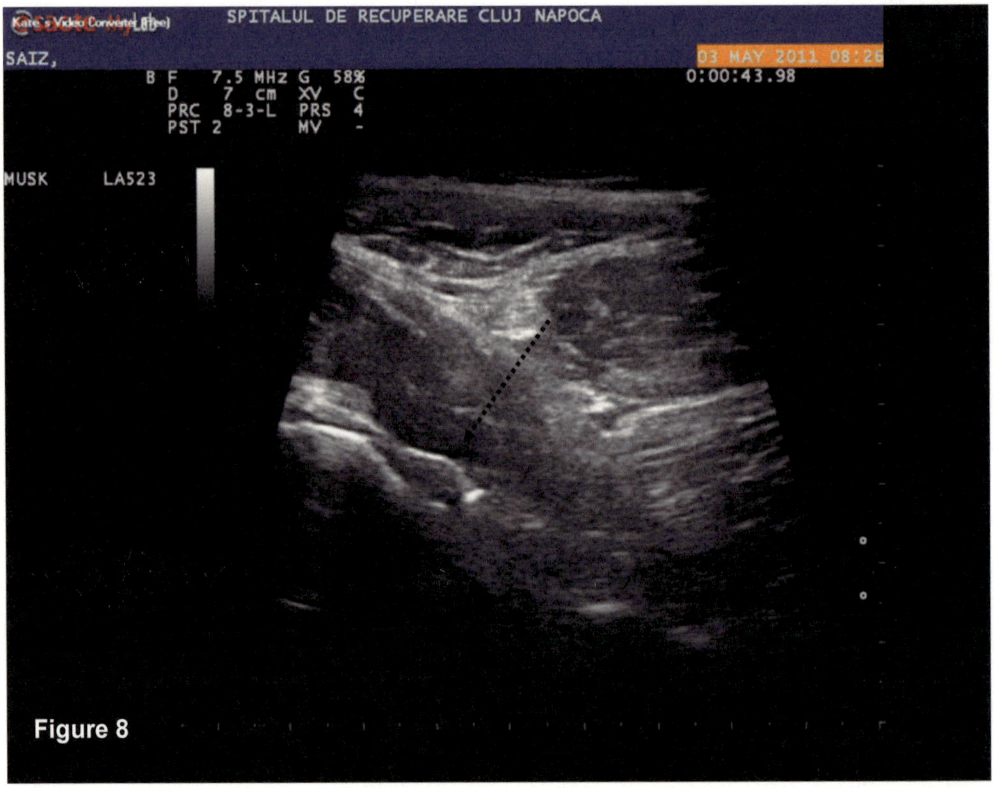

Fig. 8. Anterior longitudinal view of the hip- trapezoidal view; progressive antigravitational movement of the corticosteroid drug after intraarticular deposition (black punctured arrows) at the beginning of the injecting manoeuvre.

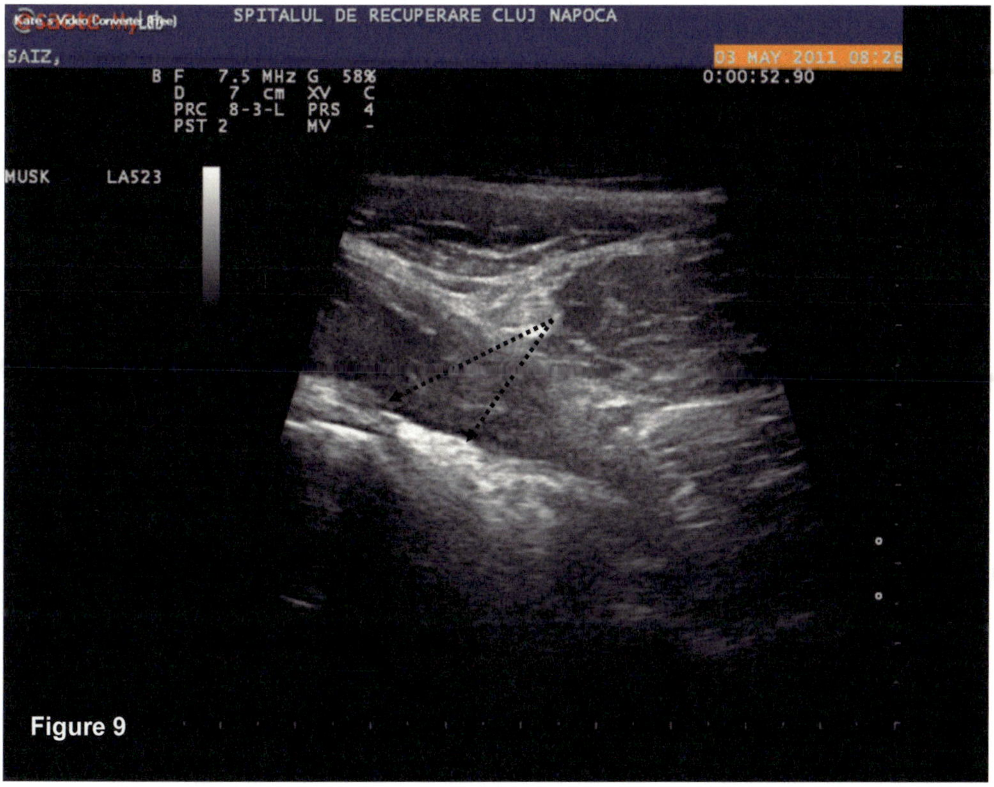

Fig. 9. Anterior longitudinal view of the hip- trapezoidal view; progressive antigravitational movement of the corticosteroid drug after intraarticular deposition generating comet tail artefact and partially blocking the ultrasound beam penetration (black punctured arrows), at the end of the injecting manoeuvre.

Sometimes, hyperechoic traces of CS can be visualized while retracting the needle, indicating the direction of previous needle penetration. Some authors suggest to flush the syringe and needle with lidocaine or saline solution at the end of the injection avoiding the reflux of corticosteroids into the shaft during the retraction of the needle (Bianchi , 2007).

10.2 Antero- superior longitudinal approach

The *antero- superior longitudinal* approach is used mainly for viscosuplementation products injection and allows deposition of the drug as close as possible to the femoral cartilage (Migliore A et al., 2004). It is not known if there is a real benefit of this kind of drug deposition and if the drug remains in the cartilage proximity after the patients regain vertical position. Other authors use also the antero- inferior approach for viscosupplementation drug deposition. (Qvistgaard E et al., 2006) The position of the patient, the scanning technique, and skin preparation procedure follow the same steps as described before and a spinal puncture needle of 22 gauge is inserted usually using a biopsy guiding device. The needle is introduced inside the anterior capsular recess at the level of the femoral head and after femoral head contact, retraction of the needle tip of 1 mm is requested and drug is injected under direct visualisation of the drug in grey scale or Doppler.

11. Patients selection criteria

The physician must be aware of the current selection criteria for diagnostic and therapeutic hip injection. For diagnostic purposes, aspiration of hip synovial fluid is important for differentiating septic arthritis from other inflammatory joint involvement, especially in monoarthritis. Aspiration can be of benefit also due to mechanical decompression and cleaning of the joint recess by pathologic fluid removal.

11.1 Corticosteroid intraarticular hip injection

The selection for corticosteroid hip intraarticular injection is made for patients with symptomatic hip OA, refractory to conventional pain killers, with synovitis and sometimes also for patients with advanced OA with contraindication for total hip replacement. (Kruse DW, 2008)

11.2 Intraarticular hip viscosupplementation

Hip intraarticular viscosupplementation is recommended in patients refractory to other non-invasive-nonsurgical treatment options, not yet candidates for hip replacement, with contraindication for NSAIDs, and refractory to corticosteroids (Migliore A et al., 2010).

11.3 Exclusion criteria

There are important exclusion criteria for hip injection techniques to be considered. Most of the contraindications are temporary and relative, such as suspected or known hip joint infection, joint fracture, anticoagulant therapy to avoid intra/ peri- capsular bleeding, extensive skin pathology in the area of injection, presence of joint prosthesis, uncontrolled high blood pressure and diabetes mellitus, glaucoma, severe congestive heart failure, some severe liver or bone marrow diseases with negative impact on coagulation. Drug(s) allergy may represent an absolute contraindication. Severe hip OA with total absence of radiological joint space contraindicates the use of intraarticular viscosupplementation drugs (Kruse DW, 2008; Migliore A et al., 2010).

12. Efficacy of intraarticular guided injections

Recent trials have demonstrated clear clinical benefit of intraarticular hip injection with corticosteroids and viscosupplementation in hip OA treatment. The imaging techniques currently used for guiding needle insertion are musculoskeletal ultrasound and fluoroscopy, in different protocols, praparates and dosage (Atchia I et al., 2011; Flanagan J et al., 1988; Kullenberg B et al., 2004; 2005; Lambert RGW et al., 2001; Leopold SS et al., 2005; Margules KR , 2001; Migliore A et al., 2004, 2010; Micu MC et al., 2010; Qvistgaard E et al., 2006; Robinson P et al., 2007; Sofka CM et al., 2005).

13. Side effects

As with any other joint injections, various and well known side effects may occur with hip intraarticular joint injection. There are three major concerns for the hip- septic arthritis, osteonecrosis and risk of joint infection after total hip replacement following pre-operative intraarticular corticosteroid injection in a close interval up to the surgical event. In fact, there are just a few cases published in the medical literature reporting the occurrence of local side effects. Intraarticular viscosupplementation drug deposition is well tolerated and without significant systemic side effects. There are by now eight reported cases of intraarticular granulomatosus inflammation developed after a series of three hyaluronic acid injection (Hyalgan GF 20). Intraarticular corticosteroid deposition may have mild systemic effects like transient facial rash, increase of blood pressure or hyperglicemia and local secondary crystalline synovitis which leads to rapid postprocedural local pain. In the literature, there are only two case reports mentioning septic hip involvement following intraarticular corticosteroid injection (Kruse DW, 2008) and four cases of hip aseptic osteonecrosis, but in three of them, corticosteroid deposition was made in another joint. (Kruse DW, 2008; Migliore A et al., 2010) Significant increase in arthroplasty revision secondary to infection in patients who received intraarticular corticosteroid injection prior to surgery is reported in a study performed in 2005 (Kaspar S & de V de Beer j, 2005), but other studies did not confirm any relationship between intraarticular corticosteroid injection prior to total hip arthroplasty. (Chitre AR et al., 2007) As caution, a gap of two months prior to the surgical event is recommended.

14. Post- procedural monitoring

Regardless of the procedure type, aspiration and/ or drug intraarticular injection, the patient must inform the performing physician if any local disturbance or fever occurs within the first 48-72 hours suggesting postprocedural infection. Musculoskeletal ultrasound evaluation for hip joint and periarticular structures can be repeated anytime during follow up without restriction.

15. Conclusions

Ultrasound guided hip injections is ideal for clinical practice because it is rapid, safe and cheap. The method allows precise aspiration even of small amounts of intraarticular fluid and accurate deposition of corticosteroids and viscosupplementation drugs increasing the treatment efficacy. The increasing evidence that musculoskeletal ultrasound is of paramount importance in the rheumatological practice is a further support for its use in guiding the intrarticular injections in order to avoid damage of the structures, misplacing of drugs and help fluid aspiration for diagnostic purposes.

16. References

Aliabadi P, Baker ND & Jaramillo D (1988). Hip arthrography, aspiration, block and bursography. *Radiol Clin North Am* ,Vol. 36, No. 4, (July 1988), pp. 673-690, *ISSN* 0033-8389

Atchia I, Birrell F, and Kane D(2007). A modular, flexible training strategy to achieve competence in diagnostic and interventional musculoskeletal ultrasound in patients with hip osteoarthritis. *Rheumatology* , Vol.46, No. 10, (October 2007), pp. 1583- 6, *ISSN* 1462-0332

Atchia I, Kane D, Reed M, Isaacs JD, Birrell FN et al (2011). Efficacy of a single ultrasound guided injection for the Treatment of Hip Osteoarthritis. *Ann Rheum Dis* , Vol. 70, No. 1, (January 2011), pp.110-116, *ISSN* 1468-2060

Backhaus M, Burmester G, Gerber T, Grassi W, Machold K, Swen W, Wakefield R, Manger B (2001). Guidelines for musculoskeletal ultrasound in rheumatology. *Ann Rheum Dis* , Vol. 60, No. 7, (July 2001), pp. 641–649, *ISSN* 1468-2060

Bianchi , BS. (2007). *Ultrasound of the Musculoskeletal System* , Springer - Verlag Berlin Heidelberg, ISBN 978-3-540-42267-9, Germany

Bierma-Zeinstra SM, Bohnen AM, Verhaar JA, et al (2000). Sonography for hip joint effusion in adults with hip pain. *Ann Rheum Dis* , Vol.59, No. 3, (March 2000), pp.178–82, *ISSN* 1468-2060

Birrell F, Afzal C, Nahit E, et al (2003). Predictors of hip joint replacement in new attenders in primary care with hip pain. *Br J Gen Pract* , Vol. 53, No. 486, (January 2003), pp.26-30, *ISSN* 0960-1643

Bradley MJ (2001). An in-vitro study to understand successful free-hand ultrasound guided intervention. *Clin Radiol* , Vol. 56, No.6, (June 2001), pp. 495-498, *ISSN* 0009 -9260

Brooks PM (2006). The burden of musculoskeletal disease- a global perspective. *Clin Rheumatol* , Vol. 25, No. 6, (November 2006), pp.778-81, *ISSN* 1434-9949

Cantini F, Niccoli L, Nannini C et al. Inflammatory changes of hip synovial structures in polymyalgia rheumatica (2005). *Clin Exp Rheumatol* , Vol. 23, No. 4, (July- August 2005), pp. 462-8, *ISSN* 0392-856X

Chitre AR, Fehily MJ, Bamford DJ (2007). Total hip replacement after intra-articular injection of local anaesthetic and steroid. *J Bone Joint Surg Br* , Vol.89-B, No.2, (February 2007), pp.166-8, *ISSN* 0301-620X

Flanagan J, Casale FF, Thomas TL, Desai KN (1988). Intra-articular injection for pain relief in patients awaiting hip replacement. *Ann R Coll Surg Engl* , Vol.70, No. 3, (May 1988), pp.156–7, *ISSN* 0035-8843

Foldes K, Balint P, Balint G, Buchanan WW (1995). Ultrasound guided aspiration in suspect sepsis of resection arthroplasty of the hip joint. *Clin Rheumatol* , Vol.14, No. 3, (May 1995), pp.327–9, *ISSN* 1434-9949

Hamper UM, Savader BL, Sheth S (1991). Improved needle-tip visualisation by color Doppler sonography. *Am J Roentgenol* , Vol. 156, No. 2, (February 1991), pp. 401-402, *ISSN*:1546-3141

Iagnocco A, Filippucci E, Meenagh G, et al (2006). Ultrasound imaging for the rheumatologist III. Ultrasonography of the hip. *Clin Exp Rheumatol* , Vol. 24, No. 3, (May- June 2006), pp.229–32, *ISSN* 0392-856X

Iagnocco A and Naredo E (2010).Ultrasound- guided corticosteroid injection in rheumatology: accuracy or efficacy? *Rheumatology*, Vol. 49, No.8, (March 2010), pp. 1427-28, *ISSN* 1462-0332

Kaspar S, de V de Beer j (2005). Infection of hip arthroplasty in previous injection of steroid. *J Bone Joint Surg Br* , Vol. 87-B, No.4, (Apryl 2005), pp. 454-7, *ISSN* 0301-620X

Komppa GH, Northern JR Sr, Haas DK, Lisecki E, Ghaed N (1985). Ultrasound guidance for needle aspiration of the hip in patients with painful hip prosthesis. *J Clin Ultrasound* , Vol. 13, No. 6, (July- August 1985), pp.433-4, *ISSN* 1097-0096

Koski JM, Anttila PJ, Isomaki HA (1989). Ultrasonography of the adult hip joint. *Scand J Rheumatol* , Vol. 18, No.2, (February 1989), pp.113–7, *ISSN* 0300-9742

Kruse DW (2008). Intraarticular cortisone injection for osteoarthritis of the hip. Is it effective? Is it safe? *Curr Rev Musculoskeletal Med* , Vol.1, No.12, (December 2008), pp. 227-233, ISSN 1935-973X

Kullenberg B, Runesson R, Tuvhag R, Olsson C, Resch S (2004). Intraarticular corticosteroid injection: pain relief in osteoarthritis of the hip? *J Rheumatol* , Vol.31, No. 11, (November 2004), pp.2265–8, *ISSN* 0263-7103

Lambert RGW, Hutchings EJ, Grace MGA, Jhangri GS (2007). Conner Spady B, Maksymowich WP. Steroid Injection for osteoarthritis of the hip: a randomized, double-blind, placebo-controlled trial. *Arthritis Rheum* , Vol. 56, No. 7, (July 2007), pp.2278–87, *ISSN* 1529-0131

Leopold SS, Battista V, Oliverio JA (2001). Safety and efficacy of intraarticular hip injection using anatomical landmarks. *Clin Orthop* ; 391: 192-7, ISSN 0009-921X

Margules KR (2001). Fluoroscopically directed steroid instillation in the treatment of hip osteoarthritis: safety and efficacy in 510 cases. *Arthritis Rheum* , Vol.44, No. 10, (October 2001), pp.2449–50, *ISSN* 1529-0131

Micu MC, Bogdan G, Fodor D (2010). Steroid injection for hip osteoarthritis: efficacy under ultrasound guidance. *Rheumatology,* Vol. 49, No. 8, (March 2010), pp. 1940-4, *ISSN*:1462-0332

Migliore A, Kristoffersen H, Terslev L, Danneskiold-Samsøe B, Torp-Pedersen S, Bliddal H (2001). Guidance by ultrasound of intra-articular injections in the knee and hip joints. *Osteoarthr Cartil* , Vol.9, No. 4, (Apryl 2001), pp.512–7, *ISSN* 1063-4584

Migliore A, Tormenta S, Martin Martin LS, et al (2004). Safety profile of 185 ultrasound guided intra- articular injections for treatment of rheumatic diseases in the hip. *Reumatismo* , Vol. 56, No. 4, (Apryl- June, 2004), pp. 104-109, *ISSN* 0048-7449

Migliore A, Giovannangeli F, Granata M and Lagana B (2010). Hyalgan G-F 20: Review of its Safety and Efficacy in the Management of Joint Pain in Osteoarthritis. *Clinical Medical Insights: Arthritis and Musculoskeletal Disorders* , Vol.3, No. 12, (December 2010), pp. 55-68, *ISSN*: 1179-5441

Naredo E, Cabero F, Cruz A, et al (2005). Ultrasound guided musculoskeletal injections. *Ann Rheum Dis* , Vol.64, No. 2, (February 2005), pp.341-344, *ISSN* 1468-2060

Ozonoff MB (1973). Controlled arthrography of the hip: A technique of fluoroscopic monitoring and recording. *Clin Ortop Relat res* , Vol.93, (1973), pp.260-264, *ISSN* 1413-7852

Picano E, Matucci-Cerinic M (2010). Unnecessary radiation exposure from medical imaging in the rheumatology patient. *Rheumatology,* on line 22 Dec, doi:10.1093/rheumatology/keq412, *ISSN* 1462-0332

Qvistgaard E, Christensen R, Torp- Pedersen S, et al (2006). Intra- articular treatment of hip osteoarthritis : a randomized trial of hyaluronic acid, corticosteroid and isotonic saline. *Osteoarthr Cartilage* , Vol.14, No. 2, (February 2006), pp. 163-70, *ISSN 1063-4584*

Qvistgaard E, Kristoffersen H, Terslev L, Danneskiold-Samsøe B, Torp-Pedersen S, Bliddal H (2001). Guidance by ultrasound of intra-articular injections in the knee and hip joints. *Osteoarthr Cartilage,* Vol.9, No. 6, (August 2001), pp.512–7, *ISSN* 1063-4584.

Richette P, Ravaud P, Conrozier T, et al (2009). Effect of hyaluronic acid in symptomatic hip osteoarthritis : a multicenter, randomized, placebo- controlled trial. *Arthritis Rheum* , Vol. 60, No 3, (March 2009), pp. 824-30, *ISSN* 1529-0131

Robinson P, Keenan AM, Conaghan G (2007). Clinical effectiveness and dose response of image-guided intra-articular corticosteroid injection for hip osteoarthritis. *Rheumatology* , Vol. 46, No. 2, (February 2007), pp.285–91, *ISSN* 1462-0332

Sofka CM, Saboeiro G & Adler RS (2005). Ultrasound-guided adult hip injections. *J Vasc Interv Radiol* , Vol. 16, No 8, (August 2005),pp. 1121–3, ISSN 1051-0443

Wakefield RJ, Balint PV, Szkudlarek M, et al (2005). OMERACT 7 Special Interest Group. Musculoskeletal ultrasound including definitions for ultrasonographic pathology. *J Rheumatol* , Vol. 32, No. 12, (December 2005), pp.2485-7, *ISSN*: 0263-7103

Zhang W, Doherty M, Arden N, et al (2005). EULAR evidence based recommendations for the management of hip osteoarthritis: report of a task force of EULAR standing committee for International Clinical Studies Including Therapeutics (ESCISTS). *Ann Rheum Dis* , Vol. 64, No.5, (May 2005), pp. 669-681, *ISSN* 1468-2060

Zhang W, Moskowitz RRW, Nuki G, et al (2008). OARSI recommendations for the management of hip and knee osteoarthritis. Part II: OARSI evidence - based, expert consensus guidelines. *Osteoarthr Cartilage,* Vol..16,No.12, (December 2008), pp.137-62, *ISSN 1063-4584*

20

Hyaluronate for the Treatment of Ankle Osteoarthritis

Shu-Fen Sun[1,2], Chien-Wei Hsu[1,2],
Yi-Jiun Chou[1], Yu-Nong Wang[1] and Mei-Chia Chou[1]
[1]*Kaohsiung Veterans General Hospital,*
[2]*National Yang-Ming University School of Medicine,*
Taiwan

1. Introduction

Ankle osteoarthritis (OA) is a degenerative joint disease that can cause substantial pain, muscle weakness and functional limitations. Due chiefly to its post-traumatic origin and appearance in young patients, ankle OA has a high impact on socioeconomics and patients' quality of life. Approximately 6% to 13% of all cases of OA involve the ankle joint (Thomas and Daniels, 2003). Recent research also identify that a larger number of patients are being diagnosed with ankle OA (Saltzman et al, 2005). Currently, no curative therapy is available for OA, and thus the overall goals of management are to reduce pain and prevent disability. Treatment options include simple analgesics, nonsteroidal anti-inflammatory drugs (NSAIDs), weight reduction, physical and occupational therapy, activity modification, orthotic devices, shoe modifications, intraarticular corticosteroid injections, and surgery. Although some cases can be treated successfully with surgery, many patients are either not good candidates for surgery or may want to avoid or delay it if possible. There is a need for a treatment that reduces chronic joint pain and improves function yet avoids toxic effects of medications and the morbidity and mortality risks of surgery. One such option for these patients may be the intraarticular injection of hyaluronate.

Hyaluronate, a high molecular weight polysaccharide, is a principal component of synovial fluid and extracellular matrix of articular cartilage. It contributes to the elasticity and viscosity of synovial fluid. In addition to providing joint lubrication and shock absorbancy, hyaluronate helps to maintain the structural and functional characteristics of the cartilage matrix. It also inhibits the formation and release of prostaglandins, induces proteoglycan aggregation and synthesis, and modulates the inflammatory response (Frizziero, 1998). In OA, the concentration and molecular weight of hyaluronate are reduced, limiting its role in maintaining normal joint biomechanics (Engström-Laurent A, 1997). Viscosupplementation with intraarticular injections of hyaluronate was approved by the Food and Drug Administration (FDA) in 1997 for treating pain associated with knee OA. Although the exact mechanism of action is not understood with certainty, recent research suggests that it exerts anti-inflammatory, analgesic, anabolic and possibly chondroprotective effects on the articular cartilage and joint synovium that reduce pain and disability and improve joint function.

There are five injectable forms of hyaluronate approved for use in the United States, including Hyalgan, Supartz, Orthovisc, Synvisc and Euflexxa (Table 1). Each of these hyaluronate products differ in their origin, method of production, molecular weight, dosing instructions, rheologic properties, cost, pharmacodynamics and possibly clinical outcomes.

Trade name	Hylagan	Synvisc	Supartz	Orthovisc	Euflexxa
generic name	sodium hyaluronate	hylan G-F20	sodium hyaluronate	high molecular weight hyaluronan	sodium hyaluronate
Year Approved	1997	1997	2001	2004	2004
Source	Rooster combs (naturally derived)	Rooster combs (chemically modified, or cross-linked)	Rooster combs (naturally derived)	Rooster combs (naturally derived)	Bacterial fermentation (naturally derived)
Molecular Weight (kd)	500-730	6000	620-1170	1000-2900	2400-3600
Amount per injection	2 ml	2 ml	2.5 ml	2 ml	2 ml
Active ingredients per injection	20mg sodium hyaluronate	16mg sodium hyaluronate derivative	25mg sodium hyaluronate	30mg sodium hyaluronate	20mg sodium hyaluronate
Number of injections per cycle	3 or 5 weekly	3 weekly (In 2009, FDA approved single-dose Synvisc-One™ 6 mL injection for the treatment of knee OA)	5 weekly	3 or 4 weekly	3 weekly

Table 1. Characteristics of five formulations of intraarticular Hyaluronans available in the United States

All products are manufactured from rooster combs except for Euflexxa, which is the only non-avian derived hyaluronan approved in the United States. Also, Synvisc undergoes additional chemical crosslinking to create hylans with increased molecular weight and increased elastoviscous properties. The differing molecular weights of the products lead to different half-lives; the half-life of Hyalgan or Supartz is estimated at 24 hours, while the half-life of Synvisc may range up to several days. There is no consistent evidence from well-controlled clinical studies that documents the superior efficacy of one product over another.

Although viscosupplementation is a well-established treatment option in knee OA and is included in the professional guidelines by European League of Arthritis & Rheumatism (EULAR) and American College of Rheumatology (ACR), evidence regarding its use in ankle OA is limited. Recently, several studies attempting to evaluate the use of hyaluronate in the ankle have been published. In this chapter, we discuss our experiences, the indications, injection technique and review the clinical outcomes on hyaluronate use in patients with ankle OA. Additionally, future directions for the use of hyaluronate in the management of ankle OA and areas of active research in hyaluronate are discussed.

2. Indications

The exact indications for viscosupplementation are still evolving, but it currently can be considered for use in patients who have significant residual symptoms despite traditional nonpharmacologic and pharmacologic treatments. In addition, patients who have gastrointestinal or renal intolerance to NSAIDs, and those who wish to postpone surgical intervention or are poor candidates for surgery can be considered for these injections.

Contraindications to hyaluronate injection include protein/avian allergy (except Euflexxa), active skin disease and joint infections at the injection site. Patients with substantial venous or lymphatic stasis in the legs, bleeding disorder or treatment with anticoagulants are relatively contraindicated. Hyaluronate is not recommended to pregnant women, lactating women and children under 18, because the safety and effectiveness have not been established.

The ideal candidate for viscosupplementation has yet to be defined. Studies are inconclusive regarding the best responders with respect to age, level of OA as defined radiographically, level of symptoms and level of physical activity. We previously reported (Sun et al, 2006a) that patients with Kellgren-Lawrence grade 1and 2 ankle OA had good response to viscosupplementation (grade 1, doubtful narrowing of joint space and possible osteophytic lipping; grade 2, definite osteophytes and possible narrowing of joint space). This suggested that viscosupplementation was effective in mild to moderate ankle OA. Whether severe cases would likely respond to viscosupplementation remained unknown. In another case series by our study group (Sun et al, 2011), we stratified patients by age and radiographic severity to determine whether these factors would influence the treatment response. Subgroup analysis results showed that there was no significant difference in outcomes between patients with grade 2 and grade 3 OA in each study period. However, we found difference in clinical balance tests between patients of the younger age-group and the older age-group at different time points. As the subgroup analysis was not sufficiently powered, definite conclusion could not be drawn.

As the treatment group increases, the ideal subgroup of patients who are best candidates for ankle viscosupplementation should be identified.

3. Injection technique

In our experience, intraarticular injection of the ankle joint is easy to perform and requires no radiologic guidance. The two approaches for performing an ankle joint injection are the anterior medial and anterior lateral (Figure 1). For the anterior medial approach, we position the patient in the supine position, with the knee flexed and the foot flat on the examination table. The ankle is placed in a degree of plantarflexion, which opens the anterior aspect of the joint. We identify the space between the anterior border of the medial malleolus and the medial border of the tibialis anterior tendon and palpate this space for the articulation of the talus and tibia to locate a suitable entry point into the ankle joint. The injections are performed in aseptic conditions. We insert a 21-23 gauge needle into the identified space and direct posterolaterally to run parallel to the upper surface of the talus, which is slightly convex . Joint effusion, if present, should be aspirated before injection. Alternatively, the

anterior lateral approach is done with the patient positioned with the foot in plantar flexion. The needle is inserted from the anterior lateral position and directed posteriorly toward the medial malleolus. The needle is advanced until there is a drop in tissue resistance confirming entry into the joint. Excessive weight bearing and strenuous activity are discouraged within 2 days following injection. Otherwise, no specific post-injection instructions are necessary.
Most injection in the ankle joint was performed without any instrumental guide in the literature. One of the limitations of hyaluronate therapy is that it can be difficult to ensure that intraarticular injections are actually given into the joint capsule. In clinical trials with ankle viscosupplementation, only one trial used a fluoroscopic guide for the injection (Cohen et al, 2008). Ultrasound has been used to guide hyaluronate injection in hip and hand OA, however, no ultrasound guide has been used in ankle OA studies. The aim for the future is to encourage the ultrasound-guided intraarticular injection because it is simple, fast, economic and safe; it does not require the use of contrast, allowing the intraarticular injection in patients intolerant to iodized contrasts. It can be repeated without limits, allows an easy visualization of fluid in the articular recess, the correct position of the needle and the distance from the vessels.

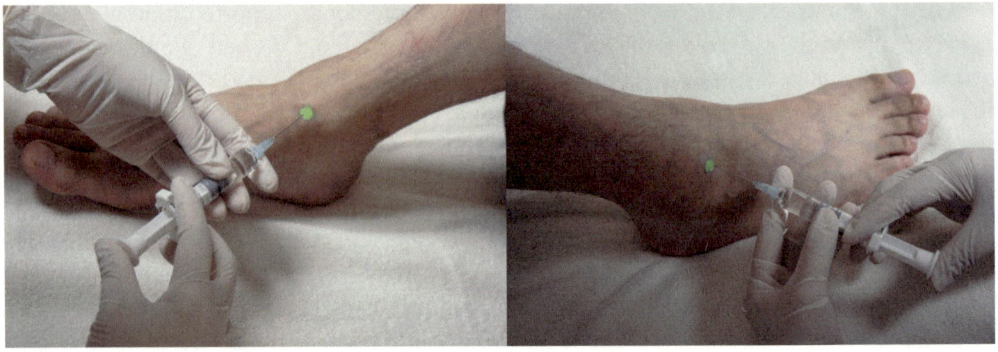

Fig. 1. The two approaches for ankle joint injection: the anterior medial and anterior lateral approaches

4. Overview of clinical outcomes

The potential for treating ankle OA by viscosupplementation has been suggested in the literature. To date, there are only 3 randomized controlled, double-blind trials (Salt et al, 2006; Cohen et al , 2008; Karatosun et al, 2008) (Table 2) and a few case series in the search of the literature on viscosupplementation therapy for ankle OA (Table 3). Two recent reviews (Migliore et al, 2011; Sun et al, 2009) have provided an overview of clinical trials with hyaluronate therapy in ankle OA.
Salk et al. performed the first randomized, double-blind, saline solution-controlled trial in patients with grade 2, 3 and 4 (Kellgren–Lawrence) ankle OA (Salk et al, 2006), assessing the efficacy and safety of hyaluronate for the treatment of ankle OA. Patients were randomized to receive 5 weekly intraarticular injections of either 1 mL of sodium hyaluronate (10 mg/mL) or 1 mL of phosphate-buffered saline solution into the ankle joint. The primary outcome measure was the ankle osteoarthritis score (AOS) pain and disability assessment (Domsic and Saltzman, 1998). At 6-month follow-up, trends toward greater improvement in

the hyaluronate group compared with sham injection control were noted. The benefit with hyaluronate in the treatment of ankle OA is consistent with previous published studies using hyaluronate in the knee.

Author Year	Viscosupplement	Study Patients	Outcome Measures	Outcomes
Salk et al (2006)	Hyalgan (5 injections), 1ml per injection	17 9 HA 8 placebo	AOS, WOMAC pain domain, Ankle ROM, Quality of life, Rescue analgesic consumption	Safe and effective at 6 months in patients with Kellgren-Lawrence grade 2-4 ankle OA
Cohen MM et al (2008)	Hyalgan (5 injections), 2ml per injection	30 15 HA 15 placebo (saline control)	AOS, WOMAC, Patient global assessment, SF-12 (short form-12)	Safe and effective for 3 months
Karatosun et al (2008)	Adant (3 injections), 2.5 ml per injection	30 15 HA 15 progressive ankle exercise	AOFAS ankle/hindfoot score, Gait quality, VAS	No statistical difference between the exercise and HA injection groups in patients with Kellgren-Lawrence grade 3 ankle OA at 12 months.

Abbreviations in the table:
HA=hyaluronic acid
AOS= ankle osteoarthritis score
AOFAS= American Orthopaedic Foot and Ankle Society
VAS= visual analog scale
WOMAC= Western Ontario and McMaster Universities Arthritis Index

Table 2. Randomized controlled trials of Viscosupplementation in the Treatment of Ankle Osteoarthritis

Author Year	Viscosupplement	Study Patients	Outcome Measures	Outcomes
Sun et al (2006)	Artz (5 injections), 2.5 ml per injection	75 75 HA N0 placebo	AOS, AOFAS ankle/hindfoot score, Ankle ROM, Patients' global satisfaction, Rescue analgesics consumption	Safe and efficacious, effects rapid at 1 week post the fifth injection, lasting for 6 months in patients with Kellgren-Lawrence grade 1 or 2 ankle OA. High patients' satisfaction rate. Significant reduction in analgesics consumption
Witteveen AGH et al (2008)	Sinvisc (1 injections), 2 ml per injection	51 one injection 24 2nd injection after 1-3 months	VAS, AOS, SF-36	Safe and effective for 6 months in patients with grade 2 ankle OA (van Dijk et al scale).
Carpenter et al (2008)	Sinvisc (3 injections), 2 ml per injection	26 14 HA post ankle arthroscopy 12 ankle arthroscopy	VAS	The mean pain score of the HA+arthroscopy group was 1, the score for the arthroscopy alone group was 3 on a 10 point VAS scale in patients with Kellgren-Lawrence grade 2-4 ankle OA at 3 months, with significant difference.
Luciani et al (2008)	Sinvisc (3 injections), 2 ml per injection	21 21 HA N0 placebo	AOS	Significant improvement in AOS from baseline in patients with Kellgren-Lawrence grade 2 ankle OA after 6 months, effect maintained at 12 and 18-month follow-ups
Mei-Dan et al. (2010)	Adant (5 injections) 2.5 ml per injection	13 13 HA N0 placebo	VAS, AOFAS ankle/hindfoot score, Ankle ROM	Improvement of 20% in the ROM, significant reduction in VAS scale and ankle-hindfoot scores in patients with Kellgren-Lawrence grade 2-4 ankle OA for 7 months

Author Year	Viscosupplement	Study Patients	Outcome Measures	Outcomes
Sun et al (2011)	Hyalgan (3 injections), 2 ml per injection	46 46 HA N0 placebo	AOS, AOFAS ankle/hindfoot score, Ankle ROM, 4 balance tests, Patients' global satisfaction, Rescue analgesic consumption	Safe and effective, improve physical function and balance with high patients' satisfaction in patients with unilateral Kellgren-Lawrence grade 2 or 3 ankle OA.

Abbreviations in the table:
HA=hyaluronic acid
AOS= ankle osteoarthritis score
AOFAS= American Orthopaedic Foot and Ankle Society
ROM=range of motion
VAS= visual analog scale

Table 3. Case Series of Viscosupplementation in the Treatment of Ankle Osteoarthritis

Cohen et al. performed a randomized, double blind, saline solution-controlled trial of patients with grade 2, 3 and 4 (Kellgren–Lawrence) ankle OA (Cohen et al, 2008). Patients were randomized to receive 5 weekly injections of either 2 mL of sodium hyaluronate (Hyalgan) or 2 mL of phosphate-buffered saline solution in the ankle joint. All injections were fluoroscopically guided. The primary endpoint was pain on movement and weight bearing using the AOS 3 months after injection. At month 3, the patients in the hyaluronate group showed a significant improvement from baseline in AOS total score than those in the control group.

Karatosun et al. performed a prospective randomized trial with 12-months follow-up, to evaluate the efficacy of intraarticular injection of sodium hyaluronate (Adant®) compared with exercise therapy (Karatosun et al, 2008). Patients with grade 3 (Kellgren–Laurence) ankle OA were randomized to receive 3 weekly intraarticular injections of hyaluronate or an exercise cycle therapy, which included a series of progressive, isometric, isotonic range of motion, resistance, closed kinetic chain and proprioceptive exercise, for 6 weeks. Outcomes, including the American Orthopaedic Foot and Ankle Society (AOFAS) Ankle-Hind Foot score(Kitaoka et al,1994), gait, pain with VAS scale were evaluated and analyzed. At 12 months, both groups improve in pain score, walking surface, gait quality and total ankle-hind foot score. The authors concluded that the patients benefit either by 3 injection of hyaluronate or by 6 weeks of exercise therapy. The advantage of exercise therapy may be its non-invasive nature being preferred by both the physicians and the patients; however, while exercise therapy last 6 weeks, hyaluronate injections stop at 3 weeks. This point may be an advantage for the preference of hyaluronate injections.

In a relatively large case series by our group (Sun et al, 2006a), we reported outcomes of 75 patients with unilateral grade 1 or 2 (Kellgren–Lawrence) ankle OA. We concluded similarly that a regimen of 5 weekly intraarticular injection of sodium hyaluronate was safe and effective in the areas of pain and ankle function. Patients expressed a high level of satisfaction, with only relatively few local adverse events. These effects were rapid at 1 week post the fifth injection and could last for 6 months. One limitation in this trial includes the absence of a control group, thus the placebo effects associated with joint injections per se were not analyzed.

In the prospective case series by Witteveen et al, patients with symptomatic grade 2 (van Dijk et al scale) ankle OA (>50 and <90 mm on a 100 mm visual analog scale (VAS), were treated with intraarticular injection of Hylan GF-20 (Synvisc, 2 mL) plus an optional second injection if pain remained at baseline level after 1, 2 or 3 months, with 6–9-months follow-up period (Witteveen et al, 2008). The primary efficacy endpoint was the change from baseline in the Pain VAS Score at 3 months. The results showed a statistically significant decrease in the mean Pain VAS score from 68.0 mm at baseline to 33.8 mm at month 3. They reported that a regimen of one single intraarticular injection of hyaluronate (Synvisc), with the option of a second injection after 1–3 months if pain relief is inadequate, is an efficacious treatment of patients with symptomatic ankle OA.

Carpenter et al. conducted a controlled trial investigating the effectiveness of Hylan G-F 20 in reducing pain following ankle arthroscopy in patients with grade 2, 3 and 4 (Kellgren–Laurence) ankle OA (Carpenter and Motley, 2008). Fourteen patients received 3 weekly injections of Hylan G-F 20 post ankle arthroscopy, while 12 patients received only ankle arthroscopy. At 3 months, the mean pain score of the Hylan G-F 20 plus arthroscopy group was 1, while the score for the arthroscopy alone group was 3 on a 10 point VAS scale, and this difference was statistically significant.

In a case series by Luciani et al, 21 patients with a grade 2 (Kellgren–Laurence) ankle OA had 3 weekly intraarticular injections of 2 ml of synvisc into the ankle joint (Luciani et al, 2008). The primary clinical outcome measurement was the AOS. The results showed significant improvement of the AOS from baseline after 6 months and this improvement was maintained at 12- and 18-month follow-ups.

Mei-Dan et al. have studied 16 patients with grade 2-4 (Kellgren-Lawrence) ankle OA who received intraarticular injections of 25mg of sodium hyaluronate for 5 consecutive weeks (Mei-Dan et al, 2010). There was a significant reduction in pain assessed by VAS scale and ankle-hindfoot scores and an improvement of 20% in the range of motion.

Previous ankle viscosupplementation studies reported that five weekly intraarticular injections of hyaluronate were safe and effective; however, the effect of three weekly injections has rarely been investigated. Our study group (Sun et al, 2011) conducted another prospective case series with a 6-month follow-up period and reported that three weekly injections of sodium hyaluronate are well tolerated, can provide pain relief, improve function and balance in patients with unilateral grade 2 or 3 (Kellgren–Lawrence) ankle OA. OA remains by far the most common disease of joints and represents a huge burden to society in terms of personal suffering and health resource utilization. The three-injection regimen may possibly represent a cost-saving therapy. Besides, pain associated with ankle OA may cause loss of balance, leading to falls, more injuries and higher costs to the patient and society. This study was the first that examined the effect of hyaluronate on balance in patients with ankle OA, as we had previously reported significant improvements in pain, physical function and balance tests after five weekly hyaluronate injections in geriatric patients with knee OA (Sun et al,2006b). Although the mechanism by which hyaluronate results in a clinical benefit in balance remains unknown and it remain an area important for future research, we thought pain reduction might be one of the major contributing factor.

5. Complications

Because use of hyaluronate in the ankle is an "off label" application of this agent, patient safety is a key issue considering this treatment. Clinical studies have demonstrated that viscosupplementation is generally safe and well tolerated. Although significant complications are rare, mild adverse effects have been reported. Because there are no known hyaluronate-medication interactions, it is a good option for patients on multiple medications, particularly the elderly. Mild injection-site pain and swelling are the most common adverse events in the injected joints. These reactions are usually transient, resolving without intervention within 1 to 3 days. Other adverse events included rash, muscle cramps, dizziness, nausea, headache, local ecchymosis and pruritus. The overall incidence of adverse reactions in knee studies has been reported to be approximately 1% to 4%. Rare cases of post-injection pseudogout with sodium hyaluronate and Synvisc have been reported. It is unclear whether these reactions were caused by the hyaluronate itself or by the injection procedure. There is growing evidence that Synvisc may be associated with an adverse event termed pseudosepsis or a severe acute inflammatory reaction. Pseudosepsis presents as severe inflammation of the joint, with a large effusion, and significant pain occurring within 1 to 3 days post injection. It requires symptomatic treatment, including use of modalities, activity modification, analgesics, and NSAIDs. Once infection has been excluded, intraarticular steroids may be of value. Despite a lack of understanding of both the etiology of pseudosepsis and the long-term effects of these local immunological reactions, such events would be expected to incur additional socioeconomic costs. Additional study is required to enable the treating physician to identify patients at risk for this injection related complication and to determine whether patients with a history of a pseudosepsis after hyaluronate injection can safely receive further hyaluronate therapy.

The safety in the treatment of ankle OA appears to be similar to the injections widely performed in the treatment of knee OA. No systemic adverse events were reported in the literature relating to ankle viscosupplementation; however, cases of local adverse reactions do exist. In study by Salt et al (Salk et al, 2006), injection site pain was noted in 5 (29%) of the 17 patients, with no significant difference between the groups. In our case series (Sun et al, 2006a), local pain and erythema at the injection site occurred in 5 of 75 patients, it was mild and resolved within 48 hours without sequela. The adverse reaction rate was 5.3% per injection and 6.7% per patient. We observed that these adverse events sometimes occurred after several injections without any reaction previously, and sometimes they did not occur in subsequent injections. Interestingly, local adverse reactions did not predict treatment failure. All of these patient received subsequent injections and they still improved clinically and reported high satisfaction. The incidence of adverse events was also low in the study by Cohen et al (Cohen et al, 2008), only one case of pseudogout, resolved without therapy, was observed in the Hyalgan group. Witteveen et al (Witteveen et al, 2008) reported 35 patients (63.6%) experienced a total of 89 adverse events in their study, which was relatively high compared with other studies. The majority of adverse events were arthralgia, injection site pain, and joint swelling, which were reported to be mild or moderate in intensity and transient in nature. Luciani et al. reported 11 patients (52%) in their case series presented transient pain and erythema in the injection site that resolved within 2 days and did not interfere with remaining injections (Luciani et al, 2008). In the case series by Carpenter et al. (Carpenter and Motley, 2008), they did not observe any local or systemic adverse events.

6. Further studies needed

Despite the fact that hyaluronate has been proposed as a useful treatment of symptomatic knee OA, its role in the treatment of ankle OA is still not clear, due fundamentally to the dearth of large, well-controlled studies and to the methodologic limitations of those that have been published. Most studies included small cohorts, short follow-up periods and an overall level of evidence is low. The clinical effects of the hyaluronate products have considerable heterogeneity and therapeutic variability, as most studies use different dosages, injection frequencies, different outcome measures, especially at different time points. Conclusions regarding the clinical effectiveness of each hyaluronate product could not be drawn. There was no evidence for differential effects according to subgroups defined by age, gender, primary/secondary disease, body mass index/weight, or disease severity. The exact mechanisms of viscosupplementation action on osteoarthritic joints are uncertain. Although recent attention has focused on the disease-modifying potential of hyaluronate, especially the chondroprotective mechanism, definitive evidence is still lacking. We believe that hyaluronate can be used as an adjunct therapy, after failure of one or more courses of oral pain medications, or perhaps as a first choice in the treatment of ankle OA before prescription of pain medications.

Future studies regarding optimal dosing regimen, injection frequency and injection technique, optimal number of injections in a course of treatment, favorable prognostic factors, duration of benefits, effectiveness and safety of repeated courses of therapy, longer term trials, head-to-head comparisons of the various hyaluronate products, as well as the biochemical, morphologic, and histopathologic effects on cartilage are warranted. Cost-effectiveness needs to be addressed. Comparison studies or combination therapies with other treatment options, such as intraarticular steroid injections, NSAIDs and therapeutic exercise, are also needed to help determine the best overall treatment plan for patients with ankle OA.

7. Conclusion

The published data suggest that viscosupplementation may potentially be a safe and effective alternative in treating patients with ankle OA. However, there are still inadequate data to provide definitive conclusions on the efficacy of hyaluronate in reducing pain or improvement of function among patients with ankle OA. The FDA has not approved intraarticular hyaluronate for joints other than the knee. To date ankle viscosupplementation should only be used under careful supervision by the clinician. Many uncertainties on the use of hyaluronate remain. The use of standardized outcome measures is encouraged to facilitate meta-analyses and between trial comparisons. Additional studies are required before viscosupplementation should be included into the treatment paradigm for patients with ankle OA.

8. References

Carpenter B, Motley T (2008). The role of viscosupplementation in the ankle using Hylan GF-20. *J Foot Ankle Surg* 47(5):377–384

Cohen MM, Altman RD, Hollstrom R, Hollstrom C, Sun C & Gipson B (2008). Safety and efficacy of intra-articular sodium hyaluronate (Hyalgan) in a randomized, double-blind study for osteoarthritis of the ankle. *Foot Ankle Int* 29(7):657–663

Domsic RT, Saltzman CL (1998). Ankle osteoarthritis scale. Foot Ankle Int 19(7):466–471

Engström-Laurent A. (1997) .Hyaluronan in joint disease. *J Int Med* 242:57-60.

Frizziero L, Govoni E & Bachin P. (1998) Intraarticular hyaluronic acid in the treatment of osteoarthritis of the knee: clinical and morphological study. Clin Exp Rheumatol 16:441-9.

Karatosun V, Unver B, Ozden A, Ozay Z & Gunal I (2008). Intraaticular hyaluronic acid compared to exercise therapy in osteoarthritis of the ankle. A prospective randomized trial with long-term follow-up. *Clin Exp Rheumatol* 26:288–294

Kitaoka HB, Alexander IJ, Adelaar RS, Nunley JA, Myerson MS & Sanders M (1994). Clinical rating systems for the ankle-hind-foot, midfoot, hallux and lesser toes. *Foot Ankle Int* 15:349–353

Luciani L, Cadossi M, Tesei F, Chiariello E & Giannini S (2008). Viscosupplementation for grade II osteoarthritis at the ankle: prospective study at 18 months' follow-up. *Chir Organi Mov* 92(3):155–160

Mei-Dan O, Kish B, Shabat S, Masarawa S, Shteren A, Mann G & Nyska M.(2010). Treatment of osteoarthritis of the ankle by intra-articular injections of hyaluronic acid: a prospective study, *J Am Podiatr Med Assoc,* 100:93–100.

Migliore A, Giovannangeli F, Bizzi E, Massafra U, Alimonti A, Lagana B, Picchianti AD, Germano V, Granata M & Piscitelli P. (2011). Viscosupplementation in the management of ankle osteoarthritis: a review. *Arch Orthop Trauma Surg* 131:139–147.

Salk RS, Chang TJ, D'Costa WF, Soomekh DJ & Grogan KA (2006). Sodium hyaluronate in the treatment of osteoarthritis of the ankle: a controlled, randomized, double-blind pilot study. *J Bone Joint Surg Am* 88(2):295–302

Saltzman CL, Salamon ML, Blanchard GM, Huff T, Hayes A, Buckwalter JA & Amendola A. (2005). Epidemiology of ankle arthritis: report of a consectutive series of 639 patients from a tertiary orthopaedic center. *Iowa Orthop J* 25:44-6.

Sun SF, Chou YJ, Hsu CW, Hwang CW, Hsu PT, Wang JL, Hsu YW & Chou MC (2006). Efficacy of intra-articoular hyaluronic acid in patients with osteoarthritis of the ankle: a prospective study. *Osteoarthritis Cartilage* 14:867–874

Sun SF, Hsu CW, Hwang CW, Hsu PT, Wang JL, Tsai SL, Chou YJ, Hsu YW, Huang CM & Wang YL.(2006). Hyaluronate improves pain, physical function and balance in the geriatric osteoarthritic knee: a 6-month follow-up study using clinical tests. *Osteoarthritis Cartilage,* 14(7):696-701.

Sun SF, Chou YJ, Hsu CW & Chen WL. (2009) Hyaluronic Acid as a Treatment for Ankle. Osteoarthritis. *Curr Rev Musculoskelet Med,* 2:78-82.

Sun SF, Hsu CW, Sun HP, Chou YJ, Li HJ & Wang JL (2011). Efficacy of Three Weekly Intraarticular Injections of Hyaluronate on Pain, Function and Balance in Patients with Unilateral Ankle Osteoarthritis—a prospective study with 6 months follow-up. *J Bone Joint Surg Am,;* 93(18):1720-1726.

Thomas RH, Daniels TR. (2003). Ankle arthritis. *J Bone Joint Surg Am.* 85:923-36.

Witteveen A, Giannini S, Guido G, Jerosch J, Lohrer H, Vannini F, Donati F, Schulz A, Scholl J, Sierevelt I & van Dijk N (2008). A prospective multi-centre, open study of the safety and efficacy of hylan G-F 20 (Synvisc®) in patients with symptomatic ankle (talocrural) osteoarthritis. *Foot Ankle Surg* 14:145–152

21

Knee Health Promotion Option for Osteoarthritic Knee: Cartilage Regeneration is Possible

S.R. Lyu[1], D.S. Liu[2], C.E. Tseng[1], H.S. Wang[3] and L.K. Chau[2]
[1]*Tzu-Chi Dalin General Hospital, Tzu-Chi University,*
[2]*Chung Cheng University,*
[3]*Yang-Ming University*
Taiwan

1. Introduction

Although articular hyaline cartilage was typically considered having no or low potential for regeneration (Zhang L et al., 2009), some still thought that it does have the capacity to grow and remodel extensively during pre- and post-natal development and after trauma (Onyekwelu I et al., 2009). Both direct and indirect evidence of articular cartilage regeneration have been observed by some authors after correction of varus deformity for osteoarthritis of the knee (Kanamiya T et al., 2002; Koshino T et al., 2003). Moreover, unlike the first impression of a more or less static tissue, articular cartilage shows a slow turnover. Anabolic and catabolic pathways were thought to be very much intermingled in articular cartilage (Aigner T et al., 2006). Thus, one of the most important questions in osteoarthritis research is to understand the balance of catabolic and anabolic factors in articular cartilage as this is the key to understand the biology of cartilage maintenance and degeneration.

Osteoarthritis (OA) of the knee is the major cause of chronic musculoskeletal pain and is ranked as a main cause of mobility disability in elderly population. It is a disease process of uncertain multifactorial etiology, which eventually affects the entire joint. Various etiologic risk factors have been proposed, but the exact pathogenesis for OA knee is still unknown. Many literatures mentioned medial compartment is more commonly involved than the lateral one and the pathogenesis may be different (Neame R et al., 2004; Nunez M et al., 2008).

In 2006, we reported that in patients with medial compartment osteoarthritic knees, the prevalence of medial plica was significantly higher than that of others and that two distinct foci of cartilaginous lesion were found on the facing medial femoral condyle in almost all of the patients who had the structure of medial plica (Lyu SR and Hsu CC, 2006). Our further study disclosed the kinematic relationship of the medial plica with the medial femoral condyle during knee motion in vivo (Lyu SR, 2007). In that study, it was revealed that all medial plicae, regardless of their size, would move reciprocally and would keep in touch with the medial femoral condyle and therefore might cause some degree of abrasion on the facing medial femoral condyle during knee motion. Another histomorphological study of the medial plica also implied the close interplay between this structure and the medial femoral condyle (Lyu SR et al., 2009). Moreover, our recent study (Wang HS et al., 2011) found that the repeated injuries elicited by this abrasion phenomenon might trigger interleukin-1β (IL-1β) production in medial plica, thus enhance the expression of matrix metalloproteinase-3 (MMP-3). Based on these findings, we developed a concept of arthroscopic medial release (AMR) for the treatment of osteoarthritis of the medial compartment of the knee joint (Lyu SR, 2008). The clinical outcome of this procedure lured us to believe that, by eradication of the abrasion phenomenon between the tight, fibrotic and hypertrophied medial structure and the adjacent medial femoral condyle, the pain of most patients could be reduced and the degenerative process in the medial compartment of some patients might be decelerated or arrested. Recently, we proposed a concept of arthroscopic cartilage regeneration facilitating procedure (ACRFP) that combines arthroscopic medial release (AMR) with conventional arthroscopic procedures including synovectomy, chondroplasty, partial meniscectomy and percutaneous lateral release (PLR) as a rationale for the deliberate arthroscopic management of OA knee. We've found that the elimination of the existing detrimental factors will provide a preferable environment for regeneration of the damaged cartilage.

The main scheme of this chapter will be a step-by-step presentation of the development of a global approach which we call "knee health promotion option (KHPO)" for OA knee. In section 2, a new entity "medial abrasion syndrome (MAS)" and the related hidden lesions will be defined. Its role in the pathogenesis of medial compartmental OA knee will be discussed based on our series of studies. The techniques and clinical outcomes of two novel arthroscopic procedures: arthroscopic medial release (AMR) and arthroscopic cartilage regeneration facilitating procedure (ACRFP) which have been developed according to the rationale conceptualized from the results of our basic research will be described in section 3 and 4. In section 5, a concept of total management of OA knee (KHPO) will be proposed. Finally, conclusions and discussions for the future prospect are presented in section 6.

2. Medial abrasion syndrome (MAS) and the hidden lesions

Medial abrasion syndrome is an unrecognized but common clinical entity caused by the repeated impingement between mediopatellar plica (medial shelf) and the opposite medial femoral condyle during knee motion. This syndrome could explain most of the symptoms and signs of the medial compartment OA knee. In this section, the definition, clinical manifestations and relavant studies to investigate the role of MAS and the correlated hidden lesions in the pathogenesis of OA knee will be presented.

2.1 Medial plica and MAS

The mediopatellar plica is a fold in the synovium representing an embryologic remnant in the development of the synovial cavity of the knee. It is found along the medial wall of the joint originating superiorly, extending obliquely and inferiorly, and inserting on the synovial lining of the infrapatellar fat pad (Dandy DJ, 1990). It is generally agreed that this structure can produce knee symptoms and could be successfully treated by arthroscopic resection when it becomes inflamed, thickened, and less elastic (Dorchak JD et al., 1991; Flanagan JP et al.).

During arthroscopic examination, different degrees of cartilaginous degeneration on the surface of the medial femoral condyle facing the medial plica has been noticed by many authors (Tasker T et al., 1982; Broom MJ et al., 1986; Dupont JY, 1997). According to a study conducted in 2006 (Lyu SR and Hsu CC, 2006), the incidence of the medial plica was significantly higher in subjects with osteoarthritis of their knees. Degenerative cartilaginous lesions on the facing medial femoral condyle were found in almost all of the patients who had the structure of medial plica. This study also found that the severity of these lesions has obvious correlation with patient's age and the severity of their plical lesions. In daily clinical practice, we likewise get an impression that the severity of the plical lesions present positive correlation with the severity of the osteoarthritis of the medial compartment as shown in figure 1.

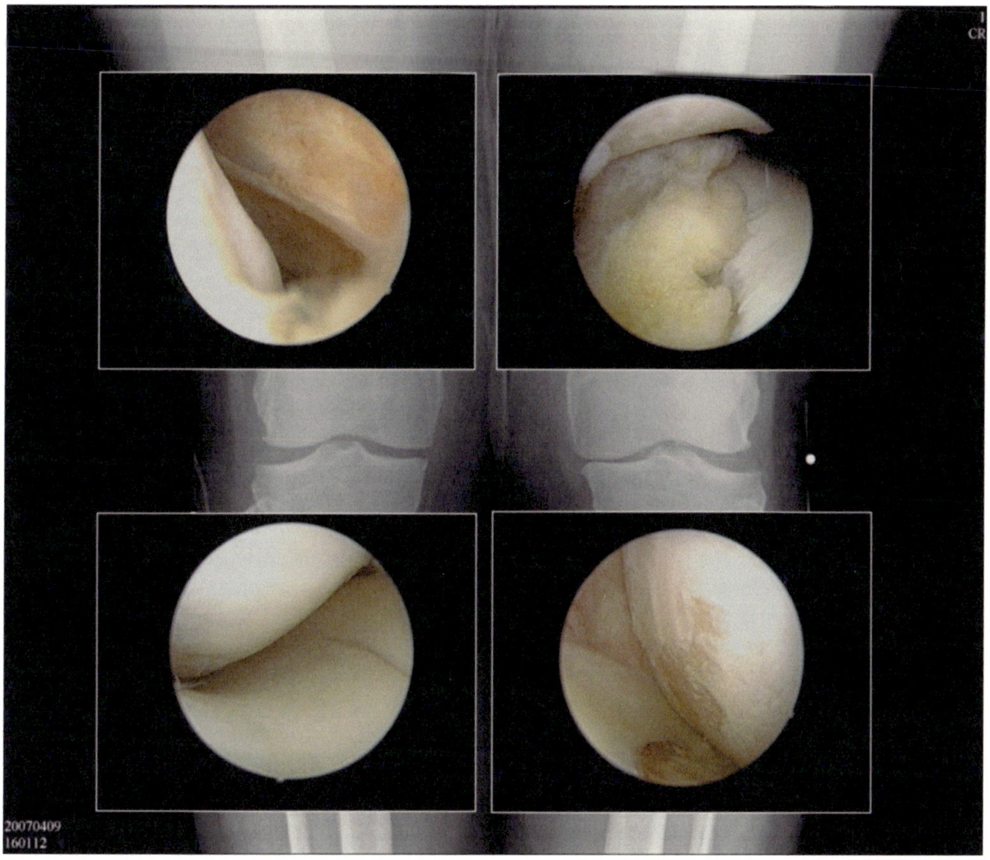

Fig. 1. Arthroscopic findings of the effect of medial abrasion syndrome, the severity of the osteoarthritis of the medial compartment seems to have positive correlation with the severity of gross appearance of the medial plica.

2.2 Clinical manifestations of MAS

In 2004, we conducted an unpublished investigation in order to find out the predisposing factors and presenting symptoms and signs of MAS in a series of 163 patients older then 40 years with 232 knees proven to have medial plica related MAS by arthroscopy. The sensitivity and specificity of each parameter about predisposing factors, symptoms and signs for the diagnosis of the medial plica related medial abrasion syndrome were analyzed. This study conceptualized the following clinical manifestations of MAS.

2.2.1 Predisposing factors

Injuries

The presentation of a single episode of injury, such as a falling down with sudden bending of the knee, direct blunt injury over the anterior-medial aspect of the knee, unexpected twisting of the knee or change of position when kneeling.

Activities need bending knee

History of repeated or prolonged bending of the involved knee, such as squatting, kneeling, climbing stairs, hiking along slopes, climbing mountains or bicycling, either due to occupational or recreational needs. Prolonged driving or riding any transportation vehicle.

Female

Females tend to bend their knee more than males do in their daily activities.

Religion

Some religious worship needs repeated squatting or kneeling.

2.2.2 Symptoms

Pain

It is always described as deep-seated, throbbing or cutting ache and would get worse when climbing stairs, sitting with the knees flexed for a long time, rising from a sitting position, or extending the knee against resistance. Night pain or soreness and difficult to find a suitable position when sleeping are also common complaints. Some patients might point out the location of pain over the anterior-medial aspect of the knee.

Crepitus

The presentation of the feeling or hearing of a click or crepitus when the involved knee is flexed or extended after prolonged sitting. It may or may not be accompanied by pain.

Snapping or locking

Patients might incidentally experience the feeling of giving way, a sense of insecurity or pseudolocking in some particular position. Mostly it occurs when the knee is partially bended during weight-bearing. Sometimes, locking will occur when patients try to walk after sitting or lying for a long time. It will get unlocked after standing for a few minutes.

2.2.3 Signs

Localized tenderness

Precise tender area could be identified over the region between the inferior-medial margin of the lower pole of the patella and the ridge of the medial femoral condyle.

Palpable band

A palpable band with snapping or crepitation might be found over the above-mentioned tender area.

Provocative test

A provocative test to reproduce the characteristic pain and snapping of the band might be conducted by compressing the tender point with the thumb of one hand and repeatedly bend the knee with the other hand.

2.2.4 Radiographic findings

Various degrees of rentgenographic manifestation of medial abrasion syndrome could be evaluated by axial view (Merchant's view) of the patello-femoral joint. In the early stage, it is always difficult to be diagnosed due to the concurrent lateral deviation or subluxation of the patella. Sometimes, narrowing of the medial patello-femoral joint space that represents as the clue of abrasion phenomenon might be found by careful evaluation. In more advanced cases, eburnation and bone attrition of the medial femoral condyle and/or medial facet of patella with obvious narrowing of the medial patello-femoral joint space could also be visualized as shown in figure 2.

Progressive narrowing of the medial patello-femoral joint space accompanied by osteophytes formation over the medial margin of patella and medial femoral condyle is the typical findings of severe cases. Subchondral cysts and hypersclerosis sometimes could be noticed over the medial femoral condyle (figure 3).

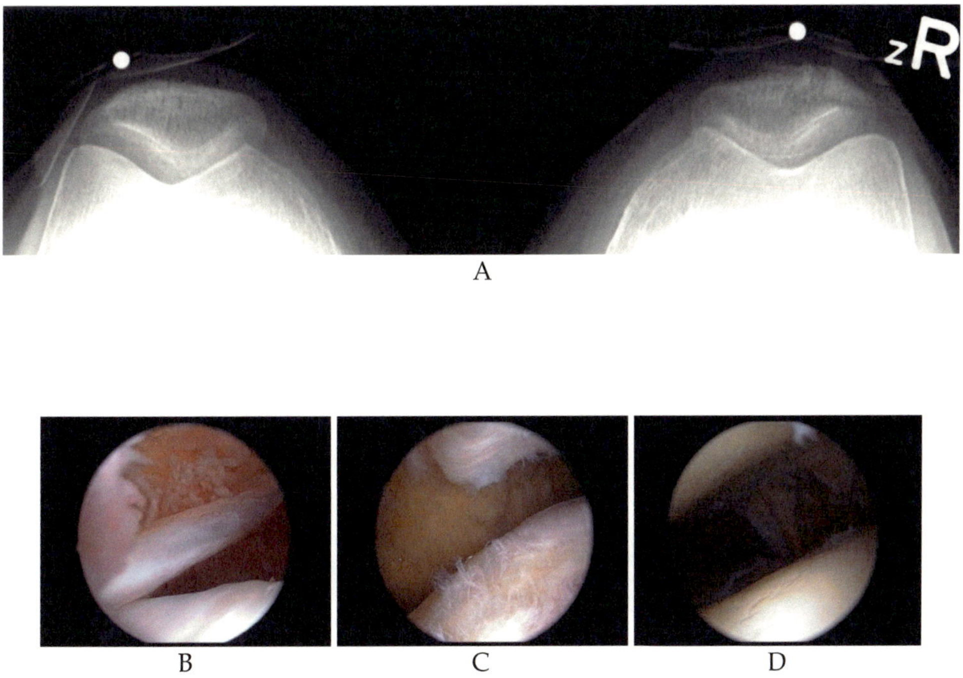

Fig. 2. A, narrowing of the medial patello-femoral joint is obvious; B, thicken medial plica with synovitis causing medial abrasion syndrome of left knee; C, after arthroscopic medial release, fibrillation of the cartilage surfaces are obvious over medial patello-femoral joint compared to that of the lateral one as was shown in D.

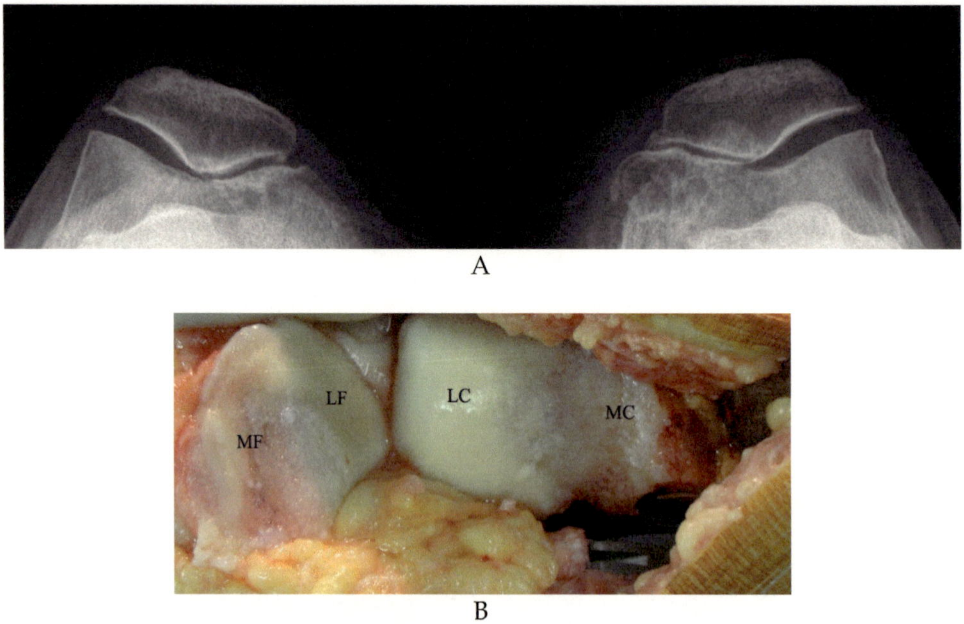

Fig. 3. Rentgenographic and gross appearance of the late effect of medial abrasion syndrome, A, marked narrowing of the medial patello-femoral joint with osteophytes, hypersclerosis and subchondral cysts; B, severe cartilage destruction over medial facet (MF) of patella and medial femoral condyle (MC) compared to lateral ones (LF and LC) could be visualized in this patient received arthroplasty.

2.3 The hidden lesions

Medial abrasion syndrome could give rise to different degrees of cartilagenous degeneration on the surface of medial femoral condyle facing the medial plica. We call it "hidden lesion" because that in most occasions, either due to synovitis or tightness of the joint space in osteoarthritic knees, these lesions are difficult to be found in routine arthroscopic examination. Only after adequate synovectomy could they be clearly visualized by special view as shown in figure 4.

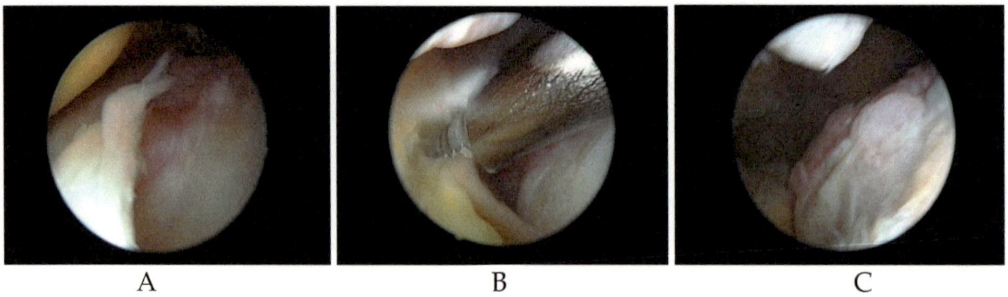

Fig. 4. The unveiling of the hidden lesion, A, the space between medial patellar facet and medial femoral condyle is obliterated by focal synovial tissue; B, during arthroscopic medial release, the hypertrophied medial plica and related tissue were debrided and removed; C, after this procedure, the "hidden lesion" could be visualized.

After proper synovectomy and release of the infero-medial area of patella and the medial gutter, two distinct foci (A and B in figure 5A) of cartilaginous lesions which we call the "hidden lesions" could be found on the edge and anterior part of the medial femoral condyle. The appearance of these focal cartilaginous lesions was unique and different from what has been described by the classical arthroscopic classification of cartilaginous lesions. We classify these lesions into five stages according to the gross appearance of their severity (figure 5). In a retrospective reviewing of the arthroscopic findings of 1587 knees, we found that the severity of the hidden lesions was positively correlated with the severity of the pathologic medial plica, total degeneration score of the knee and patient's age (Lyu SR and Hsu CC, 2006).

2.4 MAS as a cause of medial compartment osteoarthritis of the knee

The aforementioned clinical findings strongly suggest that the medial abrasion syndrome might play a role in the pathogenesis of medial compartment osteoarthritis of the knee. In 2002, we collaborated a research team and began to conduct a series of investigations focusing on the following subjects: establishment of a finite element model of the medial abrasion phenomenon for biomechanical analysis of the possible mechanical effect elicited by this abrasion phenomenon; histopathological study of the gross and histological presentation of the pathological medial plica itself; biochemical analysis of the medial plica and the related pannus-like tissue, and compartment specified joint fluid analysis. In this section, we will describe and summarize the results of these studies and make a conclusive assumption for the role of the medial abrasion phenomenon as an important etiologic factor of medial compartment osteoarthritis of the knee.

2.4.1 Mechanical factor – The finite element model

In order to establish a finite element model for the study of the relationship of medial plica with the facing medial femoral condyle, two pilot experiments were conducted.

First, an experimental study on the tensile strength of mediopatellar plica was undertaken using high precision micro-force tensile tests (Lyu SR et al, 2006). These tests were conducted with plica specimens taken from 61 knees of patients of different ages. The force-deflection curves resulting from these tests were recorded and transferred to stress-stain curves to get the Young's moduli of these specimens. In addition, pathological tissue dye tests were used to assess the fiber content ratio (FCR) of each specimen. The value of the Young's modulus was plotted versus FCR, and the relation between them was fitted properly using a quadratic regression model. The test results indicated that the value of Young's modulus sharply increased when FCR exceeded 80%. This may lead to higher contact pressure between the medial plica and the adjacent articular cartilage. This study also found that the Young's modulus of the medial plica was positively correlated with the severity of the plica lesion and the patient's age.

In the second study (Lyu SR, 2007), the inner margins of the medial plicae of 30 knees were located by inserting needles percutaneously under direct vision during arthroscopic examination. The topographic changes of the margins of these plicae during knee motion were recorded by fluoroscopy and analyzed. In all types of the medial plicae, regardless of their sizes, shifting (rubbing, sliding) medially was found when the knee was moved from extension to flexion. They remained in contact with the medial femoral condyles during the whole range of motion. This observation disclosed the kinematic relationship of the medial plica with the medial femoral condyle during knee motion in vivo. This pattern of medial-lateral motion may generate some shearing force acting on the cartilage of the medial femoral condyle.

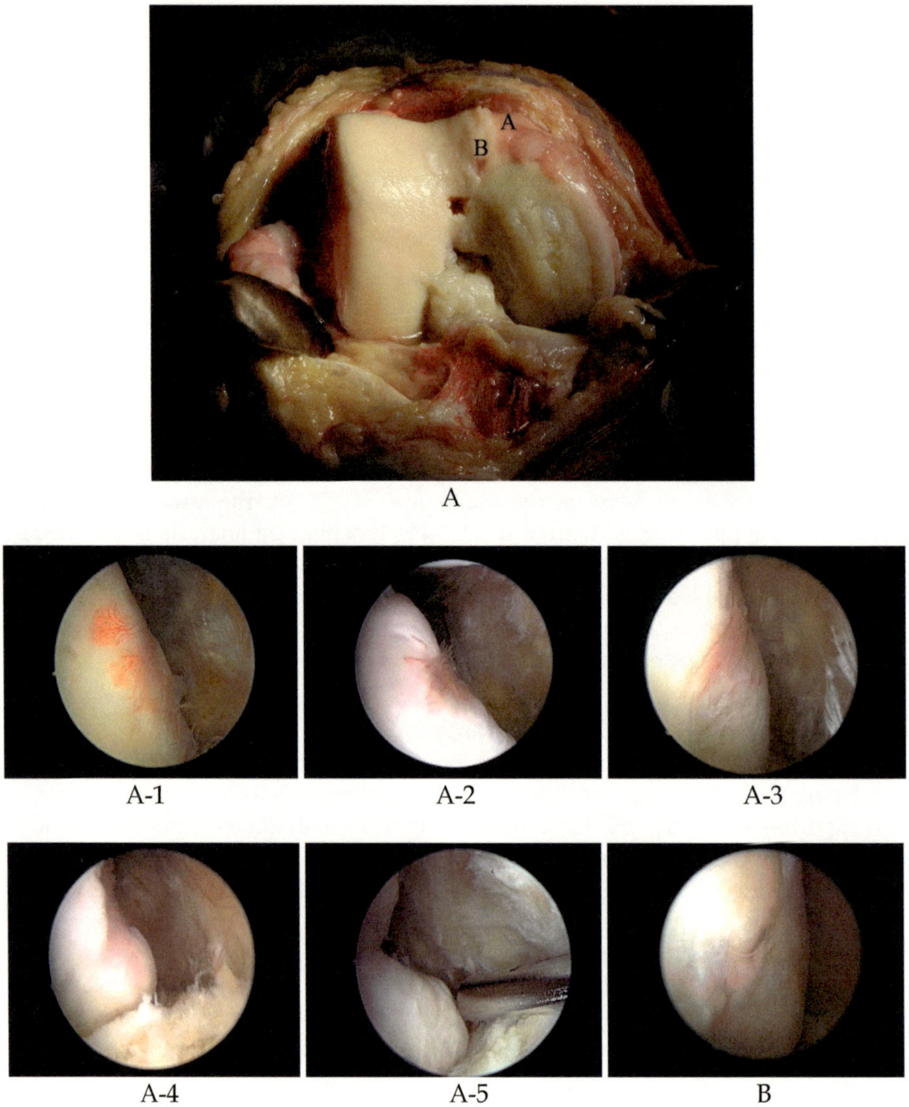

Fig. 5. The hidden lesions, A, gross appearance of the typical hidden lesions (foci A and B); arthroscopic findings of different stage of focus A lesion: A-1, in the stage I cartilaginous lesion, neovascularization and pannus formation are found over the margin of the lesion. Softening of the cartilage could be confirmed by palpation with a probe; A-2, the stage II lesion has all the findings of the stage I lesion. Moreover, flattening and indentation of the cartilage could be identified; A-3, the stage III lesion is a partial thickness cartilaginous damage. The cartilage becomes fissured and fibrillated; A-4, in a stage IV lesion, some areas of subchondral bone are exposed. A shallow gutter representing the imprint of abrasion caused by the medial plica can be identified; A-5, in a stage V lesion, the subchondral bone is completely exposed to form a deep gutter; B, the arthroscopic picture of focus B cartilaginous lesion related to medial abrasion syndrome.

Based on the findings of these pilot studies, a three-dimension dynamic finite element model composed of femur, tibia, cartilage layers and medial plica was recently developed (Lyu SR and Liu DS, unpublished). This validated model was used to investigate and compare the level of cyclic pressures acting on the cartilage of the medial femoral condyles by three different types of medial plicae with various Young's moduli. We found that all types of medial plicae remained in contact with the medial femoral condyles and shift medially when the knee moved from extension to flexion.

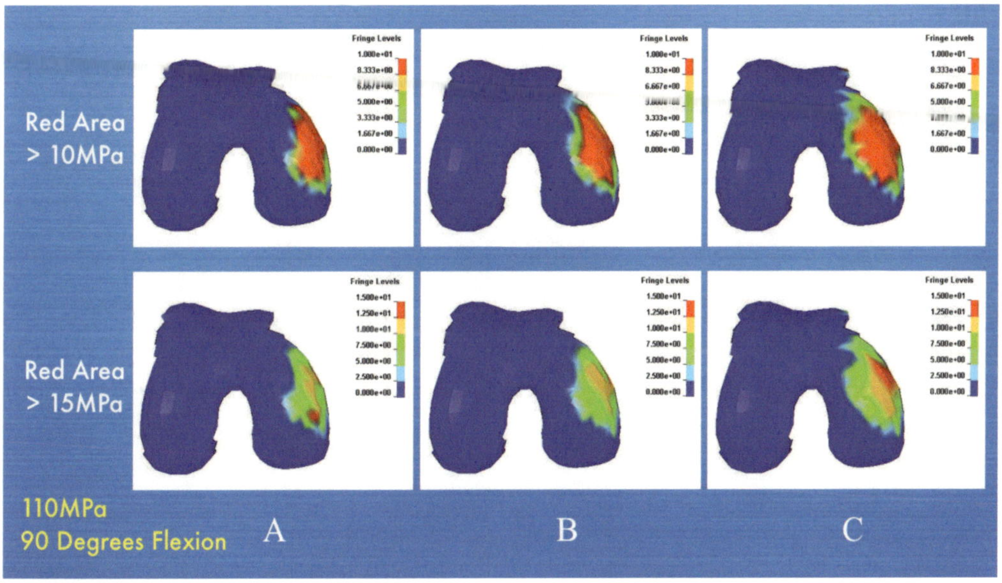

Fig. 6. The distribution of contact pressure on the medial femoral condyle elicited by different types of medial plica with Young's modulus set at 110 MPa and the knee model is flexed to 90 degrees. The high-pressure zones (red areas) are well correlated with our clinical findings.

This 3D model (figure 6) demonstrated that the contact pressures were positively correlated with the Young's moduli of the medial plicae. When the Young's moduli of the medial plicae were set greater than 40 MPa, all types of medial plicae would elicit contact pressures higher than 10 MPa on medial femoral condyles, and that is enough to cause apoptosis of chondrocytes in the cartilage tissue according to previous study using a bovine cartilage explant system to evaluate the effects of injurious compression on chondrocyte apoptosis (Loening et al., 2000).

In conclusion, according to the findings of this 3D dynamic finite element model, the close relationship and possible high contact pressure between fibrotic medial plica and medial femoral condyle during knee motion may be an crucial cause of the degenerative change of the cartilage on the medial femoral condyle.

2.4.2 MAS and abnormal gait

Successively, we have conducted an histomorphological study focusing on the gross appearance and histological features of the medial plicae removed from 48 consecutive patients who had received total knee replacement for severe medial compartment osteoarthritis of their knees (Lyu SR et al., 2010). Histologically, the majority of advanced pathologic presentation was found at the middle and distal portion of the medial plica that might abrade on the articular cartilage of the medial femoral condyle and noticeable cartilaginous lesion was found on the facing medial femoral condyle in all knees. In addition, a small branch of skeletal muscle originating from articularis genu inserting into the proximal synovial stroma of the medial plica was found in all knees (figure 7 A, B). The synovial fold of the distal part of the medial plica was disclosed to have a close relationship with the gracilis tendon sheath (figure 7 C, D).

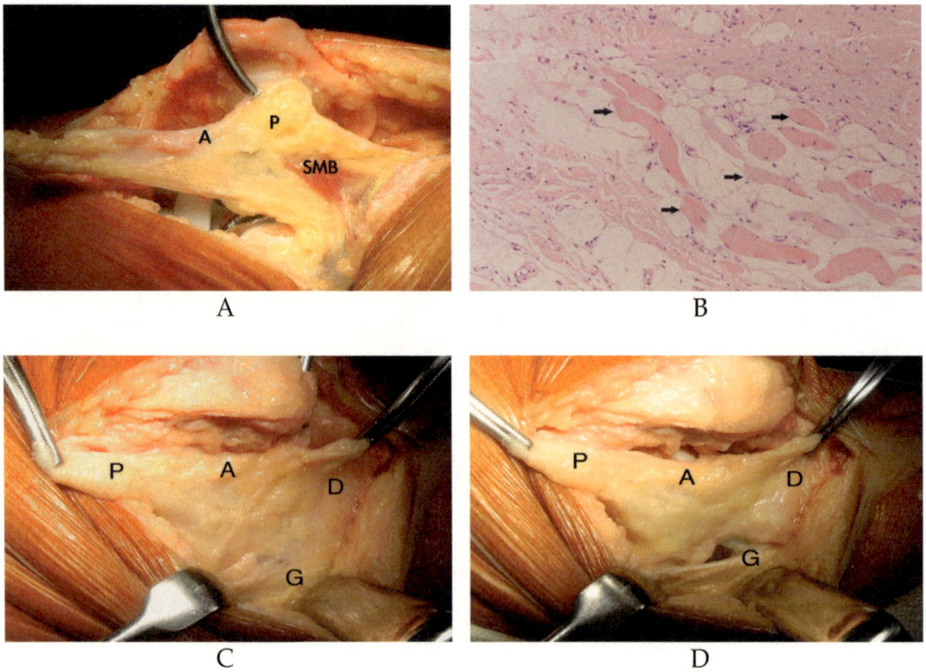

Fig. 7. A. A branch of skeletal muscle (SMB) originating from articularis genus was noticed inserting into the proximal part (P) of this medial plica. (A: abrasion portion) B. Microscopically, skeletal muscular fibers (arrows) could be found in the alveolar fibroadipose tissue of this medial plica (×40; H & E stain). C. The synovial fold of the distal part (D) of the medial plica was disclosed originating from the tendon sheath of the gracilis tendon (G). D. After the medial plica was removed, the gracilis tendon (G) could be visualized clearly. (P: proximal and A: abrasion parts of the medial plica)

It has been suggested that abnormal gait pattern may lead to the development of knee OA (Lynn SK et al., 2007). Several studies (Baliunas AJ et al., 2002; Gok H et al., 2002; Landry SC et al., 2007) have noticed that an increased knee adduction and internal rotation moment during the stance phase of gait is associated with knee OA. It was also detected that among individuals with mild radiographic knee OA, those who are symptomatic have significantly higher medial compartment loads than those who are asymptomatic (Thorp LE et al., 2007). The linkage of medial plica with the medial muscle group of the thigh found in this study might give answer to these literature findings which suggested the relationship of gaits with medial compartment OA knee. During the walking cycle, the irritation of the inflamed medial plicae by the abrasion phenomenon with the medial femoral condyle might evoke reflex contracture of the medial muscle group including vastus intermedialis and gracilis and therefore increase the adduction and internal rotation moment and the medial compartment load of the knee. This correlation could further be proven by subjective improvement of gait pattern claimed by many of our OA knee patients who have received arthroscopic resection of the inflamed medial plica.

The histomorphological findings of this study imply the close interplay between the medial plica and the medial femoral condyle that might play a role in the pathogenesis of medial compartment osteoarthritis of the knee.

2.4.3 Biochemical analysis of medial plica and pannus tissue

The most significant pathological change in OA of the knee is the progressive loss of hyaline cartilage of the articular surface. The expression of IL-1β and matrix metalloproteinase-3 (MMP-3) by pannus-like tissue in the knees of patients with advanced OA suggests that MMP-3 contributes to cartilage degradation (Shibakawa A et al., 2003; Yuan GH et al., 2004). MMP-3 is produced by both chondrocytes and synoviocytes, especially when stimulated by IL-1β (Tetlow LC et al., 2001). Synovial tissue inflammation has been predicted as a pathogenesis factor in early OA (Haywood L et al., 2003; Ayral C et al., 2005; Benito MJ et al., 2005; Ikeuchi M et al., 2005). Joint injury-induced IL-1β expression has been found to enhance MMP-3 release (Techetverikov I et al., 2005; Daheshia M and Yao JQ, 2008; Eder C, 2009), resulting in matrix degradation (van den Berg WB 2001). IL-1β levels in the knee joint were found to be associated with the severity of chondral damage (Marks PH and Konaldson ML, 2005).

In our previous study, pannus-like tissue (figures 5 and 8C) was also observed on the cartilage of the medial femoral condyle opposite the inflamed medial plica in early stage medial compartment OA of the knee (Lyu SR and Hsu CC, 2006). Further observation found that pathologic medial plica could be discovered in every patient suffering from medial compartment OA knee. This study also declared that various degrees of inflammation could be observed in the medial plicae of patients with medial compartment OA of the knee and removal of this structure by arthroscopic medial release could relieve their symptoms or even modify their disease process (Lyu SR, 2008).

In order to determine the role of medial plica and pannus-like tissue (figure 8C) in the pathogenesis of OA knee, expression of MMP-3 in the control synovial membrane, pannus-like tissue and medial plica obtained from early stage OA knee patients were investigated by immunohistochemical staining (Wang HS et al 2011). We found that MMP-3 was highly expressed in the pannus-like tissue (p in figure 8B-b) and medial plica (figure 8B-c), but not in the cartilage (ca in figure 8B-b) or control synovial membrane (figure 8B-a). Immunofluorescent staining also showed that MMP-3 was intensively expressed in medial plica tissue (figure 8C). In this study, the effect of IL-1β on cells isolated from pannus-like tissue and medial plica from early stage OA knees was also determined. Our results demonstrated that these cells expressed significant amount of MMP-3 mRNA and MMP-3 was found being released into the culture medium consequently. Moreover, similar to what were found in both medial plica and pannus-like tissue of late stage OA knees, significant high levels of IL1-β mRNA expression was found in medial plica of early stage OA knees. All of these findings suggest that IL1-β might be the triggering factor in MMP-3 expression by these tissues. Since MMP-3 plays a significant role in the progression of OA, our investigation bring to light that medial plica might be involved in the pathogenesis of medial compartment OA of the knee.

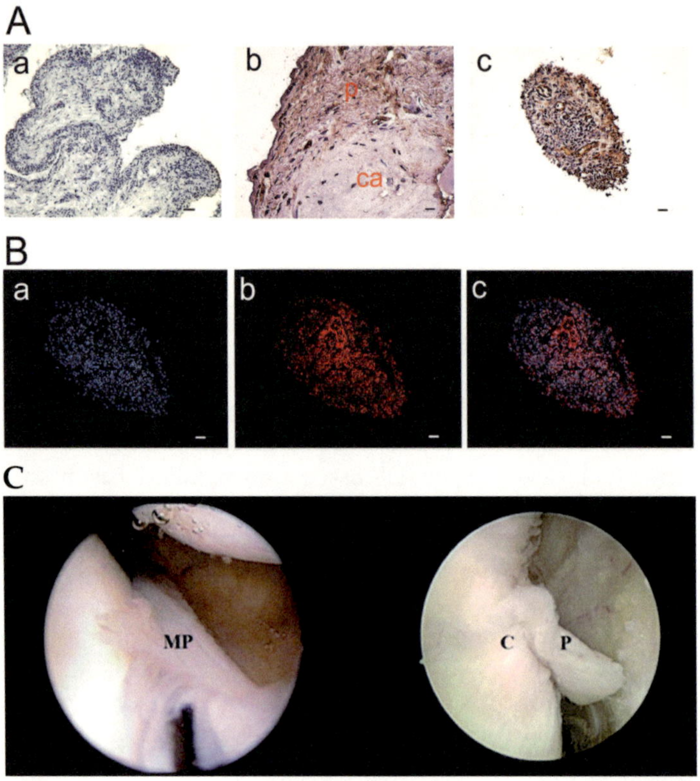

Fig. 8. A, immunohistochemical staining for MMP-3 in pannus-like tissue, cartilage and medial plica. (a) control synovial membrane, (b) pannus-like tissue ("p") or cartilage ("ca") or (c) medial plica. The bar is 20 µm in (a) and (b) and 10 µm in (c). B, Immunofluorescent staining for MMP-3 in medial plica. (a) Nuclei stained with DAPI (blue), (b) cells stained for MMP-3 (red) and (c) merged image. The bar represents 10 µm. The results are typical of those from 16 knees. C, Anatomical location of tissue biopsy in a typical right knee with stage II OA. MP is medial plica, P pannus and C cartilage. (Reproduced and adapted with permission and copyright © of the John Wiley and Sons [Wang HS et al 2011])

We propose that the abrasion between medial plica and the opposite medial femoral condyle may be the cause of inflammation in patients with medial compartment OA of the knee. This repeated abrasion injuries might trigger IL-1β production in medial plica, thus enhance the expression of MMP-3. Our finding of highly expressed MMP-3 mRNA in medial plica than in the control synovial membrane by real-time PCR analysis further supports this hypothesis. Recently, we found that inflammation in patients with medial compartment OA of the knee may also induce the production of other MMPs involved in the pathogenesis of OA knees (Wang HS et al., unpublished data). These findings agree with the observation that removal of pathologic medial plica and its related inflammatory structure by arthroscopy can be effective in symptom relief or even can modify the disease process of medial compartment OA knee (Ikeuchi M et al., 2005; Lyu SR 2008).

2.4.4 Analysis of joint fluid

There are a variety of proteins in the synovial fluid of osteoarthritic knee. These proteins include glycoprotein debris and collagen fragments derived from destructed cartilaginous tissue and enzymes such as metalloproteinase, collagenase and proinflammatory cytokines (interleukin-1α, interleukin-1β, tumour necrosis factor α, etc) (Yoshihara Y et al., 2000; Hedbom E and Hauselmann HJ, 2002; Tchetverikov I et al., 2005). All of these proteins in synovial fluid might reflect the pathological status of the knees.

Since the aforementioned abrasion phenomenon between fibrotic medial plica and the opposite medial femoral condyle may continuously produce cartilage debris and give rise to various degree of synovitis, it is interesting to see whether the concentrations of total protein, IL-1β and MMP-3 are different in medial and lateral compartments of these knees.

Recently, we have conducted a study (Lyu SR and Chau LC, unpublished) to analyze total protein, interleukin (IL)-1β and Matrix Metalloproteinase-3 concentrations in synovial fluid of medial and lateral compartments from 14 knees with medial compartment OA received unicompartmental arthroplasty due to medial compartment osteoarthritis. All of these knees were found to have fibrotic medial plica demonstrating abrasion phenomenon with the opposite medial femoral condyle. Figure 9 shows the total protein, IL-1β, and MMP-3 concentrations in the synovial fluid obtained from the medial and lateral compartments of these knees. All sets of sample analyzed revealed significant higher concentration of total protein, IL-1β, and MMP-3 in the medial compartment.

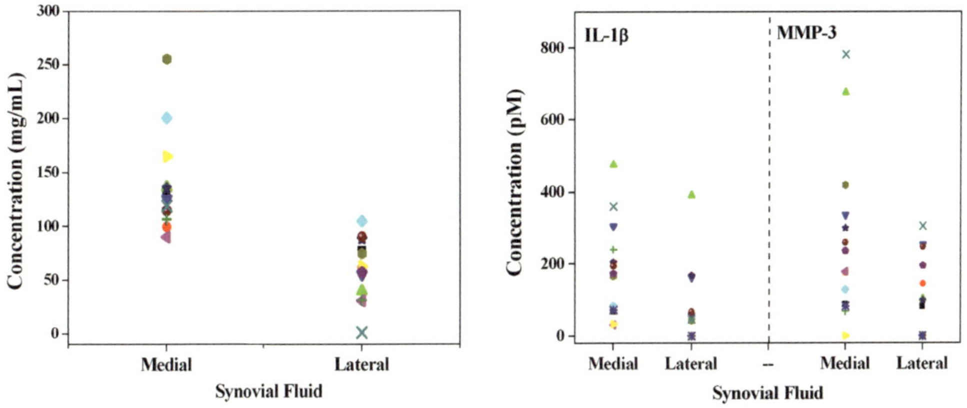

(a) (b)

Fig. 9. (a) The total protein concentration and (b) the concentrations of IL-1β and MMP-3 measured by enzyme-linked immunosorbent assay (ELISA) in samples of synovial fluid in medial and lateral compartments of osteoarthritic knees. *The difference between medial (n = 14) and lateral (n = 14) was statistically significant at $P < 0.01$ in the Mann Whitney U test.

In contrast to the common point of view that molecules should be evenly distributed within joint cavity, the above findings revealed the existence of big differences of total protein concentration, IL-1β concentration, and MMP-3 concentration between medial and lateral compartments of osteoarthritic knees. The discrepancy in the total protein distribution in synovial fluids may be attributed to the size of the protein molecules. Owing to the gravity and the contour of the tibial plateau, the debris or tissue fragments generated from the medial compartment may not pass freely between medial and lateral compartments of the knee joint and accumulate in the particular compartment. On the other hand, the local higher concentrations of IL-1β and MMP-3 are likely due to the medial abrasion phenomenon related ongoing pathologic progress in the medial compartment of these knees. Furthermore, the self-abrasion of the rough degenerated cartilaginous surfaces might also be the source of debris generation during daily activities. These findings might be important in the unveiling of pathogenesis or progression of medial compartment OA knee.

2.4.5 MAS as an important etiologic factor for medial compartment OA knee

In summary, as shown in figure 10, our series of studies have discovered the possible mechanism by which the medial abrasion syndrome cause progressive degradation of the cartilage over the medial compartment of the knee.

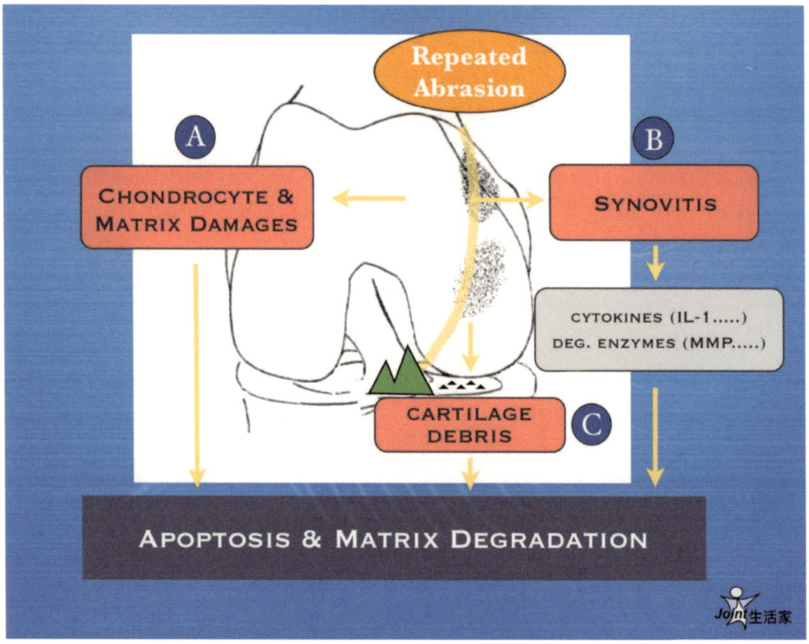

Fig. 10. Medial abrasion syndrome as an etiologic factor for medial compartment OA knee, the repeated abrasion (millions times per year) between medial plica (represented by yellow curved line) and the medial femoral condyle will cause: A, chondrocyte and matrix damage due to direct mechanical shearing force; B, synovitis around medial plica due to trauma will produce cytokines (such as IL-1β) and cartilage degradating enzymes (such as MMP-3); C, the debris and particles shedding down from the damaged cartilage accumulate in the medial compartment, further elicit third party abrasion over the weight bearing area.

Depending on the size and the severity of fibrosis of the medial plica, the abrasion itself will produce abnormal shearing force on the opposite cartilage of the medial femoral condyle and cause various degree of cartilaginous damage. On the other side, this abrasion phenomenon elicits repeated injury to the medial plica itself and results in focal synovitis that will trigger the production of cytokines such as IL-1β and then upgrades the production of cartilage degradating enzymes such as MMP-3. The continuous shedding of cartilaginous debris and production of cartilage drgradating enzymes make the whole medial compartment in a

consistently detrimental condition for the maintainance of normal cartilage metabolism and thus progressive "degeneration" results. Moreover, the painful sensation of inflammation of medial plica might evoke a reflex contracture of the pes anserinus muscle group and increase the loading of the medial compartment thus further jeopadize the cartilage.
According to our theory, medial abrasion syndrome, if present, might produce life long harmful effects on the general environment of medial compartment of the involved knee and disturb normal cartilage metabolism thus bring about the process of "degeneration".

3. Surgical treatment of MAS

In order to remove the detrimental medial abrasion syndrome, we have developed a novel arthroscopic procedure that we called arthroscopic medial release (AMR) for capsular release (Lyu SR, 2008). The target of the capsular release was the layer III, so called "true capsule" of the 3-layers medial supporting structure (Warren LF and Marshall JL, 1979). As shown in figure 11, the capsulectomy extends superiorly to the midline of suprapatellar pouch. Inferiorly, it extends to the upper margin of medial meniscus. Anteriorly, it extends to the medial margin of patella. Posteriorly, it is undertaken to remove portion of the conjoined part of layer II and III till the gracilis tendon is visualized. Only the deep medial ligament was severed by this procedure and the medial stability should not be disturbed much.

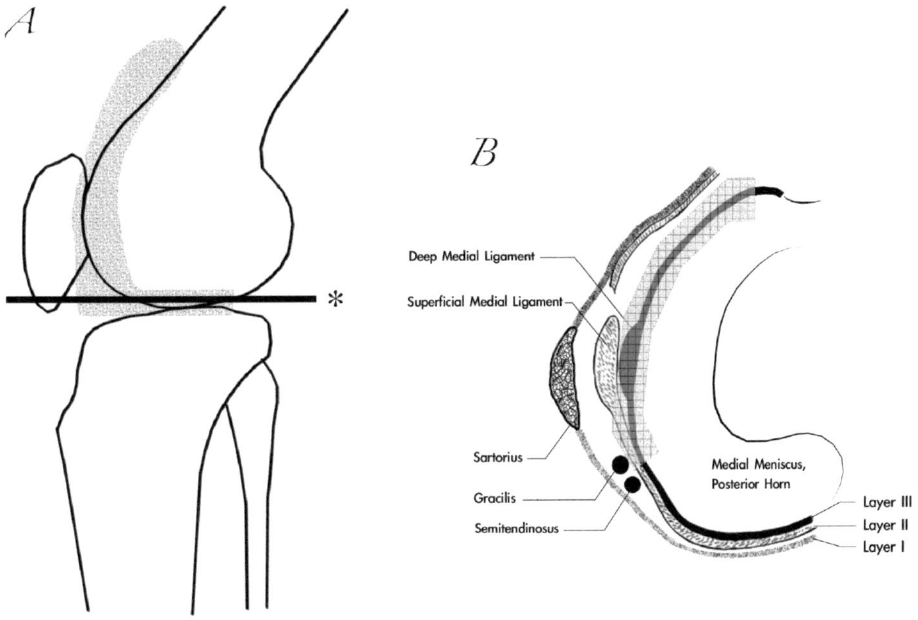

Fig. 11. A: The extent of the medial capsulectomy is shown in the hatched area of the line drawing of the lateral view of the knee joint. The line marked by * is the level of cross section above the meniscus as shown in B. B: The crossed-hatched area indicates the extent of the capsulectomy above the medial meniscus. Note that only the deep medial ligament is severed. The tendon of gracilis could be visualized after the procedure. (Reproduced and adapted with permission and copyright © of the British Editorial Society of Bone and Joint Surgery [Lyu SR, 2008])

The adequacy of the medial release could be checked by passing the scope under the patella and verified if the previously tightly closed medial patellofemoral joint space could be easily opened and the medial retinaculum visualized when the knee was put in full extension position.

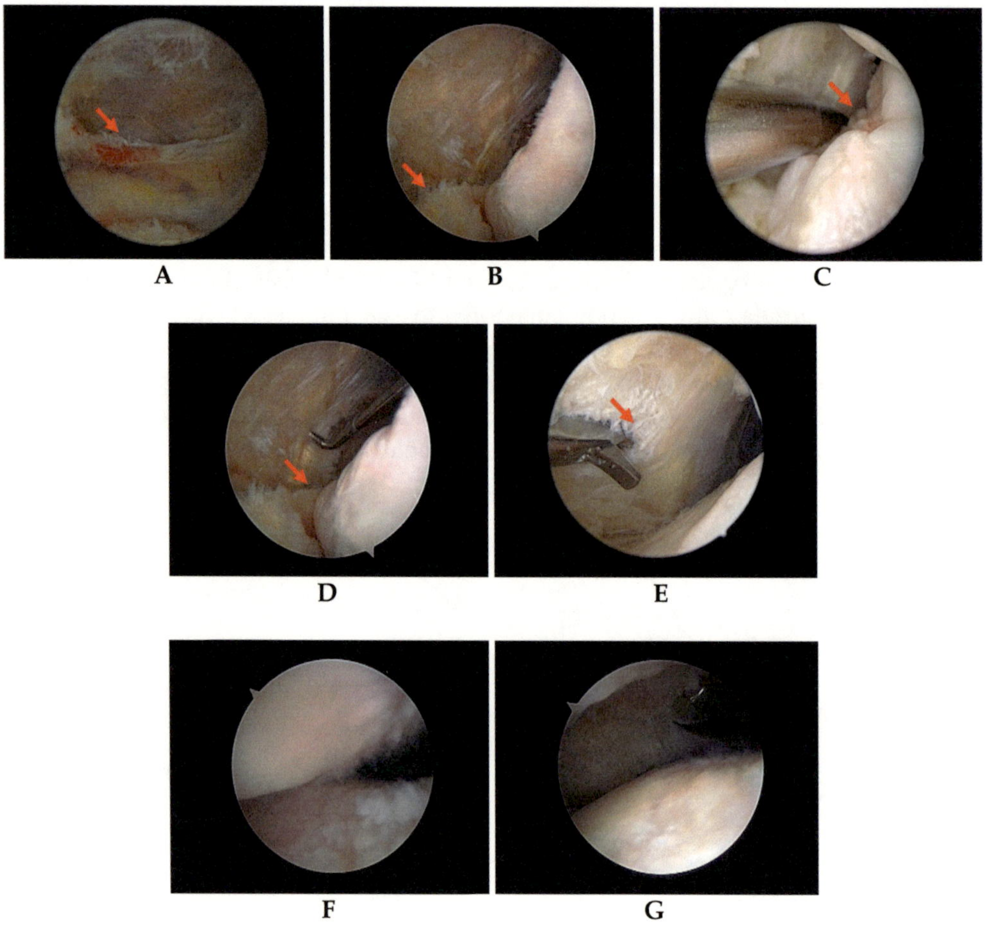

Fig. 12. For a complete arthroscopic medial release (MAS), A, proximally, the genu articularis muscle attachment (arrow) should be released; B, the anterior synoviomeniscal junction (arrow) should be release; C, the medial gutter should be cleared to its posterior corner (arrow); D, the synoviomeniscal junction of the medial meniscus (arrow) should be clearly seen; E, in some case, release of the fascia of pes anserinus (arrow) should be performed; F, before medial release; G, after medial release.

According to our experience of performing this procedure (Lyu SR, 2008), the outcome of 255 knees in 173 patients for varying stages of osteoarthritis involving the medial compartment supports our contention that AMR is a good modality for the treatment of osteoarthritis of the medial knee joint in the aspect of symptom relief. It can reduce the pain in the majority of OA patients over a period of at least 4 years. In some cases, we also found the evidence that AMR could modify the disease process and satisfied the patients.

4. Arthroscopic cartilage regeneration facilitating procedure (ACRFP)

The clinical outcome of the AMR lured us to believe that, by eradication of the abrasion phenomenon between the tight, fibrotic and hypertrophied medial plica related structure and the opposite medial femoral condyle, the pain of most patients could be reduced and the degenerative process in the medial compartment of some patients might be decelerated or arrested. Therefore, we propose a concept of arthroscopic cartilage regeneration facilitating procedure (ACRFP) that combines arthroscopic medial release (AMR) with synovectomy, abrasional chondroplasthy, partial meniscectomy or percutaneous lateral release (PLR) as a rationale for the deliberate arthroscopic management of OA knee. We believed that the elimination of the detrimental factors including medial abrasion phenomenon, focal or generalized synovitis, chondral flaps, meniscus flaps or lateral compression phenomenon will provide a preferable environment for the regeneration of the damaged cartilage.

In the year of 2005, 571 knees of 367 patients having medial compartment osteoarthritis with or without patellofemoral compartment involvement received this procedure. There were 95 (26%) male and 272 (74%) female and the mean age was 60 years (range, 29 to 82). The Knee Society score and the knee injury and osteoarthritis outcome score were used for subjective outcome study. The roentgenographic changes of femoral-tibial angle and joint space width were evaluated for objective outcome. The mean follow-up period was 38 months (range, 36 to 49). There were 505 knees in 326 patients (88.8%) available with more than 3 years follow-up. The subjective satisfactory rate for the whole series was 85.5%. For 134 knees with complete follow-up evaluation, the Knee Society score and all subscales of the knee injury and osteoarthritis outcome score improved statistically. The femoral-tibial angle improved from 1.52 degrees (95% confidence interval, 0.84~2.19) to 1.93 degrees (1.21~2.64) ($p=0.03$). The joint space width increased from 2.03 millimeters (1.81~2.24) to 2.18 millimeters (1.97~2.38) ($p=0.01$). The degeneration process of the medial compartment was found being reversed in 82.1% of these knees according to the radiographic evaluation. Examples of cartilage regeneration are shown in figures 13~16.

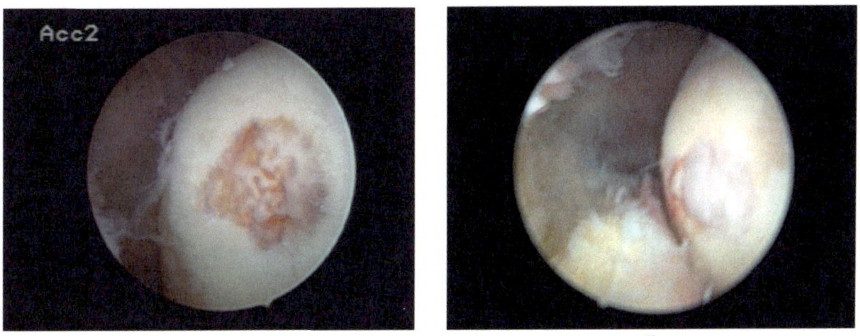

A B

Fig. 13. Cartilage regeneration demonstrated in the medial compartment of the left knee of a 56 years old lady having stage II OA; A, cartilage erosion was found over the medial femoral condyle opposite the removed pathologic medial plica; B, the defect was found regenerated during the second-look arthroscopy 3 years later when the same knee suffered from hemoarthrosis after a falling down accident.

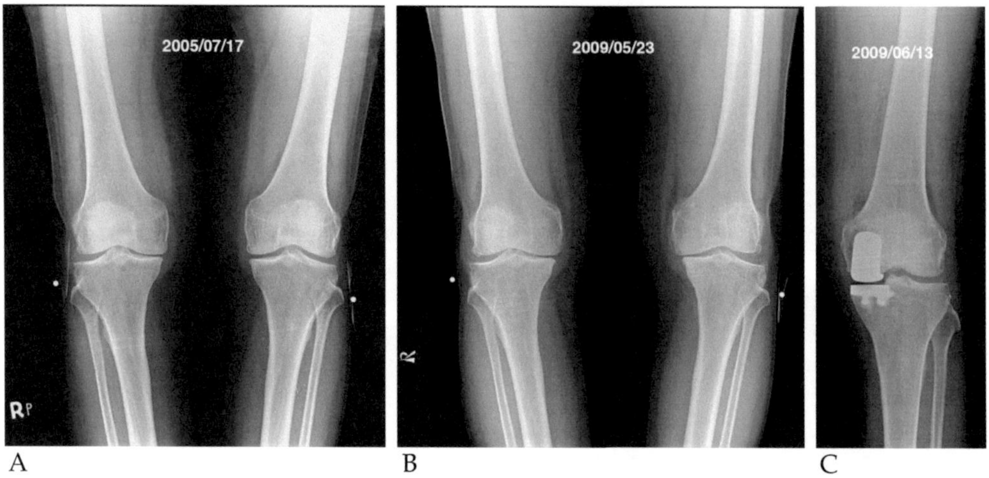

Fig. 14. A self-control example showing the benefit of ACRFP: A, pre-operative AP standing view of a 61 years old male with grade III OA over medial compartment of right knee and grade II OA over medial compartment of left knee, ACRFP was performed for his right knee; B, 46 months later, he came back due to marked disability over his left knee, the condition of his right knee was excellent and the degenerative process ceased compared to the progressively degenerated left knee; C, unicompartmental arthroplasty was necessary for his left knee that hadn't received ACRFP.

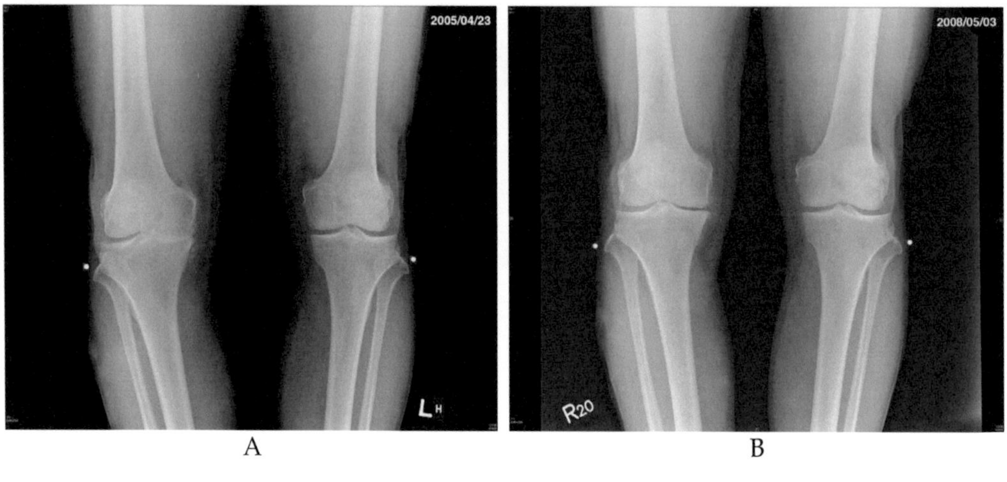

Fig. 15. An example of reversal of natural degenerative course by ACRFP in a 70 years old male patient having grade IV OA over his right knee: A, pre-operative standing AP view showing grade IV OA over medial compartment of his right knee; B, three years after ACRFP, the joint space reopened and the FTA improved from 7 degrees varus to 3 degrees varus.

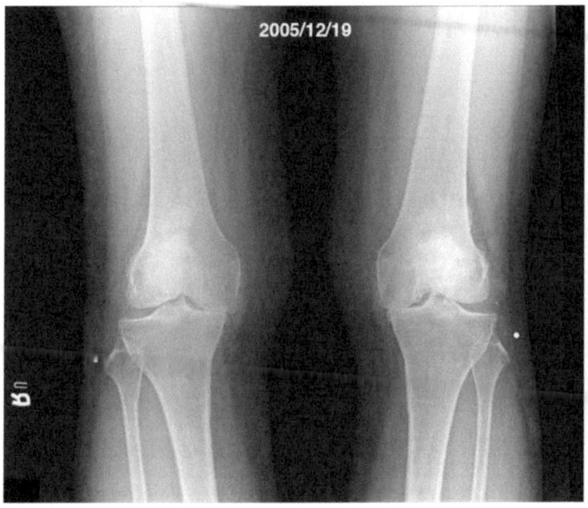

A

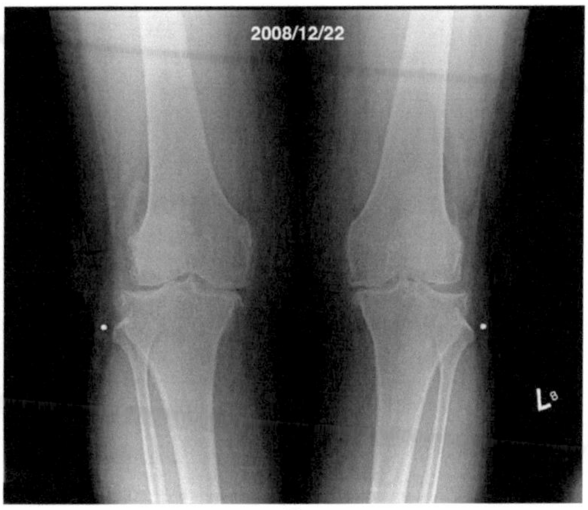

B

Fig. 16. Another example of reversal of natural course by ACRFP: A, AP standing view of a 58 years old female patient having bilateral grade IV OA with subluxation of medial femoral condyle; B, three years after ACRFP, obvious improvement of the radiographic manifestation could be observed.

Based on this constitutional study, we proposed a concept that by a purposeful eradication of all prejudicial factors in the degenerative knee, the jeopardized cartilage will have the chance to regenerate by its natural character. In comparison with the uncertain beneficial mechanism and the diversity of outcomes of current popular arthroscopic techniques for osteoarthritis of the knee, this concept of ACRFP has more precise rationale of treatment. The main theme of ACRFP is to remove any abnormal abrasion or impingement phenomenon and reestablish soft tissue balance in medial compartment and patellofemoral joint. For knees demonstrating medial abrasion phenomenon, medial release (Lyu SR, 2008) was performed to relieve the tension and abrasion between the tight, fibrotic and hypertrophied medial plica and the adjacent medial femoral condyle that have been described in previous studies (Lyu SR and Hsu CC, 2006; Lyu et al., 2006; Lyu SR, 2007; Lyu et al., 2010). On the other hand, in knees demonstrating lateral compression syndrome over patellofemoral joint, percutaneous lateral capsular release that has the benefits of tension release and denervation (Calpur OU et al., 2005; Paulos LE et al., 2008) was added.

The immediate effect of ACRFP is to release the strain caused by chronically inflamed soft tissue and to eradicate the hypertrophied synovium that may cause pain in the degenerative knees over the medial compartment and patellofemoral joint. Furthermore, this procedure might also bring forth to long-term favorable effects as a consequence of the global improvement of the environment of the knee joint for cartilaginous regeneration.

According to the experience of performing this procedure, the radiographic evaluations and clinical outcome studies have demonstrated that, by removal of all existed catabolic factors, the anabolic pathway of the damaged cartilage might become dominant and regeneration unveiled. The data support our contention that arthroscopic cartilage regeneration facilitating procedure is a good modality for the treatment of medial compartment osteoarthritis of the knee joint with/without patellofemoral joint involvement. It could modify the disease process of this common disease.

5. The future: Knee health promotion option (KHPO) for OA knee

Based on the findings of our research regarding MAS and the clinical outcome of ACRFP, an integrated protocol shown in figure 17 for the treatment of OA knee that we call "knee health promotion option (KHPO)" has been developed and put into practice in our center since 2007. The details of this protocol for global management of OA knee will be presented in this section.

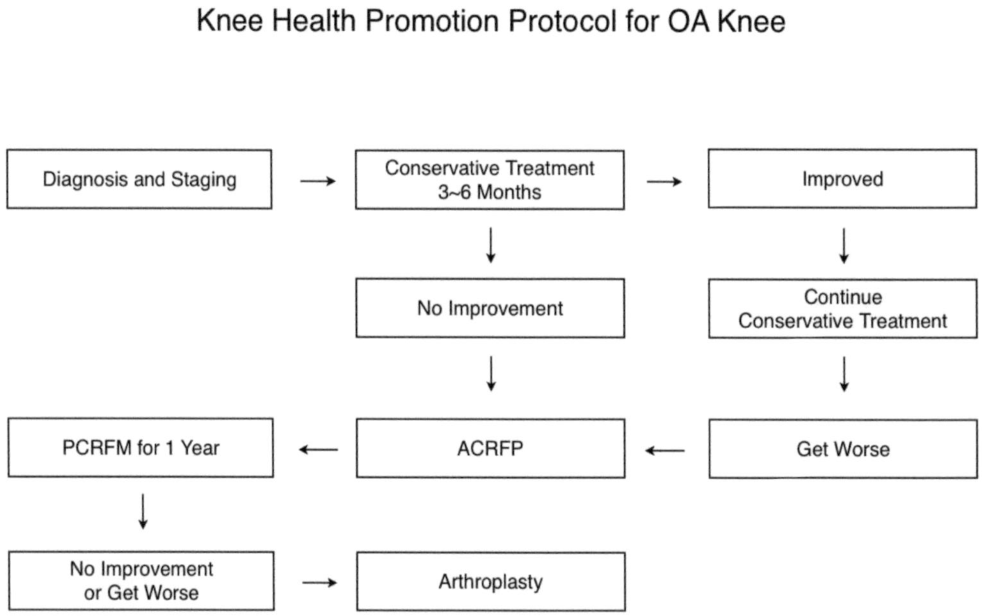

ACRFP: arthroscopic cartilage regeneration facilitating procedure

PCRFM: post-operative cartilage regeneration facilitating modalities

Fig. 17. Protocol of KHPO, the key determinant of success is to obtain complete consensus from the patient about this novel concept before enrolling him/her into this protocol. In our practice, the patients will be put under strict surveillance from case manager and nursing specialist during the whole process.

5.1 Clinical staging

The first step of knee health promotion option for the treatment of OA knee is thorough evaluation of the patient's general condition and establishing the clinical staging for each compartment of the knee by standard rentgenographic examination including standing anteroposterior, lateral, and Merchant's views. The degree of joint space narrowing, presentation of osteophytes and alignment measured by femorotibial angle were the main parameters evaluated. The staging of OA of the whole knee is given as the most advanced stage of the three compartments. We have been using this staging system since 2000 and noticed its high correlation with the corresponding arthroscopic findings (as the example of medial compartment shown in table 1).

Stage	Joint Space Narrowing	Osteophyte	FT angle	Arthroscopic findings
I	Doubtful	No	Normal	Smooth surface, loss of normal elasticity
II	Definite, no more than 1/2	Doubtful	> 0	Uneven surface, superficial to moderate cartilage damage (bubbling, fibrillation)
III	Marked, more than 1/2	Definite	Around 0	Deep cartilage damage (chondral flap, subchondral bone exposed < ½ area)
IV	Complete obliterated	Marked	< 0	Full thickness cartilage damage (subchondral bone exposed > ½ area)

Table 1. Clinical staging for medial compartment based on the rentgenographic findings and possible correlated arthroscopic findings.

5.2 Decision making for treatment option

Once the clinical staging of each compartment has been made, the decision of treatment option for idividual patient could be made according to the guideline listed in table 2. For stage I ~ III patients, KHPO is the best choice compared to osteotomy and arthroplasty. In stage IV patients, although arthroplasty is usually recommended, KHPO sometimes still has its value considering patients' preference and biopsychosocial condition.

Stage	KHPO	Osteotomy	Arthroplasty
I	++++	-	-
II	++++	-	-
III	+++	++	+
IV	++	++	++++

Table 2. Recommendation of treatment option for different stage of OA knee.

5.3 Conservative treatment before ACRFP

All of the stage I and II patients and some of the stage III patients should be recommended to encounter into this supervised conservative treatment for at least 3 months. The sine qua non for a successful conservative treatment is to make patients and the family completely understand the concept of treatment. The medial abrasion phenomenon as an important etiologic factor should be emphasized. Daily activities, job and exercise modification could then be tailored for individual patient focusing on the avoidance of the medial abrasion phenomenon. In general, activities and exercises need repeated knee bending are regarded as harmful. The following recommendation shown in table 3 for activities and exercises is an example according to this principle.

Suitable	*Harmful*
Walking Jogging Golf Swimming using freestyle or butterfly stroke	Stairs or mountains climbing Squatting (e.g. gardening) Bicycling Swimming using breaststroke

Table 3. Recommendation for suitable or harmful activities and exercises for OA knee

Home-based rehabilitation exercises including muscle strengthening and soft tissue stretching around the knee should be instructed and followed up under close surveillance from special personnels such as case managers or nursing specialists.

5.4 Post-operative cartilage regeneration facilitating modalities (PCRFM)

After the detrimental factors including medial abrasion syndrome, lateral compression syndrome, synovitis, chondral debris and meniscus flaps that have been proven as the main causes of cartilage damage are eliminated by ACRFP, the purpose of the post-operative care is to unveil and facilitate the natural repairing ability of the degenerated cartilage.

During the first 3 months after ACRFP, the aim of rehabilitation is to prevent scar contracture and consequent recurrent medial abrasion phenomenon. Gentle deep bending stretching exercise is encouraged after each session of quadriceps strengthening exercise.

To facilitate cartilage regeneration, strict rules about engaging into appropriate daily activites and exercises as listed in table 3 should be followed during the first post-operative year. The rationale of this precaution is to avoid repeated bending of the knee that might produce shearing force harmful for cartilage regeneration. Muscle strengthening and soft tissue stretching exercises around the knee should be conducted as long as possible.

6. Conclusion

The concept of knee health promotion option (KHPO) for the treatment of OA knee could be summarized in figure 18. From our series of studies and long-term clinical observation, we have defined a new entity - medial abrasion syndrome (MAS) and realized that it might be the main etiologic factor for the idiopathic medial compartment osteoarthritis of the knee joint. This syndrome could clarify most of the recognized symptoms, signs and risk factors of this common disease. Combined with other detrimental factors such as lateral compression syndrome, focal synovitis, chondral debris and meniscus flaps, the normal metabolism balance of articular cartilage is jeopadized and the knee "degenerates". If these detrimental factors could be eliminated by ACRFP in time and KHPO undertaken, the natural repairing power of the articular cartilage could be revived and the "degenerated" knee might "regenerate". In our clinical outcome study, the radiographic evaluations have demonstrated that, by removal of all existing catabolic factors, the anabolic pathway of the damaged cartilage might become dominant and regeneration unveiled.

In conclusion, we have conceptualized a novel theory for the global management of OA knee. We propose that, by a purposeful eradication of all prejudicial factors in the degenerative knee, the jeopardized cartilage will have the potential to regenerate. In comparison with the uncertain beneficial mechanism and the diversity of outcomes of current popular arthroscopic techniques for osteoarthritis of the knee, our concepts of AMR,

ACRFP and KHPO have more precise rationale for the treatment and could bring hope to the majority of patients.

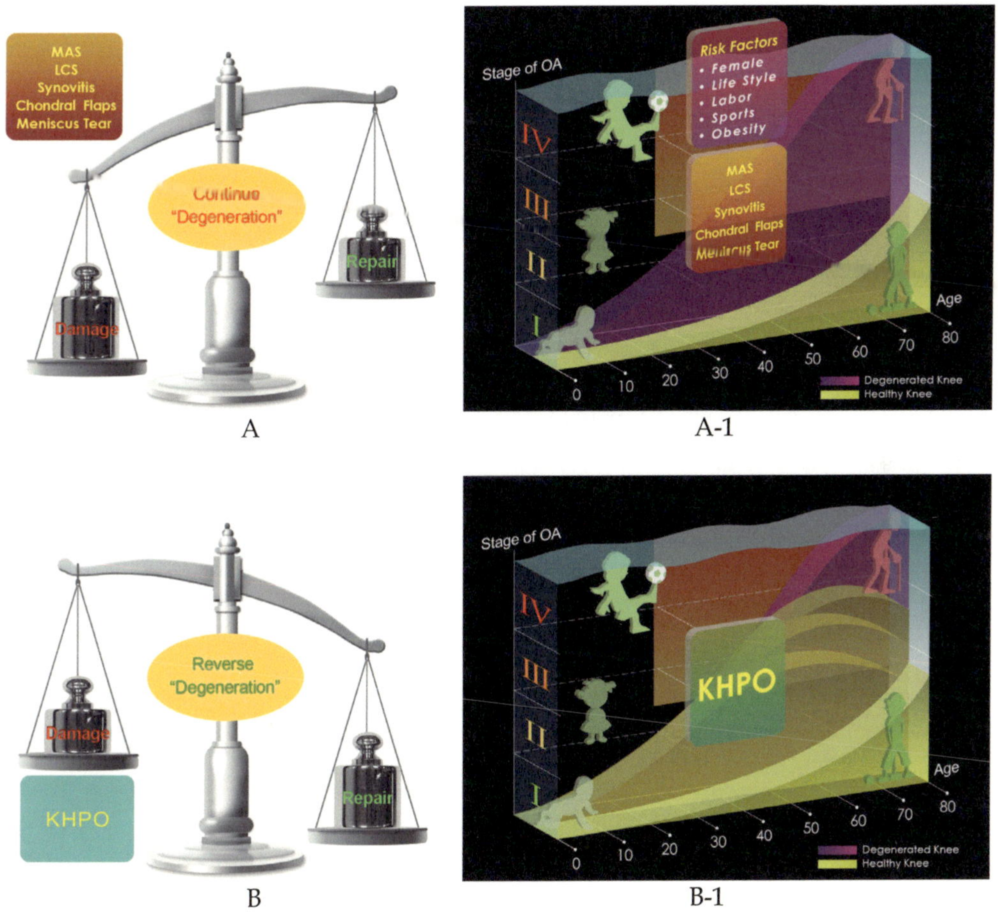

MAS: medial abrasion syndrome; LCS: lateral compression syndrom;

KHPO: knee health promotion option

Fig. 18. A, multiple detrimental factors cause imbalance of cartilage metabolism and the knee continue "degeneration"; A-1, different life span of normal (yellowish green line) and degenerated knee (purple line); B, KHPO could revive the natural repairing capacity of cartilage and "regeneration" could be anticipated, B-1, KHPO could reverse the "degeneration" process and change the direction of purple line.

7. References

Zhang L, Hu J, Athanasiou KA. The role of tissue engineering in articular cartilage repair and regeneration. *Crit Rev Biomed Eng 2009;37-1-2:1-57.*

Onyekwelu I, Goldring MB, Hidaka C. Chondrogenesis, joint formation, and articular cartilage regeneration. *J Cell Biochem 2009;107-3:383-92.*

Kanamiya T, Naito M, Hara M, Yoshimura I. The influences of biomechanical factors on cartilage regeneration after high tibial osteotomy for knees with medial compartment osteoarthritis: clinical and arthroscopic observations. *Arthroscopy 2002;18-7:725-9.*

Koshino T, Wada S, Ara Y, Saito T. Regeneration of degenerated articular cartilage after high tibial valgus osteotomy for medial compartmental osteoarthritis of the knee. *Knee 2003;10-3:229-36.*

Aigner T, Soeder S, Haag J. IL-1beta and BMPs--interactive players of cartilage matrix degradation and regeneration. *Eur Cell Mater 2006;12:49-56*

Neame R, Zhang W, Deighton C, Doherty M, Doherty S, Lanyon P, Wright G. Distribution of radiographic osteoarthritis between the right and left hands, hips, and knees. *Arthritis Rheum 2004;50-5:1487-94.*

Nunez M, Nunez E, Sastre S, Del-Val JL, Segur JM, Macule F. Prevalence of knee osteoarthritis and analysis of pain, rigidity, and functional incapacity. *Orthopedics 2008;31-8:753.*

Lyu SR, Hsu CC. Medial plicae and degeneration of the medial femoral condyle. *Arthroscopy 2006;22-1:17-26.*

Lyu SR. Relationship of medial plica and medial femoral condyle during flexion. *Clin Biomech (Bristol, Avon) 2007;22-9:1013-6.*

Lyu SR, Chiang JK, Tseng CE. Medial plica in patients with knee osteoarthritis: a histomorphological study. *Knee Surg Sports Traumatol Arthrosc 2009;18-6:769-76.*

Hwai-Shi Wang P-YK, Chih-Chang Yang, Shaw-Ruey Lyu. Matrix Metalloprotease-3 Expression in Medial Plica and Pannus-like Tissue in Knees with Medial Compartment Osteoarthritis. *Histopathology 2011;58-4:593-600.*

Lyu SR. Arthroscopic medial release for medial compartment osteoarthritis of the knee: the result of a single surgeon series with a minimum follow-up of four years. *J Bone Joint Surg Br 2008;90-9:1186-92.*

Dandy DJ, Anatomy of the medial suprapatellar plica and medial synovial shelf. Arthroscopy 1990;6(2):79-85

Dorchak JD; Barrack RL; Kneisl JS; Alexander AH, Arthroscopic treatment of symptomatic synovial plica of the knee. Long- term followup. Am J Sports Med 1991 Sep-Oct;19(5):503-7

Flanagan JP; Trakru S; Meyer M; Mullaji AB; Krappel F, Arthroscopic excision of symptomatic medial plica. Acta Orthop Scand 1994; 65(4): 408-411

Tasker T; Waugh W, Articular changes associated with internal derangement of the knee. J Bone Joint Surg [Br] 1982;64(4):486-8

Broom MJ; Fulkerson JP , The plica syndrome: a new perspective. Orthop Clin North Am 1986 Apr;17(2):279-81

Dupont JY, Synovial plicae of the knee. Controversies and review. Clin Sports Med 1997 Jan;16(1):87-122

Lyu SR, Tzeng JE, Kuo CY, Jian AR, Liu DS. Mechanical strength of mediopatellar plica--the influence of its fiber content. *Clin Biomech (Bristol, Avon) 2006;21-8:860-3.*

Lyu SR , Chiang JK, and Tseng CE, Medial plica in patients with knee osteoarthritis: a histomorphological study. *Knee surgery, sports traumatology, arthroscopy: official journal of the ESSKA 2010; 18(6):769-76.*

Lynn SK, Reid SM, Costigan PA. The influence of gait pattern on signs of knee osteoarthritis in older adults over a 5-11 year follow-up period: a case study analysis. *Knee 2007; 14:22-28*

Baliunas AJ, Hurwitz DE, Ryals AB, et al. Increased knee joint loads during walking are present in subjects with knee osteoarthritis. *Osteoarthritis Cartilage 2002; 10:573-579.*

Gok H, Ergin S, Yavuzer G. Kinetic and kinematic characteristics of gait in patients with medial knee arthrosis. *Acta Orthop Scand 2002; 73:647-652*

Landry SC, McKean KA, Hubley-Kozey CL, Stanish WD, Deluzio KJ. Knee biomechanics of moderate OA patients measured during gait at a self-selected and fast walking speed. *J Biomech 2007; 40:1754-1761*

Thorp LE, Sumner DR, Wimmer MA, Block JA. Relationship between pain and medial knee joint loading in mild radiographic knee osteoarthritis. *Arthritis Rheum 2007, 57:1254-1260*

Shibakawa A, Aoki H, Masuko-Hongo K, Kato T, Tanaka M, Nishioka K, Nakamura H. Presence of pannus-like tissue on osteoarthritic cartilage and its histological character. *Osteoarthritis Cartilage* 2003; 11; 133-40.

Yuan GH, Tanaka M, Masuko-Hongo K, Shibakawa A, Kato T, Nishioka K, Nakamura H. Characterization of cells from pannus-like tissue over articular cartilage of advanced osteoarthritis. *Osteoarthritis Cartilage* 2004; 12; 38-45.

Tetlow LC, Adlam DJ, Woolley DE. Matrix metalloproteinase and proinflammatory cytokine production by chondrocytes of human osteoarthritic cartilage: associations with degenerative changes. *Arthritis Rheum* 2001; 44; 585-94.

Haywood L, McWilliams DF, Pearson CI, Gill SE, Ganesan A, Wilson D, Walsh DA. Inflammation and angiogenesis in osteoarthritis. *Arthritis Rheum* 2003; 48; 2173-7.

Ayral X, Pickering EH, Woodworth TG, Mackillop N, Dougados M. Synovitis: a potential predictive factor of structural progression of medial tibiofemoral knee osteoarthritis -- results of a 1 year longitudinal arthroscopic study in 422 patients. *Osteoarthritis Cartilage* 2005; 13; 361-7.

Benito MJ, Veale DJ, FitzGerald O, van den Berg WB, Bresnihan B. Synovial tissue inflammation in early and late osteoarthritis. *Ann Rheum Dis* 2005; 64; 1263-7.

Ikeuchi M, Takahashi T, Tani T. Localized synovial hypertrophy in the anteromedial compartment of the osteoarthritic knee. *Arthroscopy* 2005; 21; 1457-61.

Tchetverikov I, Lohmander LS, Verzijl N, Huizinga TW, TeKoppele JM, Hanemaaijer R, DeGroot J. MMP protein and activity levels in synovial fluid from patients with joint injury, inflammatory arthritis, and osteoarthritis. *Ann Rheum Dis* 2005; 64; 694-8.

Daheshia M, Yao JQ. The interleukin 1beta pathway in the pathogenesis of osteoarthritis. *J Rheumatol* 2008; 35; 2306-12.

Eder C. Mechanisms of interleukin-1beta release. *Immunobiology 2009.*

van den Berg WB. Anti-cytokine therapy in chronic destructive arthritis. *Arthritis Res* 2001; 3; 18-26.

Marks PH, Donaldson ML. Inflammatory cytokine profiles associated with chondral damage in the anterior cruciate ligament-deficient knee. *Arthroscopy* 2005; 21; 1342-7.

Yoshihara Y, Nakamura H, Obata K, Yamada H, Hayakawa T, Fujikawa K, Okada Y. Matrix metalloproteinases and tissue inhibitors of metalloproteinases in synovial fluids from patients with rheumatoid arthritis or osteoarthritis. *Ann Rheum Dis 2000;59-6:455-61.*

Hedbom E, Hauselmann HJ. Molecular aspects of pathogenesis in osteoarthritis: the role of inflammation. *Cell Mol Life Sci 2002;59-1:45-53.*

Warren LF, Marshall JL. The supporting structures and layers on the medial side of the knee: an anatomical analysis. *J Bone Joint Surg [Am] 1979;61-A:56-62.*

Calpur OU, Ozcan M, Gurbuz H, Turan FN. Full arthroscopic lateral retinacular release with hook knife and quadriceps pressure-pull test: long-term follow-up. *Knee Surg Sports Traumatol Arthrosc 2005;13-3:222-30.*

Paulos LE, O'Connor DL, Karistinos A. Partial lateral patellar facetectomy for treatment of arthritis due to lateral patellar compression syndrome. *Arthroscopy 2008;24-5:547-53.*